# The Ancestors Diet

### Living and Cultured Foods
### to Extend Life, Prevent Disease
### and Lose Weight

By Case Adams, Naturopath

The Ancestors Diet: Living and Cultured Foods to Extend Life, Prevent
    Disease and Lose Weight
Copyright © 2013 Case Adams
LOGICAL BOOKS
Wilmington, Delaware
http://www.logicalbooks.org
All rights reserved.
Printed in USA
Front cover illustrations Irochka and Nem4a

**Publishers Cataloging in Publication Data**
  Adams, Case
The Ancestors Diet: Living and Cultured Foods to Extend Life, Prevent
    Disease and Lose Weight
    First Edition
    1. Medicine. 2. Health.
    Bibliography and References; Index

ISBN-13: 978-1-936251-41-4

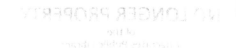

# Table of Contents

# Introduction

This book introduces a diet plan that has everything going for it. As we will illustrate in this book, this diet:

- Lowers the risk of cancer
- Reduces risk of Alzheimer's disease and other types of dementia
- Reduces incidence of arthritis
- Increases immunity and the ability to fight off disease
- Lessens the chances of autoimmune diseases
- Increases vitality and reduces fatigue
- Increases endurance
- Increases eye health – reduces risk of vision problems
- Reduces the risk of nervous disorders such as Parkinson's
- Prevents and even reverses type 2 diabetes
- Prevents and even reverses metabolic disease
- Helps reduce weight and keep normal weight
- Helps the body process fat correctly
- Prevents and even reverses intestinal disorders
- Reduces food allergies
- Reduces "bad" lipoprotein-cholesterol and raises "good" lipoprotein-cholesterol
- Prevents and even ameliorates prostate conditions

Furthermore, this is the diet our body was intended to eat. And our human ancestors, have, in fact, been eating this diet for most of our historical existence. That is, before the rise of the "Western diet" in recent centuries.

And it is for this reason that we call this the Ancestors Diet, because this diet is precisely what our healthiest ancestors ate.

No, we are not talking about the Neanderthals. We aren't talking about those of our ancestors who got holed up in some desolate part of the icy wilderness with little food to eat, facing the harshest conditions, being forced to eat food that had to be hunted down and massacred, leaving a bloody mess to try to choke down, or cook if possible.

We aren't talking about those parts of our ancestry that got stuck in inhospitable regions of the world forced to create tools of warfare in order to accomplish what their ancestors accomplished simply by reaching out and picking some nuts, fruits, berries, seeds, leaves, and grains.

We are talking about that part of our ancestry that flourished among the foods intended for their bodies – foods that were easily gathered and harvested with a minimum of tools and eaten raw, cooked minimally or

1

fermented into delicious foodstuffs that nourished the body and its microbiota.

We are talking about our early ancestors who dwelled in their natural environments: Environments providing nuts, fruits, vegetables, roots, seeds and fermented dairy foods.

These are not only our earliest ancestors: They are also the peace-loving intelligent ancestors who gave us science, math, the written word and the first and longest continual natural medicine. We are talking about those early ancestors whose diets afforded them the leisure time to develop the intelligence that eventually educated the world in culture, medicine, architecture, mathematics, science and cuisine.

Yes, certainly we can find cultures throughout the world at different times and even through today that ate opportunistically, and thus ate foods that our bodies weren't designed to eat.

This doesn't mean we need to eat those foods now.

Today most of us live in a world that allows us to select a wide range of foods. We can go to the grocery store and purchase foods that precisely fit a variety of diet plans – from a variety of cultures and traditions.

The question is, which tradition should we choose? Should we choose to eat the diet some of our ancestors ate when they were starving and there was nothing else to eat? Should we choose to eat the foods that some of our ancestors ate when they lived in the desert without the irrigation or rains to grow anything? Or foods that some of our ancestors ate because they found themselves in snowy lands in the middle of winter and nothing grew through the ice?

Why? Why should we eat those foods now? We don't have to. We can mosey on over to the fresh section of our grocery store and select from a huge assortment of the freshest, most delicious and colorful foods grown in the best conditions with the best fertilizers and best soils, given ample water to produce an array of nutrients.

Yes, most of us have the luxury to be able to select those foods our bodies were ultimately meant to eat. Those foods that prevent cancer, heart disease, diabetes, prostate conditions, obesity, arthritis, cataracts and so many other modern ailments. Those are the foods our bodies are meant to eat.

How do we know this?

Science.

In this book we provide the clear scientific evidence that shows a particular set of foods provides the healthiest diet – that diet we were intended to eat. That diet offering the most nutrition per bite. That diet offering the most delicious flavors to please our tongues. That diet offering the largest assortment of colors to please our eyes and sense of beauty. That diet offering the most benefit to the microbiota (probiotics) living within our guts. That diet offering us the least chance of dying early. That diet offering the best chances of maintaining our intelligence through our older years.

Who could refuse such a host of benefits? Possibly only the most stubborn of us – those who would prefer to continue to endanger their health and the health of our planet in order to continue the status quo.

Yes, life is full of choices.

And there sure are a lot of diet plans to choose from. It could be overwhelming. There's also a lot of confusion, and a lot of misinformation being passed around. There are diet plans for just about every possible approach to eating. There are plans that call for one food type or another food type. There are body type diets and blood type diets. There are diets that call for rationing and calorie counting, fat counting and weight control. There are diets for children, the elderly, the athletic, and the lazy couch potato. There are so many diet plans out there that each of us could take on a different one.

Most of these diet plans are too difficult to stick to. They are too restrictive in one respect or another. In some diet plans, each member of the family is eating something different at each meal. In others, meal times are so radically different that families don't eat together. In other diet plans, the food is so foreign that no one wants to eat it. Other plans are so complex that the person has to take the book where ever they go.

This is not the case with the Ancestors Diet. Why? Because this is the diet that our bodies were designed to eat. We can eat the foods of this diet anytime. Anywhere. There are no restrictions. We can eat them at midnight or every six hours. We can eat them on the run or at a nicely set dinner table.

This is the diet plan that our healthiest of ancestors ate for millions (yes, millions) of years.

This is the diet plan that gives the most flexibility because there are so many foods, preparation possibilities, combination potentials and approaches. We can eat the foods raw, out of a blender, steamed, baked or any number of combinations, as long as we don't cook the nutrients out of it.

This is the diet plan people can stick to because it contains some of the richest, great tasting foods around.

This is the diet plan people can remember because it is simple.

This is the diet plan accepted by the most peer-reviewed research to safely enable weight loss.

And as mentioned, this is the diet plan proven to provide numerous health benefits – including lowering LDL-cholesterol, preventing cancer, reducing diabetes, lowering inflammatory conditions, easing digestion and all those other items listed and more.

The Ancestors Diet is what our body knows best. It is practically intuitive. If we were sent off to the forest after weaning to eat what we wanted, we would probably eat this diet.

All the science is pointing to this diet. While one might argue the low-carb or low-fat diets, the Ancestors Diet is completely removed from these two arguments. It lies on the outskirts of these debates, because it provides healthy fats and healthy carbs.

The Ancestors Diet is also gentle on our pocketbooks. The diet uses foods readily available at every grocery store, every restaurant and hopefully, every kitchen. It is truly the human diet, and that is why those who adhere more closely to this diet have the lowest rates of heart disease and cancer.

Make no mistake: The Ancestors Diet is not the same as the raw food diet. Its not the same as the vegetarian diet, nor the vegan diet. Nor is it the same as the Mediterranean diet. While the Ancestors Diet includes many elements of these diets, it is specifically different from each in many respects.

While some might compare the Ancestors Diet to any of these, it is bigger than these diets. It is more encompassing because it hones in on eating strategies that don't just include certain foods: The Ancestors Diet also involves forgotten techniques for preparing those foods.

And the Ancestors Diet utilizes a clear category called living foods, as we'll define carefully.

Unfortunately, this book is not a recipe book, nor is it an encyclopedia of foods. There are some fabulous recipe books out there that detail how to create delicious meals from the types of foods we detail in this book.

What the book puts forth is, in my humble opinion, a convincing scientific argument validating healthy dietary choices. These are choices that science has shown will lengthen our lives, give us greater clarity of mind, help save our planet, and bring about a greater sense of compassion.

# Chapter One

# What Our Ancestors Ate

## Just Who were Our Ancestors?

Theoretically, we could define ancestors as our parents. Or our grandparents, great-grandparents and so forth. Or we might define our ancestors as our country of origin. If our great-grandparents immigrated from Italy in the 1920s we might say that our ancestry is Italian.

But we only need to ask the obvious questions. Who were our great-grandparents' ancestors – besides their parents and grandparents? Who were the ancestors of the Italians? One might say the Romans, because the Roman empire controlled what is now known as Italy.

Then we would have to ask who were the Romans' ancestors? One might say the Etruscans were the ancestors of the Romans and the Greeks, as this was the primary civilization that inhabited the Mediterranean region during what is referred to as the Iron age.

During this period we also know about the ancient civilizations of ancient India, ancient China, the Kush and Nok civilizations of the Afrikaans, along with other tribal civilizations around the world. But who were their ancestors?

Prior to these civilizations archeologists have found ancestors among the Bronze Age, including the Anatolians and Aegeans, the Minoans, the Mycenaean's the ancient Egyptians, the Punts of ancient Somalia, the Norte Carals, Olmecs and Zapotecs of the South Americas, the North American Indians, and two of the oldest advanced societies, the ancient Chinese and Indus Valley civilizations.

Yes, the ancient Chinese and Indus Valley civilizations, which gave birth to the notion of the Aryans, were the first civilizations to have organized math and science, advanced architecture, an advanced alphabet with lengthy writings, advanced medicines with Materia Medica and other advancements that were soon spread to other cultures via trade and cultural exchange. But who were their ancestors along with the rest of humanity?

Here things get a bit hazy, as records become harder to trace, but a general consensus among archeologists arrives after two centuries of focused archaeological research. This is that during the Neolithic Era – a time estimated to start about 12,000 BCE and end about 4500 BCE – the last of the nomadic tribes completed humanity's conversion to agricultural societies. They settled down to grow food and irrigate as necessary. This is also referred to as the Agricultural Revolution. Okay, different cultures converted to agriculture at different times. But who were their ancestors?

This takes us back to the famous Paleolithic Era, a time that most humans were supposedly hunter-gatherers, right?

Yet during this same era – between one and two million years ago – we find most populations of Paleolithic humans still living in Africa and Asia, with limited migrations into Europe. These excursions into Europe occurred only a few hundred thousand years ago – followed by these early northerners eventually going extinct.

This includes the *Homo heidelbergensis* and the *Homo erectus* species, who migrated to Europe from Africa. *Homo heidelbergensis* evolved into the Neanderthals (*Homo neanderthalis*). The Neanderthals, *Homo heidelbergensis* and *Homo erectus* all went extinct.

So none of these are actually our ancestors.

The assumption is that previous to this era, the ancestors of the Neolithic humans were primarily nomadic. This is based upon seeing cultures move from one region to another in periodic fashion.

What does this remind us of? Most certainly, the migration habits of animals. Many animals are also nomadic in the sense that that they travel with the seasons to regions that have more weather and food of their liking. For this reason, birds will migrate south in the winter and north in the summers (in the northern hemisphere – and opposite for the southern hemisphere), because their favorite foods also tend to be more plentiful in these regions during these seasons.

And with this migration will come seasonal mating and birthing habits, which are passed down to the next generation. Humans retain this seasonality to this day, as spring months bring increased outdoor and mating activities.

But the type of nomadic journeys these ancestors took are often described as traveling from a more hospitable environment to a less hospitable environment. The evidence shows that early humanoids traveled between the warmer comfortable climates of Africa, Asia and the Mediterranean primarily, where food was plentiful. And excursions into Northern Europe during the winters, for example, were death traps, beginning with the journey over the Swiss Alps.

Why would some early humanoids do this? Why would they travel from the lush forested, jungled and savannah regions of Africa and Asia into the icy cold regions of Europe?

Yet they did, but much later in our ancestry, some 1.5 million years after our ancestors evolved, according to the archaeology.

Why would they journey into the frozen north? This hasn't been answered. Perhaps they got pushed out of Africa as a result of territorial struggles?

A possibility, but this doesn't jive well with the scarcity of humans among the landscape. Research pegs humans at an average of one per five square kilometers even in the more populated regions. This means there was plenty of room for everyone, and at the very least, room for humans to migrate back to warmer climes as the weather got colder:

> "*Ethnographically, human forager densities were particularly low in high latitudes, a pattern attributed to low plant and mammal species diversity and high fluctuations in ungulate productivity. Human densities generally were higher in more temperate environments...*" (Morin 2007)

Or are we saying that humans are less intelligent than the vast majority of animals who migrate to Northern climates during the summer for nutritional diversity and Southern climates during the winter?

To this effect we can examine the migrating habits of any number of species of migrating animals – let's say the antelope. These and other grass-eating creatures migrate to those areas where the grasses are more plentiful, so they can eat what their bodies were designed to eat. Would they migrate into an icy snow-bound northern location? Be serious.

This is supported by archaeological finds that illustrate the early nomadic *Homo erectus* and *Homo neanderthalensis* went extinct because they were unable to survive those harsh conditions. Some recent finds have indicated some got locked in a territory struggle with other human tribes. This conflicts greatly with density issues as mentioned above. Sure, some may have been attacked by other human tribes. But this was likely related to the limited resources available in a less desirable climate rather than territory. Otherwise, the extinct tribes could surely have moved on to 'better snowy fields.'

What is known from archaeological digs in northern Europe is that one early humanoid eventually went extinct – the Neanderthals. This humanoid species didn't make it because they either died from exposure in an ice age or were slaughtered by other humanoids that also migrated north from sub-Sahara Africa and Asia Minor.

So we know the Neanderthals weren't our ancestors. That also means the cavemen were not our ancestors – as the cavemen were known to inhabit the northern regions. Humanoids didn't need caves in the warmer southern lands, but some may certainly have dwelled in caves.

Archaeology has determined that our real ancestors, the *Homo sapiens*, eventually did migrate out of Africa into Southern Europe and Asia – and on to Indonesia, Polynesia and the Americas.

Research also finds the presence of fire among hominids from about 300,000 to 400,000 years ago. This means that humans did not have fire

7

from their ascent at about two million years ago to 400,000 years ago. This means that our ancestors had no fire for over 75% of their existence – some 1.6 million years.

This means that either these groups of nomadic humans were eating raw (read bloody) flesh, or they subsisted on the diet of their own ancestors: nuts, fruits, berries, roots, barks, vegetables, seeds and grains.

In addition, we note those early hominids who seemingly utilized fire to cook flesh in their caves actually went extinct. In other words, they are not actually our ancestors.

The evidence shows that the majority of early humans maintained their ancestral diets and logical migration patterns.

The clearest evidence the archaeology presents is that our ancestors, the early *Homo sapiens*, did ascend from and eventually migrate from Eastern Africa, where the lush forests provided plentiful fruits, berries, barks, roots and other gathered foods.

But who were their ancestors?

Now we can reference some of the archaeological evidence of the oldest humanoids, living in Africa 2-3 million years ago. These are the earliest humanoids. These are our ancestors. Found in Africa, the archaeological evidence indicates that humans first arose from the taxonomy of the Family of Hominidae – which included orangutans (Pongo), gorillas (Gorilla) chimpanzees (Pan) – eventually evolving to modern humans – *Homo sapiens sapiens*.

And the direct ancestors of *Homo sapiens* evolved from their last common ancestors, the australopithecines, about four to five million years ago in eastern Africa.

Eventually one of these australopithecine species evolved to become *Homo habilis* and *Homo ergaster*. Then eventually to *Homo cepranensis, Homo erectus, Homo heidelbergensis* and *Homo neanderthalensis* (the theoretical "caveman") and other species. But it was the *Homo cepranensis* branch that eventually evolved to become *Homo sapiens*. *Homo heidelbergensis* and *Homo neanderthalensis* went extinct as mentioned. Again, we are not descendants of the cavemen. The cavemen went extinct.

This means in order to understand our true ancestry we need to look back at the earliest humanoid ancestors – our real ancestors – the australopithecines.

## The Diet of the Australopithecines

The australopithecines – which include *Australopithecus afarensis, A. africanus, A. bahrelghazali, Paranthropus robustus, Ardipithecus ramidus* and others – are our true ancestors. They stood up and walked on two feet (bipedalism) and had larger brains than their ape predecessors. They marked the distinction between the human race and its animal origins (Ruff 2010).

The latest research has discovered clear archaeological evidence of the diet of these ancestors of ours. The technologies developed over the past decade by archaeological experts have included some of the most advanced scientific instrumentation and analysis. These have discovered the diets of this earliest ancestor through careful analysis of the fossils of the australopithecines species.

By analyzing fossil teeth enamel, modern researchers have determined the primary diet of our earliest ancestors. The data has been unlocked from their teeth enamel. Basically, the teeth enamel retain carbon isotopes that identify the composition of what they were putting in their mouths to chew, digest and assimilate.

Within their teeth enamel the clarity of our original diet is found, setting the record straight and settling the debate.

But just to be sure, the data from these early teeth fossils is confirmed by analysis of abrasion patterns, along with soil analysis around the digs to confirm the composition of their surrounding food availability.

The teeth data are determined by comparing the two stable carbon isotopes – carbon-12 and carbon-13. This is because most carbon is carbon-12 (six protons and six electrons), and many plants – especially those of grasses and sedges – fix carbon-13 more heavily.

Thus by analyzing the ratio of carbon-12 to carbon-13, scientists have been able to determine the nature of the diet of the australopithecines. Much of these enamel carbon isotopes techniques were originally developed by Dr. Thure Cerling, a professor of Geology and Geophysics at the University of Utah.

The research has generally found three types of carbon photosynthesis – picked up by carbon isotope analysis from the enamel of our earliest ancestors. These include the warm-season grasses among the savannas. These take part in C4 photosynthesis, utilizing both C-12 and C-13. Trees, shrubs and herbs, along with cooler grasses like wheat, rye, barley and oats – plants which prefer C-12 over C-13 photosynthesis, but use both. The later type is referred to as C3 photosynthesis.

***Crassulacean acid metabolism*** is a carbon fixation process found among these plants as they adapt to a lack of water and an increasingly arid environment. In other words, the greater C-13 relates to the adaptation of an arid climate by these plant species.

Carbon analyses of our ancestors' teeth enamel have found that our earliest humanoid ancestors, the australopithecines, ate primarily a plant-based diet taken from bushes and trees. Carbon-wise, the ratios of their diets ranged from 75% C4 and 25% C3 to 65% C4 and 35% C3. This was contrasted by the Theropithecus, which has been found to have moved to a diet rich in C4 (Cerling *et al.* 2013).

The researchers have also been able to verify these early diets though a combination of their surroundings, teeth shape and other identifying features of their habitats, including the soils, which have a carbon footprint of their own.

This is added to analyses of the dental "microwear" of our ancestors, which confirm the type of foods our ancestors ate.

Research by Dr. Cerling and his associates have concluded that the diet of australopithecines such as *Paranthropus boisei* was:

> *"dominated by C4 biomass such as grasses and sedges."*

The researchers also stated that:

> *"the evidence indicates that the remarkable craniodental morphology of this taxon represents an adaptation for processing large quantities of low-quality vegetation rather than hard objects."*

Their research also enabled the understanding of a related species, *P. robustus*, which ate hardier plant-based foods:

> *"Carbon isotope studies of P. robustus from South Africa indicated that it consumed some plants using C4 photosynthesis such as tropical grasses or sedges, but were also consistent with most of its dietary carbon (approximately 70%) having been derived from the C3 food items favored by extant chimpanzees (Pan troglodytes) such as tree fruits."*

And the evolution to the C4 grasses and sedges (grains) by the *P. boisei* indicates what researchers suggest relate to the harvesting of roots with tools:

> *"It has recently been suggested that sedges were an important hominin resource because they are often found in the riverine woodlands favored by many savanna primates and because their tubers are a potentially high energy resource for which tool-wielding hominins would have had little competition."*

This delivers a clear understanding of our ancestors' diets on the whole. The researchers concluded:

> *"Given current evidence, however, the simplest explanation is adaptive divergence between the eastern and southern African P. aranthropus populations, with the former focusing on grasses or sedges and the southern population consuming a more traditional hominoid diet that included tree fleshy fruits, as well as variable C4 resources."*

This and other research finds that these and other early ancestors such as *Australopithecus afarensis* and *A. anamensis* primarily consumed diets consisting of fruit, roots, leaves, grasses, nuts and barks of different varieties. This diet is consistent with the last common ancestor of australopithecines – the chimpanzee, who eats primarily fruit, leaves, nuts, bark and twigs (Ströhle *et al.* 2009, Kohn *et al.* 1996; van der Merwe *et al.* 2008).

And more recent fossil discoveries have indicated that the australopithecines species were met with a warming trend that forced some to migrate from forests to grasslands. This was determined by identifying Crassulacean acid metabolism among the plant-based carbon isotopes within their teeth enamel.

The research indicates that our ancestors, the *Australopithecus afarensis* and related species, began to consume diets of grasses, sedges, roots, twigs, leaves and fruits (Ungar *et al.* 2008; Peters and Vogel 2005; Grine *et al.* 2006; Ungar *et al.* 2010; Ungar *et al.* 2011)

Grasses and sedges? What are grasses and sedges? Grains. We're talking about early grains here, along with the nutritious stalks of such grains.

This is consistent with other determinations that have found the consumption of seeds to be prevalent among early hominids (Jolly 1970).

And a study from the UK's University of Bradford (Macho and Shimizu 2010) found that the dental wear of *Australopithecus anamensis'* teeth indicates clearly that these early ancestors of ours ate considerable quantities of nuts. Yes, our ancestors consumed a diet of:

### Nuts, fruits, leaves, vegetables, roots, seeds, grains.

Yes, this is the diet of our ancestors. This is the diet that evolved though millions of years of development from apes and chimpanzees. This is the diet that propelled humanoids onto our two feet. This is the diet that helped our brains grow larger and more able to use and comprehend complex speech patterns.

And this provides the foundation for the Ancestors Diet.

This research has established scientific credibility. It has been corroborated. And it is peer-reviewed.

This position was emphatically reviewed in a 2012 Scientific American paper by Biologist Rob Dunn, entitled:

### "Human Ancestors Were Nearly All Vegetarians"

In this article we find a survey of the evidence. Here are a couple of snippets from the article:

> *"The majority of the food consumed by primates today – and every indication is for the last thirty million years – is vegetable, not animal.*

*Plants are what our apey and even earlier ancestors ate; they were our paleo diet for most of the last thirty million years during which our bodies, and our guts in particular, were evolving. In other words, there is very little evidence that our guts are terribly special and the job of a generalist primate gut is primarily to eat pieces of plants."*

Dunn puts forth further clarity on the diet of our ancestors that relates to the popular diet fad:

*"Which paleo diet should we eat? The one from twelve thousand years ago? A hundred thousand years ago? Forty million years ago? If you want to return to your ancestral diet, the one our ancestors ate when most of the features of our guts were evolving, you might reasonably eat what our ancestors spent the most time eating during the largest periods of the evolution of our guts: fruits, nuts, and vegetables — especially fungus-covered tropical leaves."*

To this last point we take up the natural extension of our ancestors' diet: As the australopithecines developed into *Homo sapiens* humans, their intelligence increased, and they figured out how to utilize the seeds of those sedges and grasses to cultivate more.

They also learned new ways to store and preserve these fruits, leaves, grasses, roots and barks. They began to utilize something we now refer to as fermentation.

It is from these origins that we have evolved. Three to four million years of existence eating a plant-based diet.

Yes, a few *Homo sapiens* who migrated out of Africa and got themselves trapped in deserts or icy regions may have been forced to scavenge animals for survival. When the snow covered the ground for several months, those not smart enough to migrate south for the winter were forced to hunt for food. Or die.

Which many did.

But the vast majority of our ancestor *Homo sapiens* in the Paleolithic era settled throughout Africa, Asia, Indonesia, the Mediterranean and other more hospitable environments where the multi-million-year-old diet of our ancestors was continued.

We cannot ignore the fact that those early societies rising from the late Paleolithic era among the world's more hospitable climes were also the most advanced human societies of those periods.

We evidence the early societies of the Indus Valley, China, Northern Africa, the Middle East, Indonesia and Polynesia: These were known for their incredible leisure time, as they became adept at survival using well-organized plant-based food gathering and cultivation strategies. Their diets included nuts, grains, fruits, vegetables, roots, seeds, kelps and a variety of fermented foods derived from dairy and grains. And it is from this core diet we find the most intelligent culinary invention – cultured foods – began to flourish.

And yes, humans are industrious and creative. Certainly those of our ancestors who landed on hard times in the wintertime in colder regions of Europe and North America, or in the desert, eventually had to figure out how to hunt down their dinners with weapons, chop them up with sharpened tools, and develop ways to cook them immediately to avoid getting intestinal infections – salmonella, parasites, campylobacter and so forth – from putrefying flesh.

Yes, this bloody mess of a diet certainly matched those harsh conditions. And certainly this diet does not represent the best case for our ancestors, but rather, desperate periods of survival in difficult circumstances.

We might compare this part of our history to what happened to those who survived the Andes plane crash of 1972 or the Donner Party of 1847 – both instances of human cannibalism. Should we all become cannibals because these people were forced by unforgiving environmental circumstances? Certainly not.

In the same vein, because we now have the luxury of choice in our diet, we should now be returning to those foods our body was best designed for – which happens to also be those foods that will keep us the healthiest.

And we find that even the extinct Neanderthals had a penchant for plant-based foods. A study from Germany (Hardy *et al.* 2012) unearthed some interesting discoveries about the Neanderthals: According to the researchers, a sophisticated knowledge of plants and plant medicines was evident:

> *"Our results provide the first molecular evidence for inhalation of wood-fire smoke and bitumen or oil shale and ingestion of a range of cooked plant foods. We also offer the first evidence for the use of medicinal plants by a Neanderthal individual. The varied use of plants that we have identified suggests that the Neanderthal occupants of El Sidrón had a sophisticated knowledge of their natural surroundings which included the ability to select and use certain plants."*

## Diet by Design

One of the most obvious and fundamental things we share with our ancestors is the human body. This is what makes researchers so focused upon the early hominids: Our similar body type, which includes the shape and design of our hands, feet, mouths, digestive tracts, and the relative metabolism of our physiology, is what undeniably links us with our ancestors.

And it is this physiology that conclusively reveals the diet of our early ancestors, confirming the technical data found by archeologists discussed above. In other words, the question is:

**What was our body designed to eat?**

There are a several aspects related to design when it comes to the human body. These include:

- Structural design – this relates to anatomy
- Functional design – this relates to metabolism
- Xenogenetic design – this relates to inheritance
- Cognitive design – this relates to mentality

These components allow us to carefully analyze the most basic elements of the human body related to our diet. These include the most and least obvious features and characteristics of the human anatomy on a comparative basis.

The discussion below thus relates to the natural design of our bodies in a comparative and relative manner. It is difficult to argue with this evidence, as it is derived from anatomy, biology and centuries of medical discovery, or is otherwise overtly and reliably visible.

**Structural design: Anatomy**

Let's start from the more macro design of our human form, and how it contrasts with those creatures that eat a predominantly animal diet:

***Gait:*** The human body is more vertical than horizontal. This tallness is especially useful for picking fruit, climbing up trees, reaching around to grab and harvest. Getting down to the level of animals proves difficult for the human gait.

As a result, our bodies are quite clumsy in terms of catching prey. A rabbit or other prey will easily slip through our legs and hands as we clumsily try to reach down and grab one. We also run particularly slow compared to most prey. This puts us at a great disadvantage. We are one of the slowest mammals around. We can't catch a deer, a rabbit, a chicken, wolf, or most other prey. We also can't fly naturally so we aren't equipped to catch birds. But our bodies are perfectly adept at reaching fruit and nuts up in the trees.

*The gait of most carnivores relates to their relative food. A tiger is longer than taller, allowing the animal to propel itself on top of its vic-*

*tims. The bird's gait is designed around catching victims from flight. The carnivore's gait is also built for speed. Sleekness creates aerodynamic design to allow the animal the ability to vault itself onto its prey. Visualize the difference between a camper van and a sports car on the highway. The camper van is so tall that it meets with a greater amount of resistance.*

*The human body would actually more closely resemble a tall, slender port-a-potty than a van in the above analogy..*

***Musculature:*** One of the reasons for our clumsiness in terms of catching animal prey is the length of our muscles. Humans have longer muscles, which allow us to reach out over a longer span – both in reach and power. Our combined arm and leg span – which can be as great as 9-10 feet – is most suited to allow us to reach branches or plants that are out of range for most other species.

But our muscles are not built for speed. Humans are particularly slow – too slow to catch practically any other animal prey with our bodies – except perhaps a cow, elephant or rhino. But these animals have intrinsic design features to help them resist tool-less human capture. These include tusks and great weight for elephants and rhinos, and horns among bulls (prior to our domestication of these animals). A human without tools – our ancestors – could easily be stomped and killed by these slower, larger animals.

Our long muscles are helpful for longer distance journeys. Our bodies are suited for taking longer trips to where the plant life may be more sustainable.

*Carnivores are designed with shorter muscles that allow them to sprint extremely fast in order to catch their prey. And these predators are typically faster than their particular prey. A falcon is faster than the rabbit. The tiger is faster than the antelope. The wolf is faster than the deer. These speedy animals are specifically equipped for speed. They can run fast naturally. They do not need to create any special tools in order to get their prey. This is because they were genetically designed for eating that particular type of prey.*

***Hair and skin:*** Our hair is mopped or curly on our heads, faces and bodies. This helps shade the skin from the sun, together with the skin's production of melanin. Our skin is also very thin – equipped for warmer climates with sweat glands.

These features aid humans in foraging for food during the daylight – when food can be carefully examined. Our thin hair and skin are not very helpful for cold regions or hunting at night.

*This contrasts baldness or thin hair among critters who hunt at night and sleep during the day in warmer climes. Carnivores with fur are typically equipped to hunt during the colder part of the night in colder climates, where they are not dependent upon plant-life.*

**Skull and brain:** Marginally thin, soft and unprotected, may be easily damaged in battle, designed for our larger brains. Large brain size provides greater intelligence for decision-making and careful analysis, and for seeking answers to the mysterious of life.

*This contrasts well-protected bony skulls with small brains among most carnivores, providing extra protection to the brain during hunting battles.*

**Eyes:** Human eyes are comparatively weak and only able to see during the daytime. This serves as a significant disadvantage, because animal meats are best caught at night, when the element of surprise is more available. Humans do not have night vision, nor can they see with focus. Humans must sleep when most prey is available for easier hunting. Our pineal glands require daylight in order to produce hormones sufficient for health.

*In contrast, most carnivores are equipped with extremely sharp vision and night vision. This combination allows them to not only spot prey at night, but spot prey far away. Pineal glands among nocturnal carnivores are quite rudimentary.*

**Ears:** Human ears are designed to hear sound that is fairly close range and with a medium frequency. The ears are located on each side of the head with little ability to 'scoop' air pressure from a single direction. Though also referred to as pinnae, our ear flaps are typically referred to as auricles because of their roundness and lack of mobility: they hence do not draw distant sound waves well.

Human ears hear with medium range – from 20 Hertz to about 15,000 Hertz in most, which declines rapidly as we age. This provides a weak combination range of hearing for defensive maneuvers, but little help in listening to events in the distance or hearing very minute sounds.

*This contrasts many carnivorous species that typically have extremely sensitive hearing, allowing them to get the jump on prey and hear predators coming in the distance. Think about how a cat can move around their ear flaps (pinnae) and perk both ears in one direction – raising their pinnae in unison toward one direction as it listens for the faint pitter-patter sounds of mice feet. Or a tiger or wolf when it comes to prey crawling along the grass in the distance.*

**Mouth:** The human oral cavity opening – our mouth – is significantly smaller than our head size. This allows only small 'bite sized' amounts of food into our mouths.

*This contrasts the mouths of predatory animals, which typically have mouth openings that are a considerable proportion of their head size. Their mouths also expand easily to enable them to envelop large portions of food in one bite.*

**Teeth:** Human teeth are made up primarily of flattened bicuspids (premolars) and molars, with a set of chopping incisors in the front and a set of dull canines on each side. Our teeth are primarily designed for grinding, with some weak ripping potential. This allows us to eat a variety of plant-based foods as opposed to a single food group such as grasses. Our molars and bicuspids are flattened with nodular cusps – perfectly designed for grinding and crushing up harder foods.

This grinding and crushing allows plant fibers and cell walls to be broken down while being mixed with carbohydrate-digesting amylase enzymes from our saliva. Our molars slide past each other sideways.

Our teeth are also very close together – allowing us to grind almost as one unit. Our incisors and canines are perfectly positioned to tear apart fleshy outer rinds of fruits and vegetables, or crack open a nut shell before we begin grinding.

*This contrasts the teeth of predatory animals, which typically have a mouth full of razor-sharp teeth with no chopping or grinding ability. Their teeth move up and down and forward and back, allowing for ripping and sheering. For this reason, carnivores cannot grind their teeth or their food. Carnivore teeth are also spaced to allow the flesh to slide through the teeth without getting hung up.*
*Toothless carnivores will have other razor-sharp equipment. These include super-sharp beaks on carnivore birds and fluorinated calcium phosphate scales among sharks. Carnivore teeth are equipped to stab and tear, allowing them to kill prey as well as rip the flesh once it is*

*dead. Once the carnivore consumes the flesh it does not/cannot chew it. It simply swallows it whole.*

**Jaws:** Human jaws use a complex joint designed for grinding, crushing and chewing foods. We have large masseters and pterygoids – as do other strict herbivores – in order to chew in multiple directions. Our jaws can move asymmetrically sideways as well as upside down. The most obvious trait among herbivores is the ability to move the jaw sideways in order to grind food. The human jaw cannot shear. This jaw type traces back to our earliest ancestors, including the australopithecines and chimpanzees (Taylor 2006).

*This jaw type contrasts the jaws of most carnivores, a simple hinge joint which typically moves only up and down, not sideways. Their jaws are equipped with huge temporalis muscles to grip onto their prey. This allows them to exert shear force and rip into flesh with significant weight and strength. This is important, because carnivore teeth must be able to not only rip into flesh, but they must be able to puncture through animal hide and kill the animal immediately. Can you imagine a human trying to kill a large animal with our little choppers?*

**Stomach:** The human stomach is a rather small sac – big enough to hold a bowl of salad and a plate of food. It comprises about 20-25% of the volume of the digestive tract. The stomach is too small to fit in a piece of meat of any size. And its pepsin and hydrochloric acid content might sterilize a few rotten pieces of fruit, but not much more.

*In contrast, a carnivore's stomach will comprise 50-70% of the animal's digestive tract potential. A carnivore stomach is expandable enough to hold practically an entire carcass. And its acidic content – dramatically more acidic than ours – allows it to digest the bones of its victims.*

**Intestines:** Here is where it gets really interesting. The human small intestines alone are about 70 feet long, some 10 to 12 times the length of our body. The colon adds another three or four feet. The intestines wind back and forth – twisting and turning to allow for complex nutrients and water trapped within plant cell walls to be adequately broken down and absorbed. Our intestines are also lined with complex cilia, which help trap and break down cellulose fibers and those nutrients that lie within. The entire digestive tract is complex, with many compartments, features and components.

This complexity is common among most herbivores and fruitarian animals. However, there is a wide range of complexity depending upon the type of food eaten. A cow's digestive tract will have multiple stomach chambers to allow them to ruminate – or ferment – grasses enabling their enzymes and probiotics to digest the plant material.

Humans are not ruminants. Humans, like many other plant-based food eaters, are *hindgut fermenters*. This means that we break down plant fibers and cell walls throughout our intestines but we finish the fermenting and digestive process in the lower small intestines and colon.

As such, human enzymes are released with saliva in the oral cavity, from the wall of the stomach and through bile ducts that empty within the small intestine. Digestion and assimilation takes place throughout the entire digestive tract.

The human colon, like many herbivores, is quite the complex fermentation facility. It is able to churn and break down fibrous quantities while extracting any remaining nutrients.

*In contrast, a carnivore's smooth intestines are very simple and short. They will only be three or four times the length of the animal's body. And this intestinal tract will be fairly straight and simple, with fewer bends and turns for meat to putrefy within. Their nutrient absorption is typically limited to the small intestine. They house no probiotics to ferment and break down food.*

*Carnivore colons are simple and short. They are not designed to assimilate nutrients – only water and salt. Because meat has no fiber, there is no fiber complexity to break down.*

*Enzymes in carnivores are typically produced from ducts connected to the liver placed within inches of the mouth. This begins the rapid digestive process early on.*

**Hands/Feet/Claws:** Human hands and feet are soft and dexterous, with rounded fingers and toes; with dull, rounded nails. We might be able to grow our nails out a half-inch or so, but they will begin curling inward or outward after that. Human fingers and their nails are suited for plying apart seeds or unpeeling fruits. They are not sharp enough to tear into the flesh of an animal. If we tried to dig our nails into the hide of an animal, we'd probably 'break a nail.'

Rather, human hands are perfectly suited for picking fruits and vegetables, harvesting roots, digging for roots or picking nuts, bark or leaves off of trees.

Human feet are designed to balance on uneven and rounded surfaces. The deep insole together with the dexterous toes allow us to grapple the bottom of a tree limb as we walk along it as we reach for that piece of fruit or leaf. Our feet also allow us to walk through fields of grasses and harvest those with a minimal of damage to the field.

It is for this reason that our early humanoid ancestors did not eat meat – as evidenced from carbon isotope studies on the teeth enamel of ancient archaeological digs. Without special tools, our bodies have little physical ability to harvest the meat – if indeed we could catch an animal. And even the first tools were related to pulling up roots and separating nutshells. They were not significant enough to rip apart an animal. To put is simply: If we were holding a dead furry animal in our hands we would be incapable of opening up that flesh in order to eat it. Without a tool of course. And even then, we'd have a bloody mess on our hands.

And even as more tools were invented by our ancestors, these tools were primarily utilized as weapons of self-defense against hungry animals that wanted to eat them – or humans that wanted to take over their territory.

*In contrast, the claws of carnivores are generally large, extremely hard and pointed at the ends of the nails. These allow them to snag onto prey as they hunt. One swipe of the claws would dig the nails in with a death grip. The sharp nails also assist in killing prey immediately (in combination with their teeth) and ripping apart the flesh (again in combination with their teeth) as needed. Carnivores will have similar claws on the feet and the hands enabling them to latch onto prey from multiple angles. Carnivores have the entire package between their teeth and claws. They require no special tools to catch an animal in their claws, and rip it apart once caught, and consume it immediately before some other predator arrives.. A carnivore's claws are not dexterous, but rather are fixed and hard, with pointed nails that allow their claws to rip through the hide of its prey.*

## Function design: Metabolism

*Saliva:* Along with immune cells, probiotic bacteria, and lysozymes, human saliva contains enzymes that begin assimilation of carbohydrates and plant fats as we chew. These are primarily amylase and lipase. Our saliva is perfectly designed to begin the process of assimilation of fruits, vegetables, nuts and seeds. In addition, humans and other herbivores maintain bacteria that break down plant cell walls. This is similar to practically every other herbivore species, whose saliva contains amylase enzymes. In addition, human and herbivore saliva has an alkaline pH.

*Most carnivores do not even have salivary glands. The juices secreted in their oral cavities also have a complete lack of enzymes, replaced by generous portions of hydrochloric acid, which reduce infectious compounds like salmonella, E. coli, parasites and others from putrefying flesh immediately upon entrance into the oral cavity. Once a carnivore gets the animal flesh into its mouth, it swallows it whole.*

*Many carnivores also have specialized secretions from different glands that allows them to either poison or paralyze their prey as they are eating them. This allows them to begin eating their prey while the prey is still alive.*

**Acid production:** This alkaline oral cavity and esophagus is followed by the human stomach, where acidic juices mixed with hydrochloric acid secreted by the stomach wall help to break down foods and bacteria before they can enter the intestines.

The human stomach pH ranges from 4 to 5 with food, and the pH of the intestines tends to be closer to 5. This rather weak acidic nature is short-lived, as the intestines are pH balanced with the entrance of bile acids from the gall bladder, together with the pH balance produced by the combination of carbohydrates, fats, enzymes and probiotic bacteria.

The human stomach produces pepsin and hydrochloric acid on this minimal basis – primarily restricted to the enclosure of the stomach. This can sterilize light pathogens, but is useless against the majority of bacteria and parasites.

For this reason we find that we find foodborne illnesses – primarily related to animal foods – one of the biggest threats to human health.

*Carnivores produce about ten times the amount of hydrochloric acid pH of the digestive juices of humans and other herbivores. The pH of their entire intestinal tract stays about 1 – some 400 to 500 times more acidic than the human stomach. This allows the carnivore to kill off the tremendous influx of bacteria and parasites that will colonize putrefying flesh.*

**Digestive enzymes:** The human stomach, intestines, liver and probiotic bacteria produce a fairly narrow range of enzymes – which we will investigate further. These include amylases that break down carbohydrates, cellulases that break down cellulose, lactases that break dairy, peptidases that break down peptide complexes (protein pieces), sucrases that break down sugars, lipases that break down fats and others. The mix of enzymes our body produces are geared towards plant-based foods.

*The carnivore's digestive enzymes are geared towards digesting animal proteins and fats. Most have no ability to digest cellulose-based nutrients. A carnivore's enzymes are suitable to digest the bones of their animal dinner. Eating a bone whole will likely kill a human.*

**Liver metabolism:** The human liver is designed to process a minimal amount of uric acid, as it processes vitamins, minerals, fats, proteins and other phytonutrients. The human liver also cannot detoxify vitamin A — which is necessary to prevent vitamin A toxicity.

*In contrast, carnivore livers are suited to process greater volumes of uric acid. Because animal flesh contains a maximum of protein, it results in huge amounts of uric acid for the liver to process. It is for this reason that meat-eating diets tend to produce a higher risk of gout and other uric acid-related conditions. Carnivore livers can detoxify vitamin A.*

**Intestinal bacteria:** The human digestive tract — typical of most herbivores — houses trillions of probiotic bacteria that secret enzymes and help process and digest our foods. This is allowed through a rather weak acidic intestinal tract, allowing the bacteria to flourish.

As we'll discuss in detail, the primary foods of these bacteria (prebiotics) are plant-based and dairy-based foods.

*In contrast, the carnivore digestive tract is so acidic that it is practically sterile. Any parasite or bacteria that survives the acidic intestines is either so virulent that it has adapted, has infested other parts of the animal's body, or the animal's production of hydrochloric acid has become faulty.*

*Curiously, this later event can happen among domesticated animals, but rarely occurs in the wild.*

## The Human Mentality

The human mentality is disposed to intelligence and compassion. Our nature is intellectual rather than violent. When we see a young cub or fawn, our minds will think about how cute and innocent those little creatures are. Instinctively, we will want to protect them rather than eat them. For this reason, even among today's slaughterhouses, it is considered immoral to slaughter a baby animal. And for this reason, humans have animal-cruelty laws.

*This contrasts the mentality of a carnivore, who sees young creatures as dessert. The mind of a carnivore is merciless when it comes to practi-*

*cally any other creature besides their own young. They look upon a young cub or deer as easy prey – delicious meat. A carnivore's mentality is geared towards seeing any living creature as potential prey.*

### Could humans be omnivores?

This has been an assumption of many nutritionists. But strictly by design, we are not omnivores.

- Omnivores – such as bears – still have the distinct ability to capture prey – humans do not. Omnivores will still have claws and razor sharp shearing teeth. Humans have neither.
- Omnivores will still have jaws that allow them to force down onto flesh to kill it. Humans do not.
- Omnivores will have large temporalis muscles to grip onto their prey. Humans have strong masseters and pterygoids – as do other strict herbivores.
- Omnivores will have sharp canines and molars. Humans do not.
- Omnivores do not have saliva with digesting enzymes. Humans do.
- Omnivores will still have a pH of 1 within the stomach to allow them to sterilize meat. Humans have 4-5 pH.
- Omnivores will have longer intestines than carnivores, but typically only one or two times body length more. Humans have twice as long intestines – like other strict herbivores.
- Omnivore livers can detoxify vitamin A. Human livers cannot.

### Disease is an indication of eating the wrong diet

Think about it. Do we see the kind of health conditions we see among modern humans within the wild? Do we see wild animals with inflammatory diseases like asthma, arthritis, Alzheimer's disease, cardiovascular disease, diabetes and the like? Hardly. Yes, we might see some osteoarthritis in some species – but only among a few.

We do see some of these maladies among our domesticated animals. But these are animals that have been taken out of the wild and away from their natural diets.

Yes, that's the point. Wild dogs – basically, wolves and foxes – will not have inflammatory diseases until they are domesticated and given processed foods.

When an animal is removed from its natural diet, that's when these kinds of inflammatory diseases are created. Given the environmental and dietary conditions that suit any physiology, until old age, inflammatory disease is practically non-existent.

And as for the natural diet for humans – the Ancestors Diet – we can provide scientific evidence for this conclusion.

As we will illustrate shortly, red meat produces an array of diseased conditions, from diabetes to cardiovascular disease to Alzheimer's to cancer and so many other maladies.

## Our Genetic Disposition

Our DNA is important because it governs all aspects of our body's design. This not only governs our body's structure and metabolism, but the ability to pass these between generations.

Our genetic disposition comes after millions of years of evolutionary development. Humans did not evolve accidentally. It wasn't as if the human body was an ecological accident – and our bodies were zapped here.

The science reveals a very long evolutionary process involved in the eventual design of the human body. This means that the bodies we have – those organs and metabolism – are the result of a gradual process of natural selection that took place over millions of years.

And it is for this reason we find the scientific evidence examined in this book that illustrates that some foods produce a myriad of disease conditions, while other foods do not. It lies within our genetic disposition, which predicts the design of the human body.

In this regard, we can consider a quote from a 2013 study by researchers from the Johns Hopkins School of Medicine (Bazzen *et al.*):

> *"Red and processed meat consumption has consistently gained a reputation as a contributor to disease, including cancer. Data is emerging that red and processed meats may influence disease recurrence and mortality as well, for example, for colorectal cancer survivors. Evidence shows that consumption of red meat can activate cancer genes in the colon such as the MDM2 and ubiquitin genes as well as the WNT gene signaling pathway which is involved in epithelial proliferation and differentiation. Such genetic modulation can facilitate cellular progression to colon cancer."*

A consistent association between a certain diet and a particular disease condition – especially related to cancer, which is related to mutation or genetic damage – clearly indicates a conflict between that particular diet and our genetic design.

To say this in the converse, if our choice of diet is consistent with our genetic design, then it should not result in genetic damage.

Some propose that our original genetic design from our ancestors has mutated, and now we have adapted to a diet different from our ancestors. However, to suddenly unwind our genetic design after millions of years of evolution is simply not possible.

Surely our bodies can learn to slowly adapt to new environments. Our bodies can also adapt to new diets. But this adaptation process is gradual, and always comes with consequences. This is what disease is. Consequence along the way toward adaptation. Yes, if we ate another diet – lets say we started eating plastic – for the next million years – our digestive tracts may adapt. But over that million years, we would be maligned with numerous disease conditions as the consequences of that diet selection.

In other words, our long, twisty intestinal tracts cannot be shortened immediately, nor can our hydrochloric acid output be pumped up to the level of carnivores right away. The latter would dissolve our intestinal tracts, for example.

The proposal put forth by some is that our recent ancestral cuisine should dictate our current diet, and after all, didn't most of our recent ancestors eat meat?

This latter assumption actually runs contrary to historical evidence. Most of the world's populations until the last few thousand years lived in regions where the climate supported humanity's primary diet of plant-based foods: nuts, fruits, berries, leaves, vegetables, bark, roots and grains.

Even evidence from the 'Old World' Europe – dating back to 5,000-10,000 years ago, indicates a human population that was primarily agricultural. Most evidence confirms that meat was rarely eaten more than once per week, and even then often less often (Flandrin 1999).

This evidence indicates that even as larger domesticated livestock farming enterprises took hold in the late Middle Ages as more humans populated the cold countries, meat consumption in Northern Europe provided less than fifteen percent of protein consumption among the pre-industrial humans. For those households with domesticated animals and even for households without animal husbandry; milk, butter and cheese were regarded as staples.

Among the more populated regions of the Middle East, Asia Minor and Africa, meat eating continued with less emphasis. In many of these cultures, meat eating was frowned upon and considered a diet for lower-class citizens, and was considered unclean. Meat eating was either forbidden or highly regulated by many ancient religious cultures.

Even among more recent Biblical times (3,000 years ago or so), among desert regions where there was little vegetation, regulations regarding meat eating included many restrictions. These included restrictions on the animal species, requirements on draining the blood before preparation, and special deity offering requirements.

Frankly, the unrestricted killing and eating of animals has historically been discouraged by most ancient religions. These cultures were for the most part nut, fruit, vegetable, leaf and root collectors. As agriculture expanded, these ancestors became crop and dairy farmers, and vegetation gatherers. Grains, tubers, berries, nuts, dairy, and fruit have formed the majority of even our more recent human ancestors.

For example, we find in the most ancient scriptures instructions that advise against eating meat. Consider this clear Biblical verse:

> *Then God said, "I give you every seed-bearing plant on the face of the whole earth and every tree that has fruit with seed in it. They will be yours for food." (Genesis 1:29 NIV)*

Whether we accept that God gave this instruction or not, we must accept that those ancient teachers who passed on this teaching certainly accepted that our bodies were designed (created) to eat a plant-based diet.

Furthermore, the oldest known religious scriptures, the *Sanskrit Vedas,* also promulgate eating a plant-based diet.

It is easy to miss the big picture of humanity while focusing on the exceptions. Sure, we can focus on the Eskimos if we want. Or how about the cannibal tribes of Papua New Guinea? As for the latter, this is how prion infections were discovered – the type that causes "mad cow disease." This has also been called Kuru disease, known to poison Papuan cannibals, and humans who've eaten infected cows (fed meat).

The point is, these cultures are exceptions to human history rather than the rule. We might add to this that there are certainly cultures today even that have resorted to cannibalism in their recent past and even present. Are we to take these exceptions and base our diet upon this?

Similarly, if we examine the larger picture of human history among the greatest and largest societies and cultures, and then trace those back to their ancestors, we find that animal diets were exceptions rather than the rule. Animal diets were limited to those groups of humans that ventured outside the human-friendly environment, where humans were forced to eat outside their normal diet.

Even if we were to accept the erroneous assumption that every human over the last 10,000 years ate meat, this would still only be a tiny blip on the screen of the 3-4 million years of humanoid existence, and the hundreds of millions of years of evolution before that, which led to the genetic disposition and physical design humans have today.

And yes, many of us are descendants of those who lived in Northern Europe for thousands of years – although most of those more Europeans descended more recently than we imagine from Middle Easterners, Asians and Aryans. But the percentage of total human population of these cultures is still only a small fraction of the total human race.

And yes, it does get cold up there in Northern Europe during the winter, forcing some cultures to develop diets with greater meat portions.

But it was either this or starve. This would properly make the animal diet more of a starvation diet. A diet that provides more of a blip in our genetic history compared to the millions of years that our ancestors ate a diet consisting of nuts, fruits, vegetables, bark, roots, seeds and grains.

And what about all those tools we invented. Were they all based upon meat eating as we've imagined? Hardly. Most of the earliest tools were digging tools and splitting tools – enabling our ancestors to dig for tubers and split open nut shells.

What about the spear then? Yes, indeed the spear, then the sword and the so-many other weapons humans have created over the past millennium must be evidence that we were out chasing down animals and spearing them.

Well, first of all, we were never fast enough to chase down many animals, and those whom we could catch up to were typically too small for spearing. Yes, spearing has been found among fishing cultures, to presumably catch fish.

But the primary reason for the spear, and then the sword, was to battle ourselves. Each group of humans carved out their own little domain, where its fruits, nuts, vegetables, roots and/or grains were plentiful, and needed to defend its territory against those groups who didn't have as much. And because humans often traveled around – migrated to where the foods were more plentiful, there were undoubtedly struggles. This was evidenced between the Neanderthals and their *Homo erectus* challengers.

The reality is that while protective and even sometimes paranoid, humans have also been pretty smart. In fact, highly intellectual writings from ancient times from Mesopotamia and the Hindus valleys – where much of early man lived – illustrated a well-thought out and organized diet of raw and fermented dairy, grains, fruits and vegetables. An everyday diet of meat for much of ancient man outside of the northernmost and colder regions has been debatable – and evidence strongly points in the other direction.

For those who did end up out in the cold diet-wise, does that blip on the human scale effect our genes much? Certainly there are effects of diet on metabolism and this can affect our genes. But the larger picture says no. Why? Because we can plainly see by the research that our ancestors' primarily plant-based diet reduces disease, and the starvation diet – that blip in human history – produces disease. This is the clearest indication that the animal diet of the colder countries has not affected our genes that much.

Yes, we find a host of inflammatory maladies related to our diets, and this also relates to our genetic disposition – our bodies' ability to digest these foods and utilize them in health.

In other words, our genes determine which foods we are genetically disposed to.

And we will show the clear evidence in this book that genetically the human body was designed for a plant-based diet.

Excuse any redundancy, but let's review the design of our physical features with respect to our genes. Just to clarify anything yet unclear.

Again, if the human body was genetically disposed for hunting and eating meat, our genes would have produced claws for ripping and tearing rather than fingers and nails able to accurately and precisely unpeel fruits, crack nuts and open plant fibers.

Human hands and feet were genetically designed for picking fruit; gathering and preparing roots; picking and prying open vegetables; cracking apart nutshells and pulling out nut meats; and harvesting seeds or honey.

Certainly if the human body was genetically designed to eat meat, we would have legs that could run at faster speeds to catch our prey. Our legs cannot even keep up with a rabbit or squirrel let alone catch an antelope or other larger "game."

Our genes would produce a mouth full of incisors instead of mostly bicuspids and molars. Our teeth are designed for grinding. Our two incisors are perfectly positioned to tear apart fleshy fruits and vegetables.

To propose these two dull incisors positioned in the middle of grinding teeth make a case for humans being carnivores is quite a reach. Our two dull incisors on each side of the mouth are positioned inside the mouth rather than at the mouth's edge. This means we cannot reach them out as we try to tear into some flesh. We have to figure out how to rip up the flesh to be small enough to fit into our mouth so that we can tear it a little.

Try, for example to reach out your teeth and rip into an animal's flesh with your incisors. It is practically impossible. The animal has to be cut up into mouth-sized pieces, and those fleshy pieces have to put into the mouth in order for us to chew it.

Meanwhile tigers, sharks, wolves and other hunters have a mouth full of razor-sharp ripping teeth and incredibly strong jaws that can reach out and chomp out a piece of flesh from the get-go. In other words, their teeth can be protruded out of the mouth to enable them to rip and tear into an animals body. They can take a chomp directly out of the side of an animal body.

Seriously, can we really expect to rip apart and fully chop up an animal's flesh and organs into small enough pieces to eat with our two rounded incisors and our weak jaws?

Our genetics have designed our mouth and teeth to certainly enable us to chomp into and take a bite out of an apple or other fruit. Those front incisors that can reach out of the mouth and take a bite out of an apple are flat and squared. They are perfectly suited for the purpose of taking bites out of apples or grinding grains – not ripping flesh out of the side of an animal.

Furthermore, if our DNA was designed to be a carnivore, our feet would have claws for tearing apart our victims instead of soft toes to walk along the soft ground harvesting food, or to balance on while we walk along limbs and climb into the trees for our fruits and berries.

If we were meat eaters, like other carnivores, our DNA would produce eyes equipped with night-vision, allowing us to track the majority of animals that roam the earth after sunset.

Rather, our DNA produces eyes with day-only vision with retinal cells equipped to distinguish bright colors of ripening fruits and vegetables. This vision allows us not only to find those fruits and vegetables ready to eat, but to distinguish between poisonous ones.

Our DNA produces ears that pick up the medium spectrum of sounds, focused on our own voices and the sounds of more dangerous animals like wolves and tigers. Our ears are not equipped to listen to the very high- and very-low pitched rhythms of the animals we are able to catch and beat up with our blunt fingers and toes, such as squirrels, mice, moles, deer and rabbits. Because of our narrow auditory skills, we have great difficulty tracking these animals.

Simply put, our DNA did not lend to humans being hunters. It had to be forced onto our lifestyle through the use of tools and extraordinary measures. And even then, our bodies are reacting in the form of numerous diseased conditions – which we'll clarify in this book.

Human DNA produces longer and slower muscles. Our leg muscles make us one of the slowest specimens on the planet. What kind of creature could we catch? Almost every creature can outrun us, from squirrels to birds to fish to wolves, tigers, horses, etc. On foot, it would be difficult for us to even catch one of the largest vegetarians, the elephant. Oh, maybe we could catch a turtle. But what then? Could we even open its hard shell with our rounded, soft fingers?

If we consider the DNA that produces the physical characteristics of species that hunt, we can easily see other drastic differences. Hunters can travel at tremendous speeds. They either are equipped to fly and swoop; jump and leap; run and snatch; or sneak up and pounce on their prey. They usually have sharp ripping claws, night vision, very quick coordination, and response, allowing them to out-maneuver or surprise other creatures during the hunt.

Our DNA has designed the human body to be slow; dull; soft; gangly; rounded; obvious; and stupid when it comes to the element of surprise. Our muscles are inflexible in comparison. We have little ability to quickly leap or jump. In comparing the length and width of our appendages, we are quite weak and slow. About the only thing we have going for us besides our problem-solving nature is a misplaced sense of pride, thinking we are so smart that we can control nature and do whatever we want without restriction.

When it comes to digestion, our DNA prevents us from easily eating meat without cooking it. Otherwise, we will likely die from salmonella, trichinosis or parasitic infections. Even if when we cook meat our enzymes are poorly equipped to digest it.

When we consider the DNA that produces the intestinal tract of hunters such as tigers or other carnivores, we find their DNA produces short, fat colons that move the non-fibrous, fleshy saturated fatty meat through faster. This allows the meat to move through their tracts within hours, while meat can take three days to get through our digestive tracts.

The DNA of herbivores has produced long digestive tracts, ranging from ten to twelve times their body length. Carnivore DNA produces shorter tracts, averaging only about three or four times their body length.

The DNA of carnivores secrete incredibly strong hydrochloric acid to enable the break down of the more complex proteins and peptides of meat. Human DNA and other herbivore DNA have hydrochloric acid strengths about twenty times weaker than meat eaters have. The DNA of humans and most herbivores produce salivary glands that produce amylase, which facilitates the digestion of plant starches. Meat eating animals do not have salivary glands.

Yes, some of these points duplicate points made previously. But we are talking genetics here. These genetic traits are not accidents. It is not as if we accidentally were given little ability to find, catch, rip open and eat flesh. Our bodies, and the bodies of our ancestors, were genetically designed to eat certain types of foods. And these foods do not include eating meat.

Yes, some of our ancestors – those who got themselves trapped in deserts, snowy mountains or glaciers, and other environments otherwise we were not intended to occupy. And once trapped in these regions, some of those ancestors had to go outside our intended diet.

And yes, our bodies were not designed to live in snowy mountains or deserts. We don't have long thick fur that keeps us warm as do bears and foxes do. We don't have thick, leathery skin and cold blood that enables us to dwell in sandy deserts as do reptiles.

But some of our less intelligent ancestors did this anyway. Whether they were chased out of their natural habitats by warring tribes or they figured they liked the solitude of the frozen mountain, this was not a smart move.

And it is for this reason that the Neanderthals and Homo erectus likely went extinct: They moved to a region their bodies were not designed to live.

The human body was designed to live in moist or arid tropical or sub-tropical regions. Those regions where fruits grow on trees and grasses (grains) grow on the plains.

And it is within these regions that humans blossomed. While the ice-men of Northern Europe were etching out primitive cave drawings, the Aryans of the Indus Valley and the ancient Chinese, along with the Egyptians of the fertile Nile basin, the Indonesians and Polynesians and the Indian cultures of South and Central America producing great writings that included a complex alphabet, mathematics, astronomy and many other scientific developments.

This is because they had plenty to eat from their environments. They didn't need to spend all day figuring out how to trap and then skin an animal. These societies that ate primarily plant-based diets were not only prosperous: They were also spiritual and intellectual, and they respected the earth.

And herein we find a critical bridge between our diet and our approach to the earth. Serious research has found that a diet that focuses upon those foods our body was designed to eat also happens to be better for our environment. This diet utilizes less water, less land and produces less environmental damage, with a smaller carbon footprint. Why? Because the design of our bodies is similar to the design of the earth: There are processes of nature that incorporate those organisms that occupy it. They are congruent and sustainable when living organisms act within nature's design.

And when they act out of nature's design, things go badly. They get out of whack. This is precisely what has happened in the case of humanity.

The human body was equipped with the perfect tools for harvesting fruits, vegetables, seeds, roots and nuts. We can eat them raw or they can easily be dried in the sun without difficulty. We have the fingers and thumb to pull the husks or peels off, or crack the hulls. Then we can just

31

pop them into our mouths and move on. We do not have to cook most vegetables, fruits and nuts. We have the digestive tools to handle these foods without any complications. Can you imagine a tiger trying to peel an orange? Certainly not. The tiger's body is not equipped for eating fruits. Its claws would shred the fruit into a mangled juicy lump.

In order to logically and scientifically determine our best diet, the focus should be on our genetic and physical traits. There are obvious foods the human body can handle without advanced or complex preparation. These are the foods we were genetically designed to eat.

Red meat would naturally fall off of this list, because most raw meat will make a human immediately ill. We simply do not have strong enough hydrochloric acids to prevent those bacteria that harbor within decomposing flesh from infecting us.

On this point, some have suggested that humans are opportunistic eaters. As if we would be harvesting fruit up in a tree, and we see a bird in the tree, and we grab the bird and chomped it down.

First of all, the bird would likely fly off before we could grab it. And if we did catch it, we couldn't choke down the bird with its beak, feathers and so forth. It would never get past our esophagus, and our stomachs could not digest it.

Instead, we'd have to pluck all its feathers, pull off its beak, feet and so forth. Then we might be able to eat it, but likely by that time it would start to decompose. Plus the bacteria – salmonella and so forth – left by the bird's feathers and its certain excrement when we killed it – would sicken us after choking it down raw.

According to archaeological evidence, humans did not invent fire until about 500,000 years ago. Humans were on the planet at least 1.5 million years prior to fire. Did these ancestors of ours eat raw flesh and drink blood? Nope.

All around, our genetics have produced physical features that make meat eating unhealthy and impractical without extensive tools and practices, such as slaughterhouses, butchers, refrigerators, frying pans or ovens and so on. And even with these extensive systems among the richest nations such as the U.S., foodborne illness outbreaks occur most often among meats – inclusive of salmonella, *E. coli*, Legionnaires disease and others.

If we had the genetics of carnivorous animals, even the most infected meats would not bother us. A carnivore can gobble down a hunk of meat from a carcass that died a week ago with no problem. This is because the genes of carnivores produce so much hydrochloric acid that practically no living organism can survive their guts.

Our genetics have produced digestive tracts too long for meat, digestive acids too weak for meat, nails are too soft, legs too long and slow, eyes and hearing too dull to find or catch an animal. Our genes simply aren't carnivorous genes.

These are the same general genes our ancestors had – which produced the same traits. They are the same traits that our ancestors had, and this is why our earliest and smartest ancestors ate a plant-based diet together with fermented dairy.

Even with this clear evidence, some still insist there are some physical traits that allow humans to eat flesh, making humans omnivores. Certainly we would be considered omnivores because this is what modern humans eat.

But outside of our harmful modern habit, eating meat was forced upon our bodies through survivalship in inhospitable environments. The only things that allow humans the ability to eat meat are those tools our bodies do not possess – the very tools that we use to kill each other and/or are killing our environment – including guns, knives, slaughterhouses, factory farms and the like.

We might compare this thesis that we are omnivores to a thesis that bicycles were designed to ride up Mount Everest. Sure, you can put a bike on a plane and take it to the base of the mountain, and then haul it up the mountain using towing equipment. Then you might be able to find a section of ice where the bike can be ridden for a few minutes without taking the rider to his death down a crevasse.

Similarly, yes, we can force the human body to eat an animal if we really want it to. We can build factory farms to imprison animals; complex slaughterhouses to trap, kill and cut up animals; employ some butchers to chop the meat up so we can take it home; and cook the meat for a an hour or two in order to eat it.

Let's compare this complicated process to eating some fruit:

*1) walk up to a tree*
*2) reach up and pick a fruit*
*3) put the fruit into the mouth and eat the fruit*

This same process is practically duplicated in the case of nuts, seeds, vegetables and roots. Some of these will require peeling or washing – able to be performed on the spot with no tools.

As alluded to above, we can dramatically see what our genes are designed for by comparing the effects between the two types of diets.

As we'll show in the next chapter, our physical response to meat – being an increase in cancer, heart disease, diabetes, high cholesterol, Alzheimer's and other conditions – is a clear indication that our genes have designed our bodies to eat a plant-based, fermented-dairy diet.

This exposes the reality that the choice to eat meat has been manufactured by those of our ancestors who decided to, for whatever reason, try to survive in environments our bodies were not designed to survive in.

Regardless of these unfortunate predecessors' experiences, most of us humans now have the freedom, where ever we may live, through the use of other modern human tools, to eat the diet our bodies were designed to eat. So unless we want to go out and chase down a rabbit and tear it apart with our bare hands and figure out how to stuff the bloody mess into our mouth and digest it, we might want to consider using the better part of our intelligence to eat those foods we were designed to eat – those foods our earliest ancestors ate.

The famous physician and botanist Dr. Carl Linnaeus (1707-1778), considered the "father of taxonomy," once stated that *"Man's structure, external and internal, compared with that of the other animals, shows that fruit and succulent vegetables constitute his natural food."*

## What About Blood Types?

Today there is a lot of interest in our more immediate ancestors due to a proposal put forth that our blood types dictate the best diet for us to eat. According to the theory, each blood type is oriented towards a different type of diet, and a different group of foods, based upon a proposal that different blood types came from different ancestries.

First off, there is no scientific evidence supporting any health benefit to a blood-type diet. In a review of research from scientists at the Belgium Red Cross published in July of 2013 (Cusack *et al.* 2013), 1,415 published medical references were reviewed for evidence, resulting in sixteen studies that looked at the blood-type diet from one perspective or another. None of them indicated any evidence that a blood-type diet has any benefit. The researchers stated:

*"No evidence currently exists to validate the purported health benefits of blood type diets."*

The thesis that foods our ancestors ate would be better for us is noble, and even a scientific approach. The problem with pegging it to blood type is that there is no scientific evidence supporting a link between blood type and unique diseases or dietary proclivities. And our blood type is not necessarily matched to our genetics.

Just the fact that one family can contain several blood types is a scientific fact. One's blood type is dictated by just one allele among our DNA – something that is determined by the combination of alleles of our parents. This creates a particular genotype. And because the blood type O is recessive, while A and B genes are co-dominant, ones blood type is not necessarily a determination of the rest of one's genetics.

Consider, for example, if one parent has type A blood, with alleles of either AA or AO, and the other parent has blood type B with alleles of either BB or BO. The child may have a blood type of AB, A, B or O. And AA of one and a BB of another will likely produce AB blood type, and a blood type of AO and BO will likely produce O, but because A and B are co-dominant, having the blood type of A or B is completely possible as well.

Historically, as we trace back nutrition among families, we arrive at the fact that these blood types have been mixing among families of different cultures for thousands of years. (The blood type connection to different cultures is still somewhat theoretical and has not been proven, and if it did occur, it occurred hundreds of thousands of years ago if not millions of years ago.) And we know that different cultures have been eating primarily the same foods within their families.

While ones blood type does have some significance to our metabolism, this importance is minimized by the fact that the human genome contains over 20,000 genes, and the blood type gene is just one of them. To this end, we can quote a recent study from scientists from the University of Chicago's Department of Human Genetics:

> "The ABO histo-blood group, first discovered over a century ago, is found not only in humans but also in many other primate species, with the same genetic variants maintained for at least 20 million years. Polymorphisms in ABO have been associated with susceptibility to a large number of human diseases, from gastric cancers to immune or artery diseases, but the adaptive phenotypes to which the polymorphism contributes remain unclear. We suggest that variation in ABO has been maintained by frequency-dependent or fluctuating selection pressures, potentially arising from co-evolution with gut pathogens. We further hypothesize that the histo-blood group labels A, B, AB, and O do not offer a full description of variants maintained by natural selection, implying that there are unrecognized, functionally important, antigens beyond the ABO group in humans and other primates."

Let's now look at this more logically. Even among variant blood types of the same cultures and families we see similar diets over hundreds, even thousands of years. A snippet of a single family might have, for example, five children, and those children might have two each, and each of those 12 people will likely eat a similar diet, based upon the diet of their parents. This is despite the fact that depending upon the blood type alleles of their parents, all of the blood types could be represented within that family of 12 people.

Now when we enlarge this picture into cultures and family lineages, we find that within many other cultures around the world all the blood types are represented yet everyone eats a similar diet. And these diets have been handed down through the families of that society for thousands of years, even with the mix of blood types.

So we must look deeper.

As mentioned by the University of Chicago researchers, primates and humans both share a mix of blood types. Yet we see that primates generally will eat a narrow selection of foods – the same foods our bodies were designed to eat. And this is regardless of their blood type.

Is this a genetic issue? Yes, certainly because certain genes express the production of particular enzymes, and these enzymes are used to break down certain foods. And as mentioned, we have over 20,000 of these genes that express the production of proteins (enzymes are proteins). So it is a very complex situation as different genes are expressed in different circumstances.

And as the University of Chicago researchers mention, our body's microbiome – the genes that make up our intestinal bacteria and the various other bacteria that cover our body, our sinuses, oral cavity, toes, vaginas, ears and so on – also must be considered if we are to match up our genes to our diets.

In fact, our microbiome – the DNA composite of all of our intestinal bacteria – is a greater determinant of what our diet should be than the rest of our DNA according to recent research. Let's delve into our microbiome in detail.

# Chapter Two

# The Diet of Our Microbiome

We can add the combination of 20,000 or so gene sequences found in the human genome to the massive number of additional gene sequences found within our microbiome.

In fact, our genome dwarfs our microbiome by many degrees. If we were to consider our entire genetic map as an apple pie, the sliver of the slice our genome would make up wouldn't be much wider than a human hair.

At evidence is the research of the Human Microbiome Project, sponsored by the National Institutes of Health. An initial study that drew samples from 242 healthy humans found 11,174 different species of commensal bacteria and yeasts among the guts, mouths, skin and vaginas (women) of the subjects.

And each of these species can have up to 13,000 gene sequences, so we can imagine the size of our microbiome.

Our bodies contain about 100 trillion of these organisms, ten times the number of cells in our body.

As researchers have investigated the variations between gut bacteria enterotypes among different ethnicities and populations, the environment and individual dietary choices have become linked with the makeup of our gut bacteria. Research from Yale University (Moeller and Ochman 2013) confirmed this. The researchers also detailed what has been discovered among chimpanzees from different locations - as common differences in gut bacteria are related to diet and environment.

This aspect was not only confirmed in this study, but in others. Multiple studies have shown that the makeup of ones gut bacteria is significantly related to ones diet. In one, University of Pennsylvania researchers (Wu, *et al.* 2011) drew fecal samples from 98 healthy people, and compared their diets and long-term diets (the diets their families had) to the makeup of their intestinal bacteria.

The researchers found that ones diet significantly correlated with the nature of their gut's intestinal bacteria. They also found an even stronger correlation between the gut bacteria and their long-term diet, based upon their ethnic cultural foods and so on. But when their diets were changed, the researchers found that the makeup of their intestinal bacteria actually changed dramatically. They stated:

> *"A controlled-feeding study of 10 subjects showed that microbiome composition changed detectably within 24 hours of initiating a high-fat/low-fiber or low-fat/high-fiber diet."*

## The Microbiome Enterotypes

The researchers also saw a pattern of two particular clusters of bacteria types, which they referred to as enterotypes. The two primary enterotypes were based upon larger populations of the genera Bacteroides or Prevotella.

Research has also found a third enterotype, Ruminococcus – based upon more of these populations – but this enterotype has been relegated as rare and not so prevalent among humans.

As the University of Pennsylvania researchers compared long-term dietary habits with each enterotype, they found that long-term Western diet and greater meat consumption was related to the Bacteroides enterotype, while the Prevotella enterotype was associated with greater long-term consumption of plant-based diets among the cultures of those being tested.

Furthermore, as reported by the researchers:

> *"Self-reported vegetarians showed enrichment in the Prevotella enterotype."*

The researchers also measured intestinal clearance – the time it takes for food to pass through the digestive tract – between the high-fiber diets with high-fat diets. They found that the transit time among high-fat diet subjects went up to a high of seven days, while the high-fiber subjects' transit time ranged from two to four days.

And changes within their gut microorganism composition occurred even within that time – as early as 24 hours from the time their diets were changed.

This enterotyping of the microbiome was also studied by Cornell University scientists (Koren *et al.* 2013), who also found the two clusters – Bacteroides and Prevotella enterotypes – prevalent among their test subjects.

And they also found that the two enterotypes were associated to the dietary habits of the subjects in the form of their recent ancestry. They found that those who were from western countries had a predominantly Bacteroides enterotype, while those who were from non-western countries were primarily Prevotella in enterotype.

This of course relates to the Yale study, as the Western diet is most closely associated with western countries – hence the term *"Western diet."*

## The Rise of *Bacteroides fragilis*

One of the most hardy and prevalent Bacteroides bacteria among the guts of humans is *Bacteroides fragilis*. When it is out of control, *Bacteroides fragilis* can be a highly pathogenic gram-negative bacteria. It has been linked to a number of inflammatory conditions within the gut and else-where.

Among scientific research on pathogenic bacteria in the gut, *B. fragilis* has been isolated the most in inflammatory infections. It has been shown to make up from 40-75% of those samples pulled from intestinal inflammatory conditions. And *B. fragilis* has been shown to be one of the most antibiotic-resistant bacteria within the gut – meaning that it will likely survive when other bacteria are killed by a course of antibiotics. These include penicillin, moxifloxacin and others (Snydman *et al.* 2010).

*B. fragilis* also has the distinction of being so hardy that it doesn't always show up in stools – especially during intestinal infections. This is because *B. fragilis* tends to be stronger than other gut bacteria, and will protect itself within colony capsules to avoid die off from competing bacteria. When *B. fragilis* escapes the confines of the intestines, infection rates skyrocket. Research has found that *B. fragilis* infections have a 19% mortality (Wexler 2007).

Intestinal-related infections known to be primarily caused by *B. fragilis* include appendicitis, irritable bowel syndrome, intestinal abscesses, polyps and others.

We should include obesity in this list as well. University of Antwerp scientists (Bervoets *et al.* 2013) tested the fecal microbiota of 26 over-weight or obese children along with 27 lean children. The data found that obese children had nearly triple the content of *B. fragilis* as the lean children (17.3% versus 6.1%). This of course is compounded by the fact that *B. fragilis* does not show up as much in fecal testing as do other bacteria. So this means that *B. fragilis* is worse of a problem in obese individuals.

One of the characteristics of many *B. fragilis* strains is that they produce a chemical called beta-lactamase, which makes them resistant to many antibiotics.

## Beta-Lactamase and Disease

In fact, beta-lactamase related infections are rising, and they have been associated with eating meats infected with beta-lactamase producing microorganisms.

Researchers from Berlin's Charité University School of Medicine (Leistner *et al.* 2013) have determined that eating pork is linked to the worldwide increase in extended-spectrum beta-lactamase positive (ESBL+) *Escherichia coli*. These multidrug-resistant bacteria can cause severe infections, and it has been seen growing among communities.

The researchers sought to determine if there was a dietary relationship with the increase in ESBL+ infections among certain communities.

The researchers studied 85 cases of ESBL+ *E. coli* infections together with 170 control patients. All of the patients were admitted to the Charité University Hospital between May of 2011 and January of 2012.

Among other risk factors, the researchers determined that eating pork more than three times a week increased the risk of acquiring the ESBL(+) *E. coli* infection by more than three and a half times. In their conclusion they stated that:

> *"frequently consuming certain types of meat like pork can be independently associated with the colonization of ESBL-positive bacteria."*

And research by Mariat (et al. 2009) and others have found that ones gut microbiota will change as we age – with an increase in *E. coli* and other pathogenic bacteria – and will be different among obese or lean individuals. Obesity has been specifically found to relate to higher levels of *E. coli* and other pathogenic bacteria such as Clostridia and *B. fragilis*.

Other studies have found a relationship between higher levels of Clostridia and *B. fragilis* with poor health.

For example, researchers from Sweden's Lund University (Karlsson *et al.* 2012) tested twenty overweight or obese children who were between four and five years old, and compared these children with twenty healthy children.

The researchers conduced a DNA analysis of the children's intestinal microbiota (using the quantitative polymerase chain reaction test). They also conducted liver enzyme tests as well.

The researchers found that the obese/overweight children had higher levels of Enterobacteriaceae – which include *E. coli* as well as Klebsiella, along with more pathogenic genus' such as Salmonella and Shigella.

Borderline but greater levels of Clostridia and *B. fragilis* species were found among obese children in another study of 26 overweight children and 27 lean children. The researchers found that overweight children had significantly higher ratios of Firmicutes (inclusive of Clostridia) than did lean children (Bervoets *et al.* 2013). This study also found higher levels of *B. fragilis* and lower levels of a Bacteroides species that balance *B. fragilis* bacteria, *B. vulgatus*.

Clostridia bacteria include *Clostridium difficile* – one of the most vigorous pathogenic bacteria, responsible for many types of infections. Growing populations are often partnered with growth of Staphylococcus – including *Staphylococcus aureus* – Bacillus species, and Enterococcus species –including numerous other pathogenic organisms.

In another study – this one comparing the gut microbiota of 16 type 1 diabetes children with 16 healthy children, researchers from Spain (Murri *et al.* 2013) found that the gut microbiota from the children with diabetes had significantly greater levels of Clostridium, Bacteroides and Veillonella bacteria – all known to be pro-inflammatory. And they had fewer populations of Lactobacillus and Bifidobacterium, which are important in a healthy gut.

Meanwhile the counts of Prevotella-type bacteria were significantly lower among the diabetes children.

They also found greater colonies of Clostridium were associated with higher levels of blood glucose – meaning problematic glucose metabolism.

Remember that the Bacteroides enterotype is associated with greater inflammation and overgrowth of *E. coli* and *B. fragilis*, while the Prevotella enterotype maintains a more balanced gut microbiota. It isn't that the Prevotella enterotype doesn't also contain plenty of *E. coli* and *B. fragilis* bacteria. In fact, the healthy gut is typically 1-2% *B. fragilis*. It is when the *E. coli* and *B. fragilis* species begin to overwhelm the gut: especially species of the hardy ESBL-producing versions of these bacteria.

When these bacteria produce greater amounts of beta-lactamase, they become stronger. This is because just as beta-lactamase helps the bacteria become antibiotic-resistant, the beta-lactamase also allows these same bacteria to become less controlled by other bacteria within the gut.

You see, bacteria control each other's populations through the production of their own unique antibiotics. And these antibiotic chemicals will allow that particular species to colonize itself into greater colonies by keeping back bacteria that compete for the same territory.

(Most antibiotic medicines are produced ultimately by microorganisms.)

Beta-lactamase is like a defense shield that allows that particular species to be impervious to the other bacterial antibiotics.

## Our Microbiome Inner World

We might compare the human gut to the world, with the various nations all competing with each other for territory. Those stable countries that are able to protect their borders (or utilize the protection of larger nations) will be able to maintain their territories. But every so often a nation of people produce a stronger weapon that endangers the borders and territories of the weaker nations. Unless those other countries figure out how to counteract that weapon, they will be taken over.

Most of the time there is a kind of stalemate between countries, as they accept each other. But if one aggressor country was to figure out how to protect itself from the bombing or nuclear threat of the rest of the countries – say with a nuclear shield defense system – that aggressor could take over other territories by gradually conquering the other nations without the threat of being controlled by the weapons of the other countries.

This is the situation with beta-lactamase. It is like the nuclear shield defense system. When pathogenic, inflammation-producing bacteria such as *E. coli* and *B. fragilis* are able to produce beta-lactamase, they suddenly have the ability to grow stronger and take over many territories of the intestinal tract normally controlled by more friendly bacteria.

And should these pathogenic bacteria escape through the walls of the intestines – infecting the intestinal walls, the appendix or the walls of the anus, they can cause serious infections. And should they enter the vagina or penis and infect the urethra, they can cause serious urinary tract infections and bladder infections.

So not only is toilet hygiene important (cleaning up what comes out), but what is put into the mouth is critical. Why? Because our diets are critical to determining the kind of bacteria our guts contain. And the longer we maintain that diet, the more likely we are to keep the Bacteroides from overgrowing our intestinal tract.

## Microbiome Enterotypes and Disease

While certainly the overgrowth of some Prevotella bacteria can cause problems – such as among dental caries – Prevotella species are known to reduce acidosis within the intestines. This was first discovered among cows, and supplementation with Prevotella species has been shown to significantly reduce and even eliminate acidosis among cows (Chiquette *et al.* 2012).

In another recent study, researchers from the University of Pittsburgh (Ou *et al.* 2013) analyzed fresh feces samples from 24 healthy Africans – 12 African Americans and 12 Native Africans between the age of 50 and 65 years old.

The researchers found that the Native Africans had predominantly Prevotella gut microbiota enterotypes, while the African Americans had predominantly Bacteroides enterotypes. The African Americans also had significantly fewer total microorganisms.

The researchers also found that the Native Africans also had higher levels of the healthier short-chain fatty acids, while the African Americans had higher levels of secondary bile acids – meaning their intestines were highly acidic compared to the Native Africans.

These relationships have been made with colon cancer: Higher levels of secondary bile acids are linked with greater incidence of colon cancer while higher levels of short-chain fatty acids – such as butyrate produced by healthy gut microorganisms – have been linked with reduced incidence of colon cancer. The researchers concluded:

*"Our results support the hypothesis that colon cancer risk is influenced by the balance between microbial production of health-promoting metabolites such as butyrate and potentially carcinogenic metabolites such as secondary bile acids."*

And the difference between the two groups of Africans? Naturally, the African Americans ate predominantly a Western diet, while the Native Africans ate more plant-based foods.

This correlation was confirmed in an earlier study by some of the same University of Pittsburgh researchers. In this study (Ou *et al.* 2012), 12 African Americans who were examined and determined to be at high-risk of colon cancer were studied and compared to 10 Caucasian Americans (who ate a high-fat diet), together with 13 Native Africans, who ate primarily a low-fat diet greater in plant-based foods.

The researchers found that the levels of components found high in colon cancer cases — notably secondary colonic bile acids, deoxycholic acid and lithocholic acid — were higher among both the Caucasian Americans and the African Americans, who both ate a higher-protein, higher-fat Western diet. These were significantly higher than those levels of the Native Africans, who ate a diet of more plant-based foods.

The researchers wrote:

*"Our results suggest that the higher risk of colon cancer in Americans may be partly explained by their high-fat and high-protein, low complex carbohydrate diet, which produces colonic residues that promote microbes to produce potentially carcinogenic secondary bile acids and less antineoplastic short-chain fatty acids."*

Again, intestinal bacteria that produce these cancer-related short-chain fatty acids are related to higher levels of the Bacteroides enterotype.

And research has shown that a switch to a plant-based diet can immediately and effectively alter the ratio of Bacteroides within the intestines. Research from the Republic of Korea's Kyung Hee University (Kim *et al.* 2013) found that changing ones diet to a strict vegetarian diet for one month dramatically changed levels of their gut microbiota, along with improvements in blood glucose levels and hypertension symptoms.

The researchers tested six adults who were obese with type 2 diabetes and/or high blood pressure. They tested their gut microbiota initially, and after a month of a strict vegetarian diet, they retested the subjects.

They found that the vegetarian diet significantly reduced levels of pathobiotics such as the Enterobacteriaceae (such as *E. coli*). They had increased levels of healthy species (type XIVa and IV) of *B. fragilis* and Clostridium (which compete with the pathogenic, beta-lactamase producing versions). They also found decreased production of the colon-cancer producing short-chain fatty acids. The month-long diet also improved fasting glucose levels, hemoglobin A1c levels, reduced triglyceride levels, reduced LDL-cholesterol levels and resulted in weight loss.

The researchers stated that:

> *"This study underscores the benefits of dietary fibre for improving the risk factors of metabolic diseases and shows that increased fibre intake reduces gut inflammation by changing the gut microbiota."*

## Probiotic Diversity and Diet

Ever wonder why some people seem to have more inflammation, fatigue and obesity than others despite their best efforts? New research has discovered the answer relates to the diversity of our gut's probiotic bacteria.

New human clinical research from France has found that the more genetic diversity our gut bacteria have, the lower our tendency for inflammation, obesity and metabolic dysfunction.

The research comes from France's Institut National de la Recherche Agronomique (National Institute of Agronomic Research or INRA). In a study that culminated from a decade of progressive research linking probiotics to obesity, over 75 prominent European researchers (Le Chatelier et a. 2013) assembled to gather and analyze the data from 292 patients.

The researchers tested 123 obese Danish people, along with 169 non-obese Danes. They conducted medical examinations on each individual, measuring not only their weight and body fat, but their level of insulin resistance, cholesterol levels, cardiovascular condition and general inflammation.

The researchers also tested the makeup of each individual's gut bacteria. This was done through DNA analysis, which tests the genetic diversity – read the number of different strains – of the probiotic bacteria living within the gut.

The researchers found that 23% of the entire group of 292 had low levels of diversity – which the researchers referred to as "bacterial richness." This 23% had an average of 380,000 genes, while the average gene count of those with more diverse bacteria had a count of 640,000 genes on average.

More importantly, the researchers found that those with lower probiotic diversity had significantly greater levels of obesity, higher cholesterol levels, more insulin resistance and a greater level of inflammatory conditions.

Those with lower levels of probiotic diversity also would struggle more with their weight. The researchers noted:

*"The obese individuals among the lower bacterial richness group also gain more weight over time."*

In their investigation of the strains of probiotics that directly lead to greater probiotic diversity, the researchers found that species of Faecalibacterium, Bifidobacterium, and Lactobacillus were associated with greater gene microbiota diversity. They also found that pathogenic microorganism genus' such as Bacteroides and Ruminococcus are linked with lower levels of genetic diversity.

It should be added that the former group of probiotic bacteria have been linked in the research as being anti-inflammatory, while those in the second (pathogenic) group have been associated in the research as being pro-inflammatory microorganisms.

Another French study (Cotillard *et al.* 2013) – a partner study within MetaHIT, a European Union-commissioned organization – focused upon solving obesity and metabolic disease among western countries – also linked lower probiotic gene diversity with greater levels of inflammation.

In this study, 49 obese or overweight patients were tested for gene diversity among their intestinal bacteria. The researchers found that 40% of the group had lower levels of probiotic gene diversity, and these individuals also had greater levels of *"low-grade inflammation"* and general *"dysmetabolism"* as compared with the rest of the group.

This study also found that a healthier diet with fewer processed carbohydrates (read junk food) led to higher scores of genetic diversity. However, the dietary intervention did not work as well for those with lower levels of genetic diversity at the beginning of the study:

*"Dietary intervention improves low gene richness and clinical phenotypes, but seems to be less efficient for inflammation variables in individuals with lower gene richness."*

In other words, a diet that aids the growth of healthy probiotics (rich in prebiotics) can also help reduce weight and inflammation, but the problem of lower levels of probiotics in the gut must also be focused upon.

## Obesity, Glucose Metabolism and Gut Bacteria

New research from New York University's School of Medicine has determined that obesity and lack of blood sugar control are associated with overgrowths of Helicobacter pylori, a species of bacteria that colonizes in the stomach.

The research, led by Yu Chen, Ph.D., MPH (et al. 2012), an Environmental Medicine professor at New York University, consisted of a cross-sectional analysis of examinations of 13,489 people tested for Helicobacter pylori bacteria and glycosylated hemoglobin – also called HbA1c.

After eliminating possible conflicting data, they found that those with former or present *H. pylori* infections had higher HbA1c levels, as well as higher body mass index (BMI) levels.

Higher HbA1c levels have been associated with glucose intolerance – also referred to as lack of blood sugar control. This is because glucose reacts with hemoglobin in the bloodstream to produce glycated hemoglobin. Higher HbA1c levels indicate abnormally high levels of blood sugar. Therefore, doctors will typically test HbA1c levels, and if they find that HbA1c levels are above normal ranges, they will suspect the patient has glucose intolerance and possibly even diabetes.

Increased HbA1c levels are also associated with obesity, as glucose intolerance increases fat storage. High HbA1c levels have also been associated with cardiovascular disease and diabetes.

The researchers noted that the greatest association with *H. pylori* occurred in those people with a combination of higher HbA1c levels and greater BMI. This correlates with other clinical data finding that many obese people also suffer from poor blood sugar control.

*H. pylori* is a bacteria that colonizes the stomach and upper intestines. Overgrowths of *H. pylori* were found to be associated with ulcers more than a decade ago.

However, the overgrowth of *H. pylori* in the stomach and intestines has also been the subject of controversy over the past few years. Third world populations with extremely low rates of ulcers and other intestinal issues related to *H. pylori* in Western countries are glaringly absent of these conditions. This is despite the fact that these same cultures have extremely high rates of *H. pylori* "infection" within the gut.

The conclusion is that these populations also have high probiotic diversity rates. This means their *H. pylori* colonies are kept in check and balanced by the activities of their other probiotics.

This is often also the case when it comes to *E. coli* and *S. aureus* populations in the gut. These bacteria can be highly pathogenic when their populations become dominant. At the same time, they are present in even the healthiest intestinal tracts. This is because the rest of the probiotic content – the microbiota of the body – are controlling and balancing their colonies and activities.

Not surprisingly, as detailed in my book, *Probiotics – Protection Against Infection*, probiotic research has found that *H. pylori* infections are reduced and controlled by probiotic supplementation. This may well be why research has also found that probiotics help weight loss and increase glucose control.

But the mystery deepens.

## The Mysterious *H. pylori*

*H. pylori* is not only linked to diabetes and ulcers. Overgrowths have also been associated with stomach cancer.

Researchers from the Vanderbilt University School of Medicine (Gaddy *et al.* 2013) may have found the missing piece to the puzzle of *H. pylori* and stomach/gastric cancer.

The mystery is that *Helicobacter pylori*, a gram-negative bacterium species typically found in the stomach, has been linked with gastric cancer – specifically stomach cancer – yet most of the population of third world countries host *H. pylori*, with extremely low gastric cancer rates.

Some studies have shown that nearly all healthy children host the bacterium throughout the third world, and those countries with the highest *H. pylori* communities have the lowest rates of gastric cancers.

Furthermore, the host rate of *H. pylori* infection among Americans has been going down dramatically over the past 50 years, and *H. pylori* infections have been are now extremely low. Those who do harbor the bacteria in America and other western countries have extremely higher risk of contracting stomach cancer. Over 800,000 stomach cancer cases occur each year worldwide.

Aside from these mysteries, the central mystery is why *H. pylori* does not have ill effects – including stomach and duodenal cancers – in over 80% of those populations infected by the bacterium.

This new Vanderbilt University study may well bring together some of the missing pieces.

The researchers found that gerbils that hosted *H. pylori* on a high-salt diet had nearly double the rate of stomach cancer than gerbils infected with the same species of *H. pylori* who ate a normal diet.

Every gerbil on the high-salt diet contracted stomach cancer – yes, 100% – while only 58% of the normal-diet infected gerbils contracted the cancer.

This led the researchers to conclude that salt somehow exacerbates stomach cancer.

The puzzle came together when the researchers found that those on the high salt diet were infected with another species of *H. pylori* – one that does not produce CagA, an oncoprotein secreted by certain species of *H. pylori* – did not contract stomach cancer.

In fact, none of the gerbils on the high-salt diet who were infected with a species of *H. pylori* that does not produce CagA came down with stomach cancer.

This meant first of all, that not only does CagA-negative *H. pylori* not cause cancer, but that a high-salt diet in the presence of a CagA-positive infection of *H. pylori* does produce stomach cancer – at an extremely high rate.

About 60% of isolated *H. pylori* species have been found to be CagA-positive among Western countries. But most of the third-world infections are of what is considered the Eastern strain of CagA-negative *H. pylori*.

This means that the Eastern species of CagA-negative *H. pylori* is actually not a pathogenic bacteria at all, but rather, a eugenic bacteria – not necessarily harmful or helpful to the host.

And it also means that the widespread infection of these hardy strains of CagA-positive *H. pylori* together with the highly processed and salty Western diet lie at the root of our high stomach cancer rates among Western countries (Krzysiek-Maczka *et al.* 2013; Chen *et al.* 2013).

A recent study from China's Jinling Hospital (Chiurillo *et al.* 2013) found that CagA-positive *H. pylori* infections are growing among children in China – especially in Eastern China where much of the urban areas are.

The infection rates of CagA-positive *H. pylori* are higher among those countries that eat a predominantly Western diet, and infections rates are growing among countries that have been increasingly eating a Western diet (Lu *et al.* 2013).

Gastritis is also associated with CagA-positive *H. pylori* infections (Jiménez *et al.* 2013).

Furthermore, researchers from School of Medicine of China's Jiaotong University (Wang *et al.* 2012) tracked 257 men and women with gastric cancer along with 514 matched control subjects. The researchers tested the *H. pylori* status along with their diet.

The researchers found that eating vegetables, fruits and soy foods significantly lowered the *H. pylori* infections. Vegetables reduced the risk by 70%, fruits reduced infection risk by 80% and soy products decreased *H. pylori* infection risk by 60%.

## Gut Microorganisms and Cancer-causing Enzymes

A number of clinical studies have proven that omnivore diets result in higher levels of mutagenic enzymes within the digestive tract. These enzymes directly damage cells and increase systemic inflammation. Their mutagenicity has been shown to contribute to cancer, particularly colon cancer.

In the early 1980s, Dr. Barry Goldin, a professor at the Tufts University School of Medicine, led a series of studies that found that certain diets promoted a group of cancer-causing enzymes. These included beta-glucu¬ronidase, nitroreductase, azoreductase, and steroid 7-alpha-dehydroxylase. The enzymes were linked with cancer in previous studies.

(Cancer is caused by the same types of cell damage that also stimulates systemic inflammation.)

A number of studies on vegetarians found lower levels of these mutagenic enzymes, while those eating animal-based diets had greater levels. Apparently, these cancer-related enzymes originate from a group of pathogenic bacteria that tend to occupy the intestines of those with diets rich in animal-based foods. It was discovered that the cancer-producing enzymes are actually the endotoxins (waste products) of these pathogenic bacteria.

Dr. Goldin and his research teams studied the difference between these enzyme levels in omnivores and vegetarians. In one study, the researchers removed meat from the diets of a group of omnivores for 30 days. An immediate reduction of steroid 7-alpha-dehydroxylase resulted. When the probiotic L. acidophilus was supplemented to their diets, this group also showed a significant reduction in beta-glucuronidase and nitroreductase.

In other words, two dietary connections were found regarding these disease-causing enzymes: animal-based diets and a lack of intestinal probiotics. The two are actually related, because probiotics thrive in prebiotic-rich plant-based diets and suffer in animal-rich diets.

Two years later, Dr. Goldin and associates (Goldin et al. 1982) studied 10 vegetarian and 10 omnivore women. He found that the vegetarian women maintained significantly lower levels of beta-glucuronidase than did the omnivorous women.

Other studies have confirmed that vegetarian diets result in a reduction of these carcinogenic enzymes produced by pathogenic bacteria. Researchers from Finland's University of Kuopio (Ling and Hanninen 1992) tested 18 volunteers who were randomly divided into either a conventional omnivore diet or a vegan diet for one month.

The vegan group followed the month with a return to their original omnivore diet. After only one week on the vegan diet, the researchers found that fecal urease levels decreased by 66%, cholylglycine hydrolase levels decreased by 55%, beta-glucuronidase levels decreased by 33% and beta-glucosidase levels decreased by 40% in the vegan group. These reduced levels continued through the month of consuming the vegan diet. Serum levels of phenol and p-cresol — also inflammation-producing endotoxins of pathogenic bacteria — also significantly decreased in the vegan group.

Within two weeks of returning to the omnivore diet, the formerly-vegan group's pathogenic enzyme levels returned to the higher levels they had before converting to the vegan diet. After one month of returning to the omnivore diet, serum levels of toxins phenol and p-cresol returned to their previously higher levels prior to the vegan diet. Meanwhile, the higher levels of inflammation-producing enzymes remained among the conventional omnivore diet (control) group.

A study published two years earlier by Huddinge University researchers (Johansson et al. 1992) confirmed the same results. In this study, the conversion of an omnivore diet to a lacto-vegetarian diet significantly reduced levels of beta-glucuronidase, beta-glucosidase, and sulphatase (more tumor-impli¬cated, inflammation-producing enzymes) from fecal samples.

Another study illustrating this link between vegetarianism, pathogenic bacterial enzymes and cancer was conducted at Sweden's Huddinge University and the University Hospital (Johansson et al. 1998) almost a decade later. Dr. Johansson and associates measured the effect of switching from an omnivore diet to a lacto-vegetarian diet and back to an omnivore diet with respect to mutagenicity – by testing the body's fluid biochemistry to determine the tendency for tumor formation.

In this extensive study, 20 non-smoking and normal weight volunteers switched to a lacto-vegetarian diet for one year. Urine and feces were examined for mutagenicity (cancer-causing bacteria and their endotoxins) at the start of the study, at three months, at six months and at twelve months after beginning the vegetarian diet. Following the switch to the lacto-vegetarian diet, all mutagenic parameters significantly decreased among the urine and feces of the subjects. The subjects were then followed-up and tested three years after converting back to an omnivore diet (four years after the study began). Their higher mutagenic biochemistry levels had returned.

In another of Dr. Johansson's studies (Johansson and Ravald 1995) – this from Sweden's Karolinska Institute – 29 vegetarians and 28 omnivores were tested. The tests revealed that the vegetarians secreted more salivary juices than did the omnivores. Salivation is critical to the health of the mucosal membranes among the oral cavity and airways.

## Heart disease and TMAO

Researchers conducting past research connecting heart disease with animal diets have pointed to the fat and cholesterol content in red meat as the central culprit. While most experts agree that saturated fat and meat's cholesterol content is a likely component, new research from the Cleveland Clinic (Koeth *et al.* 2013) has found the relationship is a bit more complicated.

The link between animal diets and heart disease relates more to our gut probiotics.

Medical researchers from the Cleveland Clinic's Center for Cardiovascular Diagnostics & Prevention determined that L-carnitine – a compound found in red meat, many energy drinks and supplements – is involved in accelerating heart disease. The interesting part is that red meat alters our intestinal bacteria, causing them to produce a lethal artery-clogging chemical called trimethylamine-N-oxide (TMAO).

The research, published in the *Journal Nature Medicine,* comes after decades of research has linked red meat consumption to heart disease and atherosclerosis.

The researchers conducted a series of studies using both humans and animals. In the human research, circulating levels of L-carnitine were tested among 2,595 patients who underwent evaluation for heart conditions. The researchers found that higher levels of L-carnitine were significantly associated with greater degrees of cardiovascular disease, and more specifically, atherosclerosis – the hardening of the arteries due to increased plaque and artery damage.

The researchers also tested and tracked the consumption of red meat and L-carnitine through the digestive tract, and found that those who ate animal diets maintained a particular type of bacteria species, which converts L-carnitine – a nutrient high in red meat, certain energy drinks and some supplements – into trimethylamine-N-oxide (TMAO).

The researchers then found that the TMAO produced by the gut bacteria was specifically linked to atherosclerosis.

Furthermore, the researchers found that meat-eaters had greater numbers of these TMAO-producing pathogenic bacteria, and thus metabolized more TMAO than did vegans and vegetarians.

To screen out the different possibilities, the researchers ran a series of additional tests that included giving L-carnitine in supplement form to vegetarians and omnivores, and compared their production of TMAO. They found that the vegetarians did not produce anywhere near the levels of TMAO that the omnivores experienced following L-carnitine supplementation.

The researchers also used antibiotics to remove intestinal bacteria, and repeated the tests. They discovered that the connection was their respective intestinal bacteria. The omnivore diet had promoted some species of bacteria that produce TMAO from L-carnitine.

The research was led by esteemed heart researcher Dr. Stanley Hazen:

*"The bacteria living in our digestive tracts are dictated by our long-term dietary patterns,"*

said Dr. Hazen in a statement.

*"Vegans and vegetarians have a significantly reduced capacity to synthesize TMAO from carnitine, which may explain the cardiovascular health benefits of these diets."*

This is not the first study that has linked "bad" gut bacteria to heart disease. A 2011 study also led by Dr. Hazen (Wang *et al.* 2011) determined that TMAO was produced by converting choline – another component typically found with L-carnitine in animal foods. Previous research established both choline and L-carnitine as precursors to TMAO production.

The pathogenic bacteria suspected among meat-eaters include Cytomegalovirus (CMV), Helicobacter, Chlamydia, and *Chlamydophila pneumoniae.* These pathogenic bacteria utilize a type of enzyme called flavin monooxygenase (FMO).

These bacteria apparently process choline and L-carnitine into TMAO utilizing the FMO enzymes. Dr. Hazen's researchers found these two TMAO precursors were predominant among eggs, shellfish, fish, red meat, liver and even to some degree, milk.

With regards to taking supplements with L-carnitine, drinking energy drinks or any other source of L-carnitine, Dr. Hazen's research has established that vegetarians will convert less of this L-carnitine to TMAO than will omnivores, due to the increased pathogenic bacteria counts resulting from a diet rich in animal foods.

Other studies – notably those conducted by Swedish researcher Dr. Gunnar Johansson (*et al.* 1990, 1992, 1997) – have also linked omnivore diets to increased pathogenic bacteria and higher levels of pathogenic enzymes. These enzymes – including beta-glucuronidase, beta-glucosidase, and sulphatase – have been associated with increased rates of colon cancer. Dr. Johansson's decades-long research has established that these pathogenic bacteria and subsequent enzymes decrease when people reduce their consumption of red meat, or convert from an omnivore diet to a vegetarian diet.

Let's discuss the evidence further.

# Chapter Three

# Diet and Disease

We know that humans certainly did eat a plant-based diet for much of our existence. For well over a million years, humanoids ate nuts, berries, fruits, roots and leaves directly off the trees. They also harvested some of these and stored and cooked or dried them later.

Humans also ate raw milks from goats, cows, donkeys and other animals. These raw milks contained many probiotic bacteria – as does all raw milk, including human breast milk. Our ancestors also made various cultured foods from these raw milks, and the passed on 'mother' cultures to make kefirs, yogurts and other ancient foods. We'll discuss all these momentarily.

There are a number of debates ongoing with respect to whether humans were meant to eat meat and whether meat is healthy.

But there should no longer be a debate, simply because the evidence is in. And it is not only convincing: it is clear.

## Mortality and Diet

Research is increasingly finding that certain diets increase the risk of early death – described in these studies as mortality.

In one, this from Harvard University (Pan *et al.* 2012) found that eating red meat increases the risk of dying from a disease such as cancer or heart disease by up to 20 percent.

The research, led by Harvard professor Frank Hu, PhD, followed nearly 38,000 men and almost 84,000 women between 1980 and 2008. During that period, 23,926 men and women died. The researchers followed their diets throughout the 28-year study period, updating them every four years.

Those who ate an average of one serving a day more of unprocessed red meat were 13% more likely to die. Those who ate one serving a day more of processed red meat had a 20% higher incidence of death.

Those who ate an extra serving per day of processed meat had a 21% higher risk of dying from heart disease, while those who ate a serving a day more unprocessed red meat were 18% more likely to die from heart disease.

Those who ate a serving a day more processed meat had a 16% higher risk of dying from cancer.

The researchers also found for every one serving of red meat replaced by other (non-red meat) forms of protein, the mortality risk dropped by between 7% and 19% – depending upon the type of protein. The researchers concluded clearly:

*"Red meat consumption is associated with an increased risk of total, cardiovascular disease, and cancer mortality. Substitution of other healthy protein sources for red meat is associated with a lower mortality risk."*

Lead researcher Dr. Hu was surprised at the impact of eating more red meat. Dr. Hu told Reuters Health:

*"The results are not really surprisingly given that previous studies have found consumption of red meat is linked to diabetes, heart disease and certain cancers. What's surprising is the magnitude… Even a small amount of red meat is associated with a significantly increased risk of mortality."*

This study confirms a similar study conducted by the National Cancer Institute (Sinha *et al.* 2009), which included a population study conducted by the National Institutes of Health and the American Association of Retired Persons. This study followed 500,000 people between the ages of 50 and 71 years old.

After ten years, those who ate more red meat had an increased death rate of 31% for men and 36% for women. Those who ate more red meat had an increased risk of death due to cancer by 22% and 20% among men and women respectively.

Those eating more red meat also had a 27% and 50% increased risk of dying from heart disease for men and women respectively.

In a twelve year study of 6,115 vegetarians and 5015 meat-eaters, vegetarians were 40% less mortality rate for cancer, and were 20% less likely to die before the age of 65 than meat-eaters. (Thorogood *et al.* 1994; West 1994).

In three studies of approximately 11,000 subjects each done at the University of Oxford, death rates among vegetarians were significantly lower than the general population (Key *et al.* 2003).

In a study from China (Takata *et al.* 2013) that followed more than 134,000 people, men who ate the most red meat and poultry had an 18% higher risk of mortality during the 3 years of the study. This study also found that red meat consumption led to a 41% increased risk of dying from ischemic heart disease. Higher red meat intake also increased risk of dying from cancer by 25% and lung cancer by 55%. Some of the associations of this study were tempered by the drastic income disparity within the populations, as well as the amount of red meat eaten – due to the higher costs of red meat among these populations. In other words, those who could afford to buy meat also tended to have better health care. This means that rates here are conservative.

Another study (Deriemaeker *et al.* 2011) found that elderly vegetarians are aging well and getting good nutrition compared to elderly omnivores. The study, published n Nutrition and Metabolism, tested 22 female vegetarians with an average age of 84, seven male vegetarians with an average age of 80; and 23 female and seven male omnivores with an average age of 84 and 80 respectively.

Both diets were found to provide nutrients such as protein, vitamin B12, folic acid, iron, and calcium at levels that resulted in healthy ranges of nutrients within the blood. All other parameters appeared in the normal range for their age.

The researchers concluded:

"This study indicates that a vegetarian lifestyle had no negative impact on the health status at older age."

The researchers also noted that epidemiological studies have shown that vegetarians tend to live longer and have fewer deaths to heart disease and cancer.

One such study was the Oxford Vegetarian Study (Appleby *et al.* 1999) that analyzed 6,000 vegetarians and 5,000 non-vegetarians. The researchers found that vegans, vegetarians and fish eaters had lower total-cholesterol and LDL-cholesterol than those on animal diets. They After they factored out smoking, body mass index and class, they found that death rates were significantly lower among the vegetarians for all causes of death, for heart disease and for cancer. The risk of mortality among the non-vegetarians was roughly twice the risk of mortality among the vegetarians.

The Oxford Vegetarian Study recruited subjects from the United Kingdom between 1980 and 1984. The researchers discovered that vegetarians and vegans had a 28% lower risk of dying from heart disease, a 39% lower incidence of dying from cancer, and a 20% lower incidence of death from any cause (balanced by deaths unrelated to diet).

The research also found that vegetarians and vegans had a 50% lower risk of appendicitis.

They concluded:

*"Thus, the health of vegetarians in this study is generally good and compares favorably with that of the nonvegetarian control subjects."*

In other words, the researchers assumed they would find – as was generally thought – that vegetarians lacked in certain nutrients. This assumption was proven wrong.

Researchers from Stockholm's Institute of Environmental Medicine at the Karolinska Institute (Bellavia *et al.* 2013), followed and studied the diets and death rates of 71,706 Swedish people between the ages of 45 and 83 years old, over thirteen years.

During that thirteen-year period, 11,439 deaths occurred – 6,803 among the men and 4,636 among the women.

The researchers gave each participant – 38,221 of whom were men and 33,485 of whom were women – a questionaire regarding their diets.

The researchers found that those who said they never consumed fruits and vegetables died an average of three years sooner than did participants who said they consumed at least five total servings of fruits and/or vegetables per day.

Those who did not eat fruits and vegetables also had a 53% higher death rate.

The researchers also broke out the mortality rates between those who ate or didn't eat fruit and those who ate or didn't eat vegetables. They found that those who did not consume fruit died an average of 19 months before those who consumed at least one fruit per day.

But those who did not eat vegetables died an average of 32 months sooner than those who ate at least three vegetables a day.

The researchers concluded rather simply:

*"Fruit and vegetable consumption of less than five servings a day is associated with progressively shorter survival and higher mortality rates."*

This study confirms a similar study that focused instead on the consumption of vegetables. Researchers from the Vanderbilt University School of Medicine (Zhang *et al.* 2011) studied 134,796 Chinese adults, and compared their diets with their death rates for ten years.

This study found that mortality rates ranged from 9% lower to 22% lower as their vegetable intake was increased, with the lowest mortality rates among those who consumed more cruciferous vegetables.

## Heart Disease and Diet

The relationship between diet and heart disease relates directly to mortality, so we've already quoted some clear evidence above. There's also clear evidence that our diet choices also relate directly to our risk of contracting heart disease.

Harvard researchers (Fung *et al.* 2001) followed 69,017 women as part of the Nurses Health Study, and found that those consuming more red and processed meats and processed foods increased the risk of coronary heart disease by 46%, and a diet rich in plant-based foods reduced the risk of coronary heart disease by 36%. This diet that increased heart disease risk was identified as the *"Western pattern,"* consisting of *"red and proc-*

*essed meats, sweets and desserts, french fries, and refined grains"*. The researchers concluded:

> *"A diet high in fruits, vegetables, whole grains, legumes, poultry, and fish and low in refined grains, potatoes, and red and processed meats may lower risk of CHD."*

In an associated study, the researchers (Fung *et al.* 2004) followed 71,768 women four fourteen years. They found that the risk of stroke increased by 58% for total strokes and 56% for ischemic stroke in those who ate higher amounts of red and processed meats. The researchers concluded that:

> *"These data suggest that a dietary pattern typified by higher intakes of red and processed meats, refined grains, and sweets and desserts may increase stroke risk, whereas a diet higher in fruits and vegetables, fish, and whole grains may protect against stroke."*

Other studies have shown similar findings. A study from the University of Western Australia School of Medicine (Burke *et al.* 2007) found that processed meat consumption more than doubled the risk of heart disease in Aboriginal Australians.

A study from Spain's University of Cordoba and the Reina Sofía University Hospital found that the Mediterranean diet improves artery health. They determined that the Mediterranean diet also reduces the risk of arteriosclerosis among elderly adults, according to the study.

Twenty healthy adults were followed. The subjects ate three diets for four weeks each: A high saturated fat diet (animal products); a low-fat, high-carbohydrate diet; and a Mediterranean diet. During and after the four weeks, the subjects were tested for the release of endothelial microparticles (EMPs) and endothelial progenitor cells (EPCs), which indicate artery damage. The Med Diet period resulted in the lowest microparticles, lowest activated EMP, and lowest apoptotic EMP concentrations than the other diets. The Med Diet also produced higher levels of antioxidants and lower levels of inflammatory activity than the other diets.

Scientists from Spain's University Rovira i Virgili Medical School (Solá *et al.* 2011) found that a traditional Mediterranean diet with either a high proportion of olive oil or nuts significantly lowers the risk of heart disease and the hardening of the arteries.

The researchers tested 551 people between 55 and 80 years old who already had signs of cardiovascular disease and hardening of the arteries. They were randomly split into three groups. The first group ate a low-fat diet for three months. The second group ate a traditional Mediterranean diet with 15 liters of virgin olive oil over the three-month period, and the third group ate a traditional Mediterranean diet plus 30 grams of walnuts, almonds and hazelnuts per day.

The research found that the two groups that ate traditional Mediterranean diets had significantly reduced levels of cardiovascular disease as indicated by the subjects' apolipoprotein levels and ratios. The women's risk dropped by nearly 17%, while the men's cardiovascular risk dropped by 5%.

The apolipoproteins are key markers the risk of cardiovascular disease because they relate directly to the hardening of arteries as a result of LDL oxidation. ApoA-1 is critical to HDL (good) cholesterol levels, while ApoB is a key constituent of LDL (bad) cholesterol.

The study showed that both traditional Mediterranean diet groups had an increase in ApoA-1 levels and decreased levels of ApoB. The Apo ratio – also called the total ApoB/ApoA-1 ratio – was also reduced among the two traditional Mediterranean diet groups.

The traditional Mediterranean diet emphasizes eating more fruits and vegetables, nuts, seeds, and other plant-based foods. It has been acclaimed as one of the most beneficial diets for weight loss and increased longevity.

The diet has also been shown to reduce heart disease risk more effectively than pharmaceutical medications.

This was stressed by Dr Miguel Angel Martínez-González, one of the researchers and a professor in the Department of Preventive Medicine at the University of Navarra. Dr. Martínez-González stated that the research has shown that:

> "a modification in the entire diet pattern managed to achieve, in just one year, results that pharmaceutical drugs did not – even after two years of treatment."

In one of the world's largest and longest studies on diet, research funded by Spain's Ministry of Health (Estruch et al. 2013) confirmed that the Mediterranean diet can dramatically reduce the risk of stroke, heart attacks and other cardiovascular-related events.

The research was in the *New England Journal of Medicine* by researchers who conducted a large scale landmark study called the Spanish PREDIMED (PREvención con DIeta MEDiterranea) trial.

The study enrolled 7,447 people between 55 and 80 years of age, of which 57% were women. In a randomized manner, the participants were given either a Mediterranean diet supplemented with mixed nuts, a Mediterranean diet supplemented with extra-virgin olive oil, or a control diet – which included advice to reduce fats according to American Heart Association guidelines.

The participants were followed for an average of 4.8 years during the trial, and their cardiovascular event histories were measured, along with a stratification (a break out) of risk factors to enable a clear understanding of the role of the diet versus other possible factors.

Those who were on the Mediterranean diet with olive oil had a 30% decreased incidence of cardiovascular events. Those on the Med diet with nuts had a 28% decreased incidence of cardiovascular events.

However, within those events were another surprising result. The Mediterranean diet with the mixed nuts – many of which were walnuts – had nearly half the incidence of strokes.

The control group was given low fat advice by physicians according to the American Heart Association guidelines. This means that the control group's diet was likely better than a typical Western diet. This of course means that the Mediterranean diet – as compared to a typical Western diet – would show even more dramatic results.

Remember that the Mediterranean diet is rich in grains, fruits and vegetables and low in red meat. This type of diet provides various phytonutrients that provide antioxidant benefits. Oxidative stress has been shown to be at the root of artery disease.

Both nuts and olive oil provide additional nutrients that are heart healthy – notably omega-3 fatty acids found in walnuts and other nuts, as well as monounsaturated fatty acids in olive oil.

Extra virgin olive oil is oil from olives that have been pressed mechanically at lower heats. This yields fewer radicals and more heat-sensitive polyphenols.

Heart and cardiovascular disease is directly related to inflammation. Our diets can either be sources of inflammation or not. Our diets can also be anti-inflammatory. This was addressed in the study mentioned earlier from Harvard (Bazzen *et al.* 2013):

> "The data also suggests that red meat, in particular, is pro-inflammatory and procarcinogenic. For example, the European Prospective Investigation into Cancer and Nutrition-Potsdam study of 2,198 men and women found that the consumption of red meat was significantly associated with higher levels of the inflammatory markers GGT and hs-CRP when adjusted for potential confounding factors related to lifestyle and diet. Another study showed that when people were given a 7-day dietary red meat intervention, fecal water genotoxicity significantly increased in response to the red meat intake. These effects included modifications in DNA damage repair, the cell cycle, and apoptosis pathways."

## Cancer and Diet

In this section we will review just a few of the major clinical studies that have been done linking cancer with our choice of diets.

The connection between cancer and red meats has also been made among recent European research studying the Mediterranean diet. The Med diet is known for its reduced intake of red meats, and increased intakes of fruits, vegetables, monounsaturated fats and low levels of saturated fats.

The association between colon cancer and diets heavy in red meat has been shown conclusively in a multiple studies over the years. For example, an American Cancer Society cohort study (Chao *et al.* 2005) examined 148,610 adults between the ages of 50 and 74 living in 21 states of the U.S. They found that higher intakes of red and processed meats were associated with higher levels of rectal and colon cancer after other cancer variables were eliminated.

According to the World Cancer Research Fund and the American Institute for Cancer Research, in a report *Food, Nutrition and the Prevention of Cancer: A Global Perspective* (1997), 25-50% of all cases of cancer can be prevented by a vegetarian diet.

In a twelve year mortality study of 6,115 vegetarians and 5,015 meat-eaters, vegetarians had a 40% lower risk of mortality from all cancers (Thorogood *et al.* 1994; West 1994).

Researchers from Uruguay's University of the Republic School of Medicine (De Stafani *et al.* 2012) found, in a study of 6,060 people that the risk of cancer of the kidneys, oral cavity, pharynx, esophagus, stomach, colon, rectum, larynx, lung, female breast, prostate and urinary bladder were significantly increased with higher consumption of processed meats. They found eating mortadella (large sausage), salami, hot dogs, ham, and salted meats even more associated with these cancers.

In a study (Kwan *et al.* 2009) of breast cancer survivors from the Life After Cancer Epidemiology Study, 1,901 patients diagnosed with early stage breast cancer were followed. Two eating patterns were found among the patients: One had greater consumption of fruits, vegetables, whole grains, and poultry (called the "Prudent pattern"). The other, called the "Western pattern – had greater consumption of red and processed meats with refined grains.

The researchers found that those who adhered the closest with the "Prudent pattern" had lower rates of death from breast cancer or any other cause. Meanwhile those in the "Western pattern" suffered higher incidence of recurrent breast cancers, greater incidence of death from their breast cancer, and increased risk of death from any cause.

French researchers (Couto *et al.* 2011) have found that greater adherence to the Mediterranean diet reduces overall cancer risk. Researchers from the International Agency for Research on Cancer in Lyons, France, analyzed 142,605 men and 335,873 women from around Europe. They monitored cancer incidence and graded adherence to the Med diet using a 0-9 score. Among the study population, 9,669 men and 21,062 women contracted cancer.

The researchers found that for every two points increase in the Med diet score, there was a 4% reduction in cancer, and nearly 5% among men. The results did not include cancers related to smoking.

This study was the first to study the association between the Med diet and cancer risk overall.

Fiber content in diet critical in preventing cancer. This was illustrated in a study from University of Alberta researchers (Sharma *et al.* 2013) who followed 146,389 people. They found that Japanese men who had consumed more grain were only half as likely to die from cancer.

While some of these above studies did focus on individual types of cancers, other research has focused on diet's relationship with individual cancers. Most of these have similar findings:

### *Pancreatic Cancer*
Pancreatic cancer has one of the worst survival rates of any other cancer. Pancreatic cancer survival rates are about 25% for one year, and 6% for five years. In the U.S. 38,000 people were diagnosed with pancreatic cancer in 2011, and about 34,000 died of pancreatic cancer. It is the fourth highest cause of cancer deaths.

Swedish researchers have found that eating red meat significantly increases a man's risk of pancreatic cancer, and eating processed meats increases both men's and women's risk of contracting pancreatic cancer.

The research, from Sweden's National Institute of Environmental Medicine in Stockholm (Larsson *et al.* 2012), analyzed eleven clinical studies that followed 6,643 pancreatic cancer patients. The study found that eating more red meat increased a man's risk of pancreatic cancer by almost 30%.

The study, published in the *British Journal of Cancer*, determined that both men and women have an increased risk of pancreatic cancer – by almost 20% – from eating more processed meats.

The study gauged red meat consumption by categorizing those who ate 120 grams more red meat a day for the red meat analysis, and those who ate 50 grams more processed meat for the processed meat analysis.

This finding was confirmed by another study (Bosetti *et al.* 2013) from Italy, of 326 pancreatic cancer patients matched with 652 healthy control subjects (people who didn't have pancreatic cancer).

The researchers found that those who at higher intakes of animal products had double the risk of pancreatic cancer, while those whose diets had more plant-based foods ("vitamins and fiber" pattern) had a 69% reduced risk of pancreatic cancer.

A recent review of research by cancer scientists from Poland found 11 case-controlled studies comparing red meat consumption with pancreatic cancer risk. Their meta-analysis of these studies found that red meat consumption increases the risk of pancreatic cancer by 48%. They also found that eating more vegetables and fruit decreases pancreatic risk by 38% and 29% respectively.

### Stomach Cancer

Researchers from Spain's Programme of Epidemilogical Cancer Research in Barcelona (Gonzalez and Riboli 2010) conducted an analysis of 519,978 human participants from 23 centers among 10 European countries in Denmark, France, Germany, Greece, Italy, the Netherlands, Norway, Spain, Sweden and the United Kingdom. They found that gastric cancer was associated with higher consumption of red and processed meats, and lower risk was evident among those with higher phytonutrient (plant nutrients) plasma levels.

They also found that lung cancer was lower among those who ate more fruits and vegetables, even among smokers. And they found that higher breast cancer incidence was related to higher saturated fat consumption.

### Colorectal Cancer

Researchers from the American Cancer Society (McCullough *et al.* 2013) studied 2,315 patients who had been previously diagnosed with colorectal cancer (colon cancer). Those who consistently ate higher intakes of red and processed meat before and after diagnosis had 79% higher risk of dying from colon cancer. Those who ate more meat also had a 63% higher risk of dying from cardiovascular disease compared to reduced consumption of meat in their diet.

Researchers from the Harvard School of Public Health (Nimptsch *et al.* 2013) followed 19,771 women for nine years (between 1998 and 2007) and tracked their diets together with the incidence of colon cancer among them.

The researchers found that replacing a serving per day of red meat with poultry or fish reduced their risk of colon cancer by 35% and 41% respectively.

### Breast Cancer

Multiple studies by cancer researchers have determined that a plant-based diet and less alcohol consumption significantly reduce the risk of breast cancer.

Most recently, researchers from Columbia University, Stanford University and UCLA (Link *et al.* 2013) followed 91,779 women for 14 years as part of the California Teachers study. The women were followed between 1995 and 2009.

The researchers tracked the number of breast cancers and tumors among the women during the women and matched these results with the respective diet patterns of the women. The researchers grouped the women into five basic diet patterns:

1) plant-based diet – high in fruits and vegetables

2) high-protein, high-fat diet – high in meats, eggs, fried foods, and fats

3) diet high in carbohydrates, processed and convenient foods, pasta, and bread products

4) ethnic diet – high in legumes, soy foods, rice, and dark-green leafy vegetables

5) salad and wine diet – high in lettuce, fish, wine, low-fat salad dressing, coffee and tea

Of these patterns, those who ate the most (highest quartile) plant-based diet pattern (1) had 15% less incidence of breast cancer and 34% less incidence of tumors that were estrogen receptor – negative and progesterone receptor – negative (ER-/PR-).

While the non-plant-based diets scored the lowest, the researchers also found that the "salad and wine diet" pattern produced a 29% higher incidence of estrogen receptor – positive progesterone receptor – positive (ER+/PR+) tumors.

With regard to the alcohol consumption, the researchers noted that alcohol was a contributing factor, but not the only contributing factor.

The researchers concluded that:

> *"The finding that greater consumption of a plant-based dietary pattern is associated with a reduced breast cancer risk, particularly for ER-/PR- tumors, offers a potential avenue for prevention."*

Other studies have shown that a plant-based diet reduces the risk of breast and other cancers.

A study from France's INSERM scientists conducted a large study that followed 65,374 women for nearly 10 years (9.7 to be exact). The researchers divided the women into two primary eating patterns:

1) The Western diet – high in meat products, fried foods, cakes, mayonnaise, butter/cream and alcohol

2) The Mediterranean diet – high in vegetables, fruits, olive oil, sunflower oil and seafood

The Western diet plan resulted in a 20% greater incidence of breast cancer among those eating the most (highest quartile) of this diet, and 33% greater risk for ER+/PR+ tumors. Meanwhile, those eating the Mediterranean diet plan had 15% incidence of all breast cancers.

This study also captured a difference of 6% greater breast cancer risk among those with greater alcohol consumption. This appears to be consistent with the UCLA study.

Specific to alcohol, another study – this from Sweden's Karolinska Institute (Cottet *et al.* 2009) – followed 51,847 women for more than eight years. This study found that those women who drank more than 10 grams of alcohol per day had a 35% greater incidence of ER+/PR+ breast cancers. This was increased among women who were taking hormones.

The researchers noted that the ER+ relationship was important, as they stated in their conclusion:

> *"The observed association between risk of developing postmenopausal ER+ breast cancer and alcohol drinking, especially among those women who use postmenopausal hormones, may be important, because the majority of breast tumors among postmenopausal women overexpress ER."*

The relationship between diet and breast cancer becomes more evident as we examine a study (Suzuki *et al.* 2008) of 51,823 Swedish women who were followed for more than eight years. Here the researchers found that those women who had the highest quartile of total fiber intake had a 34% decreased incidence of breast cancer and a 38% reduced incidence of ER+/PR+ tumors.

This study also found that among those taking hormones, the reduction of breast cancer incidence was a whopping 50%.

The researchers also found that those eating more cereal-based fiber (grains) had an even greater reduction in breast cancer incidence. A plant-based diet is naturally higher in fiber because whole fruits, vegetables and grains contain various plant fibers.

So it seems that fiber is a critical issue, and plant-based foods maintain higher fiber content, while the Western diet maintains lower fiber content.

Certainly this is compounded by the increased content of numerous anti-cancer phytochemicals.

## Alzheimer's disease, Cognition and Diet

New research is proving that Alzheimer's disease and dementia are linked to a process that occurs in the body called oxidative stress. Oxidative stress is caused by a combination of poor lifestyle choices and a diet that produces increased levels of oxidative radicals and lower levels of antioxidants.

Researchers from the Beijing Hospital of Traditional Chinese Medicine and the Capital Medical University in China (Shi *et al.* 2012) analyzed urinary biomarkers of oxidative stress among 46 patients with vascular dementia, 24 patients with vascular disease without dementia, and 26 people without symptoms of either.

They found that patients with dementia had significantly higher levels of a urinary biomarker called 8-hydroxydeoxyguanosine (or 8-OHdG). 8-OHdG is associated with significantly high levels of oxidative stress. These levels were significantly higher than both of the other groups of patients.

Another recent study, this one from Qingdao University's School of Medicine, analyzed multiple studies and two large genome studies and concluded that Alzheimer's disease patients have significantly higher levels of clusterin, also known as apolipoprotein J. Clusterin has been found to bind to amyloid-beta (Abeta) proteins, and has the ability to reduce fibril formation.

It is now thought that in an attempt to resist the formation of the Abeta proteins and fibrils, the body produces clusterin as a defense measure against oxidative stress. This has been confirmed in studies showing that clusterin lowers cell death and levels of oxidative stress.

Oxidative stress is produced with increased levels of toxin exposure, either within the diet, water or air, combined with lower levels of antioxidants and increased levels of lifestyle stressors. Toxins become oxidized and become radicals, which can damage our arteries and tissues.

Researchers from Columbia's University of Pontificia Javeriana (Albarracin *et al.* 2012) studied the connection between antioxidant intake and Alzheimer's disease in a variety of studies. They found that an increased consumption of "polyphenol-rich" foods significantly lowered the risk of Alzheimer's disease. Plant-based foods provide polyphenols.

The researchers confirmed their findings:

> *"It has been demonstrated, in various cell culture and animal models, that these [polyphenol] metabolites are able to protect neuronal cells by attenuating oxidative stress and damage."*

After fifteen year study of elderly persons, Japanese researchers (Ozawa *et al.* 2013) confirmed that ones diet can dramatically reduce our chances of Alzheimer's disease and dementia.

The researchers, from Japan's Kyushu University Graduate School of Medical Sciences, followed 1,006 people who were between 60 and 80 years old. They tracked their diets, and tracked whether they contracted vascular dementia and/or Alzheimer's disease during that period.

The researchers grouped the diets among the subjects into seven general categories. These included Western diet patterns, traditional Japanese diets and more or less vegetable intake, more or less soy intake, more or less rice intake, more or less dairy intake and more or less algae (seaweed) intake – part of the traditional Japanese diet.

Among the total population, after an average of fifteen years 144 people developed Alzheimer's disease and 88 developed vascular dementia – the second-leading type of dementia after Alzheimer's disease. (Research has estimated that 20-30% of dementia cases are vascular, and vascular dementia can also produce Alzheimer's symptoms.)

The researchers found that those whose diets had the highest intakes of vegetables, soybeans, algae, milk and dairy products, and low in rice had a 65% reduced incidence of Alzheimer's disease, 66% less incidence of any dementia, and 45% less incidence of vascular dementia.

It should be pointed out that white polished rice is the primary rice being eaten among the Japanese today. We discuss the problems with white rice and why brown rice is healthier for a myriad of reasons later on.

Other research has found that diets rich in fruits and vegetables – notably the Mediterranean Diet – decrease the risk of Alzheimer's disease and other forms of dementia. In a study from Australia's Edith Cowan University (Gardener *et al.* 2012), it was found that diets that most closely adhere to the Mediterranean Diet reduce the risk of Alzheimer's disease and mild cognitive impairment. This study followed 970 people – including 149 with Alzheimer's and 98 with mild cognitive impairment (MCI).

As to the effect of seaweed (the primary algae eaten in the Japanese diet), a recent study from Russia (Besednova *et al.* 2013) has concluded that seaweed contains compounds that prevent and possibly reverse oxidative damage to brain and nerve cells. The primary group of nutrients in seaweeds having these effects are called sulfated polysaccharides. These have been shown in laboratory and animal studies to reverse degeneration of nerve cells among the brain and central nervous system. According to the researchers:

*"Sulfated polysaccharides can arrest a number of secondary pathological effects observed in neurodegenerative diseases (oxidative stress, inflammation, the phenomenon of increased neuronal apoptosis, toxic effects etc.)."*

They also suggested that:

*"sulfated polysaccharides may be the basis for the creation of next-generation drugs for the treatment of neurodegenerative diseases."*

Or, we can simply include seaweeds in our diet. What a novel idea.

As to milk and dairy products finding, these foods contain certain long-chain polyunsaturated fatty acids that nourish nerve cells. Studies with infants have found that these type of fatty acids promote brain and nerve cell development (Koletzko *et al.* 2003). And assuming the dairy product is fermented, there is a reduction of casein and lactose – as casein has been linked in other research with increased cancer incidence. We'll talk more about this later as well.

As to soybeans, numerous studies have shown soy is heart-healthy, reduces the risk of cancer, and its phytoestrogens help balance hormone levels among the aging. Soy provides all the essential amino acids, making it a complete protein. Non-GMO, organic soybeans are not only nutritious, but they have a solid scientific basis for being healthy. This is especially true for fermented soy products such as tofu, natto and tempeh. More on soy later.

This and other studies give us a mature view of how our dietary habits today will effect our future mental health. Diets that produce high levels of oxidative free radicals have been shown to produce a higher risk of not just cardiovascular disease, but also dementia, because what damages the heart and blood vessels can also damage brain and nerve cells. And when it comes to blood flow, brain cells will suffer first when arteries become clogged.

Plant and seaweed compounds – phytonutrients – provide the opposite effect. They not only neutralize free radicals. They also provide an array of nutrients that protect the brain and blood vessels (Kelsey *et al.* 2010).

This result is confirmed by another study from Japan's Kyushu University Medical School (Ohara *et al.* 2011), which found that dementia and Alzheimer's disease are associated with type 2 diabetes. Because type 2 diabetes has also been linked to poor nutrition and lack of exercise, dementia and Alzheimer's can now be linked directly to diet and exercise.

The researchers, from the Graduate School of Medical Sciences' Environmental Medicine Department, followed 1,017 adults over the age of

60 years old for fifteen years. The elderly adults lived in an adult community and were dementia-free at the beginning of the study.

The adults were given oral glucose tolerance tests periodically. At the end of the fifteen years, those the adults whose glucose tolerance testing confirmed a diagnosis of diabetes by the end of the study were more than twice as likely to have Alzheimer's disease, and 74% increased incidence of vascular dementia.

Dementia and Alzheimer's disease risk also significantly increased among those whose two-hour post-load glucose levels were over the 7.8 mmol/Liter levels, and the highest risk was found among those with two-hour post-load glucose levels over 11 mmol/Liter.

The study was published in the medical journal *Neurology*, and has been coined the Hisayama Study.

The researchers concluded:

> *"Our findings suggest that diabetes is a significant risk factor for all-cause dementia, Alzheimer's disease, and probably vascular dementia."*

In research funded by the National Institutes of Health, Columbia University Medical Center researchers found that a diet with higher consumption of vegetables, fruits, grains and legumes, with lower saturated fat levels and higher monounsaturated fats reduced the risk of brain damage.

The diets of 712 New Yorkers were divided into three groups. They were followed up with brain scans an average of six years later. The scans indicated that 238 people had brain damage of some sort.

The group following more closely to a Mediterranean diet (primarily vegetarian and fish diet with little or no meat) had a 36% lower risk of brain damage. The group that had a closer Med-diet had 21% lower risk of brain damage than the group that ate the typical (red meat) Western diet.

In another study, Columbia University (Gu *et al.* 2010) researchers followed 2,148 elderly persons for four years, giving them dementia testing every 18 months. This research found that a diet high in nuts, fruits, cruciferous vegetables, leafy green vegetables, nuts, tomatoes and fish – and had a lower intake of red meat and high-fat dairy products – were 38% less likely to develop Alzheimer's disease by the fourth year. None of the elderly subjects had symptoms of Alzheimer's or dementia at the beginning of the study and they were all over 64 years old.

In another study from the Columbia University researchers (Scarmeas *et al.* 2009), 1,880 elderly people without dementia at the beginning of the study were followed for over five years. At the end of the study, 282 people contracted Alzheimer's disease. The researchers found that adhering to a Med diet decreased the risk of Alzheimer's by 40%.

In a study (Scarmeas *et al.* 2006) with 2,258 elderly New Yorkers, those who adhered more closely (highest third) to the Mediterranean diet had a 40% reduced risk of contracting Alzheimer's disease within four years.

In another study (Scarmeas *et al.* 2006) that compared 194 Alzheimer's patients with 1,790 healthy elderly persons, it was found that those adhering more closely (highest tertile) with the Mediterranean diet had a 68% reduced risk of Alzheimer's compared to those with the lowest adherence – the highest consumption of the Western diet.

Another study by the same researchers (Scarmeas *et al.* 2007) found that a higher adherence to the Med diet reduced the risk of dying for Alzheimer's disease patients as well.

In 2013, Researchers from the University of Athens School of Medicine (Psaltopoulou *et al.* 2013) conducted a review of research that studied the connection between the Med diet and the risk of stroke, depression, cognitive impairment, and Parkinson's disease. They found 22 well-designed studies that followed many thousands of patients. Their meta-analysis of these studies found that the Mediterranean diet reduced the risk of stroke by 29%, reduced the risk of depression by 32%, and reduced the risk of cognitive impairment by 40%. We document the one Parkinson's study below.

In one of these, researchers from Australia's Edith Cowan University (Féart *et al.* 2011) studied nearly 1,000 people – including some with mild cognitive decline and Alzheimer's. They found that those who had diets closest to a Mediterranean Diet had the least incidence of cognitive decline and Alzheimer's disease. Many other studies have confirmed these results over the past few years.

The question also arises is what are the factors of the Mediterranean diet and why does this diet help reduce cognitive decline? As stated recently by researchers from the University of Malta (Solfrizzi *et al.* 2011) – the Med Diet:

> *"is rich in the antioxidants Vitamins C and E, polyunsaturated fatty acids and polyphenolic compounds."*

What do these elements have in common with the Mediterranean diet? Yes, the Med Diet certainly does contain many of these nutrients. But the Med Diet, as pointed out by the University of Malta scientists – contains numerous nutrients that synergize with each other. And because the Med Diet is rich in plant-based foods, the Med Diet contains polyphenols.

These polyphenols are plant components that include flavonoids, proanthrocyanidins, sterols and many other types of special compounds. These compounds work synergistically within plant-based foods to provide a host of benefits, which include brain cell health, artery health, heart health, liver and kidney health and many others. The combination of these plant-based foods provide the ultimate in cognitive decline prevention, because along with other benefits they reduce damage produced by free radicals – which are ultimately at the core of cognitive decline according to most research.

The bottom line is that nature works in synergy, just as the body does. The brain does not sit in a laboratory jar isolated from the rest of the body. The brain operates as part of the rest of the whole body. The health of the rest of that body – including the arteries, heart, liver, kidneys, bloodstream and so on – directly affects the health of our brain cells.

A primarily plant-based diet and regular exercise are the key elements in keeping the whole body healthy. This is proven not only in cognitive research, but in cancer research, heart disease research, liver and kidney research and elsewhere. Turns out, those plant-based foods the Western diet relegates to a small portion at the edge of the plate are the very medicines our body needs to keep itself healthy.

After reviewing some of the same research, Dr. Gad Marshall, a Harvard Alzheimer's researcher and Assistant Professor of Medicine at Harvard concluded that ones diet can delay and even prevent cognitive decline and Alzheimer's. According to Dr. Marshall:

> *"My strongest recommendations are a Mediterranean-style diet and regular physical exercise," he says. "There's good evidence from multiple studies showing that these lifestyle modifications can prevent cognitive decline and dementia and also slow down existing cognitive decline."*

These two factors have been proven to reduce memory and cognitive decline without question. The evidence comes from numerous studies and reviews from eminent researchers around the world.

(Other research with supportive and/or similar findings: Vassallo *et al.* 2012; Wyka *et al.* 2012; Devanand *et al.* 2012; Solfrizzi *et al.* 2011; Solfrizzi *et al.* 2011).

## Parkinson's disease and Diet

Columbia researchers (Alcalay *et al.* 2012) tested 257 patients with Parkinson's disease along with 198 control subjects. They used the standardized Willett semiquantitative questionnaire to compare their diets with their disease and symptoms – or lack thereof.

The researchers scored the test on compliance with the Mediterranean diet adherence. They found that a Med diet lowered the risk of Parkinson's disease by 14%, and a lower Med diet score increased the risk of Parkinson's disease by 9%.

The researchers concluded:

> *"PD patients adhere less than controls to a Mediterranean-type diet. Dietary behavior may be associated with age at onset."*

Illustrating the effect of diet in both Parkinson's and Alzheimer's diseases, several studies have suggested that a nutrient derived from a commercially farmed green algae species may treat and even reverse cognitive impairment and conditions relating to neuron damage.

Researchers from China's Fujian Medical University (Ye *et al.* 2012) tested a nutrient called Astaxanthin with nerve cells and found that the nutrient blocked the type of oxidative stress that has been identified as the primary cause of neuron damage that result in brain and nerve damage.

The researchers found that Astaxanthin blocked the MPP+ related Heme oxygenase process implicated in nerve and brain cell damage. This type of oxidative damage has been linked to Parkinson's disease, Huntington's disease and Alzheimer's disease.

Other research has found that Astaxanthin comes with antioxidant properties from an estimated one hundred to one thousand times the antioxidant level of vitamin E. One of the richest natural sources of Astaxanthin is the algae *Haematococcus pluvialis* – which we'll discuss later.

The Fujian Medical University researchers' conclusion:

> *"ATX suppresses MPP+-induced oxidative stress in PC12 cells via the HO-1/NOX2 axis. ATX should be strongly considered as a potential neuroprotectant and adjuvant therapy for patients with Parkinson's disease."*

Clinical research has supported this finding and more. Last year, researchers from the Graduate School of Medicine at Japan's Juntendo University (Katagiri *et al.* 2012) tested Astaxanthin using 96 elderly adult volunteers. In this randomized, double-blind and placebo-controlled study, the researchers gave the subjects either a capsule with Astaxanthin extract or a placebo for three months.

Before, after and every four weeks during the study, the researchers tested the subjects' cognition, and found that those who took both dosages of Astaxanthin extract – 12 milligrams or 6 milligrams – scored significantly higher on learning and cognition testing than the placebo group.

The researchers concluded:

*"The results suggested that astaxanthin-rich Haematococcus pluvialis extract improves cognitive function in the healthy aged individuals."*

Another study from Japan (Ikeda *et al.* 2008) – this from the Life Science Institute – found among ten healthy adults that 12 milligrams a day of Astaxanthin significantly improves cognitive function and psychomotor functions.

Other clinical studies have found that Astaxanthin treatment significantly raises blood levels of carotene, and improves the health of circulating red blood cells – reducing free radical related damage that can eventually produce nerve and brain cell damage.

Carotenes are also abundantly available among a variety of vegetables and root foods.

Parkinson's disease has been linked to damage to the brain's dopaminergic nerve cells located in the motor region of the brain, called the substantia nigra pars compacta. Research has increasingly unfolded the process of oxidative stress related to radical damage.

This oxidative stress process is related to the same process that damages brain cells in the hypothalamus – causing the beta-amyloid peptide (Abeta) oxidative process linked with the memory loss associated with Alzheimer's disease.

We might also mention that a smaller study (Marder *et al.* 2013) of 211 Huntington's disease patients found that a diet with the highest consumption of dairy products resulted in more than double the risk of Huntington's disease. While this relationship is not clear, we discuss some of the issues of pasteurized dairy products later on.

## Obesity and Diet

Certainly diet and obesity are related, but many believe it is strictly a question of calories. Let's dig a little deeper. First let's look at some of the facts related to obesity.

According to the latest statistics from the Centers of Disease Control, about 36% of American adults are obese and 69% are overweight. This means that the majority of Americans are either overweight or obese.

The United States is first in the world in obesity. This is followed by Mexico, where 30% of adults are obese, and New Zealand, where 27% of adults are obese. Australia is fourth with 25% of adults, followed by the UK, where 25% is also obese. Canada is the sixth most obese country, with 24% of adults. Ireland is seventh, with 23% obesity among adults, and Chile is eighth with 22%. Iceland is ninth with 20% obesity among adults.

Other countries with higher percentages include Hungary, Greece, Germany, Finland and Poland.

The countries that are the least obese include Japan, Korea, China, India, Indonesia, Italy and others. China, for example, has 2.9% obesity, and India has about 5% obesity. Korea and Japan are close to China's rate. Italy is about 7% obesity.

What is the prevailing diet of the most obese countries versus the countries with less obesity? The Western diet, composed primarily of red meats, fried poultry and seafood, processed starchy foods, and sugary foods. Could this possibly be a coincidence that the countries that consume more of a Western diet have greater levels of obesity? Nada. Numerous universities and governmental agencies have been studying the relationship between obesity and diet for many years, and have concluded that the Western diet is by far the most fattening diet.

For example, research from China has shown that as more people eat the Western diet, obesity rates have been rising (Wang and Zhai 2013).

Most of us realize that diet and obesity are related. But do we know that toxicity and obesity are related? As we discussed earlier, many toxins – especially many dangerous ones – are fat soluble. This means that they will build up among our fat cells. This also means that the more and larger fat cells we have, the more build up of toxicity we can have.

Obesity is also associated with a disorder now called *metabolic syndrome*. According to the American Heart Association, metabolic syndrome is related to the following conditions:

> ➢ Blood sugar issues (diabetes, insulin resistance, hypoglycemia)
> ➢ Obesity (most specifically abdominal obesity)
> ➢ Cholesterol issues (high LDL, low HDL, high triglycerides)
> ➢ High blood pressure
> ➢ Chronic inflammation markers (including C-reactive protein, high white blood cell count, high eosinophils)
> ➢ Atherosclerosis (damage and hardening to the arteries – indicated by fibrinogen, circulation problems and so on.)

Metabolic syndrome is characterized by cholesterol problems, high blood pressure, diabetes or hypoglycemia, chronic inflammation, cardiovascular disease, high CRP levels, and heart disease. All of these issues add up to the same issue: systemic inflammation. Furthermore, each of these conditions have the same underlying issues: Poor dietary choices, high levels of reactive oxygen species, increased infections, an overburdened immune system, lack of exercise and other poor lifestyle choices.

It is thus not an accident that the relative intake of our fats is specific to our levels of toxicity. This has been studied by a number of researchers, who have concluded that obesity and inflammation are irreparably tied.

It is a well-known fact that obese people have higher rates of cardio-vascular disease, diabetes, kidney disorders, liver diseases, arthritis, asthma, hay fever, dementia, intestinal disorders and many, many other conditions. Just about every medical condition is worsened by obesity, and we need no scientific reference for this fact, simply because the research is so widely known.

In a recent study from Boston University's School of Medicine, led by cardiologist and medical professor Noyan Gokce, MD, fat tissues from 109 obese and lean people provided clear evidence. Tissue from none of the lean patients illustrated any signs of inflammation. In comparison, fat tissues from the obese patients showed "significant" signs of inflammation.

In addition, the lean patients showed "no sign" of poor vascular function while the obese patients showed significantly poor vascular function. This of course relates to inflammation, as we've discussed. When the blood vessel walls become damaged by free radicals and lipid peroxides. This results in scarring and artery deposit build-up, which inhibits healthy circulation and releases clots that block other arteries.

The research also illustrated that the obese persons exhibited varying degrees of inflammation, indicating that a toxic environment and intake of toxins is also associated with higher levels of inflammation. Obesity simply allows for a better 'net' to capture more filters within the fat cells.

### So other than consuming fewer calories, can a change in our diet really make a difference?

The evidence says yes. Researchers from Northwestern University's Feinberg School of Medicine (Shay *et al.* 2012) followed 1,794 adult Americans from eight different population samples. Of course, they found that lower calorie intake related directly to lower levels of Body Mass Index (BMI).

But they also found that calories equal, those who ate more fresh fruit, pasta and rice had lower BMIs. Lower BMI was also associated with less meat intake and lower saturated fat consumption, while higher dietary fiber (read plant-based foods) were associated with lower levels of BMI.

The researchers concluded:

> *"The consumption of foods higher in nutrient-dense carbohydrate and lower in animal protein and saturated fat is associated with lower total energy intakes, more favorable micronutrient intakes, and lower BMI."*

In a study from the School of Public Health of the UK's Imperial College (Romaguera *et al.* 2011) followed 48,631 men and women from five different European countries for an average of 5 and a half years. They found that those eating more meat, processed breads, margarine and soft drinks had a significantly greater risk of becoming obese. They concluded:

> *"A dietary pattern high in fruit and dairy and low in white bread, processed meat, margarine, and soft drinks may help to prevent abdominal fat accumulation."*

Another study found that a mostly-vegan diet plan with daily Greenfoods and Apple Cider Vinegar supplementation in addition to a daily supplement can result in significant weight loss and reductions of "bad" cholesterol in just three weeks.

The researchers (Balliett *et al.* 2013) gave 49 adult men and women a three week diet containing mostly vegan meals. The meals totaled 1200-1400 calories for the women and 1600-1800 calories for the men.

The men and women were also given, once daily, nutritional supplements. The daily supplement contained a greenfood drink with alfalfa, wheatgrass and apple cider vinegar. In addition, the group was given a nutritional supplement with enzymes and vitamins.

During the second week, the adult subjects – with an average age of 31 – were given a daily cleanse supplement. This supplement contained magnesium, chia, flaxseed, lemon, camu camu, cat's claw, bentonite clay, turmeric, pau d'arco, chanca piedra, stevia, zeolite clay, slippery elm, garlic, ginger, peppermint, aloe, citrus bioflavonoids, and fulvic acid. The cleanse supplement was given before every meal during the second week.

During the third week, the researchers gave the subjects supplements with probiotics and prebiotics instead of the cleanse supplement.

The average weight loss after 21 days was nearly nine pounds per person – equating to a 2-3% drop in weight per person.

And the average drop in total cholesterol was 30 mg/dL while the drop in low-density lipoprotein (LDL) – the "bad" cholesterol – was 21 mg/dL. Their average LDL levels prior to the three-week diet was 103 mg/dL, dropping to an average of 83 mg/dL, while total cholesterol went from an average of 185 mg/dL to 155 mg/dL. These are significant drops in both total and LDL cholesterol by any standard, let alone from only three weeks of a diet with natural supplements.

Triglycerides also decreased dramatically. Average triglyceride levels went from 93 mg/dL to 83 mg/dL during the three weeks.

In addition, testosterone levels among the women in the group went up significantly, from an average of 400 n/dL (nanograms per deciliter) to over 511 n/dL.

Average blood pressure went down as well. Average systolic blood pressure went from 116 to 112 mmHg during the three weeks, while diastolic pressure went from 76 to 71 mmHg.

In a large review of studies from the University of Naples (Esposito *et al.* 2011), researchers found that among the 19 studies that fit their quality standards, the Mediterranean diet resulted in significant weight loss, especially in studies lasting longer than six months.

## Diabetes, Glucose Control and Diet

Diabetes rates around the world are at epidemic levels, according to Harvard researchers. Almost 350 million adults have diabetes worldwide, and over 25 million U.S. adults or 11% of U.S. adults have diabetes – most of which is type 2.

Researchers from Harvard (Pan *et al.* 2013) followed 26,357 men for 20 years, 48,709 women for 20 years and 74,077 women for 16 years, and compared their diets with incidence of type 2 diabetes.

In a pooled multivariate analysis, the researchers found that increasing red meat consumption for at least four years increased the risk of diabetes significantly during that period.

Their data found that an average increase in ½ serving of red meat per day resulted in a 48% increased incidence of type two diabetes.

This increase in meat consumption also resulted in weight gain risk by 30%.

Meanwhile reducing red meat consumption for a four year period resulted in a 14% lower risk of diabetes. The researchers concluded that:

> *"Increasing red meat consumption over time is associated with an elevated subsequent risk of T2DM, and the association is partly mediated by body weight. Our results add further evidence that limiting red meat consumption over time confers benefits for T2DM prevention."*

Researchers at the Harvard School of Public Health found in a huge study that eating red meat regularly increases the incidence of type 2 diabetes. Furthermore, they found that replacing red meat in the diet with non-meat proteins significantly lowers incidence of type 2 diabetes.

The research was led by An Pan, PhD and Frank Hu, PhD, a professor of nutrition and epidemiology at Harvard's School of Public Health. The researchers followed 37,083 men for 20 years, 79,570 women for 28 years, and 87,504 women 14 years. In addition, they performed a meta-analysis review by combining their data with previous studies, to arrive at a massive total of 442,101 human subjects. Of this population, 28,228 developed type 2 diabetes during the period of study.

The study eliminated trends related to lifestyle and other dietary risk facts, as well as age and body mass index (BMI). In the final analysis, a average of 50 grams of processed meat per day increased diabetes incidence by 51%, while a 100 gram serving of unprocessed red meat per day increased diabetes incidence by 19%.

Dr. Hu explained the results in a press release by Harvard:

> *"Clearly, the results from this study have huge public health implications given the rising type 2 diabetes epidemic and increasing consumption of red meats worldwide. The good news is that such troubling risk factors can be offset by swapping red meat for a healthier protein."*

The Harvard press release also stated this was the largest study of its kind to link red meat with diabetes – confirming the findings of other smaller studies. The study was supported by the National Institutes of Health's National Institute of Diabetes and Digestive and Kidney Diseases, along with the National Heart, Lung, and Blood Institute.

The Harvard researchers suggested that processed red meats such as bacon, sausage, hot dogs, and deli meats, as well as unprocessed red meats should be "minimized" or "reduced." They recommended replacement with healthier protein sources.

Healthier proteins, according to the researchers, include nuts, grains, beans and low-fat dairy.

The study also found that even substituting one serving of grains per day instead of meat protein lowered diabetes incidence by 23%. Substituting one serving with nuts reduced incidence by 21%, and low-fat dairy resulted in a 17% reduction.

This study confirms another Harvard study done in 2010 (Micha et al.), which found that meat consumption increased the risk of diabetes along with coronary heart disease and strokes. This study analyzed 20 clinical studies that met their quality review, which included 1,218,380 total human subjects. Among other findings, they found that red meat increased incidence of coronary heart disease by 42%.

Dr. Pan stated in a followup interview:

> *"Our study clearly shows that eating both unprocessed and processed red meat – particularly processed – is associated with an increased risk of type 2 diabetes,"*

He also suggested that it was unfair to lump other healthier sources of protein together with the unhealthier red meats.

Other research has found that type 2 diabetes is associated with a lack of exercise, obesity and diet.

In one, researchers from Simmons College in Boston (Fung *et al.* 2004) followed 69,554 women between 38 and 63 yeas old for ten years. They found that for every single serving increase in red meat resulted in a 26% increased risk of diabetes. The risk increased to 38-43% for processed meats, 73% for bacon, and 49% for hot dogs.

In a study of 42,504 men by researchers from the Harvard School of Public Health (Van Dam *et al.* 2002), it was found that the frequent consumption of processed meat was associated with a 46% higher risk of type 2 diabetes.

Another study from Harvard (Schulze *et al.* 2003) that followed over 91,000 women between 26 and 46 years old found that eating processed meat for more than five times a week increased the risk of type 2 diabetes by 91%.

Dutch researchers van Woudenbergh *et al.* 2012) analyzed 4,366 participants who did not have diabetes initially. After 12.4 years, the researchers reviewed the diets and the incidence of diabetes among the study group.

The research determined that eating 50 grams more processed meat per day increased the incidence of type 2 diabetes by 87%. Eating 50 grams more meat in general increased the incidence of type 2 diabetes by 42%, and 18% after adjusting for BMI levels.

The researchers also looked into the connection between C-reactive protein levels and diabetes, since other research has recently linked meat consumption with increased levels of CRP. Higher CRP levels are associated with heart attacks and cardiovascular disease.

While the research confirmed the link between meat consumption and CRP, they found that increased CRP seems to be unrelated to diabetes when considering meat consumption. In other words, they are independent associations with meat consumption.

Other studies have linked type 2 diabetes with diet.

In a study from the Britain's University of Bristol (Andrews *et al.* 2011) studied 593 type 2 diabetes patients, and found that while the control group (no diet or exercise regimen) worsened over a six month period, those who underwent diet therapy had 28% increased glycemic control, and those who underwent diet and exercise therapy had 31% increased glycemic control after six months.

A study from Italy (Panunzio *et al.* 2011) shows that the Mediterranean diet significantly improves metabolism, glycemia, insulin levels, C-reactive protein levels and body mass index.

All of these factors present the issues related to metabolic syndrome. Metabolic syndrome is symptomized by cardiovascular disease, being overweight and a tendency for type 2 diabetes.

The study followed 80 volunteers who were between 51 and 59 years old. They were randomly split into two groups, and one group ate the Mediterranean diet and the other ate a Western diet. Before and after six months, the subjects underwent extensive testing.

After 25 weeks on the diet, the Mediterranean diet subjects had an average of 12.4% lower body mass index, 8.3% less weight, 9.2% lower fasting glycemia and 32% lower fasting insulin. The Med diet group also had 34% lower levels of C-reactive protein.

C-reactive protein is a marker for inflammation. High CRP levels indicate systemic inflammation, often accompanying the hardening of the arteries, also called atherosclerosis, coronary artery disease and a higher risk of heart disease and stroke in general.

Lower fasting glycemia levels means lower levels of blood sugar, related to a lower risk of diabetes.

Lower fasting insulin levels are also a marker that is associated with a reduced risk of diabetes.

The diets of the Med diet group proved consistent with these in this study. The Med diet group showed 39% higher levels of fruit, 30% higher levels of vegetables, 18% higher cheese and 38% higher levels of fiber.

## Respiratory Conditions such as Asthma, and Diet

Medical researchers from Britain's University of Nottingham (McKeever *et al.* 2010) researched the relationship between diet and respiratory symptoms, including forced expiratory volumes. Their data was derived from 12,648 adults from the Monitoring Project on Risk Factors and Chronic Diseases in The Netherlands. They also included dietary patterns and lung function decline over a five-year basis.

They found that diets with higher intakes of meat and potatoes, and lower levels of soy and cereals, was linked to reduced lung function and lower expiratory levels (FEV1) levels. They also found that the heavy meat-and-potatoes diet produced higher levels of chronic obstructive pulmonary disease. They also found that a "cosmopolitan diet" with heavier intakes of fish and chicken (both of which are commonly fried) produced higher levels of wheeze and asthma.

In a study of 460 children and their mothers on Menorca – a Mediterranean island – medical researchers from Greece's Department of Social Medicine and the University of Crete (Chatzi *et al.* 2008) found that children of mothers eating primarily a Mediterranean diet (a predominantly plant-based diet) produced significantly lower rates of asthma among the children.

They found that mothers with a high Mediterranean Diet Score during pregnancy reduced the incidence of persistent wheeze among their children by 78%. Their children also had 70% lower incidence of allergic wheezing; and a 45% reduction in allergies among their children at age six (after removing other possible variables).

In a study of 460 children and mothers on Menorca – a Mediterranean island in Spain – medical researchers from Greece's Department of Social Medicine and the University of Crete (Chatzi *et al.* 2008) found that children of mothers eating primarily a Mediterranean diet (a predominantly plant-based diet) produced significantly lower rates of asthma among the children.

Mothers with a high Mediterranean Diet Score during pregnancy reduced the incidence of persistent wheeze among their children by 78%. Their children also had 70% lower incidence of allergic wheezing; and 45% reduced allergies among their children at age six (after adjusting out other possible variables).

Another study by researchers from the University of Crete's Faculty of Medicine (Chatzi *et al.* 2007) surveyed the parents of 690 children from ages seven through 18 years old in the rural areas of Crete. The children were also tested with skin prick tests for 10 common allergens. This research found that consuming a Mediterranean diet reduced the risk of allergic rhinitis by over 65%. The risk of skin allergies and respiratory conditions (such as wheezing) was also reduced, but by smaller amounts. They also found that more consumption of nuts among the children cut wheezing rates in half, while consuming margarine more than doubled the prevalence of both wheezing and allergic rhinitis.

Researchers from the Harvard School of Public Health (Varraso *et al.* 2007) studied the effects of nitrites in the diet and lung health. They analyzed 111 diagnosed cases of COPD (Chronic obstructive pulmonary disease) between 1986 and 1998 among 42,915 men who participated in the Health Professionals Follow-up Study. The average consumption of high-nitrite meats (processed meats, bacon, hot dogs) was calculated from surveys conducted in 1986, 1990, and 1994. They found that consuming these meats at least once a day increased the incidence of COPD by more than 2-½ times over those who rarely ate high-nitrite meats.

These same Harvard researchers used a similar analysis of 42,917 men, but with more dietary parameters. This research found that the *"Western diet"* consisting of refined grains, sugary foods, cured and red meats, and fried foods, increased COPD incidence by more than four times. Meanwhile, a *"prudent"* diet, rich in fruits, vegetables and fish, halved COPD incidence.

The same researchers from the Harvard School of Public Health studied lung function, COPD and diet among 72,043 women between 1984 and 2000 in the Nurses' Health Study. Diets that had more fruit, vegetables, fish and whole-grain products reduced the incidence of COPD by 25%. Meanwhile, a diet heavy in refined grains, cured and red meats, desserts and French fries increased the incidence of COPD by 31%.

## ADHD and Diet

Attention deficit and hyperactivity disorder (ADHD) incidence is growing, particularly among western industrialized societies. Research has found that about 5% of children between 9 and 17 have been diagnosed with ADHD, while possibly 2-4% of adults have it. Some research has estimated that up to 10% of the U.S. population may be affected by ADHD.

Boys have more ADHD diagnosis than girls, at a rate of nearly 5 to 1. Some have suggested that this is the result of girls having different symptoms than boys.

Research from the University of Western Australia (Howard *et al.* 2011) found that ADHD in children is linked to diet, and more specifically, to the Western diet.

The study reviewed the dietary patterns of 1,799 children. The children's diets were followed for fourteen years. The researchers divided the children into two basic groups based on their diet habits: A "Healthy" group and a "Western" group.

Of the 1,799 children, 115 were diagnosed with ADHD.

Those children who ate a Western diet were more than twice as likely to have ADHD, or 2.21 times more likely.

Dr. Wendy Oddy, a professor at the University of Western Australia, was the lead author of the study. Dr. Oddy commented about the study for Perth's Telethon Institute for Child Health Research, which participated in the study:

*"We found a diet high in the Western pattern of foods was associated with more than double the risk of having an ADHD diagnosis compared with a diet low in the Western pattern, after adjusting for numerous other social and family influences."*

In this study, the "Western pattern" was categorized as the higher intake of red meats, fried foods, fast foods, sweets and processed foods. The "Healthy pattern" diet pattern was associated with a diet high in whole grains, fresh fruit, vegetables and fish.

The ADHD group also were more likely to eat certain foods.

*"When we looked at specific foods, having an ADHD diagnosis was associated with a diet high in takeaway foods, processed meats, red meat, high fat dairy products and confectionary," Dr Oddy said.*

For those who doubt the connection between diet and ADHD, there are other studies to consider.

For example, the ADHD Research Center in Enhoven, Netherlands (Pelsser *et al.* 2011) studied 100 children aged 4-8, who were randomly assigned to either a control group or an elimination diet group. The control group was instructed to eat a healthy diet, while the elimination group eliminated particular foods according to food challenge tests. This study found that many children's ADHD was indeed induced by certain foods.

## Arthritis and Diet

Numerous studies have connected arthritis to the Western diet.

Let's consider just a few of these.

Pro-inflammatory messengers involved in arthritis are created by two conversion processes of arachidonic acid—a fatty acid. The critical enzymes used for this conversion to prostaglandins, thromboxanes, and leucotrienes are cyclooxygenase (COX) and lipoxygenase (LOX). A significant amount of research over the past decade has confirmed that a disproportionate amount of arachidonic acid in the diet will produce increased levels of inflammation (Calder 2008 and many others) due to an oversupply of these messengers.

In fact, research headed up by Dr. Darshan Kelley from the Western Human Research Center in California illustrated that diets high in arachidonic acid stimulated four times more inflammatory cells than diets low in arachidonic acid content. And this problem actually increases with age. In other words, the same amount of arachidonic acid-forming foods will cause higher levels of arachidonic acid the older we get (Chilton 2006).

This also relates to many other health-related problems as people age. For example, higher arachidonic acid levels in the bloodstream correlate with greater platelet aggregation. This creates a higher risk of blood clots. Higher levels of arachidonic acid can also cause difficulties with glucose utilization, lung efficiency, intestinal health and so many other disorders related to inflammation.

According to the USDA's Standard 13 and 16 databases, animal meats and fish produce the highest amounts of arachidonic acid in the body. Diary, fruits and vegetables produce little or no arachidonic acid. Grains, beans and nuts produce none or very small amounts. Processed bakery goods produce a moderate amount of arachidonic acid.

Hundreds of studies have now confirmed that an increase in long-chain fatty acids such as DHA, EPA, ALA and GLA in the diet slows down inflammation in the body. How do they do that? Because these fats convert to other compounds—such as phospholipids used for cell membranes—leaving less fat available to convert to prostaglandins, leucotrienes and thromboxanes.

In a study from Germany published in Rheumatology International (Adam et al. 2003), sixty-eight patients with diagnoses of rheumatoid arthritis were divided into two groups. For eight months, one group maintained a typical Western diet (meat diet high in arachidonic acid), while the other group ate a diet low in arachidonic acid for eight months. Parts of each group also supplemented DHA/EPA oil or a placebo.

The Western diet caused no reduction in pain and swelling. The placebo (no DHA oil) group in the low arachidonic acid group had a 14% reduction in pain and swelling. The DHA supplemented-Western diet group had 11% reduction in joint pain and 22% reduction in joint swelling. The DHA supplementation, low-arachidonic acid group had a reduction in joint pain of 28%, and a reduction in joint swelling of 34%. Therefore, while taking a DHA oil supplement can reduce pain and inflammation, the Western diet—high in arachidonic acid—will continue to contribute to chronic inflammation: Like taking a few steps forward while taking a few steps back.

Saturated fats have also been connected specifically to arthritis. In a study at the Loma Linda University School of Medicine, 23 people with rheumatoid arthritis ate a low fat diet of 10% calories from fat. They were compared to a control group eating an unregulated diet high in saturated fats. The low-fat group experienced a 20-40% reduction in joint inflammation as a group. Dr. Edwin Krick, the study leader and professor at the medical school, recommended a diet low in saturated fats for arthritic sufferers.

We will discuss the science of fats in more detail later.

Plant-based antioxidants have been shown to significantly reduce the severity of a number of disorders, including atherosclerosis, heart disease, liver disease, diabetes and others. This is because they support the immune system's process of removing toxins before they do any further damage. This was illustrated in a study (McAlindon et al. 1996) at the Boston University School of Medicine.

The study revealed that people consuming more than 200 milligrams a day of vitamin C were one-third less likely to experience a worsening of their osteoarthritis. Dr. Timothy McAlidon, a professor at the University suggested that the reduction in free radicals by the antioxidant vitamin C was the likely mechanism.

A team of leading medical researchers (Scher et al. 2013) more recently determined that new cases of rheumatoid arthritis occurs following intestinal dysbiosis and the overgrowth of a particular gut microbe.

The researchers – from the New York University School of Medicine, Cornell Medical College, Italy's University of Trento, Harvard School of Public Health, Spain's University of Valencia, Oxford and the Howard Hughes Medical Institute – found that the overgrowth of a bacteria called *Prevotella copri* within the gut was linked with newly onset rheumatoid arthritis.

The researchers used DNA analysis of the microbiome (the gut's total bacteria load) together with specific analyses to relate the overgrowth of this particular bacteria.

But the growth of the bacteria didn't happen in isolation. In a predominance of the cases, the bacteria overgrowth was related to the loss of colonies of healthy probiotic colonies – an event called dysbiosis.

The researchers based their findings upon DNA sequencing of 114 stool samples from patients with rheumatoid arthritis and healthy control subjects. This indicated the total DNA of the gut's microbiome: The general species make up of intestinal bacteria. The researchers then took 44 of the samples and analyzed them with more detail to isolate the particular species of bacteria at the root of the dysbiosis.

Using further analysis of the genetic composition of the patients' microbiome together with the patients' own DNA, it was established that rheumatoid arthritis is linked with the overgrowth of this *Prevotella copri* bacteria combined with dysbiosis.

While the Prevotella enterotype is related to plant-based diets, the condition of dysbiosis is related to the Western diet. This is because the Western diet has a reduced compatibility with healthy probiotic bacteria within the gut.

A healthy microbiota consists of a balance of many many organisms. An overgrowth of any of these species leads to dysbiosis and the risk of inflammation.

This pro-inflammatory condition relates to several variables, as we'll discuss further. With regard to intestinal bacteria, the Western diet maintains a lack of prebiotic conditions. That is, a lack of complex prebiotics as we will describe in detail. Plant-based prebiotics feed our healthier species of intestinal bacteria.

Meanwhile, the Western diet promotes the growth of pathogenic organisms. As these pathogenic organisms gain in colony strength and territory, they begin to push aside the probiotic organisms that support intestinal health.

Healthy probiotic organisms also support the immune system and thus are anti-inflammatory in nature.

Contrasting this, pathogenic organisms facilitated by the Western diet produce an array of waste products, which can find access to the blood stream, where they can promote inflammatory responses.

These waste materials from pathogenic organisms are typically called endotoxins. Why? Because as they find their way into the blood stream, they become toxins within the body – which is why they are described with the word *"endo."*

# Chapter Four

# Anatomy of Dead Foods

## How We Take the Life Out of Our Foods

Eating is a common denominator for all organisms. We all need fuel to drive metabolism. But what is the best fuel, and how best do we assimilate it? The body's fuels must meet its substance. The body as a pulsing array of living organisms: Yes, our body contains trillions of cells. But it contains even more living microorganisms in the form of bacteria, yeasts, viruses and fungi.

In a healthy person, most of these microorganisms are beneficial or at least harmless. In an unhealthy person, most of these are pathogenic.

In other words, our bodies are chock full of microbes. Our skin is covered with microorganisms. Our mouths, nasal cavities and sinuses are swarming with microorganisms. Our airways are teeming with microorganisms. Our digestive tracts are lined with even more microorganisms. It doesn't stop there either. Our vaginas, urinary tracts, toes, nails, ears and eyes are also populated with billions of organisms.

Over the past century, our diets have become increasingly sterile. The advent of pasteurization, sterilization, chlorination and hydrogenation has all but decimated our sources of beneficial microorganisms.

To this we add the devastating effects of antibiotics and other pharmaceuticals, which have progressively killed off colonies of probiotics that have been inhabiting the bodies of our ancestors since the dawning of humankind.

Yes, our sterile society is killing our bodies slowly from the inside, by killing off our probiotics.

This is causing an epidemic of diseases.

The western world is finally beginning to understand the connection between diet and health. Still, our understanding of food is still in its infancy. Mesmerized by the scientific names of food constituents like *lycopene* or *phytosterols,* we might think we understand food because we know the names of a few active constituents. However, do we know the true nature of food; and how food really works to nourish the body?

During the latter half of the twentieth century, the western world became mesmerized by a food manufacturing disaster of massive proportions – driven by the profit motive. Our free enterprise economy somehow created a food system that put profits before nutrition. Huge food manufacturer concerns with large pubic investment began to proliferate as a result. Perhaps this was innocent enough. But the nutritional quality of the food simply was not on the agenda – due largely to human-kind's ignorance of nature's sophistication.

After World War II, this manufacturing environment spawned increasingly efficient machinery for efficient food processing. Various refining and pasteurization techniques allowed for longer shelf lives, creating the opportunity for shipping food all over the world from fewer facilities. This centralized not only the operations of food production, but also focused the profitability among fewer companies – giving them greater control over our food choices.

This industrialized food economy resulted in the proliferation of highly refined foods, peeled and strained to remove important fiber, and heated to extreme temperatures to increase shelf life. They also resulted in foods with various toxic additives and preservatives, and that ever-addicting ingredient – refined sugar.

Ironically, at the same time, three decades of research have conclusively shown that fermented foods, fresh fruits and fresh vegetables lower cancer rates, lower heart disease rates, increase longevity, decrease various other illnesses and increase energy. Why is this? What is it about these foods that give this extraordinarily high level of health-giving properties?

While we answer this we might ask the counterpart: What is it about overly-cooked, salted, fried and preserved foods that seem to increase rates of cardiovascular disease, cancer and other illnesses? And why do some of these foods taste so good? And are not some cooked foods good for us?

In most of our health information books and science journals, these questions are answered by describing certain molecules or constituents existing in foods, and how these molecules either protect, nourish, or damage the various cells of the body. Our science literature is intently focused on the molecular particulates contained in foods, rather than the matrix or combinations of these constituents. We are told lycopene in tomatoes gives tomatoes many of their healthy qualities. As a result, we extract or even synthesize lycopene in an attempt to capitalize on those qualities.

Another example is garlic. We are told allicin gives garlic its antimicrobial and antioxidant qualities. As a result we extract the allicin, putting it into little pills to get more into one sitting.

Why not just pull the nutrients out of our foods and forget about all the bulk? Certainly freight charges are less if we can extract out just the essential parts. This will also make eating easier too, right? We can just take the extract pills and then have cake.

It is certainly commendable that biochemists and nutritionists have broken down the elemental contents of our favorite foods in an attempt to figure out which parts cause the negative or positive effects of that food. Unfortunately, this process has not always led to positive results, however.

This process of breaking down the health-giving qualities of fresh foods has led to a flurry of fake foods, made up of devitalized, overly processed recipes with a few fortifications of seemingly beneficial constituents. Sugar water with vitamin C added? Stuff like that. How about cake with vitamins? Or a donut made with fortified flour, fried in non-trans-fat oil?

This kind of food masquerade is simply cheating. It is an attempt by food and supplement manufacturers to create the false need to eat their devitalized processed recipes. Forget about spending time making complex flavors from nourishing foods. That is too expensive. That is for the "health food industry."

The real focus for mainstream food manufacturers is making money – not health. As a result, their food only has something to do with health if it is profitable. While we applaud those food companies foraging into the healthy food category, we propose their responsibility is to combine whole foods in such a way to deliver nutrition and taste first, and the profits will come.

This is not to say that there are not many food companies trying to package natural and organic foods with minimal processing. We commend these attempts, and hope that they continue their efforts to put nutrition first and profits second.

Healthy foods are fermented foods, fresh fruits, fresh vegetables, raw nuts, minimally cooked grains and legumes processed minimally. As for grains and legumes, soaking and cooking are required to convert many of their elements to digestible. By far the greatest and healthiest foods that arise from grains, beans and the seeds of fruits and vegetables are sprouts, however. Research has confirmed the nutritional content of a sprouted seed is vastly greater than the nutritional content of the original seed or bean. We will discuss this further later.

As for fermented foods, we will dive into this topic in depth later as well. Suffice for now that humans have been fermenting foods for thousands of years, because this was the primary means to preserve fresh foods after harvest. Fermenting means that we are allowing probiotic yeasts and bacteria to colonize the food. While they colonize, they culture it. They partially digest it, allowing us to further absorb those nutrients later. They also provide their own nutrients, again as we'll define later.

A good example is vitamin K. We are just beginning to discover that most people on a Western diet are chronically deficient in vitamin K. Why is that? Because vitamin K1 – which makes up about 90% of our needs of vitamin K – is abundant in nature's living foods such as broccoli, spinach, lettuce and other green leafy vegetables. Put quite simply, most Western diets simply do not contain much in the way of fresh leafy vegetables.

This was evidenced from research at the University of Maastricht (Cranenburg *et al.* 2007), indicating that not only are most apparently healthy adults sub-clinically vitamin K deficient, but the current European dietary recommendations of 1 microgram per kilogram of body weight per day is likely too low for maintaining health. As stated by one of the study's authors, the biological half-life of vitamin K is very short. As a result, vegetables must be eaten daily, as deficiencies take will yield symptoms within only a few days.

The western world has a hard time understanding the balance of nature for some reason. This may be because the western world has been trying to avoid nature and conquer it for so long. Our culture likes to remove ourselves from nature by hiding out in our square boxes most of the time. Being removed from nature allows us to forget how nature works harmoniously, within a finely tuned balance. It is like a building made of bricks. The entire building structure will be damaged if we were to remove some bricks in the lower walls or foundation.

Our culture is so removed from nature that we actually consider it a coincidence that foods furthest removed from their natural states are those foods that give us atherosclerosis, cancer, diabetes and so many other degenerative diseases. We are so surprised when we discover that natural foods prevent these diseases. We publish major headlines with statements like: *"Vegetables Prevent Cancer."* When our research indicates natural food constituents like lycopene (in tomatoes) and sulforaphane (from cruciferous vegetables) prevent disease, everyone is amazed.

## The Problems with Processed Foods

Let's now connect how processed foods contribute to these. Food processing consists of one or a combination of the following actions on food:

> ➢ chopping or pulverizing
> ➢ heating to high temperatures
> ➢ distilling or extracting its constituents
> ➢ otherwise isolating some parts by straining off or filtering
> ➢ clarifying or otherwise refining

Most consider food processing a good thing, because we humans like to focus on one or two characteristics or nutrients within a food. The idea is that we want the essence of the food, and don't want to fool around with the rest. In most cases – in terms of commercial food – it is a value proposition, because all the energy and work required to produce the final food product must equal or be greater than the increase in the processed food's financial value. Therefore, the more concentrated or isolated the attractive portion is, the more financial value is added.

Typically, this increase in financial value is due to the food being sweeter, smoother or simply easier to eat or mix with other foods. In the case of oils or flours, the food extract is used for baking purposes, for example. In the case of sugar – which is extracted and isolated from cane and beets – it is added to nearly every processed food recipe.

Ironically, what is left behind in this extraction is the food's real value. The healthy fiber and nutrients are stripped away in most cases. Plant fiber is a necessary element of our diet, because it renders sterols that aid diges-tion and reduce LDL cholesterol. Many nutrients are also attached to and protected by the plant's fibers. Once the fiber is stripped away, the remain-ing nutrients are easily damaged by sunlight, air, and the heat of process-ing.

What is being missed in the value proposition of food processing is that nature's whole foods have their greatest value – nutritionally – prior to processing. When a food is broken down, the molecular bonds that attach nutrients to the food's fibers and complex polysaccharides are lost. As these bonds are lost, the remaining components can become unstable in the body. When these components – such as refined sugar and simple polysaccharides (starches) – become unstable, they can form free radicals in the body. They thus add to our body's toxic burden because they can damage our cells.

In other words, whole foods provide the nutrients our bodies need in the combinations our bodies recognize. Nutrients are bonded within a matrix of structure and fiber, rendering their benefits as our bodies re-quire them.

In some cases, we might need to physically peel a food to get to the edible part. In other cases, such as in the case of beans and grains, we may need to heat or cook them to soften the fibers to enable chewing and digestion. In the case of wheats, we can mill the whole grain (including the bran) to deliver the spectrum of fibrous nutrients. In other words, the closer we match the way our ancestors ate foods, the more our bodies will recognize them, and the better our bodies will utilize them.

Because many of our processed foods have been in our diet for many decades, it is difficult to prove that our modern diet of overly-processed foods produces greater levels of systemic inflammation. This doesn't mean that it is impossible, however.

To test this hypothesis, French researchers (Fremont *et al.* 2010) stud-ied the effects of processed flax. Foods containing processed flax are a new addition to our diet – although our ancestors certainly ate raw or cooked whole flax. So they studied the introduction of modern processed flax into the French diet. In a study of 1,317 patients with allergies, they found that those who were allergic to flax could be identified by their sensitivity to extruded, heated flax, rather than raw flax seed. This of course indicates that the increase in flax allergies among the French is due to the increase in *processed flax* rather than the increased availability of flax. Certainly, over time, as flax allergies proceed, there will be more crossover allergies to raw flax. But now, while flax exposure is fairly recent, allergies to processed flax but not raw flax indicate that it is the extrusion processing that causes the identification of flax protein as an allergen.

What does processing do to create more inflammatory sensitivity? Our digestive enzymes and probiotics have evolved to break down (or not) certain types of molecules. Imbalanced or denatured molecules can be considered foreign.

We can also see how processing increases diseases when we compare the disease statistics of developing countries with those of developed countries.

For example, like many developing countries, India has more heart disease in recent decades because of increased consumption of processed and fried foods. In the same way, the Chinese thrived for thousands of years on a rice-based diet. But when modern processing machines introduced degermed white rice, malnutrition diseases began to occur. This is because the degerming and bleaching process results in the loss of important lignans, B vitamins E vitamins and others.

Processed and refined foods damage intestinal health and promote free radicals. They are nutrient-poor. They burden and starve our probiotics. Frying foods also produces a carcinogen called acrylamide (Ehling *et al.* 2005).

## Salt

Salt is included in this section because not only is most modern salt refined: Processed salt is stripped of important mineral nutrients. And processed foods typically contain incredible amounts of refined salt.

Salt is sometimes also referred to as sodium. However, it is not technically sodium. It is actually sodium chloride. Sodium is an essential trace element that helps balance blood pressure and the kidneys. Guidelines for maximum salt levels range from 2,200 milligrams a day to 2,300 milligrams. Adults who eat processed foods at every meal can consume from 3,000 milligrams to 5,000 mg per day.

An overload of processed salt has been implicated in high blood pressure, cardiovascular disease, kidney disorders and lung disorders.

Researchers from Indiana University (Mickleborough *et al.* 2005) found that dietary salt among 24 patients caused higher levels of pro-inflammatory neutrophils, eosinophils, eosinophil cationic protein (ECP), leukotrienes, prostaglandins, and inflammatory cytokines interleukin (IL)-1beta and IL-8 among the high-salt diet group, compared with the lower-salt diet group.

As we discussed earlier, the earth provides natural living salts in the form of rock salts and unprocessed sea salts. These provide a matrix of up to 80 different trace elements in addition to sodium. This broad spectrum of trace elements, according to some clinical findings as discussed earlier, lower the imbalances created by processed sodium chloride salts.

## Glycation

The rates of peanut allergies nearly doubled during the 1990s (Sicherer *et al.* 2003), and have continued to slowly rise among industrialized nations. As discussed earlier, peanut allergies are associated with inflammation, and cause one of the deadliest forms of inflammation – anaphylaxis.

So what changed during the 1990s? Did industrialized counties eat more peanuts during the 1990s? There is no evidence of that.

What changed during this period was the way peanuts are produced and packaged. Dry-roasted and sugar-coated ("honey roasted") peanuts became more popular among consumers in Western industrialized countries due to the fact that manufacturers developed new technologies for dry-roasting processing.

While trying to understand the associations, researchers from the Mount Sinai School of Medicine (Beyer *et al.* 2001) determined that even though the Chinese also eat a significant amount of peanuts, there are significantly fewer peanut allergies in China. Since the Chinese primarily eat boiled or minimally fried peanuts – while Western countries are now eating mostly dry-roasted peanuts – the researchers decided to compare the allergenicity of dry-roasted peanuts with boiled and fried versions.

First they found that the *Ara h1* protein content in peanuts – a primary allergen – was significantly reduced when peanuts are fried or boiled, as compared with the dry-roasted. Secondly, they found that the IgE binding ability of the *Ara h2* and *Ara h3* proteins was reduced when peanuts were boiled or fried – again compared with dry-roasting. This protein-IgE binding affinity is directly associated with the allergenicity of a food, as we discussed earlier.

A couple of years later, researchers from the USDA's Agricultural Research Service (Chung *et al.* 2003) confirmed these findings when their tests revealed that mature dry-roasted peanuts produced an increase in IgE binding – along with glycation end products.

This research was also duplicated later by other USDA researchers (Schmitt *et al.* 2004). However, in this study, the researchers also established that all three methods – frying, boiling and dry-roasting – increase the allergenicity of peanuts when compared to raw peanuts.

One of the leading researchers in the 2001 Mount Sinai study was Dr. Hugh Sampson. Dr. Sampson has since commented:

> *"The Chinese eat the same amount of peanut per capita as we do, they introduce it early in a sort of a boiled/mushed type form, as they do in many African countries, and they have very low rates of peanut allergies. All the countries that have westernized their diet are now seeing the same problem with food allergy as we see. Countries that have introduced peanut butter are now starting to see a rise in the prevalence of peanut allergies akin to the high rates already found in the UK, Australia, Canada and some European countries."*

We would add to his point regarding peanut butter that many peanut butter producers use dry-roasted peanuts. Additionally, there are generally two ways to manufacture peanut butter. Many commercial peanut butters are produced through a complex heating and blending process that includes blending the peanut butter with sugar and hydrogenated oils.

Alternatively, peanut butter can simply be made using a natural grinding process where the whole peanuts are ground and packed into jars without heating or blending. This process typically produces a separation of the oil on top, which is why so many manufacturers over-process and blend their peanut butters. However, the oil stirs back in quite easily.

Researchers from France's University of Burgundy (Rapin and Wiernsperger 2010) have confirmed that protein or lipid glycation produced by modern food manufacturers is linked to allergies.

In general, food manufacturing glycation is produced when sugars and protein-rich foods are combined and heated to extremely high temperatures. This is a typical process used for the manufacture of many commercial packaged foods on the grocery shelves today. During the process, sugars bind to protein molecules. This produces a glycated protein-sugar complex and glycation end products, both of which have been implicated in cardiovascular disease, diabetes, some cancers, peripheral neuropathy and Alzheimer's disease (Miranda and Outeiro 2010).

With regard to Alzheimer's disease, one of the end products of the glycation reaction is amyloid protein. Amyloid proteins have been found among the brain tissues and cerebrospinal fluids of Alzheimer's disease patients. Glycation is implicated in the amyloid plaque buildup found in Alzheimer's.

Glycation also takes place within the body. This occurs especially with diets with greater consumption of refined sugars and cooked or caramelized high-protein foods.

## Too Much Protein

The Western diet contains extraordinary levels of processed protein compared to traditional diets. Americans eat far beyond the amount of protein required for health. Studies indicate that Americans eat an average of 80-150 grams of protein a day. This is significantly higher than the 25-50 grams of protein recommended by nutritionists and health experts (Campbell 2006; McDougall 1983).

This amount of protein in the American diet is also significantly higher than even U.S. RDA levels. The U.S. recommended daily allowance for protein is 0.8 grams per 2.2 lbs of body weight. This converts to 54 grams for a person weighing 150 pounds. Americans eat on average nearly double that amount.

Too much protein produces a state of proteinuria. This produces excess uric acid in the tissues and joints, leading to a state of acidosis toxemia. Remember that amino acids are acids, and too many of them can overload the body. Conditions that have been linked with proteinuria include gout, bile stones, kidney stones and others.

## Too Much Refined Sugar

The Western diet is also laden with refined sugars. Today, nearly every pre-cooked recipe found in mass market grocery stores contains refined sugar. Many brands now try to white-wash the massive sugar content of their products by calling their sugar content "all natural." This is a deception, because nature in the form of fiber has been unnaturally stripped away from their refined sugars. This is hardly a "natural" proposition.

Research has linked refined sugars to diabetes, obesity, kidney diseases, Candida and many other conditions. This is hardly news to those who have investigated natural health literature.

Nature attaches sugars to complex fibers, polysaccharides and nutrients in such a way that prevents them from easily attaching to proteins. Sugars that are cooked and stripped of these complexes are assimilated too quickly, and drive the pancreas to produce and even overproduce insulin. This has the effect of stressing the pancreas. Refined sugars also stress the liver that feeds the pancreas, and stresses the detoxification processes that must metabolize the insulin, glucose and glycogen byproducts. All of this slows down the body's immunity and detoxification processes.

Refined sugars also feed pathogenic microorganisms. While our probiotics feed on oligosaccharides such as FOS, GOS and others, pathogenic microorganisms tend to feed on refined sugars. This is the case for *Candida albicans,* a virtual sugar fiend.

Refined sugars also become immediate unnatural glycation candidates within the body.

As our digestive system combines refined sugars with proteins, many of the glycated proteins are identified as foreign by IgA or IgE antibodies in immune-burdened physiologies. Why are they considered foreign? Because glycated proteins and their AGE end products damage blood vessels, tissues and brain cells. In this case, the immune system is launching an inflammatory attack in an effort to protect us from our own diet!

There is no surprise that glycation among foods and in the body is connected with systemic inflammation. It is also no accident that the increased consumption of overly-processed foods and manufacturing processes that pulverize and strip foods of their fiber; and blend denatured proteins and sugars using high-heat processes has increased as our rates of inflammatory diseases have increased over the past century.

In fact, this connection between inflammatory diseases and processed foods has been observed clinically by natural physicians over the years. They may not have understood the precise mechanics, however. Many of these reputable health experts have categorized the effect of processed foods as one of acidifying the bloodstream. The concept was that denatured and over-processed foods produced more acids in the body.

This thesis did not go over too well among scientific circles, because the acidification mechanism was not scientifically confirmed, and there was no concrete mechanism.

Well this can now change, as we are providing the science showing both the mechanism and the evidence that glycation end products do produce acidification in terms of peroxidation radicals that damage cells and tissues.

We should note that a healthy form of natural glycation also takes place in the body to produce certain nutrient combinations. Unlike the radical-forming glycation formed by food manufacturing and refined sugar intake, this type of glycation is driven by the body's natural enzyme processes, resulting in molecules and end products the body uses and recognizes. When glycation is driven by the body's own enzyme processes, it is termed *glycosylation,* however.

**Hydrolyzed Proteins**

Proteins are composed of very long chains of amino acids. Sometimes hundreds and even thousands of amino acids can make up a protein. The body typically breaks apart these chains through an enzyme reaction called *proteolysis.*

Proteolysis breaks down proteins into amino acids and small groups of aminos called polypeptides. This is also called *cleaving.* As enzymes break off these polypeptides or individual amino acids from proteins, they replace the protein chain linkages with water molecules to stabilize the peptide or amino acid. This process is called *enzymatic hydrolysis.* Breaking away the peptides or amino acids allows the body to utilize the amino acid or polypeptide to make new proteins within the body.

The body then assembles its own proteins from these amino acids and small polypeptide combinations. The body's protein assembly is programmed by DNA and RNA. For this reason, the body must recognize the aminos and polypeptide combinations. The body produces a variety of enzymes to naturally break apart multiple proteins and polypeptides. Protein-cleaving enzymes are called *proteases.*

For this reason, strange or large polypeptide combinations can burden the body, especially if the body does not have the right enzymes to break those peptide chains apart.

Food manufacturers can synthetically break down proteins by extrusion, heating and blending with processing aids – including commercially produced enzymes. These enzymes force the break down of the proteins in the food. As water is integrated into the process, synthetic hydrolysis occurs. This produces foods that contain hydrolyzed proteins. These synthetically hydrolyzed protein foods may not be recognized by the body's immune system, and may stimulate an inflammatory response.

Illustrating this, French laboratory researchers (Bouchez-Mahiout *et al.* 2010) found by using immunoblot testing that hydrolyzed wheat proteins from skin conditioners produced hypersensitivity, which eventually crossed over to wheat protein food allergies. In other words, hydrolyzed wheat proteins in skin treatments are not necessarily recognized by the immune system. Once the body becomes sensitized to these hydrolyzed wheat proteins from skin absorption, this sensitivity can cross over to sensitivity to similar wheat proteins in foods.

Researchers from France's Center for Research in Grignon (Laurière *et al.* 2006) tested nine women who had skin contact sensitivity to cosmetics containing hydrolyzed wheat proteins (HWP). Six were found to react with either skin hives or anaphylaxis to different products (including foods) containing HWP. The whole group also had IgE sensitivity to wheat flour or gluten-type proteins. The tests showed that they had become sensitive to HWP, and then later to unmodified grain proteins. As they tested further, they found that reactions often occurred among larger wheat protein peptide aggregates. The researchers concluded that the use of HWP in skin products can produce hypersensitivity to HWP, followed by a crossover to inflammatory responses to the wheat proteins in foods.

Spanish researchers (Cabanillas *et al.* 2010) found that enzymatic hydrolysis of lentils and chickpeas produced allergens for four out of five allergic patients in their research.

The commercial enzymes used by many food manufacturers can also stimulate allergic responses. Danish researchers (Bindslev-Jensen *et al.* 2006) tested 19 commercially available enzymes typically used in the food industry on 400 adults with allergies. It was found that many of the enzymes produced histamine responses among the patients.

Hydrolyzing proteins through manufacturing processes can create epitopes that the immune system does not recognize. Once the immune system launches an immune response to the epitope, it will remember those as foreigners, and possibly allergens, even if they are part of foods once accepted by the body.

## Toxins Consumed

A considerable amount of research has illustrated that selenium deficiencies are common among those who have muscle fatigue, thyroid issues, reproductive issues, lung disorders, immune disorders and cognitive issues. While many diets might be lacking in selenium, it should be noted that selenium deficiency is dramatically *more common* among those with these issues than the general population.

Significant research confirms that selenium deficiency relates directly to systemic inflammation:

Researchers from the University of Alabama's School of Public Health (Stone *et al.* 2010) reviewed the association between low levels of selenium and higher rates of AIDS, HIV infections and other immune diseases. They found that HIV-infected persons who have low selenium levels have a faster progression of their disease to AIDS, and higher rates of mortality.

Selenium is a key ingredient in the liver's production of glutathione peroxidase. Glutathione peroxidase neutralizes toxins and free radicals, especially those relating to lipid peroxides.

In one of the early studies that established this link, researchers from Stockholm's Karolinska Institute (Hasselmark *et al.* 1993) gave 24 intrinsic asthma patients either placebo or 100 micrograms of sodium selenite per day for two weeks. The selenium group had higher glutathione levels and activity, and their asthma significantly improved as compared with the placebo group.

Researchers from Slovakia's Institute of Preventive and Clinical Medicine (Jahnova *et al.* 2002) also gave 20 asthmatic adults either a placebo or

200 micrograms of selenium per day for six months, in addition to inhaled corticosteroids and beta-agonists. They found that the selenium blocked IFN-gamma adhesion molecules, reducing inflammation.

Researchers from Britain's Imperial College (Shaheen *et al.* 2007) tested 197 patients with 100 micrograms of a selenium-yeast formula or a placebo for 24 weeks. Quality of life increased among the selenium patients but in this study, there was little difference between the selenium group and the placebo (yeast only) group. It should be noted, however, that the patients were all taking regular steroid medication and this study only used 100 micrograms of a blend of selenium and yeast.

So the selenium dosage was substantially (less than half) the dosage of the studies that showed reductions in inflammation symptoms and improvement in lung function.

Certainly these studies roughly replicate a diet containing whole natural foods – which is rich in selenium.

The recommended daily allowance for selenium is 55 micrograms. One ounce of Brazil nuts contains over 540 mcg.

The critical component in this mystery is glutathione peroxidase – an enzyme produced in the liver. Glutathione peroxidase is the leading enzyme responsible for the breakdown and removal of lipid hydroperoxides. Lipid hydroperoxides are oxidized fats that damage cell membranes. As they do this, they create pores in the cell. The resulting damage eventually kills most cells. Lipid hydroperoxides are one of the most damaging molecules within the body. They are responsible for many deadly metabolic diseases, including heart disease, artery disease, Alzheimer's disease and many others.

When lipid hydroperoxides accumulate in the body, they can also damage the cells of the airways, causing irritation and inflammation. The damage from lipid hydroperoxides stimulates an inflammatory response. Researchers have called the initial signal from the cell that initiates this inflammatory response *lipid peroxidation/LOOH-mediated stress signaling*. In other words, the cells are stressed by lipid peroxidation, and this initiates a distress signal to the immune system.

This distress signal stimulates the contraction of the smooth bronchial muscles while stimulating leukotriene activity – which delivers cytotoxic (cell-destroying) T-cells and eosinophils into the region. This stimulates the production of more mucous, which drowns the cilia and restricts breathing.

The production of more mucous is intended to clear out the damaged cells. In other words, much of the increased mucous that drowns the cilia and produces wheezing is caused by the influx of dead cell matter from lipid hydroperoxide damage.

By virtue of removing lipid hydroperoxides, glutathione peroxidase – not to be confused with glutathione reductase – regulates pro-inflammatory arachidonic acid metabolism. In other words, glutathione regulates the release and populations of those pro-inflammatory mediators, the leukotrienes. Leukotriene activity is directly associated with the damage created by lipid hydroperoxides. Thus, when lipid hydroperoxide levels are reduced by glutathione peroxidase, leukotriene density is reduced.

Selenium is required for glutathione peroxidase production. Should the body be overloaded with lipid hydroperoxides, more glutathione is required to clear out the damage. As more glutathione is produced, more selenium is utilized, which runs selenium levels down.

This issue was illustrated by research from Britain's South Manchester University Hospital (Hassan 2008). The researchers studied 13 aspirin-induced asthmatics and a healthy matched control group. They found that the asthmatics maintained higher levels of selenium in the bloodstream – especially among blood platelets. This high selenium content in the blood-stream correlated with higher glutathione peroxidase activity. The research illustrated how selenium is used up faster in by those with inflammation through this glutathione peroxidase process.

## Lipid Peroxidation

As we touched on earlier, lipid peroxidation means that the lipids that make up the cell membrane are being robbed of electrons. This 'robbery' results in an unstable cell membrane. Let's take a closer look at the process of lipid peroxidation.

The first step takes place with the entry of a reactive oxygen species into the proximity of the cell. Reactive oxygen species are elements that require an electron – such as hydrogen ($H+$) – in order to become stable.

Fatty acids that make up the membranes of cells are the likely candidates for peroxidation. Remember, the name "lipid" refers to a fatty acid. Fatty acids include saturated fats, polyunsaturates, monounsaturates, and so on (see fatty acid discussions later on).

Several types of lipids make up the cell membrane. Fatty acids will combine with other molecules to make phospholipids, cholesterols and glycolipids. Saturates and polyunsaturates are typical, but there are several species of polyunsaturates. These range from long chain versions to short versions. They also include the cis- configuration and the trans- configuration. Cell membranes that utilize predominantly cis- versions with long chains are the most durable. Those cell membranes with trans- configurations can be highly unstable, and irregularly porous. This is one reason why trans fats are unhealthy. The other reason is that trans fats easily become peroxidized.

Cell membranes with more long chain fatty acids are more stable and are less subject to peroxidation. Shorter chains that provide more double bonds are less stable, because these are more easily broken. Also, mono-unsaturated fatty acids such as GLA are more stable.

Once the fatty acid is degraded by an oxygen species, it becomes a fatty acid radical. The fatty acid will usually become oxidized, making it a peroxyl-fatty acid radical. This radical will react with other fatty acids, forming a cyclic process involving radicals called cyclic peroxides.

This becomes a chain reaction that results in the cell membrane becoming completely destroyed and dysfunctional. This forces the cell to signal to the immune system that it is under attack and about to become malignant. The T-cell immune response will often initiate the cell's self-destruct switch: TNF – tumor necrosis factor. Alternatively, the cell may be directly destroyed by cytotoxic T-cells. The combined process stimulates inflammation. As these cells are killed or self-destruct, they are purged from the system – provoking increased mucous formation.

While this peroxidation and cell destruction is taking place, the immune system is not simply standing by. The body enters a state called *systemic inflammation*. As we discussed earlier, during systemic inflammation, the immune system launches an ongoing supply of eosinophils, neutrophils and mast cells, which release granulocytes that inflame the airways.

In other words, due to this ongoing peroxidation, the immune system is on a hair-trigger. Imagine a person at work who is stressed from being buried in work and a myriad of problems. You walk into their office and they immediately react: "And what do *you* want?" they ask.

If they were not overloaded with work, problems and deadlines, your coming into their office would probably be met without such a frantic response. But since they were overloaded, they reacted (hyper reacted is a better word) more defensively than needed, *because they thought you were going to add to their workload.*

In other words, inflammation is simply a defense measure by an immune system that is overwhelmed.

Typical associations with inflammation include artery damage and plaque build-up, obesity, diabetes, a sedentary lifestyle, and a diet high in saturated fats and/or fried foods. High blood pressure and fast or irregular heart rate, especially in persons over 40 years old, are also strong markers.

Along with these associations come higher levels of total cholesterol, low-density lipoprotein (LDL) and very low-density lipoprotein (VLDL) cholesterol, and total triglycerides are also key markers. The link between small LDL particle size and atherosclerosis is a key factor, and the oxidation of LDL particles is the match that lights the fuse. These involve hyperperoxides, as they readily form oxidative radicals. The cascade towards LDL oxidation also seems to be accelerated by lipooxygenases like 15-LOX-2 along with cyclooxygenases. The process as a whole is lipid peroxidation.

In addition to launching systemic inflammation due to widespread cell damage, the body also produces processes that attempt to halt the peroxidation cycle. One of these components is the glutathione peroxidase enzyme discussed earlier, formed by the body using selenium as a substrate. Depending upon the rate of lipid peroxidation, however, this could be like trying to blow out a forest fire. There is simply too much fire spreading too quickly.

## Reactive Oxygen Species

Let's take a wider perspective on the problem. The initiation process of the lipid peroxidation is started by a reactive oxygen species. What is this?

This is also often called a free radical. A free radical is an unstable molecule or ion that forms during a chemical reaction. In other words, the molecule or ion needs another atom, ion or molecule to stabilize it. Once it is stable, it is not reactive.

While a free radical is unstable, it can damage any number of elements it meets. These include the cells, organs and tissues of the body.

Nature produces many, many free radicals. However, nature typically accompanies radicals with the molecules, atoms or ions that stabilize the radical. In the atmosphere, for example, radicals become stabilized by ozone and other elements. In plants, radicals become stabilized by antioxidants from nutrients derived from the sun, soil and oxygen. In the body, radicals are stabilized by antioxidizing enzymes, nutrients and other elements. These include glutathione peroxidase, as we discussed earlier.

Confirming this, the research from South Manchester University Hospital mentioned earlier concluded with a comment that the increased glutathione peroxidase activity related to radical oxidation: *"administration of aspirin to these patients increases the generation of immediate oxygen products..."*

Another anti-oxidation process within the body utilizes the *superoxide dismutase* (SOD) enzyme. The SOD enzyme is typically available within the cytoplasm of most cells. Here SOD is complexed by either copper and zinc, or manganese – similar to the way selenium is complexed with the glutathione peroxidase enzyme. Several types of SOD enzymes reside within the body – some in the mitochondria and some in the intercellular tissue fluids. SOD neutralizes superoxides before they can damage the inside and outside of the cell – assuming the body is healthy, with substantial amounts of SOD. The immune system produces superoxides as part of its strategy to attack microorganisms and toxins.

Another broad anti-oxidation process utilizes *catalase*. Here the body provides an enzyme bound by iron to neutralize peroxides to oxygen and water. It is a standard component of many metabolic reactions within the body.

Yet another enzyme utilized for radical reduction is *glutathione reductase*. This enzyme works with NADP in the cell to stabilize hydrogen peroxide oxidized radicals before they can damage the cell.

Notice that all of these antioxidizing enzymes require minerals. We have seen either selenium, copper, zinc, manganese or iron as necessary to keep these enzymes in good supply. Many other minerals and trace elements are used by other antioxidant and detoxifying enzyme processes. These minerals, and many of the enzymes themselves, are supplied by various foods and supplements, as we'll discuss further.

Another tool that the healthy body utilizes to stabilize radicals are the antioxidants supplied by plant foods. Plants produce antioxidants to protect their own cells from radical damage. Thus, their plant material contains a host of these oxidation stabilizers, which our bodies use to neutralize radicals.

The antioxidant capacity of a food is often measured with an ORAC (oxygen radical absorbance capacity) assay. This test specifically measures the ability of the food to neutralize quantities of peroxyl radicals. By measuring this capacity to reduce the number of peroxyl radicals in a solution, that food is judged for its antioxidant capacity. The theory behind this is that if a molecule has *unpaired electron* then those electrons must become paired somehow, so they in effect "steal" electrons or donate their unpaired electrons to another molecule. In effect, this donating or stealing process is thought to be what damages biological tissues.

Investigation on antioxidant capacity reveals that there are many assays used besides ORAC assays. There is the *Total Radical Trapping Antioxidant Parameter* assay (TRAP), the *Crocin Bleaching* assay, *Folin-Ciocalteu Reagent* assay (RCR), the *Trolox Equivalence Antioxidant Capacity* assay (TEAC), *Ferric Ion Reducing Antioxidant Power* (FRAP) and a *Total Antioxidant Potential* assay which uses copper as an oxidant. While some of these assays apparently measure the ability of some molecules to transfer hydrogen atoms, others are thought to measure electron transfer only. While ORAC is considered one of the more reliable measurements of antioxidant capacity, it is rendering only a narrow window of what happens within a (living) biological system (Huang *et al.* 2005).

In reality, radicals are not bad guys in themselves. The biological system produces radicals through normal metabolic activities, and they are necessary for many physiological functions. As energy is produced through the Krebs cycle, oxygen is a necessary part of the process, and oxidative radicals are part of the byproduct. Superoxide can both accept electron moments or donate electrons. Even though superoxide is considered a radical, it is a necessary species for other metabolic functions. It is part of the feedback-response regulating mechanism within cells. Superoxide reacts either independently or through catalytic conversion with *superoxide disumutase* to form the biological version of the natural antibiotic, hydrogen peroxide along with oxygen. This 'free radical' superoxide is thus an important component working within the body's immune functions.

Interestingly, research indicates the body's own production of melatonin neutralizes reactive singlet oxygen. While not providing the classic antioxidant identity, melatonin production appears to substantially reduce reactive oxygen species and other harmful radicals such as the *peroxynitrite anion* – caused by the consumption of nitrites. Trytophan – another molecule naturally produced in the body – also appears to stimulate radical neutralization. In fact, both tryptophan and melatonin not only neutralize radicals, but they also provide protective mechanisms, preventing cells from being damaged. They assist in the production of various enzymes. They will even entering cells and line cell membranes. These wonderful biochemicals of rhythm protect the body against oxidative radical and other types of free radical damage (Reiter *et al.* 1999; Tax *et al.* 2000).

Now should the body not properly manufacture these protective biochemicals, radical species such as singlet oxygen can invade cell membranes, disfiguring and genetically damaging the cell. This is especially true if the lipid quality of the cell membrane is not structurally sound (i.e. through the eating of trans fats, etc.). The radicals themselves can damage the cell membrane. This will allow other radicals to pour into the cytoplasm and damage proteins, organelles and more importantly, the body's DNA. Should radicals interfere with the precise spiraling bonding sequences of DNA within the cell dangerous mutations can develop. While cells have a tremendous capacity to repair genetic damage, a large population of radicals can overwhelm this capacity. This is the mechanism most thought to instigate metastasizing and invasive cancers.

Should an radical encounter the electromagnetic structure of a stable molecule such as triplet oxygen, there will be a change in the biochemical aspects and characteristics of that molecule. As the body's personal defense systems recognize that capacity for damage, various neutralizing biochemicals are drawn in to neutralize it. We have discovered in our research on antioxidants that tremendous neutralizing biochemicals are produced through the process of the conversion of chlorophyll. While this process, plants produce a various phytochemicals such as sterols, anthocyanidins and others.

In the case of devitalized foods over-processed and/or blended with chemicals, these foods are chemically imbalanced. The bonds that tie together the various minerals, vitamins and amino complexes – have become serrated. The resulting molecular structure is homogenized. The bonds have been robbed of much of their capacity though processing (notably heat, freezing and reheating). Electromagnetic waveforms interact with the bonds of the nutrient factors, creating instability. The instability breaks apart many of the cofactors, releasing ions and breaking bonds. A fractured and minimized array of nutrients is now available.

When we cook at home we can retain much of this nutrient release by cooking with the lid on at lower temperatures. Studies out of Britain's University of Warwick (2007) and the American Chemical Society (2007) illustrate that while boiling and frying reduces the nutritional content of vegetables, steaming vegetables will not only retain nutrient content, but may even – as in the case of anti-carcinogenic glucosinolates – be increased with steaming. Whatever heat remains in the food can also assist in a recombant molecular bonding, retaining some of the energy released with the breaking of bonds.

This is especially the case when food is lightly cooked in water. The water will absorb many of the nutrients as they are released from the food. This occurs in slow-cooked soups. Hot soup more nutritious than after it is cooled down (careful, do not burn the tongue) as well.

In overly processed food, both the heat and the nutrients are gone by the time it reaches the shelf of the store. Only a fraction of the covalent nutrient bonds will remain in the food. The complex high-energy bonds are broken. Many of the fat- and water-soluble nutrients that were once part of the whole food will have either evaporated or broken up into denatured fractions. The complex oscillating bonding binding the various nutrients to their carbon chain skeletons (often polysaccharides or glycerides) have been separated.

What we slowly discovered from the refining of cane, beets and wheat will also be what we learn about the rest of nature's nutrients: We cannot separate the nutrient from its surrounding matter and achieve the same effects. This goes for the concept of antioxidants and free radicals. Nature produces antioxidants like polyphenols and sterols within a molecular field of components derived from living organisms. These bond the nutrients to elements such as fiber, carbohydrates, glycosides, minerals, phytosterols, fatty acids, lignans, and even special polysaccharides like beta-glucans. All of these components and many others we have yet to discover come together within living organisms. Once we denature them, free radical species are created.

## Inflammatory Choices

Systemic inflammation indicates that the immune system is overburdened. The extent or combination of the elements mentioned simply overwhelms the immune system. Typically, the immune system can resolve most of these problems when it is presented with a small amount or a few of them at a time. But when an avalanche of them becomes too great, the immune system goes on alert, resulting in systemic inflammation.

Systemic inflammation is the immune system's version of all-out war. The immune system begins to launch the nukes. These can include fever, vomiting, diarrhea, swelling and pain.

The rest of this chapter will more specifically discuss lifestyle choices that produce or worsen systemic inflammation within the body. In other words, these are all *contributing causes*. This means that just one of these factors may not in itself cause systemic inflammation. But any one of these, in addition to others, can overwhelm the immune system – producing systemic inflammation.

### Systemic Inflammation Factors

While toxin overload is the primary condition, the following list summarizes conditions that collectively contribute to systemic inflammation:

1) *Toxemia:* An overload of toxins that produce radicals.
2) *Infections:* Infection with microorganisms that produce mutagenicity, toxins and radicals: viruses, bacteria, yeasts and parasites.
3) *Antioxidant enzyme deficiencies:* An undersupply of antioxidizing enzymes that stabilize radicals, including glutathione peroxidase, glutathione reductase, catalase and superoxide dismutase.
4) *Dietary antioxidant deficiencies:* An undersupply of antioxidants from our foods to help stabilize radicals.
5) *Barriers to detoxification:* Lifestyle or physiological factors that block our body's ability to rid waste products and toxins. Detoxification requires exercise, fresh air, sweating, sunshine and so on.

6) ***Poor dietary choices:*** A poor diet burdens the body with toxins, unstable fatty acids, refined sugars and overly processed foods.

7) ***Immunosuppression:*** A burdened or defective immune system.

## The Rotten Core of the Western Diet

Let's discuss some of the issues with the most core element of the Western diet - red meat. This might be a topic of debate around the dinner table, but the research is clear: Red meat shortens lives and produces greater incidence of numerous disorders. We have discussed some of this research so far, but there is much, much more evidence illustrating this.

Here we will lay out some of the reasons and mechanisms for this. Some of this is caused by how red meat must be prepared. In order to eat meat, we must substantially overcook it. Should we not cook meat enough, we risk the ingestion of multiple species of pathogenic bacteria and parasites, which quickly accumulate in dead flesh.

This is a natural occurrence, as formerly living tissue undergoes biological decomposition. And the process is very difficult to curtail, even with refrigeration. After the long haul between the slaughterhouse and the market, the process will surely begin, despite refrigeration and even freezing.

As a result, meat typically has to be cooked intensely for quite some time. This process destroys many of the heat-sensitive nutrients available in meat. And cooking means charbroiling or frying, both of which create various trans-fats, altered saturated fats, nitrites and various other toxic byproducts such as the deadly heterocyclic amines (or HCA). Let's discuss some of the other mechanisms related to this fundamental part of the Western diet.

### Dysbiosis

Animal foods facilitate the growth of colonies of pathogenic microorganisms in the intestines. These produce endotoxins that damage cell membranes and tissues, stimulating inflammation, again through peroxidation. Let's discuss how this occurs.

While meat typically has higher levels of protein, animal proteins are typically complex, with amino acids bound tightly into complex and lengthy molecules.

The bonds of these molecules are quite difficult for our peptidase enzymes to break down into the more digestible amino acids. As a result, the digestive system must work extra hard to break down those complex proteins. This significantly slows down the digestive process. As a result, a meat meal takes about twice the amount of time to digest than a vegetarian meal.

Yes – at least twice as long. This means a meat diet will result in a greater tendency of constipation, diverticulosis, colorectal cancer and irritable bowel syndrome. In a study published in the *Journal of the American Medical Association,* those who ate more red meat had twice the risk of colon cancer and 40% chance of rectal cancer (Chao 2005). While a typical vegetarian meal takes 24-36 hours to turn around food from meal to stool, a meat meal may take from 48-72+ hours to complete the cycle.

What happens to food matter sitting for this long in the intestines or colons? It putrefies. It stagnates. It rots. We might compare the process of decomposition through a 2-3 day cycle to a compost heap. During the composting process, various species of pathogenic bacteria accumulate. As the composting time increases, pathogenic bacteria accumulate in larger numbers, causing dysbiosis. As a result, not only do meat-eaters have more colon cancers, but they burden their immune systems and are thus more susceptible to infections.

### A Question of Proteins

When we compare animal proteins to vegetable proteins, we find a vast difference in terms of digestive affinity. The amino acid composition in plants is far easier to assimilate. Our peptidase enzymes easily break down the various peptides available from plants.

Because the body builds its own protein complexes from amino acids and simple peptides, plant protein is easier for the body to digest and assimilate. A healthy vegetarian diet will easily supply every essential and non-essential amino acid.

Contrary to information presented several decades ago, the body does not require every amino acid is present in each meal to form the appropriate proteins. The body does store and utilize various amino acids and peptides, and as long as all are available in the diet the body will make the appropriate protein molecules just fine.

Ironically, while Americans have been fixated on getting enough protein in the diet, research has been revealing that typical meat-eating diets contain too much protein.

The overloading of amino acids into the bloodstream a condition called *protein metabolic stress:* Animal proteins require significant effort by the body to break them down into useable amino acid and smaller peptide form. The body utilizes single amino acids and small amino acid chains (peptides). Animal proteins contain hundreds, even thousands of amino acids in a single molecule. This requires significantly more energy and enzyme production to break down and process these complex proteins.

To counter this situation, the body releases calcium from bones and tissues to neutralize this overly acidic situation. The loss of calcium contributes to osteoporosis, weakened bones, joints, and muscles. This precious body calcium is excreted out through the kidneys.

After two studies of 72 women, Purdue University researchers (Campbell and Tang 2010) concluded:

> *"Consumption of higher protein omnivorous diets promoted decreased bone mineral density after weight loss in overweight postmenopausal women."*

Unusable protein is broken down in the liver and converted to urea. Urea stimulates urination, which works the kidneys harder and stimulates the excessive loss of water. This can cause sub-clinical dehydration and kidney disorders. The combination of excess calcium and urea can also create painful and even lethal kidney stones.

Animal foods also contain high levels of purines. Purines are part of RNA and DNA. Purines are converted to uric acid by the body. Circulating uric acid can cause a common problem among heavy meat-eaters: Gout. Circulating uric acid will find its way into the joints, where it can cause extreme pain and stiffness.

Nutritional experts like James McDougall, M.D. state that healthy protein consumption should range from 30 to 60 grams per day. The average American consumes more than 100 grams a day. Populations who eat greater quantities of meat (Eskimos and Americans, for example) have shown higher levels of many of the illnesses discussed above (McDougall and McDougall 1983) than lower-protein consuming regions such as Africa and Asia.

### Acidic Plasma

Amino acids – the building blocks of protein – are acids at the end of the day. This means they exert a general acidic pH upon the body's tissue fluids. A healthy plant-based diet provides a number of phytonutrients and minerals that are alkaline – which will neutralize the acidic nature of protein.

The excess proteins in animal foods produce greater levels of acids in the bloodstream and tissues because of their greater protein content and the complexity of their peptide combinations. This has been implicated in proteinuria and albuminuria issues and kidney problems.

### Hormones

Like any mammal, animals circulate extensive amounts of hormones through their bodies in order to regulate their various organ systems. Notable among these are the steroid hormones such as cortosteroid, which speeds up metabolism and sparks the stress response. Included in these steroids is adrenaline.

When an animal is about to be killed, it pumps these corticoids through its bloodstream in a "fight or flight" stress response. These steroid hormones will saturate the tissues, especially the muscles, in preparation for a physical response to the fear.

In other words, these same hormones are present in the meat that is eaten, even if the blood is partly drained from the animal before butchering.

The relationship between hormone availability among meat foods has been made through the testing of growth hormones. Research has found that growth hormones injected into the body of an animal will be consumed in the meat (Epstein 1991).

### Bacteria and Parasites

Dangerous bacteria such as E. coli and L. monocytogenes (listeria) are common and prevalent in most red meats. Salmonella and campylobacter are also quite common infectious agents found in meat. Consumer Reports found 50-75% contamination levels among meat and chicken and 25% of meat had listeria between two studies done in 1997 and 2003 in 60 U.S. cities. To make matters worse, one study showed that 42% of meat-eaters did not cook their meat enough to remove these sorts of pathogens.

### Toxins

Animal foods typically contain a greater number of toxins compared to plant foods. This is because animals are bioaccumulators: They accumulate toxins from the environment and from the foods they eat. For this reason, pesticides in the foods they eat will accumulate within their tissues.

Animals also harbor viruses and pathogenic bacteria, and these produce toxins. These are called mycotoxins.

Many toxic chemicals are fat-soluble: The toxins thus accumulate among fat cells, and those fat cells will be amongst the meat that is eaten.

Animals also produce and circulate their own waste products, and their waste production increases during slaughter.

Plant-based foods, by contrast, provide various antioxidants.

Dr. Walter Willett, a professor at the Harvard School of Public Health puts it clearly after reviewing the evidence – a fair amount coming from Harvard researchers over the years:

> "At most, it [meat] should be eaten only occasionally. And it may be maximally effective not to eat red meat at all."

### Nitrosamines and Nitrites

Red meats have greater levels of nitrites. This is especially true for processed and fried meats. As nitrites enter the body, they produce reactive nitrogen species. These damage cells and cell membranes, producing inflammatory peroxidation.

Processed meats also contain additional sodium nitrite, used as a preservative.

When nitrites and amines from meat peptides are cooked at high temperatures, nitrosamines are formed.

Nitrites can also disrupt our metabolism, especially related to the blood's ability to carry oxygen.

The real danger in nitrates relates to the formation of nitrosamines. There are several nitrate metabolites, and these are called N-nitroso compounds. These may also form hydrazines.

Nitrosamines and hydrazines have been identified as carcinogens.

The highest levels of nitrosamines have been found among red meat, fish, beer and tobacco smoke.

UK researchers (Silvester et al 1997) tested fecal matter from high-meat diets and found that such a diet leads to significant amounts of metabolites that damage DNA (creating mutations). They stated:

> *"ATNC produced in the large bowel in association with a high-meat intake could represent an important source of DNA-damaging alkylating agents in the human large bowel."*

The relationships here are not happenstance. In a series of three studies from Scotland (Holtrop *et al.* 2012), researchers found that:

> *"red meat intake was positively correlated with the fecal log N-nitroso compounds concentration."*

### Iron

The levels of iron found in meat can be dangerous for other reasons. The body does not need the quantity of iron present in many meats. About 3 or 4 grams is probably the max that a healthy adult body should retain. Meanwhile the body probably loses about 1 gram a day in sweat or through the kidneys. Healthy systems should absorb just enough to replace that amount. Any more has the possibility of accumulating in the tissues.

Additionally, should we have an iron-absorption disorder such as *hemochromatosis,* we may find our iron overloading synovial membranes, organs and other tissues of the body.

### Saturated Fats

Animal foods provide increased levels of saturated fats, which lead to greater levels of LDLs (low density lipoproteins). LDL-carried cholesterol is considered "bad" cholesterol because the LDLs are more susceptible to lipid peroxidation. Lipid peroxidation results in the release of free radicals that damage the walls of our arteries and other tissues.

Most meats have about 50% of their calories as fat — much of it saturated. A number of studies have confirmed meat-eaters suffer more heart disease — we've quoted a few earlier. One study showed that meat-eating four or more times a week had twice the risk of congestive heart disease. This reduces the heart's ability to circulate blood throughout the body, causing various functional organ and tissue problems stemming from a build-up of blood and a lack of circulation and nutrition. Today close to 5 million people live with this condition, with over a half million new cases developing each year.

### Beta-glucuronidase and other cancer-causing enzymes

We discussed the research on this topic in detail earlier. The research of Tufts University School of Medicine professor Dr. Barry Goldin determined that omnivore diets produced numerous disease-causing enzymes, including beta-glucu-ronidase, nitroreductase, azoreductase and steroid 7-alpha-dehydroxylase. These were found to be implicated not only in intestinal inflammatory diseases, but also colon cancer.

### Trimethylamine-N-oxide (TMAO)

We discussed TMAO at length in the last chapter. Remember TMAO is a chemical that is produced by intestinal bacteria when people eat animal diets, and therefore consume a greater amount of L. carnitine

TMAO has been shown to directly produce heart disease and atherosclerosis, as it damages the blood vessel walls.

### Arachidonic Acid

Added to these issues is the problem of consuming too much arachidonic acid in the diet. Arachidonic acid is a fatty acid converted from other fatty acids by the body. However, diets rich in arachidonic acid can directly overload the body with too much of this fatty acid, producing a pro-inflammatory condition within the body.

Red meats and oily fish provide higher levels of arachidonic acid. Increased arachidonic acid levels in the body push the immune system towards inflammation.

This subject has been studied extensively by researchers from Wake Forest University School of Medicine, led by Professor Floyd Chilton, Ph.D. Dr. Chilton has published a wealth of research data that have uncovered that foods high in arachidonic acid can produce a pro-inflammatory metabolism, especially among adults. Dr. Chilton's research also confirmed that a pro-inflammatory metabolism is trigger-happy and hypersensitive: creating the systemic inflammatory conditions prevalent in many degenerative diseases.

In research headed up by Dr. Darshan Kelley from the Western Human Research Center in California, diets high in arachidonic acid stimulated four times more inflammatory cells than diets low in arachidonic acid content. And this problem increases with age. In other words, the same amount of arachidonic acid-forming foods will cause higher levels of arachidonic acid as we get older (Chilton 2006).

According to the USDA's Standard 13 and 16 databases, red meats and fish produce the highest levels of arachidonic acid in the body. Diary, fruits and vegetables produce little or no arachidonic acid. Grains, beans and nuts produce none or very small amounts. Processed bakery goods produce a moderate amount of arachidonic acid.

### Phytanic Acid

Another association we can make between inflammation and diets rich in animal-based foods relates to phytanic acid. Phytanic acid (tetramethylhexadecanoic acid) is a byproduct of plant food digestion inside the intestinal tracts of ruminating animals such as cows, goats, sheep and so on. While phytanic acid can be derived from plant-based foods, greater concentrations of nonesterified phytanic acid are formed in animals when chlorophyll is degraded within the stomachs of ruminants, along with mammalian peroxisomes. This is the result of these animals' unique multiple-stomach digestion process of grasses and other plant material. Humans, of course, do not digest food in the same manner, so we do not produce these concentrated levels of nonesterified phytanic acid from plant-based diets.

Otto-von-Guericke University (Germany) professor Dr. Peter Schönfeld has showed that the nonesterified phytanic acids from ruminants directly damage the membranes of our cell's mitochondria. The end result, his research found, is a corruption of the mitochondrial ATP energy production process (Schönfeld 2004).

This corruption in turn damages cell function, stimulating inflammation.

### Heterocyclic Amines (HCA) and Polycyclic Aromatic Hydrocarbons (PAHs)

HCAs and PAHs are formed when meat is cooked. HCAs have been linked with colon cancer in a number of studies. Research has isolated seventeen different types of toxic HCAs that have been linked with cancer. For example, a seven-year study of 2,719 colon cancer patients found that colon cancer risk was linked with greater consumption of fried and grilled meats, which were associated with greater levels of HCAs (Cross *et al.* 2010).

Another study also found this association, as part of the European Prospective Investigation into Cancer and Nutrition, which followed 21,462 people (Rohrmann *et al.* 2007).

We can quote the National Cancer Institute Fact Sheet on HCAs and PAHs:

> *"Heterocyclic amines (HCAs) and polycyclic aromatic hydrocarbons (PAHs) are chemicals formed when muscle meat, including beef, pork, fish, or poultry, is cooked using high-temperature methods, such as pan frying or grilling directly over an open flame (1). In laboratory experiments, HCAs and PAHs have been found to be mutagenic – that is, they cause changes in DNA that may increase the risk of cancer. HCAs are formed when amino acids (the building blocks of proteins), sugars, and creatine (a substance found in muscle) react at high temperatures. PAHs are formed when fat and juices from meat grilled directly over an open fire drip onto the fire, causing flames. These flames contain PAHs that then adhere to the surface of the meat. PAHs can also be formed during other food preparation processes, such as smoking of meats."*

# Chapter Five

# Whole Living Foods

Our ancestors ate whole living foods. Living foods are those foods that are picked or cut from living plant organisms. They also include cultured foods – foods prepared with bacteria and yeasts.

This contrasts animal meats. Animals have to be slaughtered, and their meat has to be separated from their former living metabolism. Typically this means cooking it at high temperatures. Doing so is necessary to avoid bacteria and parasite poisoning. But it also leaves us with a food devoid of many nutrients our bodies require: Those nutrients considered phytonutrients.

Plant foods can also be made dead. This is done through overcooking, extraction and isolation of certain components while leaving or evaporating others. Think white sugar, white flour, high fructose corn syrup.

## The Healthier Diet

We have presented a fair amount of evidence so far – actually only a slice of the large body of research confirming and re-confirming the basis for the Ancestors Diet.

Yes, the research shows – just as our body design, our genetics, our disposition and the diseases related to the Western diet show – that our bodies were not designed to eat an animal-food rich diet. Yes, our bodies could adapt to such a diet out of necessity, and certainly survive. But our chances of healthy survival are minimized by this choice of diet.

Some would put forth that there are other variations outside of these two general choices – the plant-based diet versus an animal-based diet. Yes, indeed, there are. Among animal diets there are several. And among plant-based diets there are several. But we're not splitting hairs in this book. We are laying out the bigger picture. We can each take the picture back to our kitchens and decide for ourselves.

But we can also continue to learn the specifications of our foods. Here these are presented with a scientifically validity. This diet is delicious and generous with lots of choices. And the Ancestors Diet is not stingy. Certainly there is room for graduation and moderation. Life is really never black or white. It is typically shades of all types of colors.

With this, I leave a few additional studies for you to ponder regarding the plant- and cultured food-based Ancestors Diet.

After reviewing a multitude of studies, the American Dietetic Association and the Dietitians of Canada published an extensive report in 2003 regarding vegetarian diets.

The report found that vegetarians have lower body mass indices, lower levels of prostate and colorectal cancer, healthier cholesterol levels, lower blood pressure, lower levels of type 2 diabetes, and lower death rates from heart disease. Other studies have revealed that people on vegetarian diets experience lower cancer levels, lower osteoporosis, lower rates of urinary diseases, less dementia, lower rates of diverticulosis, fewer gallstones, and lower rates of rheumatoid arthritis (Leitzmann 2005).

In another review of 4,500 studies, fifteen international scientists suggested a primarily vegetarian diet consisting of fruits, vegetables, cereals and legumes could reduce cancer risk by 40 percent (Rice, 2003).

Research has also confirmed that vegetarians have higher levels of circulating antioxidants such as lutein, xanthins, carotenoids, and corresponding higher levels of glutathione and superoxide dismutase (Rauma 2003).

This is no accident. What goes in must come out. It is not as if all the junk that decomposed, overcooked flesh contains will just evaporate once inside our bodies. Our bodies will have to process what we eat. That's where things can go seriously wrong.

Living plant-based foods, on the other hand, produce a myriad of immune-boosting phytonutrients that, as long as we don't cook them or extract them out during processing, will extend our lives, reduce healthcare costs and increase our vitality.

## Phyto Foods

The benefits of natural foods are not simply their vitamin and mineral content. The constituents of natural food are much more complicated than a few vitamins and minerals. Tomatoes for example, are thought to contain some 10,000 different phytochemicals. Every year researchers are discovering new nutrients in food. While we assume we only need what our vitamin pills give us in nutrients, we are slowly discovering diets without natural plant phytochemicals create weakened immune systems and a host of deficiencies. These include sulforaphanes, xanthenes, carotenes, beta-glucans, lignans, anthocyanins and many others. While many consider only the RDI or RDA of vitamins as important, in reality a lack of hundreds if not thousands of phytochemicals in the diet may certainly create a variety of deficiencies.

This reality illustrates a deeper relationship between our food sources and our bodies: They are both alive. For example, certain phytochemicals increase levels of glutathione peroxidase, glutathione S-transferase, and superoxide dismutase – all understood as part of the body's own detoxification and cleansing systems. The word *phyto* refers to plants that produced these nutrients when they were alive.

Flavonoids serve as a good example of this. There are six major types of flavonoids. These include isoflavonoids, flavones, anthocyanidins, flavanones, flavanols and flavonols.

Some types of flavonoids – most specifically those in citrus – have been dubbed 'bioflavonoids' but the broader term flavonoid has a greater specificity among the various food groups.

Flavonoids have a variety of health benefits. Most flavonoids are free radical scavengers – antioxidants. They reduce inflammation and many have been found to prevent cancers of different types.

Some of the more well known flavonoids include quercetin – a nutrient found in apples, onions, garlic and other foods; hesperidin and rutin from citrus products; epicatechins from vegetables, green tea, herbs and cocoa; kaempferol from cabbage, Brussels sprouts, kale, leeks, grapes and apples; and proanthocyanidins from oats, barley and flax.

Diets that contain significant quantities of these constituents are typically diets high in fresh foods – as many flavonoids are heat sensitive. Diets high in fresh foods also have many other benefits, because these foods are nutrient-dense and rich in fiber.

In a large study from ten European countries, Italian researchers (Zamora-Ros *et al.* 2012) found that diets containing higher levels of flavonoids significantly reduce the incidence of gastric cancer.

In this subset of the European Prospective Investigation into Cancer and Nutrition study (EPIC), the researchers from the Catalan Institute of Oncology followed 477,312 people – the majority of whom were women. The subjects answered extensive diet and lifestyle surveys, and they were followed for ten years. The compositions of their diets were compared to the USDA's database on food-composition along with the Phenol-Explorer database to determine their flavonoid content.

Those women who had diets with greater amounts of total flavonoid content had nearly 20% lower incidence of gastric cancers than those women with lower flavonoid diets. The inverse association was even greater among intestinal tumors. And specific flavonoid types also had greater association with cancer prevention – anthocyanidins, flavonols, flavones, and flavanols.

The researchers' study confirmed this. Their conclusion:

*"Total dietary flavonoid intake is associated with a significant reduction in the risk of gastric cancer in women."*

Another study – a review of research that included nearly 400,000 people from China's National Center of Colorectal Surgery (Jin *et al.* 2012) determined that the phytonutrients flavonoids and flavanols reduce incidence of colorectal cancer.

The researchers narrowed the research down to eight studies, which included 390,769 people. These included a range of protocols, including large population studies as well as controlled randomized studies.

The research found that foods containing flavanols – more technically referred to as flavan-3-ols – resulted in a significant reduction in incidence in colorectal cancer. The greater the flavanol consumption, the greater the association. More specifically, they found that greater consumption of epicatechin – a flavanol – significantly decreases the risk of colorectal cancer.

Flavanols include the category of catechins, which includes epicatechin, gallocatechin and epigallocatechin. Depending upon the molecular classification, they can also include kaempferol. Collectively these and others are also referred to as polyphenols. Plant polyphenols like catechins are found in many fruits and vegetables and vinegar. They are also found in herbal teas and green tea, as well as cocoa (from *Theobroma cacao*). Significant flavanol content has also been found in apples, onions and some beans.

The research also found that the consumption of procyanidins and phytoestrogens also reduced colorectal cancer incidence. The researchers characterized the association of these as "medium quality," meaning there was a definite association between the consumption and colon cancer, but not as strong as the polyphenol association.

Two other phytocompounds have been found to reduce colorectal cancer: Genistein and formononetin. These are considered isoflavonoids but also phytoestrogens because they have the ability to bind to the body's estrogen receptors. This can be significant because as people age – especially women – estrogen availability slows and this can be pro-inflammatory. When phytoestrogens are in the diet, these can help dampen the effects of estrogen reduction as we age.

The phytoestrogens genistein and formononetin are significantly found in beans, soy, red clover and some whole grains.

The number of plant compounds – phytonutrients – available from a plant-based diet is gigantic. The researchers described more than 5,000 individual flavonoids that have been divided into more than ten different categories. The big six categories include isoflavonoids, flavones, anthocyanidins, flavan-3-ols, flavonols (note the "o" instead of a second "a"), and flavanones.

One of the studies included in the review was from the U.S. National Cancer Institute (Bobe *et al.* 2008). The study followed 1,905 people and their diet with an average age of 61. The researchers compared the consumption of 29 different flavonoids together with the incidence of the occurrence of adenomatous polyps – a frequent symptom of colorectal cancer. The research used colonoscopies to determine polyp incidence. This study also showed that switching to a high-fiber diet also significantly reduced polyp incidence and subsequent colorectal cancer.

Furthermore, the study found that colorectal cancer prevention occurred most significantly among those who consumed the higher levels of flavonol foods. In other words, just adding a few veggies to the diet won't necessarily tip the scale in terms of preventing cancer.

## Nutritional Consciousness

Nutrients are not simply chemicals we can synthesize in the lab. Nutrients are manufactured in the bodies of living organisms. Certainly if we were to scoop up some dirt, we'd get a fair amount of inorganic minerals like calcium and phosphorus. We would not be getting much in the way of organic, life-giving nutrients however. By "organic," we are not talking food free of chemical fertilizers and pesticides – which is important. We are talking about nutrients connected to life. In strict chemical terms, "organic" also means any molecule containing carbon. Incidentally, this is also a function of living organisms – connecting atoms to carbon backbones.

Once an organism connects a molecule to carbon, the resulting nutrient can sustain a number of biochemical functions. It will be more easily assimilated and utilized by the body. Some refer this process – molecules becoming bound to carbon – as *chelation*. Recent research on the assimilation of minerals has confirmed that chelated minerals are assimilated at higher rates than inorganic minerals, for example.

A lab scientist may be able to mix a variety of ingredients, including organic compounds, and force a chelation process. In fact, this is done in a few popular supplements to increase absorption rates. While we might compare this process to the organic process of chelation (it is after all driven by living organisms), it is simply a weak attempt to replace the complex process living organisms already perform billions of times daily as they produce organic vitamins, proteins and mineral matrixes. A living organism is nature's nutrient manufacturing plant.

During digestion, our bodies also use living organisms – our probiotics – to help break down these nutrients. Along with colonies of probiotics, we produce a number of enzymes to further break apart food molecules into forms our bodies can easily use. We then combine (or chelate) these nutrients with others, and our body's own biochemicals.

These combinations enable our bodies to escort them into the bloodstream to be used by the body. While most descriptions of this process emphasize the "breaking down" of nutrients into their simpler molecules for absorption, the reality is, not only do nutrients require breaking down, but they require a process of bonding with the digestive elements produced by the body.

This bonding process allows the body to absorb the nutrients through the mucosal brush barrier of our intestinal wall. The intestinal mucosal membrane forms a protective surface medium over the intestinal epithelium. It also provides an active nutrient transport mechanism for nutrients and toxins. This mucosal layer is stabilized by the grooves of the intestinal microvilli. It contains glycoproteins, mucopolysaccharides and other ionic transporters, which attach to amino acids, minerals, vitamins, glucose and fatty acids – carrying them across intestinal membranes.

This mucosal layer is policed by billions of probiotic colonies, which help process and identify incoming food molecules; excrete various nutrients; and control toxins and pathogens. These are accompanied by immune cells such as IgA and IgE, along with T-cells and B-cells. These enable the body to identify nutrients as they enter our body and begin their journey through the body.

As these integrated molecules wander through the liver, the bloodstream and the cells, they continue to be monitored by the body's immune system. If the nutrients were broken down and chelated correctly in the digestive tract, they will be "approved" by the immune system throughout their journey. One might compare this "approval" process to traveling through the airport security systems, where there are cameras, x-ray scanners and metal detectors, all positioned to pick up specific problems as we travel through them. Molecules traveling through the body are not only scanned for intrusion, but they are also matched with the molecular and genetic needs of the body as a result of their configuration.

During digestion, enzymes like amylase, lipase, trypsin (along with other proteases), lactase, and many others are secreted through the membranes of the digestive tract to affect this process of break down and chelation. Some of these arrive via the pancreas. Some, like amylase and some proteases, are secreted through the salivary glands and the pyloric glands of the stomach – arrive earlier in the process.

The combination of food processing by our probiotics and enzymes not only breaks down our foods. It also prepares the food for use by the body. Without this process, the food particles will be identified by the body as being "foreign." They will be molecularly wrong, and their molecular 'fingerprints' will cause those molecules to be flagged and removed by the immune system. This removal process is a casual process for the immune system under ordinary conditions, but for many – especially those with compromised or burdened immune systems – it can result in allergies, hives or other inflammatory mechanisms.

The probiotic-enzymatic digestion-chelation process done in our guts is extremely complex. It takes place with the ultimate in precision and timing. Once nutrients are properly 'fingerprinted' by proper breakdown, chelation and absorption, they are ready to be utilized for the body's complex cellular mechanisms.

There are a number of biochemical terms associated with these sequential breakdown and chelating mechanisms performed by the body: These include conjugation, debranching, phosphorylation, glycolysis, methylation, gluconeogenesis and many others. Most biochemical processes taking place within the body require a specific staged or cascading mechanism, where enzymes and substrates are formed through different steps, creating new molecules, which in turn convert to other substrates and enzymes and so on.

Often these cascades create looping or cyclic conversions, where the enzymes and catalases are supplied first and drive the reaction. These cyclic processes will exchange ions and electrons between molecules, and push off various byproducts, including heat, energy, waste products, antioxidants, immune system substrates and others. Each of the resulting biochemicals will maintain the molecule 'fingerprints' of the body due to this cyclic reaction. The body thus knows precisely how to handle these various biochemical byproduct streams.

However, this cyclic process of biochemical 'fingerprinting' by the body through these cascading mechanisms require the specific nutrient inputs. These nutrient inputs most comply with the specifications of the body's biochemical processing requirements.

Should food be harshly processed or be infused with chemical additives that substantially change these specifications, that "food" will not result in right molecular structures. This will throw off the entire probiotic-enzymatic chelation process, and supply nutrients to the intestinal wall that are unrecognizable by the body's cyclic biochemical processes.

In other words, our body's systems will not accept these adulterated 'foods.'

The critical issue presented by this text is the need for receiving nutrition is by eating byproducts of the cascading mechanisms of other living organisms. Vegetables, fruits, nuts, seeds, dairy, grains, and so on all are produced by living organisms utilizing some of the same cascading probiotic-enzymatic-substrate processes existing within the human body. Those cyclic biochemical reactions taking place in other living organisms render those nutrients identifiable by the processes taking place in our bodies.

We might compare this to how we comprehend language. We will not understand the speaking of another language, but we will readily understand what someone is saying to us in the English language – assuming we are an English speaker. In the same way, nutrients obtained directly from a living organism have the right biomolecular 'language' to be recognized by our bodies. Those foods that have been adulterated in ways that are outside the confines of living organisms and their natural potentials are not readily recognized by the body.

Because these foods are not readily recognized by the body, they are not chemically neutralized through the forms of chelation discussed above. Because they are not readily neutralized by the body's natural processes, they must become neutralized by 'stealing' something from the body's tissues or cells. This produces imbalances, which leads to degeneration and disease.

Nutrients are the byproducts of the energy created by living organisms. All of life on our planet is interconnected. We are feeding off of each others' nutrient streams and waste streams. A plant will utilize the sun to produce energy for its activities, and the byproducts of that process become the nutrients we eat for our nourishment. Subsequently, these nutrients produced by living organisms contain the molecular 'fingerprints' recognized by the body's immune systems and biochemical energy cycles.

## So What Exactly are Living Foods?

There are a variety of fad diets and gimmicks out there, some using incredibly restrictive protocols and clever approaches. Some call for relatively complex combinations of foods or restrictive diets. Some tie foods to blood type. Some say we have to become hunters. Some say we need lots of fats and proteins, while others say we need lots of carbohydrates.

One popular diet is called the raw food diet. In fact, many raw food advocates have called their foods "living foods" to indicate that they are 'alive' with enzymes and various nutrients.

We in no way criticize the raw food diet. Certainly this diet is incredibly healthy, and someone who can maintain such a diet should be commended for their discipline and determination to be healthy.

However, we are not recommending the raw food diet here simply because it is too restrictive, and very few people can maintain such a diet for long. In addition, there are many foods that are better when they are minimally cooked. These include grains, beans and a variety of vegetables that have fibers that need to be softened in order to adequately digest them and extract their nutrients. In addition, there are many other that are most nutritious when they are cultured or fermented. This, in fact, is how most of our healthier ancestors ate.

Thus our definition of 'living' is radically different than raw foods. 'Living foods' in this text refers to:

122

✓ Foods that are cultured or fermented with probiotic micro-organisms, whether yeasts or probiotic bacteria.

✓ Foods that are mixed with cultured or fermented foods.

✓ Grains or beans that have been sprouted.

✓ Plant-based foods that have been harvested whole and prepared as whole foods, with no or minimal cooking and processing.

✓ Supplements that contain probiotics and/or plant-based whole foods, with no or minimal cooking and processing.

While the strict definition of 'living' might eliminate those foods that are no longer alive – such as are cultured foods with live probiotics – it is essential that we be practical. Certainly many animals – deer for example – can cruise through a forest and directly eat from living plants, few of us have the luxury of being able to eat as we walk through the woods. Modern humans are stuck with having others collect and harvest our foods before storing them and shipping them to our local food stores.

A diet high in living foods will:

➤ increase antioxidant levels
➤ increase detoxification
➤ lower the burden on the body's immune system
➤ provide a host of bioavailable nutrients
➤ provide fiber, reducing LDL lipid peroxidation
➤ increase liver activity and strengthen of the liver
➤ alkalize and help purify the blood
➤ provide the body with trace and macro minerals
➤ lower inflammation
➤ increase our body's resident probiotics

All of these effects work together to cleanse the body of toxins and reduce the body's toxic burden. When the body's toxic burden is reduced, our immune system's ability to remove toxins is increased. This is the secret to a life-long purification: A long-term reduction of toxins.

The more we honor and respect the natural state of those living organisms that produce our nutrients, the more nutrition we will derive from them. Consider our garden. If we carefully water and fertilize the plants in our garden, they will produce a splendid array of nutrients.

That care must continue after their fruits are harvested. The stripping of hulls, peels and rinds, the overcooking and mixing with denatured, isolated sweeteners and fats ruins the biochemical orientation of the nutrients the plants produced. This is why even bananas shipped from South America can still have much of their nutrition intact. They have been shipped inside of nature's packaging, which naturally keeps nutrients like potassium locked within. Even with fumigation and a long journey by boat, bananas can still be tasty and nutritious. This is because the packaging provided by the living plant – the peel – protects the fruit from damage by insulating it.

Peels, rinds and hulls have been designed to protect the plant's procreative efforts – which provide our nutrients. by the Creator to insulate the tender inner fruit or nut from a host of environmental insults. This can be easily seen by microscope and touch: A peel or hull is typically extremely fibrous, waxy and in many cases extremely hard. This is the result of a very cohesive and stable bonding structure within the biochemical matrix of that substance. Manufacturing this stable bonding structure requires intense organization and effort by the plant. For many peels, their softness and flexibility provide additional protection for the fruit's nutrients. It is like comparing a pillar to a tree in an earthquake or strong wind. The pillar is solid and does not move until it breaks in a strong wind or earthquake. Meanwhile the plant is more flexible, waving back and forth yet difficult to break.

Picking many plant foods early – as is done on many commercial farms – not only prevents the complete peel from forming, but also prevents a number of nutrients from developing. This later point was illustrated by a recent study done at the University of Innsbruck in Austria. Researchers identified some of the mechanisms that give fruit their antioxidant levels, revealing that as fruit ripens, chlorophyll is converted to *nonfluorescing chlorophyll catabolytes* (or NCCs). This is the effect noticed as fruits turn from green to their ripened colors. These NCCs become powerful antioxidants when eaten (Krautler 2007). When a food is picked green, much of this conversion does not take place.

The most nourishing parts of most natural foods are the parts of plants produced for procreation. These are the fruits, the nuts, the seeds, the beans, the grain, and so on. The delivery of nutrition during plant procreation provides nutrients because this is a conscious expression. This is why fruits, nuts, seeds, beans, and grains are so healthy for us, providing a host of vitamins, minerals, protein and various micronutrients. Our bodies become intimately connected to the nourishment provided by living organisms during their procreative expression.

A molecule is like a small band of musicians. While each atom is comparable to an individual musician with a particular instrument, a molecule together produces a song produced from the coherence between the atoms.

Say we have a quartet band made up of a flute, cello, oboe and violin and the quartet is playing a concerto in a concert hall. During the performance, a heavy metal rock band barges in and stands besides our quartet, with their amps plugged in. Certainly, their music will clash with the chamber music of the quartet. This is because the coherent quality of the metal band conflicts with the coherent quality of the quartet. They are not complementary. They do not resonate together. They are not in harmony. As a result, people get upset. Some storm out. Some try to kick out the heavy metal band. An inflammatory reaction takes place.

This is almost precisely why chemically-infused and/or devitalized foods are rejected by the body's immune system. They simply do not resonate with the body.

## About Enzymes

Living foods contain enzymes and their catalases, as well as the ingredients for our body to make our own enzymes.

If we are deficient in a particular enzyme, the food will not be properly broken down. This can create a macromolecule that may be exposed to the cells and tissues of the intestines. If the intestinal barrier is weakened, the immunoglobulins within the intestines can mark the macromolecule as an invader. Worse, the macromolecule can get into the internal tissues and bloodstream – where the immune system can launch an immune attack against it – often resulting in allergies.

The body has a very exacting way it breaks down proteins. This requires specific protease enzymes and the process of natural enzymatic hydrolysis. This of course means that the body also needs to have plenty of water on hand as well.

Confirming the relationship between food allergies and digestive enzymes, researchers from the Medical University of Vienna (Untersmayr *et al.* 2007) studied the effects that incomplete digestion of fish proteins has on fish allergies. Healthy volunteers and those with diagnosed codfish allergies were challenged with codfish. They were also tested with fish proteins incubated with varying degrees of digestive enzymes. The subjects were tested for histamine release from fish allergen sensitivity with each type.

The researchers found that the inadequate breakdown of fish proteins produced more allergic responses, while a more complete breakdown by enzymes produced fewer allergic responses among both groups. Inadequate digestion produced allergens that the body sensitized to.

Here is a short list of the body's major digestive enzymes:

**Major Digestive Enzymes**

| Enzyme | Foods it Breaks Down |
|---|---|
| Amylase | Starches |
| Bromelain | Proteins |
| Carboxypeptidase | Proteins (terminal) |
| Cellulase | Plant fiber (cellulose) |
| Chymotrypsin | Proteins |
| Elastase | Proteins and elastins |
| Glucoamylase | Starches |
| Isomaltase | Isomaltose and Maltose |
| Lactase | Lactose |
| Lipase | Fats |
| Maltase | Maltose |
| Nuclease | Protein nucleotides |
| Pepsin | Proteins |
| Peptidase | Proteins |
| Rennin | Milk |
| Steapsin | Triglycerides |
| Sucrase | Sucrose |
| Tributyrase | Butter Fat |
| Trypsin | Proteins |
| Xylanase | Hemicellulose (plant fiber) |

We can see from this list that there are many different protein enzymes. This is because there are so many different types of food molecules to break down. There are numerous enzyme sub-types and others that break down specific food constituents and particular foods. The body makes some of these; some are drawn from plant-foods; and some are produced by our colonies of intestinal probiotics.

## The Protein Solution

We've discussed how too much protein in the diet can be problematic. Let's illustrate this a bit further before we get to the solution.

Research from Denmark's National Food Institute (Pedersen *et al.* 2013) concluded that eating too much protein causes early mortality and a higher incidence of cardiovascular disease, type II diabetes and possibly more kidney diseases.

The Denmark government researchers reviewed 5,718 scientific research abstracts as well as 412 complete studies. They landed on 64 scientific studies that had clear and conclusive results regarding the consumption of high protein low carbohydrate diets. These studies included over 200,000 people from a number of health studies and large population studies.

The purpose of this study was to review the Norwegian nutritional recommendations for protein requirements and determine whether or not a low carbohydrate, high-protein diet was safe.

The high-protein diet was qualified by the parameter of one gram of protein per kilogram of body weight. This would convert to about .45 grams of protein per pound of bodyweight. This means a person who weighs 150 lbs would be eating more than about 67 g of protein per day. Many Americans eat upwards of 100 grams of protein a day, and high-protein diets can be as high as 150 grams per day.

The scientists systematically compared results of these 64 studies and concluded that a high-protein, low carbohydrate diet – those over 1 grams of protein per day per kilogram of body weight – had a direct correlation with early death, greater cardiovascular disease, and greater incidence of type II diabetes.

However, the research also concluded that diets high in vegetable protein had a lower risk of cardiovascular disease and early death compared to those who ate predominantly animal-protein high-protein diets. And in some studies high vegetable protein diets decreased the risk of early death and cardiovascular disease significantly.

In other words, those diets particularly high in animal protein suffered more early death, cardiovascular disease and type II diabetes.

While the study populations were two large to formulate clear statistics in terms of the exact amount of mortality in years or percentage increased risk, they could clearly identify the associations through the large population studies.

The researchers concluded that protein intake should not exceed 20 to 23% of one's overall energy intake.

Diets that have particularly high protein intakes – often called "Low Carb Diets" – include the South Beach Diet, the Atkins Diet and others. These have also been known to produce ketosis, which can result in dizziness, mood issues and other side effects. The American Heart Association, the American Cancer Society and the National Cholesterol Education Program have all suggested our diets should include a lower percentage of protein.

Most people think the body absorbs and utilizes protein from our foods. Not true. The body utilizes amino acids and short chains of aminos, and assembles its own protein complexes as needed for our tissues. The reason we each have slightly different genes is because we each assemble slightly different arrangements of aminos.

Aminos are called peptides and the simple amino chains are called polypeptides. The process of complex protein assembly is orchestrated by our RNA, and driven by special enzymes – which also happen to be proteins.

Each one of the body's countless unique proteins will contain thousands of peptides strung together to form a unique combination. Myosin – the muscle contraction protein – contains about 6,100 peptides, for example.

The body makes these incredibly long protein chains from only 22 amino acids. So the better our access to these single peptides, the more efficient our body's protein production will be.

Meanwhile, only 8-10 of these amino acids are considered "essential." The "core" eight essential aminos are isoleucine, leucine, lysine, methionine, phenylalanine, threonine, tryptophan and valine. Without these in our diet, we can become protein deficient.

What about the other aminos? The body has the ability to produce the other amino acids using the essential eight.

Nevertheless, a diet containing all of the 22, or at least the essentials, is required to maintain the body's cell structures and enzymes.

The question becomes, how can we guarantee we are getting all of these, and how can we best get the most efficient forms – the single peptides and simple polypeptides?

## The power of plant protein

The most efficient form of peptides comes from plant foods. Most plant foods have from 10% to 50% peptide or polypeptide-form protein by weight. These simple polypeptide or single peptide forms allow the body to quickly assimilate proteins. This sets up the RNA to more efficiently organize and string together these peptides into the body's unique protein combinations.

Protein quality outranks protein content. Plant-based proteins provide excellent quality because they typically contain a full spectrum of simple peptides.

While the body can store the eight essential aminos for a week or two, they all need to be available in the diet. As the body degrades its protein structures, most of the aminos are degraded and run out of the body.

Many plant foods contain all eight essential amino acids in their most efficient forms. A mixed diet of plant foods will assure us of getting all essential aminos as well as most if not all of the non-essentials. A mixed green salad with some sunflower seeds will supply practically every amino acid, including the essential eight. Sunflower seeds contain 19 amino acids, including all of the essential aminos, and 22-27% protein content by weight.

So how much protein do we need?

The American Heart Association and several research studies – as we documented earlier – have suggested that 50-60 grams of amino-protein per day is adequate for most adults, and World Health Organization research has found that even 30-40 grams of good quality amino-protein per day is adequate.

Most Americans easily eat 100-200 grams of rich, complex protein per day. Some body builders and low-carb dieters consume two or three times that amount. As a result, Americans experience phenomenally high levels of gout, gallstones, cardiovascular disease and kidney stones – all related to excess uric acid produced by excessive protein intake.

Again, quality is better than quantity. The key is eating good quality protein foods with easily assimilable peptide forms. As a percentage of calories, no more than 15% of daily calories should be protein according to several notable nutritional experts.

It is very easy to get enough protein with plant foods. Just one cup of lentils will supply 18 grams of good quality protein. A cup of black beans will contain 15 grams. A cup of baked beans will contain 12 grams. A cup of soybeans will contain 29 grams, while four ounces of tofu will contain nine grams. A half-cup of cashews contains 10 grams.

Other healthy plant-based foods contain good efficient protein content. Whole wheat bread will contain five grams. A cup of broccoli will contain four grams. Two teaspoons of peanut butter will contain eight grams. A cup of brown rice will contain five grams, as will a cup of spinach.

While milk whey is also a great way to include all the essential aminos into our diet, most of the foods mentioned above also have all eight essential aminos and more. In general, good quality, high-protein plant foods include all the beans, nuts, whole grains and leafy greens. A dinner that contains beans, a few nuts, some grains and/or leafy greens will supply all the protein we will ever need to assemble great protein combinations.

## Whole versus Isolated Nutrients

We cannot replace the orange with vitamin C. While we may eliminate scurvy with synthetic vitamin C – ascorbic acid – we also find its absorption is limited and thus laxative at higher levels. This is because efficient vitamin C absorption requires bioflavonoids and other phytonutrients to stabilize, buffer and balance the vitamin C.

Sugar is another example. We can certainly gain energy from refined sugar isolated from beets or cane. However, our bodies will quickly become out of balance, due to the spiking of blood sugar levels. This results in the spiking of insulin, glucose absorption and resulting sugar low characteristic of refined sugar foods. Some call this the *sugar-high-rebound* effect.

We find this situation repeatedly when we consider other isolated nutrients. While we might take plenty of isolated calcium in a supplement, researchers have discovered the only way it will be properly utilized is with plenty of vitamins A, D and K as well as boron and silica available in the diet to help process and resorb the calcium into bones and other tissues.

Folate and folic acid provides another lesson:

A study from Seattle's Fred Hutchinson Cancer Research Center (Zschäbitz *et al.* 2012) has confirmed that synthetic folic acid supplementation may increase the risk of colorectal cancer.

This conclusion was determined using the Women's Health Initiative Observational Study, which included 88,045 postmenopausal women who were tested and studied between 1993-1998, just following the mandated folic acid supplementation requirement in the United States.

Most of the folate supplementation to foods was synthetic folic acid, rather than nature's molecule, which is called folate.

The research found 1,003 colorectal cancer incidences among the study population as of 2009. When nutrient consumption was analyzed, the researchers found that those women in the top quarter of folic acid consumption had higher incidence of colorectal cancer between three an nine years after the folic acid mandate.

The researchers could not determine whether the cause was too much supplementation or due to the supplement being the synthetic form of the nutrient. The two are indelibly tied, however, because a healthy diet that supplies the natural form of folate has been connected with reduced cancer incidence.

Other research has found that high supplementation of synthetic folic acid can increase malignant tumor proliferation and increase cancer risk in general.

The folic acid mandate was instituted in 1995 in order to combat a series of birth defects in children, including spina bifida and other neural tube issues.

The fortification requirement came from the U.S. Food and Drug Administration, which required 40 micrograms of folic acid be added to every 100 grams of grains and flours, including noodles, pasta, corn meals and other refined grain products. In 1998, the FDA added the folic acid fortification requirement to breads, cereals and other foods that contained refined flour.

Whole grain flours and foods do not require folic acid supplementation because they already maintain natural folate content.

Research has found that spina bifida and other defects may be reduced up to 70% should women of child-bearing age consume at least 400 micrograms of folic acid per day.

Now the research is showing there is a price to pay for the extensive folic acid supplementation by women. Increasingly, nutritionists are warning against folic acid supplementation over 400 mcg per day. Pregnant women are often advised to double this dose, to 600-800 mcg per day (Williams *et al.* 2005).

Too much folic acid supplementation can also mask a vitamin B12 deficiency (Strickland *et al.* 2012).

Folate and folic acid are also called vitamin B9. The natural form, folate, can be found in a large number of natural, unprocessed foods, including most leafy green vegetables including romaine lettuce and broccoli; many fruits including citrus, banana, raspberries, cantaloupe, honeydew; peas; beans; beets; seeds including sunflower seeds; and many whole grains including whole wheat and oats. Most nutritionists agree that a whole-foods, mostly raw diet with plenty of these foods will supply sufficient folate. For those with a questionable diet, there are whole food supplements available that supply natural folate.

In addition, certain probiotic bacteria naturally produce folate, which include *Lactobacillus plantarum*, *Bifidobacterium adolescentis* and *B. pseudocatenulatum* (Rossi *et al.* 2012).

The research by the Fred Hutchinson Cancer Research Center also found that other B vitamin supplementation reduced colorectal cancer incidence. These included vitamin B6 and riboflavin. Both of these B vitamins are also available in whole foods and also supplied, to a marginal extent, by probiotic bacteria.

We see a similar issue with calcium supplementation.

Just when the medical institution was convinced that more calcium in the diet was the answer to osteoporosis, recent research has confirmed a short-term effect of calcium-supplementation but no long-term improvement of osteoporosis rates or broken hips. In an 18-year study of 72,337 women, done at the Harvard Medical School and Brigham and Woman's Hospital (Feskanich *et al.* 2003), calcium supplementation or greater milk drinking did not decrease the likelihood of osteoporosis or breaking a hip.

There are other factors. The above research indicated that vitamin D with greater sunlight did significantly reduce osteoporosis and broken hip occurrence. Other studies have confirmed that exercise contributes significantly to a reduction of these occurrences as well. In other words, a full spectrum of wholesome food together with sunshine and exercise are the key to strong bones – not just calcium.

When we take a whole array of vitamins, we may be obtaining some phytonutrient elements of foods with enough biochemical structures to provide some nutrients missing in our diets. If those nutrients were chemically manufactured however, it is far less likely that these nutrients will do more good than harm. The bonding angles of the molecules will likely different from natural food nutrients. There may be various non-nutritive chemicals added to the tablet as preservatives, binders or fillers – collectively called *excipients*. All of these will have to processed through the liver and broken down as if they were toxic chemicals (and many might be at large-enough quantities). Some of the nutrients of these synthetic vitamins might be useable. Most will be processed through the liver and exit the body as metabolites – putting extra pressure on both the liver and the kidneys.

Should the vitamins have been grown on yeasts or other natural substrates, we may find that they will provide a level of nourishment similar to eating natural foods. This is because they were produced from consciousness. The key issue is how they were produced. When we go to the store and shop for vitamins, we should look for vitamins that are whole-food based and grown on yeast and/or spirulina. There are some wonderful food-based supplements on the market now.

## Methylation

Our bodies conduct an interesting process called *methylation*. To simplify a very complex biological process, this is a process where methyl groups replace hydrogen atoms on larger molecules. The critical biological methylation process is called DNA methylation. In this process, methyl donors convert the DNA component cytosine to 5-methylcytosine using a special enzyme called methyltransferase. This CpG-to-Me-CpG is an important gene expression, which is related to adapting to various stress-factors. Should there be a lack of methyl groups available to construct this exchange, the likelihood for cancer and nervous disorders increase substantially. Another type of methylation is called protein methylation, which will modify proteins for biological processes. Lysine and arginine are usually the amino acid portions of the proteins where methylation typically occurs.

Methylation is a critical mechanism for the body. It is a key process for energy production and detoxification. Through methylation, the body can produce Co-enzyme Q. It is the key mechanism for the repair of tissues and neutralizing toxic elements. It is critical to neurotransmitter production, stimulating the production of dopamine, melatonin, norepinephrine and others. Methyl transfer also enables the body to produce SAM-e and DMG, critical to our moods and our energy levels. Homocysteine processing is also dependent upon methyl transfer. High homocysteine levels have been linked with cardiovascular disease. Methyl transfer is what the body uses to neutralize homocysteine levels.

B vitamins are known methyl donors. For this reason, B12 and folate are critical for health, as are choline and S-adenosyl methionine (SAM) – which is derived from the amino acid methionine. Methionine is one of only two sulfur amino acids (cysteine is the other, which can be converted by methionine and is the precursor for the all-important glutathione) that the body uses for protein synthesis. Methionine is a powerful chelating agent, which through the trans-sulfuration pathway assists in the production of carnation, cysteine, and taurine. It is also an important component of fatty acid synthesis. Methionine is critical for phosphatidylcholine production as well – critical for brain cell function.

A lack of methyl groups in the diet causes a state of *hypomethylation*. This may produce imbalances among our DNA, stimulating possible mutation as the cells attempt to adjust to the lack of methyl donors. The resulting genetic adjustment to too few methyl groups can result in a *neoplasm*, or a tumor. Should this neoplasm begin to replicate the mutated DNA, an aggressive form of cancer can result. At the very least, a chronic lack of methyl donors may result in various degenerative diseases.

For this reason, it is important to have a wide selection of foods in the diet containing B vitamins and methionine. Probiotic living foods produce B vitamins and other methyl group donors. Foods like whole grains, lentils, sesame seeds, garlic, onions, sunflower seeds, Brazil nuts, spinach, peppers and dairy foods are great sources of methionine.

The planet also undergoes a process of methylation. This is conducted through various bacteria within the seabed, converting toxic elements like lead, arsenic and mercury into their innocuous methyl forms such as dimethyl mercury and trimethyl arsine. This process speeds up the detoxification process while rebalancing the environment to the extent possible – just as methylation does in the body. The earth's methylation process helps to convert toxins into useable molecules.

The biochemicals natural to our environment undergo constant recycling. A single biochemical may be eaten by one organism, excreted by another, inhaled by yet another and become the skin of yet another organism. At the same time, an intricate chemical balance is kept through these changes, making biochemical a vital source for nutrition. In other words, the earth's natural biochemical recycling maintains its nutritional nature on a consistent basis. While one organism's waste may be another's food, that food/waste still maintains its nutritional content.

What we have then, is a living biochemical system.

## Synthetic versus Natural

The assumption of modern chemistry is there is no inherent difference between a chemical synthesized in a lab or manufacturing facility from one made in nature by living processes. This assumption has led humankind to haphazardly invent new synthetic chemical combinations with reckless abandon. Blinded by patents and profits, the industrial chemical complex has assumed there is no environmental cost.

When we interfere with any one part of nature's cycling of molecules, we can interrupt the balance of the rest of the cycle, often causing reverberations on an exponential basis. This is precisely what humans have unfortunately arrived at after two hundred years of industrial technological development.

Let's look at some interesting examples.

Consider the delicate chemical pathway of nitrogen. Animals and humans consume nitrogen from the atmosphere and through nutrition — by breathing, eating plants, root nitrogen fixing, and so on. When an organism dies, *ammonifying bacteria* decompose the body and release ammonia into the soil. *Nitrosifying bacteria* oxidize the ammonia, converting it to nitrites, and *nitrifying bacteria* then oxidize the nitrites to soil nitrogen and ammonia ions. Plants utilize these to form amino acids and proteins. Nitrogen is also released into the air with *denitrifying* bacteria. As plant protein is eaten by animals and humans in plant food, these nitrogen amino acids become part of the proteins that make up our bodies. When our bodies die, the cycle begins again.

Throughout the nitrogen cycle, there is a precise balance of nitrogen in the atmosphere, the soils, and within each organism: Just enough to serve the combined purpose of all involved. Every species then gets a balanced dose of nitrogen, from the soil microbes and earthworms all the way up to humans.

Enter chemical fertilizer. The beneficial addition of nitrogen chemical fertilizers into the soil has increased crop production for agribusiness-based farms. While adding something already available in nature seems innocent enough, the dumping of pure nitrogen without the balance of nutrients provided by living organisms produces an imbalance throughout the nitrogen cycle.

Without the complex of nutrients produced by nature's nitrogen-fixing process, the soil begins to erode and thin. The heavy load of unused nitrogen leaches through the soil, settling into the ground water. This nitrogen leaching creates a build-up of dangerous nitrates within the ground water. Nitrate build up has been poisoning ground water in agricultural areas throughout the world. In areas of heavy fertilizer use, undrinkable ground water is reaching increasingly deeper wells. Nitrate levels above about 50 parts per million can make a person sick. Higher levels have been known to be fatal.

In addition, nitrogen-fertilizer-rich soils choke rivers and oceans with extra nitrogen, causing abnormal blooms of algae, cutting off oxygen supplies and leading to dead ocean zones with high toxicity levels.

The use of nitrogen fertilizers illustrates how the precise rhythms of nature – the use and recycling of natural biochemistry – can so easily be disrupted. Now why couldn't we simply have supplied the nitrogen produced by compost, as degraded by soil organisms and earthworms?

Consider fats. When palm and coconut oils are cooled, they become hardened. This makes them good thickening agents for cooking and good for frying. In an attempt to match nature, in 1902 German Wilhelm Normann patented the first hydrogenation process, which was eventually purchased by Proctor and Gamble, leading to Crisco® oil and eventually margarine. When nutritionists convinced us that *"all saturated fats are bad"* in the sixties and seventies, margarine sales took off. Processors also found that frying oil had a better shelf life and was cheaper if cottonseed oil and soybean oil were *partially hydrogenated*. Because these oils do not normally harden at room temperature as does palm, coconut and lard, hydrogenation allowed processors to use the less expensive oils for frying, spreading and cooking.

Hydrogenation means to *saturate* hydrogen onto all of the available bonds of the central molecule. Whereas a natural substance might have a double bond between carbon and other atoms, hydrogen gas can be bubbled through the substance – using a catalyst to spark the reaction – to attach more hydrogen to the molecule. To saturate carbon bonds with hydrogen, catalyst is added, and the oil undergoes the bubbling of hydrogen within a heated catalytic environment. This saturation synthetically changes the oil's melting point, giving it more versatility at a lower cost.

Let's review. Food scientists took real foods – oil extracted from soybeans or cottonseed – and synthetically converted it into what appeared to be the same molecular structure, but with a different melting point. Harmless, yes? Think again. After decades of use and millions of heart attacks and strokes later, health researchers began realizing that partially hydrogenated oils have damaging effects upon the cardiovascular system.

While the saturated or partially saturated molecule was the same formula, the synthetic process of hydrogenation created an unusual (transversed) molecular structure called a *trans-fat*. Trans-fat is now implicated in a various degenerative disorders, including atherosclerosis, dementia, liver disease, irritable bowel syndrome, and Alzheimer's disease among others. While the epidemic increase in cardiovascular disease has focused billions of dollars into research, the consumption of trans-fats was altogether overlooked. Why? Because researchers assumed that hydrogenated soybean oil was harmless because its molecularly-identical cousin – raw soybean oil – was harmless, and even healthy because it was a polyunsaturated oil.

The mechanism whereby trans-fats produce damage in the body – as we'll discuss later – is called lipid peroxidation. Because trans-fats are less stable than cis-fats, and because fats make up our cell membranes, trans-fats become more readily damaged, producing what is called lipid peroxides. Lipid peroxides damage blood vessel walls and other tissue systems, producing cardiovascular disease and other degenerative disorders.

So now researchers realize that the orientation – polarity and spin – of a molecule can have altogether different effects from the same molecule rotated in the orientation nature designed.

Nature normally orients healthy oil molecules – and many other nutrients – in *cis* formation: They are oriented so that the hydrogens are on the same side with the other molecular bonds. A *trans* configuration has hydrogens on the opposite side of the bonds.

This *cis* and *trans* orientation issue is also evident from the opposite perspective in the case of resveratrol. Resveratrol is a phytochemical constituent of more than seventy different plant species, including many fruits such as berries and grapes. Studies have shown natural resveratrol has many biological properties important to health. These include antioxidant, anti-bacterial, anti-viral, anti-fungal, liver-cleansing, mood-elevation, and amyloid-plaque-removal properties. Resveratrol also activates an enzyme-protein called sirtuin 1, which appears to promote DNA repair.

However, these effects are exclusive to the natural form: *trans*-resveratrol. Not surprisingly, pasteurization and other processing will convert the *trans*-resveratrol molecule to its less effective cousin, *cis*-resveratrol.

Another example of human meddling is vitamin E. While natural vitamin E is d-alpha-tocopherol, the synthetic version is dl-alpha-tocopherol. While d-alpha-tocopherol has one isomer, dl-alpha-tocopherol has eight. One of those eight is similar to the one natural isomer. The difference is that the natural version is more readily bioavailable than the dl-alpha version.

Illustrating this, in one study (Burton *et al.* 1998), subjects took either natural vitamin E or the synthetic vitamin E. Natural vitamin E levels in the bloodstream for all subjects were at least twice as high as levels of the synthetic versions. After twenty-three days, tissue levels were also significantly higher for the natural vitamin E group, compared to the synthetic vitamin E group. These tests illustrated that nature's form of vitamin E is more readily absorbed and utilized than the synthetic version.

Furthermore, Oregon State University researchers (Traber *et al.* 1998) found that humans excrete synthetic vitamin E three times faster than natural vitamin E. So not only does the human body not readily absorb the synthetic version, but it wants to rid the body of this version three times faster.

This ratio was confirmed in another test (Kiyose *et al.* 1997) showing that it took three times the quantity of synthetic vitamin E to reach the same levels achieved by natural vitamin E among seven women.

Vitamin C provides another example. Gas chromatography has revealed several structural differences between synthetic vitamin C (isolated ascorbic acid) and natural forms of vitamin C. While many people supplement with isolated ascorbic acid, nature provides a completely different structure. Not only is the molecule itself different, but natural vitamin C is naturally bonded – or *chelated* – to other natural compounds called biofactors. These include bioflavonoids, minerals, rutin, and other biochemicals produced by living organisms or nature's ecology. These are often referred to as *ascorbates*.

Synthetic vitamin D – referred to as vitamin $D_2$ or ergocalciferol – is also molecularly different from naturally produced cholecalciferol. In a study published in 2004 by Armas *et al.*, twenty healthy male subjects were given single doses of 50,000 IU of either vitamin $D_2$ or nature's form, vitamin $D_3$.

After supplement, their 25-hydroxyvitamin D (25-ODH) levels in the blood were measured over a twenty-nine day period. 25-ODH is the metabolite of vitamin D utilized by the body. The measured 25-ODH levels were the same between the $D_2$ and $D_3$ in subjects for the first three days. However, blood levels of 25-OHD fell dramatically after that for the $D_2$ subjects. The $D_3$ group's 25-OHD levels continued to rise, and peaked fourteen days after the initial dose was given.

After 29 days, the subjects taking $D_2$ had concentrations of less than a third of the levels of the $D_3$ subjects. Using a calculation called the *area under the plasma curve* (AUC), this translated to the synthetic $D_2$'s potency being about one-tenth of the potency of the nature's vitamin $D_3$.

Illustrating this further, in a recent study from Washington University's School of Medicine (Nicola *et al.* 2007), 168 healthy postmenopausal women were tested for supplemented calcium versus dietary (natural) sources of calcium. Women whose calcium intake was primarily from supplementation – even though their dosages were higher – had lower bone mineral density levels than the women whose calcium intake was primarily from dietary sources. Those taking supplements plus good dietary sources had the highest totals.

Naturally occurring nutrients are electromagnetically different than synthesized chemicals. The resulting quanta of spin, angular momentum and so on will vary between nature's version and a version synthesized in a lab or processed beyond nature's intended course.

Spectroscopy tests show that when two different ions with different atomic character are brought together, the resulting compound will display different spectra than either did independently. The combination's waveforms are not necessarily a composite of the two. It is a new waveform combination resulting from the resonating interference of the combining elements together with its natural catalysts and environment.

Most biological combinations require a catalyst (a facilitator) to complete. These catalysts may supply or borrow electrons in an oxidizing or reducing mechanism to assist in the combination. They will also supply the needed electromagnetic energy to speed up the reaction. Nature's catalysts provide specific changes in molecular structure – creating a unique *fingerprint* of sorts.

Synthetic catalysts will produce a different molecular combination, even if the original ions or compounds are the same as found in nature. Even if the combination may be similar to nature's version, often the molecular orientation – as with trans-fats – will be subtly different.

Because it is not cohesive – or stable – with the body's components, a synthetically combined compound throws off the balance between oxidizers and reducers in the body. This produces increased levels of oxidized or oxidative radicals, which will rob electrons or ions from the molecules that make up our tissues – notably our cell membranes, and the membranes that make up our mitochondria.

This later point – damage to the membranes of our mitochondria – is now implicated as the functional event that causes dementia, chronic fatigue and fibromyalgia. When the mitochondria within our brain cells is damaged by free radicals, these brain cells begin to shut down.

In chronic fatigue and fibromyalgia – often considered the same condition – damage to the membranes of mitochondria shuts down the energy production of muscle cells.

This is because mitochondria is where are energy is produced. The mitochondria house the Krebs cycle, which converts glucose and oxygen to heat and energy. As they become damaged and dysfunctional, we experience fatigue.

While our bodies are built to handle moderate levels of free radicals, our synthetic world is overloading our body with synthetics, which produce these oxidized or oxidative radicals within the body. This oxidizing potency of toxins leads to an overload of acids (H+), causing excessive acidosis, and the subsequent degeneration of our tissue systems.

## Alkaline Nutrition

This discussion of nutrients should also include the reflective effects of a healthy diet: The proper acid-alkaline balance among the blood, urine and intercellular tissue regions. The reference to acidic or alkaline body fluids and tissues has been made by numerous natural health experts over the years. Is there any scientific validity to this?

Many nutritionists condemn an acidic metabolism and loosely call appropriate metabolism as a *state of alkalinity*. Strictly speaking, however, an alkaline environment is not healthy. The blood, interstitial fluids, lymph and urine should be *slightly acidic* to maintain the appropriate mineral ion balance. Let's dig into the science.

Acidity or alkalinity is measured using a logarithmic scale called pH. The term pH is derived from the French word *pouvoir hydrogene,* which means 'hydrogen power' or 'hydrogen potential.' pH is quantified by an inverse log base-10 scale. It measures the proton-donor level of a solution by comparing it to a theoretical quantity of hydrogen ions (H+) or $H_3O+$.

The scale is pH 1 to pH 14, which converts to a range of $10^{-1}$ (1) to $10^{-14}$ (.00000000000001) moles of hydrogen ions. This means that a pH of 14 maintains fewer hydrogen ions. It is thus *less acidic* and *more alkaline* (or basic).

The pH scale has been set up around the fact that water's pH is log-7 or simply pH 7 – due to water's natural mineral content. Because pure water forms the basis for so many of life's activities, and because water neutralizes and dilutes so many reactions, water was established as the standard reference point or neutral point between what is considered an acid or a base solution. In other words, a substance having greater hydrogen ion potential (but lower pH) than water will be considered acidic, while a substance with less H+ potential (higher pH) than water is considered a base (alkaline).

Now the solution with a certain pH may not specifically maintain that many hydrogen ions. But it has the same *potential* as if it contained those hydrogen ions. That is why pH is hydrogen power or hydrogen potential.

In human blood, a pH level in the range of about 6.4 is considered healthy because this state is slightly more acidic than water, enabling the bodily fluids to maintain and transport minerals. It enables the *potential* for minerals to be carried by the blood, in other words. Minerals are critical to every cell, every organ, every tissue and every enzyme process occurring within the body. Better put, a 6.4 pH offers the appropriate *currency* of the body's fluids: This discourages acidosis and toxemia, maintaining a slight mineralized status.

Acidosis is produced with greater levels of carbonic acids, lactic acids, and/or uric acids among the joints and tissues. These acids are readily oxidizing, which produces free radicals. However, an overly alkaline state can precipitate waste products from cells, which also floods the system with radicals. For this reason, *toxemia* results from either an overly acidic blood-tissue content or an overly alkaline blood-tissue content. In other words, pH *balance* is the key.

Ions from minerals like potassium, calcium, magnesium and others are usually positively oriented – with alkaline potential. But to be carried through a solution, the solution must have the pH potential to carry them.

Besides being critical to enzymatic reactions, these minerals bond with lipids and proteins to form the structures of our cells, organs and tissues – including our airways, nerves and mucosal membranes.

Natural health experts over the past century have observed among their patients and in clinical research that an overly acidic environment within the body is created by a diet abundant in refined sugars, processed foods, chemical toxins and amino acid-heavy animal foods. More recently, research has connected this acidic state to toxemia. The toxemia state is a state of free radical proliferation, which damages cells and tissues. It is also a state that produces systemic inflammation, because the immune system is over-worked as it tries to remove the cell and tissue damage.

As mentioned earlier, animals accumulate toxins within their fat tissues. They are bioaccumulators. Thus, animals exposed to the typical environmental toxins of smog and chemical pollutants in their waters and air – along with pesticides and herbicides from their foods – will accumulate those toxins within their fat cells and livers. And those who eat those animals will inherit (and further accumulate) these accumulated toxins. In addition, animals secrete significant waste matter as they are being slaughtered.

Plants are not bioaccumulators. While they can accumulate some pesticides and herbicide chemicals within their leaves and roots, they do not readily absorb or hold these for long periods within their cells. This is because many environmental toxins are, as mentioned, fat soluble. Because plants have little or no fat, they can more easily systemically rid their tissues of many of these toxins over time.

Further, as the research has shown, a diet heavy in complex proteins – which contain far more amino acids than our bodies require – increases the risk and severity of inflammation. Amino acids are the building blocks of protein. A complex protein can have tens of thousands of amino acids. While proteins and aminos are healthy, a diet too rich in them will produce deposits in our joints and tissues, burdening our immune system.

As we discussed in the last chapter, research also reveals that diets rich in red meats discourage the colonization of our probiotics, and encourage the growth of pathogenic microorganisms that release endotoxins that clog our metabolism and overload our immune system. Diets rich in red meats also produce byproducts such as phytanic acid and beta-glucuronidase that can damage our intestinal cells and mucosal membranes within the intestines. Greater levels of cooked saturated fats also raise cholesterol levels, especially lipid peroxidation-prone low-density lipoproteins (LDL).

The complexities of digesting complex proteins produce increased levels of beta-glucuronidase, nitroreductase, azoreductase, steroid 7-alpha-dehydroxylase, ammonia, urease, cholylglycine hydrolase, phytanic acid and others. These toxic enzymes deter our probiotics and produce systemic inflammation. Not surprisingly, they've been linked to colon cancer.

By contrast, plant-based foods contain many antioxidants, anti-carcinogens and other nutrients that strengthen the immune system and balance the body's pH. Plant-based foods also discourage inflammatory responses. Plant-based foods feed our probiotics with complex polysaccharides called prebiotics. They are also a source of fiber (there is little fiber in red meat) – critical for intestinal health.

The Mediterranean diet does not completely eliminate meat, but it is focused on more plant-based foods, healthier oils and less red meat. However we configure our diet, there are choices we can make at every meal. The research shows that the greater our diet trends toward the Mediterranean diet, the lower our toxic load will be and the stronger our immunity will be. This will allow us to better combat and eventually lower systemic inflammation.

This also not a condemnation of dairy. Milk is a great food, assuming it contains what nature intended: probiotics. Real milk is inseparable from probiotics, and when probiotics are killed off by pasteurization, milk becomes a dubious food.

Nature's food packages as delivered by living organisms are better than the stripped down, refined and purified versions we produce. This seems just too complicated for us. We cannot seem to understand this. Why cannot we just isolate those constituents contained in the healthy food versions and just add them into our unhealthy foods and make them healthy? Perhaps it might help to consider that food scientists have found more than 10,000 phytochemicals in tomatoes, and more than 27 medicinal constituents in garlic (and most likely hundreds more phytochemicals).

# Chapter Six

# Our Ancestors' Foods

Real foods are not only nourishing, they are medicinal. In this chapter we'll discuss strategies to arm and boost the body's nutrient levels naturally. Without taking vitamins or mineral supplements, we should be able to keep our nutrient levels up if we consume nature's whole nutrient resources.

Here we will lay out the foods that we should incorporate into our diets. Certainly it may be difficult for some to completely give up eating certain foods. And certainly, some of those foods may be toxic to our body (such as deep-fried foods) because they release lipid peroxidation into our bodies. Still, this protocol does not necessarily require us to fully give up our current diets – though it might be healthier to do so.

Rather, this protocol is about *adding* certain foods and nutrients to our diet. We can incorporate these foods as best we can, while making selections among the foods that we outline here. In other words, we can add the foods and nutrients that are more available to us, and can more easily be blended into our diets.

For this reason, this book will not outline extensive recipes. Recipes can be awfully restrictive. And restrictive diets do not last long. Rather, this chapter will lay out a number of foods in each category, and the reader can choose the foods to add to their current recipes. This may require a bit of substitution for some, but there are many natural food recipe books on the market today that will outline how to have most of the standard dishes we might eat today, but with the foods we outline here.

It should be added that doing this will have an interesting effect: Because most of the foods outlined here are tasty and delicious when added to our recipes, and because they have a positive benefit upon our moods, our immunity and our energy levels, it is likely that we will naturally add more and more of these foods to our diet. As we do that, we will experience even more of the benefits that these living foods provide – without having to undergo either a restrictive diet or a maddeningly disciplined protocol.

## Antioxidant Foods

When we harvest a fresh plant-based food and eat it with minimal storage, processing and cooking, we are deriving significant benefits from the living organism that produced the food. Because living organisms defend themselves against toxins throughout their lives, by eating fresh whole foods or whole foods minimally cooked, our bodies can utilize the same elements the plant utilized to protect itself against toxins.

This in turn stimulates our immune systems, and also provides direct free radical protection. This is because antioxidants are designed to neutralize toxins.

As we've discussed, a plethora of research has confirmed that damage from free radicals is implicated in many health conditions. Free radicals from toxins damage cells, cell membranes, organs, blood vessel walls and airways – producing systemic inflammation – as the immune system responds to an overload of tissue damage.

Free radicals are produced by synthetic chemicals, pathogens, trans fats, fried foods, red meats, radiation, pollution and various intruders that destabilize within the body. Free radicals are molecules or ions that require stabilization. They reach stabilization by 'stealing' atoms from the cells or tissues of our body. This in turn destabilizes those cells and tissues – producing damage.

Antioxidants serve to stabilize free radicals before our cells and tissues are robbed – by donating their own atoms. A diet with plenty of fruits and vegetables supplies numerous antioxidants. Although antioxidants cannot be considered treatments for any disease, many studies have proved that increased antioxidant intake supports immune function and detoxification. These effects allow the immune system to respond with greater tolerance.

Antioxidant constituents in plant-based foods are known to significantly repeal free radicals, strengthen the immune system and help detoxify the system. These include *lecithin* and *octacosanol* from whole grains; *polyphenols* and *sterols* from vegetables; *lycopene* from tomatoes and watermelons; *quercetin* and *sulfur/allicin* from garlic, onions and peppers; *pectin* and *rutin* from apples and other fruits; *phytocyanidin flavonoids* such as *apigenin* and *luteolin* from various greenfoods; and *anthocyanins* from various fruits and oats.

Some sea-based botanicals like kelp also contain antioxidants as well. Consider a special polysaccharide compound from kelp called *fucoidan*. Fucoidan has been shown in animal studies to significantly reduce inflammation (Cardoso *et al.* 2009; Kuznetsova *et al.* 2004).

*Procyanidins* are found in apples, currants, cinnamon, bilberry and many other foods. The extract of *Vitis vinifera* seed (grapeseed) is one of the highest sources of bound antioxidant *proanthocyanidins* and *leucocyanidines* called *procyanidolic oligomers* or PCOs. Pycnogenol® also contains significant levels of these PCOs. Blueberries, parsley, green tea, black

currant, some legumes and onions also contain PCOs and similar proanthocyanidins.

Research has demonstrated that PCOs have protective and strengthening effects on tissues by increasing enzyme conjugation (Seo *et al.*
2001). PCOs have also been shown to increase vascular wall strength
(Robert *et al.* 2000).

Oxygenated carotenoids such as *lutein* and *astaxanthin* also have been
shown to exhibit strong antioxidant activity. Astaxanthin is derived from
the microalga *Haematococcus pluvialis,* and lutein is available from a number of foods, including spirulina.

Most of these phytonutrients specifically modulate the immune system. For example, the flavonoids *kaempferol* and *flavone* have been shown
to block mast cell proliferation by over 80% (Alexandrakis *et al.* 2003).
Sources of kaempferol include Brussels sprouts, broccoli, grapefruit and
apples.

Furthermore, *resveratrol* from grapes and berries modulate nuclear
factor-kappaB and transcription/Janus kinase pathways – which strengthens immunity. Good sources of resveratrol include peanuts, red grapes,
cranberries and cocoa (wine is not advisable for cleansing as we'll discuss
later).

Nearly every plant-food has some measure of phytonutrients discussed above and more. These phytonutrients alkalize the blood and increase the detoxification capabilities of the liver. They help clear the blood
of toxins.

Foods that are particularly detoxifying and immunity-building include
fresh pineapples, beets, cucumbers, apricots, apples, almonds, zucchini,
artichokes, avocados, bananas, beans, collard greens, berries, casaba, celery, coconuts, cranberries, watercress, dandelion greens, grapes, raw honey,
corn, kale, citrus fruits, watermelon, lettuce, mangoes, mushrooms, oats,
broccoli, okra, onions, papayas, parsley, peas, whole grains, radishes, raisins, spinach, tomatoes, walnuts, and many others.

These plant-based foods are also our primary source of soluble and
insoluble fiber. Diets with significant fiber help clear the blood and tissues
of toxins, and lipid peroxidation-friendly LDL cholesterol. Fiber is also
critical to a healthy digestive tract and intestinal barrier. Fiber in the diet
should range from about 35 to 45 grams per day according to the recommendations of many diet experts. Six to ten servings of raw fruits and
vegetables per day should accomplish this – which is even part of the
USDA's recommendations. This means raw, fibrous foods should be present at every meal.

Good fibrous plant sources also contain healthy *lignans* and *phytoestrogens* that help balance hormone levels, and help the body make its own natural corticoids. Foods that contain these include peas, garbanzo beans, soybeans, kidney beans and lentils.

Plant-based foods provide these immune-stimulating factors because these vary same factors make up the plants' own immune systems. For example, the red, blue and green flavonoid pigments in plants and fruits help protect the plant from oxidative damage from radiation. The proanthocyanidins in grains like oats, for example, help protect the oat plant from crown rust caused by the *Puccinia coronata* fungus. So the same biochemicals that stimulate immunity in humans are part of plants' immune systems.

These same whole food phytonutrients also neutralize oxidative radicals in our bodies – the reason they are called antioxidants. How do we know this? Scientists can measure the ability of a particular food to neutralize free radicals with specific laboratory testing. One such test is called the *Oxygen Radical Absorbance Capacity Test* (ORAC). This technical laboratory study is performed by a number of scientific organizations that include the USDA, as well as specialized labs such as Brunswick Laboratories in Massachusetts.

Research from the USDA's Jean Mayer Human Nutrition Research Center on Aging at Tufts University has suggested that a diet high in ORAC value may protect blood vessels and tissues from free radical damage that can result in inflammation (Sofic *et al.* 2001; Cao *et al.* 1998). These tissues, of course, include the airways. Research has confirmed that consuming 3,000 to 5,000 ORAC units per day can have protective benefits.

### ORAC Values (100 grams) of Selected (raw) Fruits (USDA, 2007-2008)

| | | | | |
|---|---|---|---|---|
| Cranberry | 9,382 | | Pomegranate | 2,860 |
| Plum | 7,581 | | Orange | 1,819 |
| Blueberry | 6,552 | | Tangerine | 1,620 |
| Blackberry | 5,347 | | Grape (red) | 1,260 |
| Raspberry | 4,882 | | Mango | 1,002 |
| Apple (Granny) | 3,898 | | Kiwi | 882 |
| Strawberry | 3,577 | | Banana | 879 |
| Cherry (sweet) | 3,365 | | Tomato (plum) | 389 |
| Gooseberry | 3,277 | | Pineapple | 385 |
| Pear | 2,941 | | Watermelon | 142 |

There is tremendous attention these days on two unique fruits from the Amazon rain forest and China called *açaí* and *goji berry* (or wolfberry) respectively. A recent ORAC test documented by Schauss *et al.* (2006) gives açaí a score of 102,700 and tests documented by Dr. Paul Gross gives goji berries a total ORAC of 30,300. However, subsequent tests done by Brunswick Laboratories, Inc. gave these two berries 53,600 (açaí) and 22,000 (goji) total-ORAC values.

In addition, we must remember that these are the dried berries being tested in the latter case, and a concentrate of açaí being tested in the former case. The numbers in the chart above are for fresh fruits. Dried fruits will naturally have higher ORAC values, because the water is evaporated – giving more density and more antioxidants per 100 grams.

For example, in the USDA database, dried apples have a 6,681 total-ORAC value, while fresh apples range from 2,210 to 3,898 in total-ORAC value. This equates to a two-to-three times increase from fresh to dried. In another example, fresh red grapes have a 1,260 total-ORAC value, while raisins have a 3,037 total-ORAC value. This comes close to an increase of three times the ORAC value following dehydration.

Part of the equation, naturally, is cost. Dried fruit and concentrates are often more expensive than fresh fruit. High-ORAC dried fruits or concentrates from açaí or goji will also be substantially more expensive than most fruits grown domestically (especially for Americans and Europeans). Our conclusion is that local or in-country grown fresh fruits with high total-ORAC values produce the best value. Local fresh fruit offers great free radical scavenging ability, support for local farmers, and pollen proteins we are most likely more tolerant to.

By comparison, spinach – an incredibly wholesome vegetable with a tremendous amount of nutrition – has a fraction of the ORAC content of some of these fruits, at 1,515 total ORAC. Spinach, of course, contains many other nutrients, including proteins lacking in many high-ORAC fruits.

Dehydrated spices can have incredibly high ORAC values. For example, USDA's database lists ground Turmeric's total ORAC value at 159,277 and oregano's at 200,129. However, while we might only consume a few hundred milligrams of a spice per day, we can eat many grams – if not pounds – of sweet colorful fruit every day.

Red tart cherries have even higher levels of ORAC than most other cherries. That's not all. Montmorency (red tart) cherries also have a number of other powerful phyto-nutrients, including melatonin, anthocyanins 1, 2 and 3, perillyl alcohol, quercetin, SOD (super oxide dismutase) and many others.

Melatonin has been connected to relaxation, sleep and healthy circadian rhythms. Anthocyanins have been linked to helping protect arteries from plaque build-up and other tissues from oxidative damage. Perillyl alcohol and ellagic acid have been studied for their cancer-protective qualities, while quercetin and SOD have been shown to support detoxification and healthy immune function.

## The Need for Chlorophyll

Chlorophyll is a primary constituent of green vegetables. It is the pigment that makes plants green. Plants use chlorophyll to help convert the sun's energy into nutrition in a process called photosynthesis.

Nutritionists and traditional doctors have long held that chlorophyll provides numerous health benefits. Besides the array of vitamins, minerals and other phytonutrients, new research illustrates that chlorophyll protects against the formation and growth of tumors.

The study, from Oregon State University (McQuistan et al. 2011), first analyzed a number of studies that have been done testing chlorophyll for cancer prevention, including those involving rainbow trout, mice and humans. In the human study, cellular uptake of the carcinogen aflatoxin was blocked by chlorophyll.

The researchers then focused on what is called the dose-response relationship between chlorophyll and the prevention of tumor-genesis – or cancer formation.

The research utilized 12,360 rainbow trout, treated with chlorophyll after exposure to dibenzochrysene – a toxic carcinogen. Those trout given chlorophyll had from 29 to 64 percent fewer liver tumors, and 24 to 45 percent fewer stomach tumors. The mechanism involved again appears to be that chlorophyll blocks carcinogen absorption and use by the cells.

However, when carcinogen exposure was significantly increased, chlorophyll did little to reduce tumors, and even accompanied an increase in the number of tumors. However, the researchers characterized this level of toxin exposure as "unrealistic."

In other words, when considering the typical exposure to toxins, and the healthy inclusion of vegetables in the diet – within the parameters that resulted in chlorophyll's ability to reduce tumors – there is a clear cancer prevention benefit from eating dark green leafy vegetables and other chlorophyll sources.

The researchers concluded:

> *"These results show that chlorophyll concentrations encountered in chlorophyll-rich green vegetables can provide substantial cancer chemoprotection, and suggest that they do so by reducing carcinogen bioavailability."*

## Quercetin Foods

A number of foods and herbs that reduce inflammation and toxicity contain quercetin. This is no coincidence. Multiple studies have shown that quercetin inhibits the release inflammatory mediators histamine and leukotrienes. Foods rich in quercetin include onions, garlic, apples, capers, grapes, leafy greens, tomatoes and broccoli. In addition, many of the herbs listed earlier contain quercetin as an active constituent. Many of the herbs listed in the herbal section also contain quercetin. Onions, garlic and apples contain some of the highest levels.

Quercetin stimulates and balances the immune system. In an *in vivo* study, four weeks of quercetin reduced histamine levels and allergen-specific IgE levels. More importantly, quercetin inhibited anaphylaxis responses (Shishehbor *et al.* 2010).

Cairo researchers (Haggag *et al.* 2003) found that among mast cells exposed to allergens and chemicals in the laboratory, quercetin inhibited histamine release by 95% and 97%.

Over the past few years, an increasing amount of evidence is pointing to the conclusion that foods with quercetin slow inflammatory response and autoimmune derangement. Researchers from Italy's Catholic University (Crescente *et al.* 2009) found that quercetin inhibited arachidonic acid-induced platelet aggregation. Arachidonic acid-induced platelet aggregation is seen in allergic inflammatory mechanisms.

Researchers from the University of Crete (Alexandrakis *et al.* 2003) found that quercetin can inhibit mast cell proliferation by up to 80%. Onions have also been shown *in vivo* tests to reduce bronchoconstriction.

Organic foods contain higher levels of quercetin. A study from the University of California-Davis' Department of Food Science and Technology (Mitchell *et al.* 2007) tested flavonoid levels between organic and conventional tomatoes over a ten-year period. Their research concluded that quercetin levels were 79% higher for tomatoes grown organically under the same conditions as conventionally-grown tomatoes.

## Root Foods

It is no coincidence that many antioxidants are roots, such as ginger, turmeric, onions garlic, beets, carrots, turnips, parsnips and others. These root foods are known for their ability to alkalize the bloodstream and stimulate detoxification. They are also known to help rejuvenate the liver and adrenal glands.

Beets, for example, contain, among other nutrients, betaine, betalains, betacyanin and betanin. They also contain generous portions of folate, iron and fiber. One of the primary fibers in beets is pectin, which is also found in apples. Pectin has a unique soluble and insoluble fiber content that maximizes the attachment of radical-producing LDL cholesterol in the intestines. Pectin also attaches to many other toxins, drawing them out of the body as well.

Meanwhile, betaine is known as stimulating liver health. Betaine has been shown to reduce liver injury (Okada *et al.* 2011). Betaine is also considered healthy for the bile ducts, because it helps draw out toxins. Beets are delicious foods that can be grated into salads, juiced, steamed, baked and simply eaten raw. Red beets are typically considered the healthiest, but pink and white beets also contain betaine.

We should note that while beets contain significant amounts of betaine, other betaine-rich foods include broccoli, spinach and some whole grains.

Each of the root foods listed above contain unique constituents that support liver health and detoxification.

Consider for a moment, beets.

Several recent studies have proven that beetroot increases not only athletic endurance and stamina, but also increases cardiovascular health by lowering blood pressure and reducing free radical damage.

One of the more recent studies comes from the UK's University of Exeter Sport and Health Sciences department (Kelly *et al.* 2013). The research tested team sport players in a double-blind study. Fourteen of the athletes were given 490 milliliters of beet juice and a matched group was given the same beet juice but without the nitrate content.

They found that the beet juice with nitrate group performed at significantly greater levels than the other group and had faster recovery rates. The researchers concluded:

*"Dietary nitrate supplementation improves performance during intense intermittent exercise and may be a useful ergogenic aid for team sports players."*

Another study, this from the University of Exeter (Wylie *et al.* 2013) found in testing nine athletes with cycling tests, that 250 milliliters of beet juice twice a day significantly increased endurance during intense exercise. Several other studies from the same university have confirmed these findings.

As researchers have struggled to find the mechanism and active constituent, it appears beets supply some complex biomolecules that fuel the cell's energy producers – the mitochondria.

A study from Mexican researchers (Alcántar-Aguirre *et al.* 2013) found that beet juice stimulates the voltage-dependent anion channels within the mitochondria. This creates a more streamlined production of energy in a pathway called oxidative phosphorylation.

This mechanism proves out in practical endurance situations as well. Researchers at the Saint Louis University (Murphy *et al.* 2013) studied 11 athletes (men and women). The subjects were either given placebo or 200 grams of baked beets prior to being tested.

Those who ate the baked beets ran 0.4 kilometers faster than the athletes who ate the placebo on average for a five kilo run, but during the last mile, the beet eaters rant 5% than those who did not eat the beets.

The researchers concluded:

> *"Consumption of nitrate-rich, whole beetroot improves running performance in healthy adults."*

Mid Sweden University researchers (Engan *et al.* 2012) also found that the nitrate content in beets may help sleep apnea as well.

Research from the University of Reading (Hobbs *et al.* 2012) found that beetroot juice and even bread infused with beets significantly lowered both systolic and diastolic blood pressure among 32 adults.

Research from The Netherlands' Maastricht University Medical Centre (Engan *et al.* 2012) found that 140 milliliters of concentrated beet juice a day significantly improved the times and speeds in cycling tests on cycling athletes.

Meanwhile, Polish university researchers (Zielińska-Przyjemska *et al.* 2012) found that the betanin in beets stimulated developing immune cells – neutrophils – and reduced free radicals.

Other studies have found that the nitrate content in beetroot juice increases muscle efficiency and exercise intolerance (Cermak *et al.* 2012).

Beets also contain lutein, which has been shown to slow down age-related macular degeneration.

A study from Texas (Włodarek *et al.* 2011) showed that beets and other nitrate-containing foods can increase endothelial function.

Perhaps those cyclists and other athletes who want to somehow increase their performances might consider beets over steroids?

Other root foods have high nitrate levels, because roots typically fix nitrogen. Roots also contain numerous medicinal compounds. Other root foods to include in our diet are potatoes, carrots, onions, ginger, peanuts, turnips and others.

## Cruciferae

The Cruciferae family, often termed cruciferous, includes broccoli, cabbage, bok choy, watercress, cauliflower, collards, kale, turnips, rutabaga, mustard seeds, radish, daikon, wasabi, arugula, komatsuna, cress, horseradish and even rapeseed (canola is a rapeseed hybrid).

Cruciferous veggies contain numerous constituents that improve liver function and stimulate the immune system. These include sulforaphane and allyl isothiocyanate – which was shown in a study from the University of Pittsburgh to inhibit prostate cancer cells (Xiao *et al.* 2003).

Besides glucoraphanin, these include indoles, glucosinolates, dithiolthiones, sulfoxides, isothiocyanates, sulforaphane and indole-carbinol.

Here we will discuss broccoli and cabbage, but the Cruiferae family shares most of these benefits.

## Broccoli

Researchers from Italy (Riso *et al.* 2013) have determined that eating broccoli for just ten days will cut inflammation in more than half. Other studies find it prevents and repairs DNA damage and may even curb osteoarthritis.

For ten days, the researchers – from Italy's University of Milan – gave 250 grams of broccoli to a group of young smokers.

Before and after the study the researchers collected blood from the subjects and conducted an extensive analysis of the blood. They measured the subjects' various immune cell status, including C-reactive protein (CRP) levels, tumor necrosis factor alpha (TNF-α) levels, interleukin 6 (IL-6) and adiponectin. They also analyzed levels of folate and lutein in the blood.

After the 10-day broccoli-enriched diet the subjects were re-tested and the researchers found that their CRP levels went down by 48%. This is a significant drop in CRP levels, indicating the smokers' inflammatory levels went down by over a half.

The researchers also found that circulating levels of lutein and folate went up as well. The drop in CRP levels was found independent of lutein and folate levels, and the researchers found that lycopene increases also accompanied a drop in IL6 levels – indicating a relationship between lycopene and inflammation factors – as other studies have confirmed.

This study confirms an earlier study done at the same university in 2010 (Riso *et al.* 2010). In this study the researchers tested 27 young smokers who were otherwise healthy, and gave them either 250 grams of steamed broccoli per day or a control diet. In this study the researchers tested mRNA and DNA enzyme levels – which relate directly to the repair of DNA. They also measured DNA strand breaks within the blood.

In this study, the researchers found that those eating the broccoli had 41% drop in strand breaks of DNA, and other changes in enzyme levels associated with DNA protection.

Meanwhile, researchers from the UK's University of East Anglia (Roberts 2013) are conducting a study of 20 patients with osteoarthritis by serving them 100 grams of broccoli for two weeks. The researchers believe, based upon mice studies, that broccoli – and perhaps this super-strain of broccoli being tested with more glucoraphanin levels – will help reduce inflammation associated with osteoarthritis.

In a number of laboratory studies, broccoli has been shown to be anti-carcinogenic as well as helpful for heart and cardiovascular disease.

Broccoli is also a significant source of tocopherols, magnesium, selenium, thiamin, riboflavin and pantothenic acid.

Broccoli sprouts have been shown to have more of these anti-inflammatory and anti-cancer nutrients than conventional broccoli.

## Cabbage

Nature also provides nutrients from whole foods that can help rebuild our mucosal membranes. One of the more productive whole foods applicable to rebuilding our body's mucosal membranes is cabbage. Cabbage contains a unique constituent, s-methylmethionine, also referred to as vitamin U. Through a pathway utilizing one of the body's natural enzymes, called Bhmt2, s-methylmethionine is converted to methionine and then to glutathione in several steps.

In this form, glutathione has been shown to stimulate the repair of the mucosal membranes within the stomach, intestines and airways. Glutathione has also been shown to increase the health and productivity of the liver.

Raw cabbage or cabbage juice has been used as a healing agent for ulcers and intestinal issues for thousands of years among traditional medicines, including those of Egyptian, Ayurvedic and Greek systems. The Western world became aware of raw cabbage juice in the 1950s, when Garnett Cheney, M.D. conducted several studies showing that methylmethionine-rich cabbage juice concentrate was able to reduce the pain and bleeding associated with ulcers.

In one of Dr. Cheney's studies, 37 ulcer patients were treated with either cabbage juice concentrate or a placebo. Of the 26-patient cabbage juice group, 24 patients were considered "successes" – achieving an astounding 92% success rate.

Medical researchers from Iraq's University Department of Surgery (Salim 1993) conducted a double-blind study of 172 patients who suffered from gastric bleeding caused by non-steroidal anti-inflammatory drugs (NSAIDs). They gave the patients either cysteine, methylmethionine sulfonium chloride (MMSC) or a placebo. Those receiving either the cysteine or the MMSC stopped bleeding. Their conditions became *"stable"* as compared with many in the control group, who continued to bleed.

Plants use s-methylmethionine to help heal cell membrane damage among their leaves and stems. This is reminiscent of antioxidants: Plants produce antioxidants to help to protect them from damage from the sun, insects and diseases. In other words, the very same biochemicals that protect plants also help heal our bodies.

Note that MMSC or cabbage juice does not inhibit the flow of gastric juices in the stomach to produce these effects as do acid blocking medications. Rather, they stimulate the body's natural production of mucous, which serves to protect the stomach's cells from the effects of acids.

## Watercress

Watercress contains a host of antioxidant nutrients, including xanthophyll, beta-carotene, alpha-tocopherol and gamma-tocopherol (two forms of vitamin E), each of which have been shown to slow free radical formation in the body.

Strenuous exercise typically produces DNA damage, which a healthy body will hopefully repair. Watercress has been shown to reduce DNA damage and cancer growth.

Research from Britain's Edinburgh Napier University (Fogarty et al. 2012) found that watercress reduces DNA damage and oxidative stress induced by exercise, confirming other research showing watercress inhibits cancer.

The researchers studied ten healthy young men (average age 23) for four months. The men were tested before and after the study, and on a daily basis, before an after exhausting aerobic exercise. During one eight-week period, the subjects took watercress supplements daily, two hours before exercise. During the other eight-week period, they were given 85 grams of watercress two hours before their workouts.

When given the watercress supplement, the men showed a significant reduction in reactive oxygen species levels, and the damage to their DNA as a result of exercise.

Blood samples revealed that levels of lipid peroxidation – the major cause for artery disease – were also significantly lower when taking the watercress.

The researchers commented on this aspect of the study:

> "The study demonstrates that exhaustive aerobic exercise may cause DNA damage and lipid peroxidation; however, these perturbations are attenuated by either short- or long-term watercress supplementation, possibly due to the higher concentration lipid-soluble antioxidants following watercress ingestion."

Previous research has established that watercress contains a nutrient called phenethyl isothiocyanate or PEITC. Georgetown University researchers (Wang et al. 2011) established that PEITC inhibited the growth of cervical cancer and breast cancer cells.

## Living Greens

A greenfood is a category of foods that are considered nutritionally superior than the typical fruits and vegetables. Greenfoods include the wheat grasses, sprouts, algae, and sea vegetables.

Greenfoods provide practically every nutrient imaginable, including enzymes, minerals, trace elements, essential and non-essential amino acids, vitamins, antioxidants and various phytonutrients. Many will provide over 1,000 nutrients.

A big benefit of greenfoods is their alkalinity. This gives them the ability to neutralize radicals and lipid peroxides.

Much of this alkalinity comes from greenfoods' bioavailable mineral content. Many of these minerals are also are colloidal. They tend to be hydrophobic, and maintain a positive electrical charge – rendering them alkaline.

### Leafies

Leafy greens include lettuce, kale, spinach, chard, beet leaves, cabbage, mustard greens and turnip greens. They are nutrition powerhouses, containing folates, antioxidants, minerals like iron, potassium and calcium, and a whole array of vitamins including vitamin K. They also contain beta-carotene, lutein, zeaxanthin and others.

The need for vitamin K is critical to immunity, as it helps regulate inflammation, healing and blood clotting.

But there's more.

Australian researchers (Rankin *et al.* 2013) determined that green leafy and cruciferous vegetables stimulate the immune system of the intestines by donating a gene that regulates the gut's defense mechanisms.

The research comes from the University of Melbourne and Melbourne's Walter and Eliza Hall Institute of Medical Research. The researchers studied the ingestion of leafy and cruciferous vegetables along with other foods. They measured and analyzed intestinal levels of interleukin 22 – a critical element that regulates intestinal immunity through an immune cell called NKp46+. This is also called an innate lymphoid cell – or ILC.

IL-22 and the innate lymphoid cells play a critical part of the intestine's control of inflammatory conditions and food allergies. Low levels have been seen amongst various inflammatory diseases.

The genetic factor which stimulates these innate lymphoid cells from greens is called T-bet. T-bet is a genetic transcription factor that stimulates the a type of signalling gene called a Notch gene. These Notch genes stimulate the conversion of from lymphoid tissue-inducers to innate lymphoid cells, according to the research.

The research was led by Dr. Gabrielle Belz from the Walter and Eliza Hall Institute. Dr. Belz commented on the research:

> *"we discovered that T-bet is the key gene that instructs precursor cells to develop into ILCs (innate lymphoid cells), which it does in response to signals in the food we eat and to bacteria in the gut. ILCs are essential for immune surveillance of the digestive system and this is the first time that we have identified a gene responsible for the production of ILCs."*

The research illustrated that leafy and cruciferous greens apparently donate key proteins. "Proteins in these leafy greens could be part of the same signalling pathway that is used by T-bet to produce ILCs," added Dr. Belz.

The green vegetables apparently interact with cell surface receptors, which switch on the T-bet gene.

## Celery

The Romans awarded wreaths of celery to winners of sporting events. Ancient Asian cultures harvested wild celery and brewed it to produce a tonic used for stomach difficulties and general vitality. Celery garlands were found inside tombs of ancient Egyptian pharaohs. While many other cultures used wild celery as a medicinal herb, cultivated celery is mentioned being grown in France in 1623, and celery began being grown commercially in the U.S. in the 1880s.

The famous Naturopath, Dr. Paavo Airola, recommended celery for blood purification, detoxification and for building immunity. Dr. Bernard Jensen has recommended it for neutralizing rheumatic acids within the body, detoxification, fevers, nervous conditions and cardiovascular conditions.

Celery is a member of the parsley family. It contains a host of nutrients, including potassium, vitamin K, vitamin A, folate and vitamin B6. It also contains a number of phytonutrients. Notably celery is also rich in sulfur, which has been shown to be useful for joint conditions.

One Chinese remedy celery has been used for is to lower blood pressure. Dr. Quang Le and Dr. William Elliott from the University of Chicago found that one of celery's phytonutrients, 3-n-butyl phthalide, reduced blood pressure by 13-14% by eating the equivalent of four stalks per day. Dr. Le also tried this remedy himself and found that his blood pressure went from 158/96 to 118/82.

Celery also contains compounds called acetylenics. Acetylenics have been shown in several studies to inhibit tumor growth (Siddiq and Dembitsky 2008).

Celery also contains phenolic acids. Phenolic acids provide protection against free radical oxidative damage, and slow inflammation. Oxidative free radical damage is what causes arteriosclerosis, stroke, liver damage and heart disease in general.

In a study done by researchers from the Chinese Academy of Agricultural Sciences (Yao et al. 2010), 11 cultivars of celery from two different species were examined for their phenolic acid composition. The phenols found in the celeries included caffeic acid, p-coumaric acid, and ferulic acid. P-coumaric acid was the most abundant phenolic acid found amongst the samples. They also found several flavonoids, including apigenin, luteolin, and kaempferoland.

Furthermore, the researchers found that the phenols and flavonoids in celery exhibited significant antioxidant potency. Of the 11 cultivars studied, Shengjie celery had the highest antioxidant activity, and the Tropica variety had the lowest levels of antioxidant potentcy.

Just as proposed by Dr. Airola decades earlier, the phenolic acids in celery stimulate phenolsulfotransferases (PSTs) within the body. PSTs are detoxifying metabolic enzymes that stimulate the removal of toxic compounds, including pharmaceutical chemicals and environmental chemicals.

In a study by researchers from Taiwan's National Chung Hsing University (Yeh and Yen 2005), phenolic acids were shown to directly increase the levels and activities of PST-P within the body. In a study using 20 different vegetables, celery was among the top five (along with asparagus, broccoli, cauliflower, celery and eggplant,) that stimulated PST-P the most among human HepG2 cells.

Celery is best eaten raw, but it can also be juiced and put into soups. Each of these methods will preserve most of the phytonutrient levels. A vegetable-barley soup with sliced celery is also delicious. Put the sliced fresh celery into the pot only after the barley has been cooked enough to be soft. After 10 more minutes on a low flame, the celery will be softened enough to eat, but not overcooked.

Celery also makes a fun and great snack for kids when combined with peanut butter and/or cream cheese. Just spread unsweetened natural peanut butter and/or fresh cream cheese into the chamber of the stalk to the brim and hand it over. It makes a delicious, satisfying and nutritious snack that your child will never forget.

**Parsley**

Parsley is rich in numerous antioxidant nutrients, including vitamin A, vitamin C, vitamin E, beta carotene, lutein, cryptoxanthin, zeaxanthin, folate and is one of the greatest sources of vitamin K, with 1640 micrograms per gram – over 12 times the U.S. DRI (dietary reference intake) of 90-120 micrograms per day. One hundred grams of Parsley also contains more than double the RDA for vitamin C and almost triple the RDA of vitamin A.

These antioxidant nutrients have been shown to reduce the effects of oxidation of lipids, relating directly to reducing vision disorders, heart disease, dementia and other inflammation-related conditions.

Hungarian researchers (Pápay et al. 2012) confirmed that parsley (*Petroselinum crispum*) contains significant anti-inflammatory properties, boosts liver health, is antioxidant and even anti-carcinogenic. It also supplies numerous nutrients and relaxes smooth muscles.

The research found that parsley contained numerous nutrients and bioactive constituents, including several flavonoids and cumarins. One flavonoid called apigenin has been shown to provide significant anti-tumor properties, as well as the ability to slow inflammation and neutralize oxidative radicals (free radicals). Its ability to stop tumor growth lies in its ability to block tumors from creating blood vessels.

Research published from China's Jiangsu Polytechnic College of Agriculture and Forestry (Liu et al. 2011) found that apigenin also blocked the action of MEK kinase 1, which in turn prevented bladder cancer cells from migrating and thus inhibited tumor growth.

The ability of Parsley to relax smooth muscles appears to come from its blocking of the polymerization of actin. This has significant importance to asthmatics, as a severe asthmatic attack will accompany the over-contraction of the smooth muscles around the lungs. Relaxing those smooth muscles is one key component of urgent care in asthmatic attacks.

Other bioactive constituents in Parsley include eugenol, crisoeriol, luteolin and apiin. Eugenol has been used by traditional doctors as an antiseptic and pain-reliever in cases of gingivitis and periodontal disease, and has been shown to reduce blood sugar levels in diabetics.

Parsley's ability to encourage healing has also been shown in numerous studies.

For example, a study published from Turkey's Hacettepe University Faculty of Medicine (Tavil et al. 2012) found that increased parsley consumption was associated with fewer complications after hematopoietic (bone marrow) stem cell transplantation in children.

In this study, the diets of 41 children who underwent the stem cell transplantation were analyzed. Improved outcomes were seen among those eating more Parsley, as well as those children who ate onions, bulgur, yogurt and bazlama (a Turkish yeast bread).

## Sprout Power

Sprouts and their powders are nutritional powerhouses. They have exponential nutritional value, well above the nutrient content of their seeds or the fully-grown plants. This was confirmed in 1970s experiments by former Hippocrates Health Institute Director of Research, Viktoras Kulvinskas, M.S. Kulvinskas, who found that ascorbic acid levels in soybean sprouts increased from zero to 103 milligrams per 100 grams by day six – about the ascorbic acid content found in lime juice. These levels fall off significantly within days.

Each plant has a different nutrient peak. Ascorbic acid content in broad bean sprouts – used to cure scurvy during World War I – peaks in three days, after which the levels fall off.

Many believe that sprouts produce this greater antioxidant content to defend themselves against threats from the soil.

During germination beans and seeds undergo a natural enzyme-intensive process, converting protein peptides and surrounding inorganic minerals to highly digestible chelated amino acid-mineral complexes. Various other nutrient levels increase during soy germination. Levels of vitamin C, riboflavin, niacin and biotin increase from 25% to 150% during germination (Kulvinskas *et al.* 1978). Highly antioxidative phenolic compounds also develop during sprouting according to recent research (Lin *et al.* 2006).

Great nutritional sprouts include wheat grass sprouts, barley, oats, beans, broccoli and cabbage. The latter two provide a class of nutrients called glucosinolates. These glucosinolates yield sulfur compounds and indole-3 carbinols. Both have shown to have significant anticarcinogenic and anti-inflammatory effects in the body.

Researchers from Mexico's prestigious Monterrey Institute of Technology (Guajardo-Flores et al. 2013) determined that black bean sprouts are anticarcinogenic against breast cancer, liver cancer and colon cancer cells.

The researchers sprouted black beans (Phaseolus vulgaris) and then tested them and their constituents against cancer cell lines of various types of cancers. The researchers found that after three days and five days of germination, the phytonutrient extracts isolated the sprouts were able to inhibit the growth of all the cancer cells tested.

They also tested the same sprout isolates against non-cancerous (healthy) cells as controls, and found no negative impact upon these healthy cells.

The sprouts only inhibited the growth of the cancer cells.

The researchers then isolated some of the constituents of the sprouted beans, and found that the saponins and flavonoids had the greatest inhibition against liver and colon cancer cells. Meanwhile the genistein content of the sprouts was found to inhibit the breast cancer cells.

The researchers also found the black bean sprouts to be particularly high in antioxidants.

Early sprout research as documented by Hofsten (1979) and others has determined that during the germination process many nutrients are increased or made more available for assimilation. Other research (Chen and Pan 1977) found that phytic acid in soy beans decreased 22% while the enzyme phytase increased 227% after five days of soybean germination. Because phytic acid/phytate will bind minerals, nutrients like calcium and zinc are more assimilable. Also the oligosaccharides that produce flatulence are hydrolyzed during germination, making bean sprouts easier to digest.

A study last winter from the Complutense University of Madrid (López et al. 2013) found that raw, cooked and germinated black beans (Phaseolus vulgaris) all had anti-tumor effects, particularly with colorectal and breast cancer as well as melanoma cancer cells. The raw beans had the most anti-tumor effects in this research.

Seed or bean selection for sprouting is critical. A good quality seed or bean will germinate at least 50%. Heirloom seeds often germinate at much higher rates.

## Sea Vegetables

The ocean's plant kingdom provides an incredible source of nourishment for sea creatures and humans alike. For us, most ocean botanicals are either cultivated in ponds or sustainably wildcrafted from the ocean. Sea vegetables are not as sensitive to over-harvesting and bycatch issues. Because ocean plants rely upon photosynthesis rather than filtering, they are also less likely to contain environmental toxins like mercury and DDT.

There are about 70,000 known algae of three general types: Chlorophyta or green algae, Phaeophyta or brown algae and Rhodophyta, or red marine algae. These range from single-celled microalgae to giant broadleafed kelps. Sea vegetables trump all other food sources for protein production. While an acre of beef production yields about 20 pounds of useable protein, an acre of soybeans yields about 400 pounds. Seaweeds like nori can yield 800 pounds per acre of tidal zone, and spirulina can yield a whopping 21,000 lbs of useable protein per acre of pond cultivation.

Commercial spirulina is harvested from huge dedicated ponds in sunny areas and typically freeze-dried. Spirulina is a good source of carotenoids, vitamins, minerals, and important fatty acids like gamma linolenic acid—known to help reduce inflammation. Spirulina also contains all the essential and most non-essential amino acids, with 55-65% protein by weight. It also has a variety of phytonutrients such as zeaxanthin, myxoxanthophyll and lutein. Clinical studies have indicated spirulina can increase brain cell health, reduce inflammation, and help prevent cancer.

Chlorella pyrensoidosa, or simply chlorella, is also cultured in outdoor ponds. Over 800 published studies have confirmed its safety and efficacy for various health issues. Chlorella's ability to detoxify heavy metals and other toxins make it a favorite of natural health practitioners. Chlorella's phytonutrients include beta-carotene, various vitamins, and a substance called Chlorella Growth Factor—which seems to increase cell growth. Chlorella is also a complete protein at 40%-60% by weight with every essential and non-essential amino acid. Clinical studies have shown that chlorella stimulates T-cell and B-cell activity and increases macrophage activity. Chlorella has been shown to help fibromyalgia, hypertension, and ulcerative colitis. Its cell wall is tough, but most producers crush it. This releases polysaccharides and fiber, giving chlorella its unique ability to bind to toxins in the body.

Aphanizomenon flos-aquae—or simply AFA—is an alga that grows on the pristine volcanic waters of the Klamath Lake of Oregon. AFA's nutrients are readily available because of its soft cell wall. The rich volcanic lakebed of Klamath Lake renders it an available source of vitamins, minerals, phytonutrients, and all the essential and non-essential amino acids. Like spirulina and chlorella, AFA is a complete protein with 60% protein by weight. AFA also contains up to 58 trace minerals.

Another exciting pond-grown microalga is Haematococcus pluvialis, noted for containing astaxanthin. Astaxanthin is an oxygenated carotenoid with significant antioxidant properties, some hundreds of times the antioxidant value of vitamin E. Recent studies have shown astaxanthin to be effective in reducing inflammation and stimulating the immune system. Studies have shown astaxanthin's ability to prevent and treat retinal oxidative damage and macular degeneration, with activity greater than beta-carotene. Reports from marathoners and tri-athletes also reveal that astaxanthin increases recovery rates from rigorous exercise.

There are about 1,500 species of kelp-like brown algae, many of which flourish in the cold waters of the North Pacific and Atlantic oceans. Well known kelp-like sea veggies include nori, wakame, dulse, kombu, Irish moss, sea palm, and several species of laminaria. Kelps are harvested periodically and managed carefully—easy to do since kelp beds are stationary. Out of necessity, kelp farmers maintain a sustainable supply.

Kelps have an impressive array of vitamins—more than most land-based vegetables, with A, B1, B2, B5, B12, C, B6, B3, folic acid, E, K, and a steroid vitamin D precursor. Nori and dulse have beta-carotene levels as high as 50,000 IU per 100 grams. Certified organic kelps show 60 minerals at ppm levels. They are also good sources of calcium and magnesium. Most brown algae also contain all the essential amino acids. Nori is 30% protein by weight and other kelps average about 9%. Laminaria also produces the sugar substitute mannitol.

Kelps also contain a number of beneficial polysaccharides and polyphenols. One such sulfated polysaccharide, fucoidan, has been shown to have anti-tumor, anticoagulant and anti-angiogenic properties. Research shows it also inhibits allergic response, inhibits beta-amyloid formation (linked to Alzheimer's), and decreases artery platelet deposits.

Red marine algae research has confirmed some potentially amazing health benefits. Dumontiae, a larger-leaf Rhodaphyte typically harvested in colder oceans by either wildcrafting or rope farming, has been shown to inhibit growth of several viruses, notably herpes simplex I and II, and HIV. Most studies have pointed to their heparin-like sulfated polysaccharide content for antiviral effects, which blocks DNA and retroviral replication.

Michael Neushul, Ph.D. from University of California Santa Barbara's biology department has reported antiviral properties among all of the 39 California red marine algae varieties tested. Sulfated polysaccharides such as carrageenan are considered the central antiviral constituents, along with dextran sulfate and other heparinoids. Retrovirus inhibition has also been illustrated by the research.

Some algae also produce a potent and pure form of docosahexaenoic acid, or DHA—a fatty acid recommended by medical doctors and naturopaths alike for reducing inflammation and increasing cardiovascular health. Commercial DHA-producing microalgae are cultured in tanks, so their DHA is harvested without the risk of mercury or DDT toxicity. Algal DHA doesn't put pressure on fish populations. The two algal DHA microorganisms commercially produced are Crypthecodinium cohnii and Schizochytrium spp. They are now used in many supplements and infant formulas. Eicosapentaenoic acid or EPA is produced in the human body from DHA, so no need to add EPA.

While vegetables from the sea are often overlooked as viable food and supplement sources, they are some of the most nutritious foods on the planet. They can be used to increase well-being and stamina, rendering a stronger, healthier body and mind.

## Fruits, Fructose and Diabetes

While all the science illustrates that fruit is one of the keys to extending life and increasing vitality, there are still naysayers. We still find blogs and books saying that fruit is somehow bad for us – that it contains too much sugar and drives up our glucose levels.

There are even some diets that swear off of fruit, because they say the sugar in fruit – mostly fructose – is not good for us. Even some medical doctors contend that fruit is not good for a diabetic.

Well, that's just plain wrong.

A recent study by Danish hospital (Christensen *et al.* 2013) researchers has disproven the efficacy of this awful advice often given by conventional doctors and nutritionists – that type 2 diabetics should lay off the fruit.

The research comes from the Department of Nutrition of Denmark's West Jutland Regional Hospital. The researchers tested fruit consumption on 63 men and women who had been recently diagnosed with type 2 diabetes. The researchers randomized the participants into two groups. One group was given the advice to eat at least two fruits a day, while the other was given the more common conventional medicine advice to eat no more than two fruits a day. This advice accompanied the other typical medical and nutritional advice typically given to diabetics.

The participants then recorded their fruit consumption each day for three months. Before and after the trial began the patients were tested for HbA1c status, body weight and waist circumference. Because many of the patients were overweight, their diet plan also included strategies for weight loss.

The HbA1c test shows the mean glucose levels over the past three months. It illustrates glucose control among diabetics. Less than 5.6% or lower is considered normal, while 5.7 to 6.5 is considered pre-diabetic, and more than 6.5% is considered diabetic. The patients studied were all over 6.5%.

After the three months on their new diets, the patients were all retested, and their fruit consumption was analyzed together with their HbA1c results, weight and waist size.

The researchers found that those on the high fruit diet had little difference in their relative HbA1c levels, amount of weight loss or waist size as compared to the group that consumed less fruit.

The researchers concluded that:

> *"A recommendation to reduce fruit intake as part of standard medical nutrition therapy in overweight patients with newly diagnosed type 2 diabetes resulted in eating less fruit. It [consuming less fruit] had however no effect on HbA1c, weight loss or waist circumference. We rec-*

*ommend that the intake of fruit should not be restricted in patients with type 2 diabetes."*

In fact, when the data is looked at more closely, those who ate more fruit had slightly more weight loss and lower ending waist circumference than those who ate less fruit.

The high-fruit diet group had an average weight reduction of 2.5 kilos while the low-fruit diet group had a 1.7 kilogram average loss in weight. Meanwhile, the high-fruit diet group had an average waistline shrinkage of 4.3 centimeters, while the low-fruit diet had an average shrinkage of 3.0 centimeters.

The reason why this nutritional advice of lower fruit consumption has been erroneous is that conventional medicine has failed to understand the importance of consuming the fibers within fruits: They have assumed the sugar levels of fruit without the fiber. Whole fruits contain a number of long-chain polysaccharides – such as pectin and others – which have been shown to reduce glycemic levels and balance blood sugar.

This reality – that fruits pose no threat to type 2 diabetics – has been in front of conventional medicine for over two decades. Research at the Veterans Affairs Medical Center in Minneapolis (Ercan *et al.* 1993) – published in the *Journal of the American College of Nutrition* – tested seven diabetic men with bananas of various ripeness. Their testing illustrated that the ripeness of the bananas had no effects upon the patients' levels of glucose, insulin, C-peptide and glucagon. This should have led to the immediate abandonment of this notion that fruit is not advisable for diabetics.

In fact, the precisely opposite is true.

Just about every whole fruit will contain both soluble and insoluble fiber – often at precisely the perfect levels for our digestive tract. Fiber levels among popular fruits range from a low of about three grams for every 100 calories to a high of seven to over eight grams per 100 calories – among raspberries, blackberries (about a cup), prunes and figs. An apple or pear will contain close to four grams each.

Fruit juices, on the other hand, present the sugar of fruits without their fiber. Thus fruit juices are a quite different thing altogether.

Scientific data has determined that between 30 and 40 grams a day of fiber is best, while some suggest as low as 25 is okay. Most Americans eat between 10 and 15 grams per day. Fiber is critical to maintaining blood sugar balance.

Soluble fiber – also called water-soluble – has been shown to lower cholesterol because it prevents bile from resorption – as bile acids are produced from cholesterol. Fiber will attach bile acids and escort them out of the body. Soluble fiber also slows carbohydrate absorption and decreases insulin requirements. These together help balance blood sugar levels. Insoluble fiber attaches to toxins and waste material in the digestive tract and escorts them out of the intestines.

Fruits make up one of the best ways to get both soluble and insoluble fiber. Other ways to add beneficial fibers to the diet include whole grains and seeds. Psyllium husks and flaxseeds are some of the best supplemental forms of fiber.

Plus, whole fruits are delicious. There are a myriad of super nutritious fruits, melons and berries high in antioxidants and various phytonutrients, including kiwis, plums, peaches, pears, strawberries, blackberries, watermelon, cantaloupe, cherries, blueberries and of course the king of fruits – the apple.

Better blood sugar control also leads to better weight management along with good nutrition.

This conclusion was confirmed in a 2011 study (Keast *et al.* 2011) that analyzed dried fruit consumption among 13,292 U.S. adults. The research found that those who eat more dried fruit have on average lower weight, lower obesity levels, and higher nutrient levels in vitamin A, vitamins C, vitamin K, calcium, phosphorus, fiber, magnesium and potassium than those who consumed less dried fruit.

These studies illustrate that fructose, the primary sugar within fruits and concentrated in dried fruits, is not unhealthy as supposed by some. The theory that fructose from fruits and fruit juices has negative consequences thoroughly ignores that these healthy foods contain a balance of not only fructose, but also a myriad of other healthy components, including pulp, pectin, vitamins, minerals, polyphenols and other healthy nutrients. These balance and slow the absorption of the fructose – rendering the whole fruit supremely healthy, just as nature designed it.

## The Amazing Citrus Fruits

As we'll discuss further later, drinking fruit juices devoid of their pulp is not the best approach to fruit, as it stresses the body's glucose controls. While most commercial fruit juices have been pressed devoid of their fibers, most commercial 100% orange juices will retain the orange pulp.

Researchers from Louisiana State University's Agricultural Center (O'Neil *et al.* 2011) determined that children who drink 100% orange juice have less weight gain per consumed calories, and significantly better overall nutrient levels and better diets in general. In a related study, the consumption of dried fruit also resulted in less weight gain.

While the results might not be surprising to some, the orange juice research further contradicts the notion that fructose is an unhealthy sugar, and that drinking 100% fruit juices are just as bad as drinking sodas and other drinks high in sugar content. This has been an argument made by some, claiming that fructose from fruit juices produces obesity and other negative health factors.

This notion is contradicted by research that studied 7,250 children between 2 years old and 18 years old from the National Health and Nutrition Examination 2003-2006 Survey. This was cross-referenced with diet quality indices such as the Healthy Eating Index of 2005 and MyPyramid data.

Of this total group of 7,250 children, 2,183 children drank 100% orange juice regularly, or 26% of the children. The average amount of orange juice consumed by each OJ consumer was a little over 10 ounces a day.

The research found that children who regularly drank orange juice consumed an average of 523 calories a day more than children who did not drink orange juice regularly. Yet surprisingly, there was no difference in the weight levels between the orange juice consumers and the non-orange juice consumers.

In other words, drinking orange juice regularly helps prevent weight gain among children.

Not so surprisingly, the researchers also found that children who drank orange juice regularly also had significantly higher nutrient levels of vitamin A, vitamin C and magnesium than those children who did not drink orange juice regularly. The children who drank orange juice regularly also ate better in general than children who did not.

One eight ounce glass of 100% (non-fortified) orange juice contains 137% of the U.S. Daily value of vitamin C, 35% of the Daily Value of calcium, 18% of the Daily Value of thiamin, 14% of the Daily Value of potassium, 11% of the Daily Value of folate, 7% of the Daily Value of magnesium and 7% of the Daily Value of vitamin B6.

The study also reveals that it is not so much the number of calories, but the type of calories we eat. Calories from diets that contain healthy plant-based foods are better than calories from diets heavily laden with over-processed foods and sugary foods.

In fact, two ingredients commonly found in many citrus fruits, naringin and neohesperidin, will effectively reduce blood sugar. And as we've shown throughout this book, weight loss is directly linked to glucose control.

Studies (Zhang *et al.* 2012; Lu *et al.* 2006) have identified these and tested the two citrus constituents using human liver cells. The scientists found that the two natural compounds increase the uptake of glucose among the cells.

This study confirms previous research that pointed to the possibility that these citrus constituents may be helpful for reduce blood sugar for those with or at risk for type 2 diabetes and suffer from poor glucose control and/or heightened glucose tolerance.

Other research (Jung *et al.* 2004) has found these compounds also regulate liver enzymes phosphoenolpyruvate carboxykinase and glucose-6-phosphatase – helping glucose uptake regulation and increasing liver efficiency.

The researchers extracted the two flavonoids from the Chinese citrus fruit called Huyou (*Citrus changshanensis*). This citrus, as well as others such as Grapefruit and related species – has been used as an anti-diabetic agent in Traditional Chinese Medicine, Ayurveda and other traditional Asian medicines.

The naringin and neohesperidin compounds were found throughout the fruit part of the citrus, including the juice sacs and the segments. Another Chinese study found that the Huyou peel contained the highest naringin and neohesperidin content.

Several other citrus fruits contain naringin and neohesperidin. This doesn't mean that orange juice necessarily contains naringin and neohesperidin.

A study from the Citrus Research and Education Center (Widmer 2000) tested a number of orange juices using liquid chromatography. The analysis found that the two 100% orange juice samples tested contained neither naringin nor neohesperidin. However, juice samples that contained orange juice together with small amounts of grapefruit juice, sour orange (*Citrus aurantium*) juice and K-Early citrus juice did contain naringin and neohesperidin.

Other research (Peter *et al.* 2006) has determined that the common sweet orange (*Citrus sinensis*) will typically contain naringin, but very small amounts, and will typically not contain neohesperidin. Sour oranges (*Citrus aurantium*) – especially when picked early, will contain considerable amounts of naringin and neohesperidin. Mandarin oranges (*Citrus reticulata*) are also good sources for both naringin and neohesperidin. Grapefruit contains naringin and neohesperidin, but its neohesperidin content is typically smaller.

Lemons and limes typically do not contain either compound in lieu of their hesperidin content, but a few species – such as the Bergamot – will contain naringin and possibly small amounts of neohesperidin.

In addition to its anti-diabetic properties, naringen has been found in laboratory studies (Kumar *et al.* 2006) to be neuro-protective (helps protect brain tissue). It appears to protect against the effects of 3-nitropropionic acid, which has been found to be one of the primary

167

agents that produce nerve damage in Huntington's disease and other nerve disorders.

Both of these weight-related studies illustrate that fructose, the primary sugar within fruit juices like orange juice and concentrated in dried fruits, is not unhealthy as supposed by some. The theory that fructose from fruits and fruit juices has negative consequences thoroughly ignores that these healthy foods contain not only fructose, but also a myriad of other healthy components, including pulp, pectin, vitamins, minerals, polyphenols and other healthy nutrients.

This of course does not apply to high-fructose corn syrup – a highly refined form of fructose.

But that's not all citrus can do for our health. Citrus can also reduce our risk of stroke.

Researchers from the Norwich Medical School of the UK's University of East Anglia (Cassidy et al. 2012) found that higher consumption of citrus is associated with a reduction of stroke and ischemic stroke among women.

The researchers studied 69,622 women for 14 years. There were 1,803 strokes among the women during that period. The researchers found that those who consumed the highest amounts of citrus fruits or juice had a nearly 20% lower incidence of in ischemic strokes, and a 10% lower incidence of all strokes.

An ischemic stroke is caused by a blockage of blood flow that feeds the brain. This can produce a loss of physical, nervous or cognition function. The source of the blockage can be caused by a blood clot somewhere else in the bloodstream, causing thrombosis. This is often related to atherosclerosis of an artery – the build of plaque within the artery walls.

The researchers attributed the effect to the increased level of flavanones from the citrus. Flavanones are a type of flavonoid that typically contain glycosides. Examples of flavanones are Hesperetin, Hesperidon, Naringin and Naringenin – all of which are contained in citrus fruits.

However, the research also found that flavanone consumption did not specifically relate to stroke reduction.

Why? Because citrus contains a variety of bioactive substances other than flavanones.

In a study published in the *Journal Agricultural Food Chemistry* (Gironés-Vilaplana et al. 2012), researchers found that lemon juice combined with berry fruits are potent antioxidants that break down a variety of free radicals.

Plaque build up is associated with an increase in oxidative radicals in the form of oxidized LDL cholesterol. The ability of antioxidants to neutralize oxidized LDL has been shown in numerous nutraceutical studies.

The researchers also found that lemon juice in particular inhibits cholinesterases such as acetylcholinesterase and butyrylcholinesterase. The ability to reduce these cholinesterases gives lemon therapeutic properties against neuromuscular disorders and chronic nervous issues.

### Don't Squeeze the Lemons (and other Citrus)

Lemons have been recognized as healing, anti-microbial food fruits for thousands of years. They were cultivated well over 2,500 years ago, and used extensively to preserve foods and purify the blood in sickness. Traditional healers have used lemons for the treatment of arteriosclerosis, bleeding gums, ulcers, arthritis, gingivitis, warts, ringworm, skin irritations, varicose veins and other issues. Lemon also stimulates appetite and increases metabolism.

Lemon is highly acidic, but it is known for its alkalinity effects once within the body. This is because its acids, oils and antioxidants neutralize free radicals produced by toxins and lipid peroxides. Lemon also appears to stimulate elimination of toxins at a faster rate.

A lemon will contain about 5% vitamin C, more than oranges and grapefruits. This natural form of ascorbic acid, together with bioflavonoids, provides a superior form of vitamin C.

Lemons also contain calcium, phosphorus, vitamin A, protein and iron. In fact, a pound of lemons can contain as much as 274 milligrams of calcium and 3.3 grams of protein.

Lemons also contain the oils limonene, beta-pinene, citral, alpha-terpinene and alpha-pinene. These oils are known to stimulate the immune system and help clear toxins. Lemon oil is also highly antibacterial, and it has been shown to inhibit pneumococcus and meningococcus bacteria.

For this reason, it is important not to extract the juice from the lemon and leave behind other nutrients that are embedded into the fiber and inside peel portions.

Most people do just that. They extract the acidic juice, leaving behind those alkaline portions that balance its acidity. Those alkaline fibers and calcium are important in terms of the benefit that lemons bring.

For this reason, squeezing out the lemon juice and throwing away the peel and fiber is not advised. The best way to eat a lemon is to peel the outer rind off, leaving a good portion of the inner rind – where most of the oil resides – and then putting the entire fruit into a blender. And don't worry about the lemon seeds. Some of them will be chopped up, and a few partial whole seeds might have to be spit out or swallowed (better if swallowed). The end result will be delicious and nutritious.

A whole lemon minus the rind, together with other fruits and some kefir is simply delicious. The tartness usually reserved for lemons is surprisingly absent, simply because of the wholeness of the lemon addition.

This nutritional point applies to all citrus fruits. Oranges, mandarins, grapefruit and other citrus fruits all contain limonene in the peels, along with other healthy components.

A new study has found that a polymethoxylated flavonoid called nobiletin reduces very low density cholesterol (LDL or VLDL) levels. The researchers, from the Robarts Research Institute of London and Ontario (Mulvihill *et al.* 2011), found that the secretion of LDL and VLDL by human liver cells was significantly inhibited by nobiletin.

They also found that the polymethoxylated flavonoid, with a chemical structure of 3'4'5,6,7,8-hexamethoxyflavone, reduced VLDL levels found in insulin resistance and atherosclerosis.

Remember that LDL and VLDL are implicated in cardiovascular disease, because they promote lipid peroxidation, which damages the arteries and many other tissue systems.

Agricultural Research Service (ARS) scientists (Manthey and Bendele 2008) who found that 3'4'3,5,6,7,8-heptamethoxyflavone (HMF), another citrus polymethoxylated flavone found in citrus peels, inhibited a precursory protein called apoprotein B found within low-density lipoprotein (LDL).

Citrus peels contain several polymethoxylated flavonoids (PMFs). Nobiletin is a O-methylated flavone. It renders a hydroxyl group that mediates a reaction called O-methylation. Methylation allows for the donation of methyl groups, which provide radical-neutralizing effects, as well as the inhibition of lipid peroxide-friendly LDL cholesterol apoprotein B. Other O-methylated flavones include tangeritin (first found in tangerine oil), wogonin (found in the herb *Baikal scullcap*), and sinensetin, found in the Java tea herb *Orthosiphon stamineus.*

Citrus peels can contain as much as 70% oil. The oil contains a number of other healthful components including limonene and linalool. Limonene is monoterpene known for its antimicrobial and radical-scavenging abilities.

Most of us remove the peel and toss it out. Maybe this information will get us thinking twice about that. While the outer rind of an orange or lemon may taste a little bitter, the middle of the peel under the outer rind is quite mild tasting, and again, it will help balance the acidity of the citrus juice.

## The Awesome Apple

The humble apple has had a glorious and romantic history. It is also has become domesticated in many countries around the world. The Greeks considered the apple as sacred. The ancient Egyptians used the apple as both a medicine and food. After a rich history of use throughout Europe and the Middle East, apple trees began to their domestication into the US from England by Captain Simpson of the Hudson Bay Company. It is said that Capt. Simpson's first imported tree still stands. In the nineteenth century, the famous Johnny Appleseed – often considered North America's first nurseryman – focused upon the planting of apple trees throughout the country. From these humble beginnings, those trees – many of which still stand – led to further propagation, and today the US is a leading producer of apples, with millions of boxes of fresh apples being produced throughout the US every year.

At some point, the apple rightfully gained that famous adage of "an apple a day keeps the doctor away." While often said in jest now, there is a considerable amount of truth and history to this expression. The fact is, the apple is one of the healthiest foods we could choose to eat. Apples were used for many decades by traditional country doctors for a variety of different complaints. It is reputed that apples were once part of treatments for skin eruptions, gout, biliousness, nervous disorders, diarrhea, constipation, and jaundice.

Again, fiber is critical to our diet. We need between 30 and 45 grams of it per day for healthy digestion and elimination. Apples contain one of the highest levels of fiber, with a pound (two large apples or three medium apples with skin) delivering up to 10 grams. The apple also contains an almost perfect combination of both soluble fiber and insoluble fiber. We need both kinds. The apple's soluble fiber comes in the form of pectin. Pectin is important for a number of reasons.

Pectin helps reduce cholesterol because it absorbs and binds with bile and low density fatty acids in the intestine and colon, escorting these out through the colon prior to their entry into the blood stream. The insoluble fiber in apples helps keep the intestines and colon clean, providing a natural scrubber to the intestinal wall, and along the spaces between the villi – those tiny digestive fingers of the intestine. The fiber in apples keeps the colon running smoother: helping to prevent colon polyps and irritable bowels. Apples have also been known to help regulate bowel movements.

Research from Russian scientists (Chelpanova *et al.* 2012) determined that pectin slows the activity of the enzymes that break down starches and sugars.

While the research tested a variety of drug compounds, and was intended to show how pectin slows down the absorption of pharmaceuticals, the results fill in one of the gaps in understanding how fiber slows the absorption of carbohydrates and sugars, and thus helps prevent the spiking of blood sugar known to provoke glucose intolerance, diabetes and weight gain.

The research tested pectin from three different sources, including sweet pepper (*Capsicum annuum*), onion bulbs (*Allium cepa*), carrot (*Daucus sativus*), and white cabbage (*Brassica oleracea*). They found that all the pectins, extracted using two methods and with different concentrations, slowed down the activity of alpha-amylase enzymes produced by human pancreatic cells.

The measurements took place in an environment that mirrored the human stomach. The pectin slowed down the enzyme activity, which in turn slowed the absorption of several pharmaceutical drugs.

The glycemic benefits of pectin are undeniable. The fact that pectin slows glycemic response has been proven in other research. For example, researchers from Tokyo's Metropolitan Komagome Hospital studied gastric emptying and glycemic rates following eating among ten healthy men.

The researchers (Sanaka *et al.* 2007) gave the men either agar (from seaweed), pectin or a control meal at different mealtimes and tested their glycemic responses and gastric emptying rates following the meal. They found that both the agar and pectin significantly reduced the glycemic responses following the meals compared with the control meals among the men.

Besides the effect of leveling off blood sugar levels, these benefits include the reduction of low-density lipoproteins ("bad" cholesterol). Pectins also help prevent atherosclerosis, and provide prebiotics that feed our digestive probiotics. Promoting our intestinal probiotics in turn produces a myriad of digestive benefits, including helping to prevent various bowel and liver infections.

Significant sources of pectin include apples, bananas, legumes, cabbage, apricots, onions and carrots. These foods also happen to be some of the best prebiotic foods as well. Many of these pectin-rich foods also happen to contain one of the most potent prebiotic of all: fructooligosaccharides.

Several of these foods – apples in particular – have been the subject of weight loss programs. The "Three-Apple-a-Day" diet was created by registered dietician Tammi Flynn when she observed some of her clients having significant yet healthy weight loss results after eating more apples.

She recommends eating one apple prior to each meal to create a more speedy feeling of fullness. This anecdotal result meshes quite well with this newfound mechanism that pectin slows amylase enzyme activity.

Incidentally, regulating the breakdown and absorption of sugars and carbohydrates has also been observed with increased supplementation of probiotics. This illustrates the synergy between our probiotics, fibrous prebiotics and healthy blood-sugar levels – helping to prevent conditions such as diabetes.

Apples are a rich source of a number of vitamins. A pound of apples (1-2 medium-to-large apples) has up to 360 IU of vitamin A, 15-20 mg of vitamin C, and 24 grams of calcium. Apples also contain decent amounts of vitamin B6, vitamin K, B2 and B6, along with smaller amounts of B1, B3 and B5. Apples are also a great source of potassium and manganese, with respectable amounts of iron, magnesium, copper and manganese. Organic apples may contain more. Several studies have confirmed that organic fruits contain more nutrients than their conventionally-grown counterparts.

Surprisingly apples contain a number of amino acids, the building blocks for protein. Apples contain a notable amount of leucine, lysine, valine, alanine, aspartic acid, glutamic acid, glycine, proline, and serine, along with smaller amounts of tryptophan, threonine, isoleucine, methionine, cystine, phenylalanine, tyrosine, arginine and histidine. That makes up 18 of a total of 20 possible amino acids, and all nine of the "essential" amino acids. Who would have thought of the apple as a good source of protein?

Apples contain several key antioxidants, which are known to reduce the effects of aging, promote healing, decrease inflammation, boost the immune system and help detoxify cells, blood and organs. Outside of its active antioxidants vitamin C and A, apples contain flavones such as quercitin that have a much more powerful effect in the body. Apples also contain lutein and zeaxanthin, both powerful antioxidants. These healthy range of antioxidants in apples have been attributed to helping reduce inflammatory issues such as arthritis and allergies, while helping to prevent infection and cancer cell growth.

Because the apple has so much fiber, it is a great way to lose weight. An apple or two or three will provide an experience of fullness with only about 200 calories in a pound. The fiber and the high nutrient level make apples a great diet food because it takes a greater amount of energy to digest than other foods. A fair amount of the apple's calories is "eaten up" by its own digestion. That makes the lowly apple one of the best diet foods around.

Since many nutrients are disbursed under heat, cooking apples should be done in stainless steel or glassware at low heat. Apple juice should be approached with discrimination as well. Those with blood sugar issues might want to avoid apple juice on an empty stomach. The fructose and glucose content of apple juice is highly absorbable – not unlike white sugar. This is especially a concern with filtered apple juice, which has most or all of the pulp removed by filtration and heating. The heating and filtration process can also rob the juice of many nutrients. Fresh pressed whole apple juice with all the pulp is the best guarantee for preserving the nutrient content of the apple in juice. Second best would be unfiltered and pasteurized. Apple juice made from concentrate has probably the least desirable. The heat needed to evaporate the water reduces much of its nutrient content not to speak of its pulp and fibers.

Best eaten 'in the nude' and unpeeled, the apple is quite simply an incredible source of vitamins, minerals, protein, antioxidants and fiber. An apple a day is, well, as healthy as they say.

## The Antimicrobial Plum

The plum (*Prunus spp.*) and its various hybridized relatives is an ancient food known for its incredible healing properties. It is known in Asia as a special food used for medicinal properties. Those same properties are available among most hybrid plum varieties grown in Europe and North America.

*Prunus mume* (Seib et Zucc) is also referred to as *Fructus pruni mume* in Chinese medicine. It is also called *Omae* in Korea, *Ume* or *Umeboshi plum* in Japan, which translates, quite simply, to 'Dark plum' or 'Black plum.' It is also referred to as Mume. It is, quite simply, an ancient medicinal fruit.

Wu Mei – Fructus mume/Prunus mume – has been used traditionally in Chinese and Asian medicine for a number of different disorders, most of which are related to infections. Wu Mai has been used to treat dysentery, diarrhea, nausea, abdominal pain, roundworms, lung infections and others. It is a remedy that is often combined with other Chinese Medicine herbs for ailments such as diabetes and liver issues.

This plum is treasured for its immune-stimulating properties. The Chinese *Materia Medica* describes it as able to alleviate coughing and lung deficiencies. It has a strongly astringent property, and thus helps to cleanse the digestive tract and halt diarrhea. Research documented in the *Medica* has indicated that it stimulates bile production, is anti-microbial, and has been able to relieve fever, nausea, abdominal pain and vomiting.

*Prunus mume* is indigenous to Asia – China, Japan, Vietnam and Korea. It is a summer fruit that is baked or dried in the sun until the skin darkens

– giving it its characteristic name. Today different varieties of Prunus mume are grown in Western countries. These include the Bonita, Kobai and Dawn cultivars.

Prunus mume contains a number of constituents, including rutin, benzoic acid, isorhamnetin, quercetin, kaempferol, isoquercitrin and hypericin.

Research from the School of Chinese Medicine and Taiwan's Hung-kuang University (Tien-Huang *et al.* 2013) has determined that an ancient Chinese remedy often referred to in English as Black Plum or Wu Mei has the ability to inhibit the growth of multiple-drug resistant *Klebsiella pneumoniae*.

Multiple-drug resistant *Klebsiella pneumoniae* has expanded its ability to infect over the past decade and is now one of the most lethal hospital-acquired infection (HAI). Klebsiella is spreading quickly via something called a carbapenemase – an enzyme giving the organism the ability to adapt to different surroundings and resist different antibiotics.

*Klebsiella pneumoniae* is a gram-negative bacteria that will often produce what is called sepsis – body-wide infection – that will eventually infect and damage the liver, causing severe liver disease. And should *Klebsiella pneumoniae* get into the lungs, it can cause significant damage to the lungs and respiratory system – producing pneumonia, bronchitis, lung abscess, empyema and cavitation.

Even when treated with aggressive antibiotics, *Klebsiella pneumoniae* lung infections have been known to kill 50% or more of those infected (Nordmann *et al.* 2002).

Wu Mei found to inhibit one of the most fatal superbug infections

The researchers tested the Black plum against two different serotype strains of *Klebsiella pneumoniae*. They found that the *Fructus mume* significantly inhibited the growth of both serotypes. They also found that the *Fructus mume* stopped the process of mRNA expansion which is necessary for the Klebsiella to colonize. This also affects the bacteria's capsular polysaccharides – which allow the bacteria to adhere onto different surfaces.

Plums have other benefits as well.

Several recent studies have confirmed what traditional oriental medicine has known for centuries – that dried plums have the capacity to prevent and even reverse bone loss that often follows menopause.

One study, done at Florida State University (Hooshmand *et al.* 2011) using 236 women who were one to ten years into menopause.

The women were randomly divided into two groups. One group was given 100 grams of dried plums per day while the other group was given 100 grams of dried apples per day for a year. After doing bone scans at

175

three months, six months and twelve months, the researchers found that the dried plum group showed significantly greater bone mineral density than those women consuming the dried apples over that same period.

Other studies have found that dried plums prevent and even reverse bone loss among post-menopausal women. This research has included scientists from the Medical College of the University of California, San Francisco (Rendina *et al.* 2013).

Another study found that fructooligosaccharides (FOS) – a prebiotic nutrient found in bananas, chicory root, garlic, wheat, barley, leeks, onions and other foods – along with the dried plums and a soy-based diet was successful in reversing bone loss in animal research (Arjmandi *et al.* 2010).

In addition to dried plums, researchers are increasingly finding that diets rich in plant nutrients (phytonutrients) have the effect of reducing and preventing bone loss. A review of research from Switzerland found that consuming polyphenols helps prevent bone loss, including those from tea, grape seed, citrus fruits and olives in addition to dried plum. They also found that the Mediterranean diet – a diet that maintains a significant amount of plant foods along with olive oil and tomatoes – apparently helps prevent bone loss as well (Sacco *et al.* 2013).

Researchers from Texas Tech University also found in their research that phytonutrients provide the best strategy to prevent bone loss among post-menopausal women. The researchers found that phytonutrients such as pectin, lycopene, flavonoids, resveratrol, phenolics and phloridzin – nutrients that are contained in many fruits as well as tomatoes, contribute to preventing bone loss among aging women (Hooshmand and Arjmandi 2009).

While vitamin D and calcium certainly should not be left out of the equation, recent research brings into question the safety of consuming too much supplemental calcium – linking calcium supplementation to increased risk of cardiovascular conditions. The broad swath of research on bone loss combines vitamin D with natural calcium sources – from foods – along with a healthy plant-based diet.

## The Potent Tomato

A tomato has at least 10,000 phyto compounds according to various biochemical analyses. This is an incredible amount of nutrition. A tomato is one of the most nutritious foods available. The phytonutrients in tomatoes include flavonoids, phenolics, phenylalanines, numerous minerals and citric acid. Tomatoes also contain carotenes, the most famous of which is lycopene.

Research (Riccioni et al. 2011) has confirmed that lycopene, the primary carotene that makes tomatoes red, lowers the risk of hardening of the arteries. A study from researchers at the San Camillo de Lellis Hospital Cardiology Unit in Foggia, Italy determined using ultrasound that those with higher blood levels of lycopene have significantly reduced levels of atherosclerosis in the carotid artery.

The study examined 120 human subjects. After complete physical exams and blood testing, ultrasonic testing determined their level of thickening of the artery walls in the carotid artery. The carotid artery travels from the heart to the brain, and is the hardening of that artery can lead to strokes and heart attacks.

The analysis found that 58 of the subjects had progressive carotid atherosclerosis. Those with carotid atherosclerosis had higher concentrations of triglycerides, LDL-cholesterol, and total cholesterol in their bloodstreams. They also had lower levels of lycopene.

The researchers concluded:

> *"These data suggest that higher serum levels of lycopene may play a protective role versus cardiovascular diseases, in particular carotid atherosclerosis."*

Lycopene is a potent antioxidant. Antioxidants reduce the hardening of the arteries because they neutralize lipid oxidizing radicals that harm the cells of the artery walls.

## Medicinal Tropical Fruits

The tropical sun beats down on those regions closest to the equator with daily onslaught. This combined with year-round pests, volcanic soils, good rainfall and long daylight hours work together to produce plants rich in nutrients and hardy immune systems.

The tropics maintain a host of other astonishing fruits and medicinal plants. The rain forests of the tropics provide a combination of volcanic soil with plenty of rainfall and a year-round climate for plant growth.

Yet our rain forests are disappearing at a rate of 6,000 acres a minute according to the California Institute of Technology. The Amazon rain forests alone are disappearing at 200,000 square miles a year. Land developers are clear-cutting old growth tropical rain forests and converting the lands into cattle grazing and resort developments.

This "progress" is destroying the habitats for these incredible plants. Many of the important medicinal species of the tropical rain forests are disappearing, and this is forever.

On top of that, we are eliminating the oxygen production from these great rain forests, thereby speeding up the process of global warming and hastening our own demise.

For the near-term, many of us have access to tropical foods, as first-, second- and third-world countries alike complete to sell their tropical foods abroad.

And research is making us aware of how tremendously rich tropical foods are in nutrients and medicinal constitutions. Let's talk about just a few of them.

## Papaya

The papaya is also an intense food, as is contains large amounts of minerals such as potassium, magnesium and calcium. Its potassium level is superior to many foods, with a good 360 milligrams in about half an average size papaya (about a cup of cubed papaya).

Papaya also contains significant vitamin A in the form of beta-carotene. So it is beneficial as not only an antioxidant, but great for the eyes – with 1531 IU per average papaya. Papaya also provides folate and choline – two important brain nutrients.

One of the most beneficial elements of papaya is its enzyme content. Papayas contain an enzyme called papain, which is a proteolytic and fibrinolytic enzyme. This means the enzyme will not only help break down protein, but it will also reduce the build up of fibrin in the body. Fibrin will form in an inflammatory process – such as atherosclerosis or fibrosis.

Papayas with their papain content also help soothe upset stomachs. The papain along with phytonutrients provide a myriad of antioxidant benefits. And the polysaccharides in papaya provide nutrients that nourish the gut's probiotic microorganisms.

Papaya also contains some secret weapons.

In a recent study of 90 human subjects, Italian researchers found that fermented papaya significantly stimulates the immune system after six weeks. In another study, an extract of papaya leaf was shown to stop cancer growth among human cancer cells.

Papaya fruit contains linalool, benzylisothiacyanates, chitinase and alkaloids such as carpaine and benzyl-glucosides. Chitinase has been found to have antibacterial activity, and carpaine and carpasemine have been shown to inhibit parasites.

One warning about papaya is that most of the Sunrise papayas now grown in Hawaii are from genetically modified seeds. For this reason, many countries, including Japan, will not import them. Best to choose either organic papayas from Hawaii or papayas from other countries.

## Pineapple

Pineapple also contains a powerful fibrinolytic, proteolytic enzyme, called bromelain. This enzyme is very powerful, and has been shown to significantly reduce fibrin buildup and reduce artery plaque. A study published this month in the journal Alternative Therapies has found that bromelain eases the airways for asthmatics. Bromelain has also been shown to help ease arthritic issues, again due to its strong fibrinolytic powers.

Pineapple maintains one of the highest sources of vitamin C, with more than the U.S. daily value at nearly 80 milligrams in a cup of cubed pineapple. Pineapple also supplies a considerable amount of choline, folate and other B vitamins. It also contains 2% protein by weight and supplies good quantities of calcium, magnesium, potassium and manganese.

Several studies – most recently a study from Spain – have found that pineapple contains an aggregated cellulose-copper nutrient that has proven antifungal properties. Another study, this one from India, showed that bromelain inhibits the tuberculosis bacteria.

Pineapple also contains a special type of sugar called xylooligosaccharide. This is a prebiotic, meaning it feeds our intestinal probiotics.

The best way to get all these incredible nutrients from the tropics is in their natural raw forms. Even most mass supermarkets will carry raw coconuts, papayas and pineapples. However, convenient forms will also maintain many of these nutrients, including coconut water, papaya juices and canned pineapple. These forms may lose some of their fragile enzyme and phytonutrient content, but they still will rank head and shoulders above high fructose corn-sweetened sodas and junk foods.

## Mango

Mangoes (*Mangifera* spp.) grow in many tropical locations, especially those in the Pacific, Mexico, Central America, as well as India and Thailand. Mango is one of the world's most popular fruits outside of the U.S.

Mangos contain more than 20 vitamins, minerals and antioxidants.

Recent research has discovered that mangoes have a phytonutrient called mangiferin. Mangiferin has been shown to have significant anti-inflammatory and anti-cancer benefits.

Detroit's Karmanos Cancer Institute found in 2012 that mangiferin inhibits cancer cell growth. A metabolite of mangiferin is called norathyriol. University of Minnesota researchers found that norathyriol inhibits the growth of skin cancer. They found that UV radiation skin cancers were suppressed.

How ironic is it that eating tropical mango helps protect the skin against UV radiation – more significant for those living in the tropics.

Cuba's Center for Pharmaceutical Chemistry found that mango contains another anticancer compound called gallic acid. It seems that gallic acid and mangiferin cooperatively in the body.

Scientists at the 2012 conference of the Federation of American Societies for Experimental Biology (FASEB) presented research showing that people who regularly eat mangos have fewer health issues.

Their research compared the diets of over 13,000 individuals participating in the National Health and Nutrition Examination Survey (NHANES) between 2001 and 2008 to the Healthy Eating Index (HEI). Those who ate mangos regularly scored higher on the HEI than those that did not.

Compared to non-mango consumers, mango consumers had increased intake of vitamin C, magnesium, potassium and dietary fibers, and had a lower average body weight.

Mango eaters also had lower levels of the inflammatory marker C-reactive protein.

## Mangosteen

Despite the name, mangosteen (*Garcinia mangostana*) is not related to the mango. Outside of being native to some of the same tropical regions, the fruit looks and tastes completely different. Also, mangosteen's central medicinal benefits are derived from its thick rind – the pericarp.

Once the rind is taken off, the fruit also contains significant antioxidants – as many fruits do. But its rind contains an important antibacterial agent called mangostin, as well as at least 16 xanthones. Xanthones are potent plant nutrients that provide an array of protection for cells, including inhibiting inflammation and cancer.

Recent research from Australia's Flinders School of Medicine has found that mangostin inhibits the metastasizing of skin cancer cells, and other research has found it inhibits the growth of MRSA infections.

These results are consistent with mangosteen's traditional uses, which have included using the rind to heal wounds and skin infections, as well as some digestive infections.

## Noni

Noni (*Morinda citrifolia*) also grows throughout the tropics, including Hawaii, Tahiti, Fiji, Philippines, Indonesia and parts of Australia and Asia. In India, it is called Tamil Nadu or Indian mulberry. The fruit has been reputed to have significant medicinal properties, some of which have been exaggerated by suppliers.

Nonetheless, noni has some significant levels of potassium, niacin, vitamin C and vitamin A, which may provide some of its abilities.

Noni also has a tradition of medicinal use among Polynesians and Indians, who have used it for various liver issues, urinary tract infections, gastrointestinal issues, painful menstrual cramping and blood sugar issues. A recent study from the University of Illinois has found that noni can reduce cholesterol and decrease inflammation among smokers.

Some of noni's medicinal constituents include flavonoids, scopoletin, catechin, beta-sitosterol, damnacanthal, iridoids, glycosides and alkaloids.

Researchers from the University of Illinois College of Medicine (Wang *et al.* 2012) found that Noni juice significantly reduces inflammation and corrects poor cholesterol levels.

The researchers gave 132 adults who were heavy smokers either 29.5 or 188 milliliters of Noni (Morinda citrifolia) juice per day for thirty days. Another group drank a placebo. The clinical trial was randomized, double blind and placebo-controlled.

The researchers chose heavy smokers as subjects because heavy smoking has been shown to significantly increase levels of inflammation, increase triglycerides, increase low-density lipoprotein (LDL) levels and reduce HDL-cholesterol. High levels of LDL-c and triglycerides have been associated with greater incidence of artery and heart disease.

Furthermore, these two indicators are easily tested with blood testing. Inflammation was tested by way of high-sensitivity C-reactive protein (hs-CRP) levels and homocysteine levels.

Smoking causes greater levels of oxidative stress, due to the greater influx of oxidative radicals from the toxins contained in tobacco and cigarettes. One review of research studied 54 clinical trials and found smokers will maintain 3% higher cholesterol levels, 9% higher triglycerides, and almost 6% reduced HDL-cholesterol (the good cholesterol) than non-smokers.

According to the U.S. Centers for Disease Control, cigarette smoke contains over 4,000 chemicals, of which more than 250 have been found to produce disease.

After the 30 days, those in the Noni groups showed significantly lower levels of inflammation and corrections in their respective cholesterol levels. The hs-CRP levels went down by 15% among the Noni groups. Homocysteine levels decreased by 24% among the Noni group. The triglyceride levels of the noni groups went down from 29% to 41%. The LDL-cholesterol levels of the Noni group went down by 9-28% after the thirty days, and HDL-c levels went up by 49 to 57 mg/dL.

Interestingly, the researchers found no significant difference in the results between the Noni group that drank 29 mL versus the group that drank 118 mL per day of Noni. The researchers commented that "this may indicate a possible threshold of antioxidant activity."

This notion of "antioxidant threshold" has been found in other studies, where there is a certain point the phytonutrients seem to reach a point of diminishing returns with increased doses. This is not a surprise to natural health experts, who understand that the body must maintain balance.

Consider these results carefully: This is only after thirty days of Noni consumption of as little as 29.5 mL per day, drank on an empty stomach in the morning. Note that 29.5 mL is one ounce.

Now compare these results to the kind of reductions seen with statins, which come with significant adverse side effects. Statin use has been shown to increase HDL-c ("good" cholesterol) by as much as 5-15%, decrease triglycerides by up to 7-30% and decrease LDL-c by a range of 18-65% according to multiple-study reviews. The higher levels have been found with significantly higher dosages – such as 80 milligrams a day.

Side effects from statins include liver damage, muscle pain, nausea, diarrhea, constipation, rashes, diabetes, possible memory loss and confusion. No side effects were seen in this study on Noni.

## Açaí

The purple berries of the açaí (*Euterpe oleracea*) palm tree have received much acclaim over the recent years, specifically for their high antioxidant values. The ORAC (oxygen radical absorbance capacity) value of açaí berries has been measured at an astonishing 161,400 units. To give you a gauge of how high this is, the ORAC value of pomegranates is 2,860, and blueberries is 6,552. A food's ORAC value relates to its ability to neutralize and reduce free radicals in the body. Free radicals damage cells and tissues, and are the cause for many inflammatory diseases.

This tall palm grows throughout the tropics, and it is a staple for many in the Amazon region. This is because the fruit has significant protein content, at 8% by weight. It also contains significant calcium and vitamin A.

In addition, the fruit contains procyanidin oligomers, which have been shown to reduce the risk of heart disease and diabetes. Açaí also contains several other potent phytonutrients, such as ferulic acid, a potent antibacterial agent.

## Coconut Health

Botanically speaking, the "nut" of a coconut tree is not a nut: It is a drupe, as it is a palm fruit. Coconut trees sway in the tropical breeze do more than present good ambience for vacations. They are mining rich volcano- and ocean-fed nutrients and depositing them into their copra, water and meat.

Coconut water contains a variety of minerals, trace elements and vitamins. These include minerals magnesium, calcium, potassium, zinc and phosphorus, a host of B vitamins, and various antioxidants. The various trace elements contained in coconut water are often called electrolytes, making coconut water one of the best exercise partners around.

Coconut meat will contain these nutrients together with over 3% protein and a considerable quantity of a special type of saturated fat termed MCFAs – middle-chain fatty acids. MCFAs have been shown to significantly reduce LDL-cholesterol and help unclog arteries.

Coconut meat is often pressed into oil, and the oil is known not only for its MCFA content, but also for its caprylic acid and lauric acid content. These two fats have been shown to be antimicrobial and immune-enhancing when eaten.

The health community has been stirred by reports of Coconut oil being a cure-all for Alzheimer's disease. Many report it is simply "anecdotal evidence." Is there really any scientific evidence for the notion that late-stage Alzheimer's disease can be reversed by coconut oil? Surprisingly, yes, but the evidence also points to an important caveat.

In 2001, at the age of 51, Dr. Steve Newport began making memory mistakes. His memory and cognitive functions spiraled downward over the next eight years. By 2008, Steve's Alzheimer's had become severe.

So Dr. Newport conjured up a formula to mimic the 60% middle chain triglyceride (MCT) product used in a study called AC-1202. She gave Steve seven teaspoons of coconut oil per day – or 3-4 servings per day of MCT oil. During the first month, Steve's tremors resolved and his cognition difficulties improved. His cognitive test scores increased dramatically during the first few weeks of the coconut oil. And over the next few years, Dr. Newport reported that her husband "came back."

And his scores proved it. His cognition scores improved by 6 points of 75 point scale on cognitive, and 14 points of 78 on daily living activity tests.

Dr. Newport has since collected about 250 testimonies, about 90% of which were positive – though admittedly improved people would most likely write a testimony.

So is there any scientific evidence for taking coconut oil for Alzheimer's disease?

Dr. Newport's personal research established that Steve's early Alzheimer's disease was related to the inability of his brain cells to process glucose, or its alternative, ketones, for energy.

And shutting down that energy supply naturally shuts off those brain cells – spiraling a person into Alzheimer's disease.

183

But does this happen for everyone who is experiencing Alzheimer's disease? In a word, no.

Yet the ketonogenic diet – replacing glucose with ketone esters – has been shown to help epilepsy and other nervous disorders among those who have difficulty processing ketones from foods such as breast milk or dairy milk.

Breast milk, for example, contains 10-17% medium chain triglycerides (MCTs), which are converted to ketones in the form of Beta-hydroxybuterate. This is why MCTs are now added to any good baby formula.

The ketones are taken up by brain cells. Breast milk contains 10-17% medium chain triglycerides, which are converted to ketones in the form of Beta-hydroxybuterate

Enter Dr. Samuel Henderson – who patented a product called AC-1202, made up of primarily medium chain triglyceride oil processed from either palm oil or coconut oil.

Like Coconut oil, AC-1202 is taken up by the liver and released as ketones, which can be identified in the bloodstream as beta-hydroxybutyrate.

Research over the past 20 years has shown that beta-hydroxybutyrate reduces symptoms of Parkinson's, epilepsy and other nerve-related disorders, because these ketones are utilized for energy by glucose-starved brain and nerve cells (Zheng et al. 2012).

One study of children with epilepsy showed that a beta-hydroxybutyrate-rich ketogenic diet reduced seizures by as much as 75% (Neal et al. 2008).

The relationship between Alzheimer's and the need for ketones in brain and nerve cells has been related to a genetic variation, the epsilon-4 (E4) variant of the apolipoprotein E gene – also referred to as ApoE4. Because this variation seems to block the ability of the body to convert fats to ketones, the brain and nerve cells can become starved for energy.

Having a genetic variant of the ApoE4 does not always result in Alzheimer's disease, but having one E4 allele can increase the risk of AD by three times and having two E4 alleles can increase the risk of AD by 12 times.

Yet Alzheimer's is not always the result of the ApoE4 gene variant, but it has been seen among those with vascular damage – damage to the tiny blood vessels in the brain. As we've discussed with other AD research, diet is one of the greatest determinants for Alzheimer's. And vascular damage is also seen without the E4 gene variant.

But this E4 variation has provided the key to unlocking – at least for those who have this genetic variation and have some issue with processing ketones in the liver – the potential link between Alzheimer's disease and coconut oil.

The science is related to neurons being powered by ketones in the form of beta-hydroxybuterate, being taken up by brain cells that are starving for energy. For those who have difficulty producing ketones and/or have glucose resistance, mild ketosis has been shown to improve cognition, not only in animal and laboratory studies, but also in clinical research.

Over a decade ago Dr. Samuel Henderson (Henderson et al. 2009) patented a product called AC-1202 – a medium chain trigliceride oil. The AC-1202 product contains glycerin with caprylic acid – a middle chain triglyceride, with a chemical name of 1,2,3-propanetriol trioctanoate.

The AC-1202 product underwent a clinical trial published in the Medical Journal Nutrition and Metabolism in August of 2009. This study followed 152 Alzheimer's patients for 90 days using randomized, double-blind and placebo controls.

The Alzheimer's patients took the AC-1202 or the placebo for 90 days, and were given cognitive tests at 45 days and after the trial period. This included the gold standard ADAS-Cog test.

The research found that the AC-1202 significantly increased levels of beta-hydroxybutyrate, meaning they now had ketone-rich blood. As a whole, the AC-1202 group scored significantly higher in cognitive test scores compared to the placebo group. But this significant improvement took place primarily among those patients who had the ApoE4 variant. Those E4 variant patients saw a 5.73 point difference between the placebo group on the ADAS-Cog testing, while there was little difference among those patients without the ApoE4 gene variant.

*"While the cognitive effects were not significant in the overall sample, a pre-defined examination of cognitive effects stratified by genotype yielded significant effects in E4(-) participants," wrote the researchers in their discussion of the study.*

The results of this clinical study clearly indicates that the potential for dramatic positive effects of coconut oil or any other source of MCT should take place primarily for those with the ApoE4 variant – or those having another form of glucose or insulin resistance that affects brain cells' receiving glucose or ketones from our diet.

This later condition – having glucose or insulin resistance – may well be a looming issue that relates the ApoE variant to our diet. There is a growing epidemic of type 2 diabetes in modern society, due to the ravages of the Western diet.

Yet jumping to the conclusion that Coconut oil is a cure-all for Alzheimer's Disease is short sighted. It is important to understand the science and the physiology of the process, and see the relationship between the ApoE4 variant and the need for inducing mild ketosis with MCT or Coconut oil.

In their discussion of the MCT study, the researchers said:

*"While we cannot entirely rule out the role of C8 fatty acids in mediating some of the cognitive effects seen in the study, the correlation of cognitive performance with circulating beta-hydroxybutyrate suggests that ketosis plays a prominent role in MCT therapy."*

In other words, while coconut oil or MCT oil might help someone experiencing mild cognitive impairment due to glucose or insulin resistance, its more likely benefit to Alzheimer's disease will be for those with the APOE-E4 gene variant and thus cannot process triglycerides in the liver normally – combined with a diet that produces glucose and/or insulin resistance among brain cells.

This last point is the likely key that ties the diet link between AD and the ApoE4 link. Those with the ApoE4 variant who also develop glucose or insulin resistance through poor dietary habits may experience cognitive issues and Alzheimer's due to their brain cells being energy-starved – having no energy source. The research evidence illustrates that these folks may have the greatest likelihood of benefiting from a MCT-rich supplementation of diet.

Sources of middle chain triglycerides (MCTs) include palm kernel oil, coconut oil, and the milk fat of goat milk, cow's milk and breast milk. Note that non-fat milk has had the MCTs removed. The NeoBee 895 MCT oil is another source of MCTs.

Today we can find a flurry of coconut products on the market, and this is a boon for health. Coconut oil can replace butter as a meltable spread for toast, vegetables and more. It can also be used to pop popcorn and as a oil added to soups, pasta and many other cooking oil applications.

## The Wonders of Avocado

Most consider avocado a delicacy but few realize the nutrient density of avocados. Even fewer realize that avocados prevent heart disease.

The avocado grows in primarily warm climates with little risk of frost. This makes southern and central California, along with Mexico, Central America and parts of Australia prime avocado growing regions.

### The nutrient dense avocado

One medium avocado has about 500 milligrams of potassium. This makes avocados one of the richest sources of potassium available – over 50% more potassium than a banana contains.

A medium avocado will also contain a considerable amount of fiber—approximately five grams, or about one gram of fiber per ounce. About 75% of this fiber is insoluble—making it one of the best sources of this important cancer-preventative, cholesterol-reducing type of fiber.

The avocado also contains a significant amount of B vitamins: almost a third (28%) of the RDA of vitamin B5, about 20% of RDA for vitamin B6. 20% of RDAs for folate (B9), about 12% of RDAs for niacin and almost 10% of RDA for vitamin B2. This makes the avocado one of the best natural sources of B vitamins available.

Avocados also contain significant amounts of vitamin E, magnesium, coper, iron, zinc and magnesium.

### Healthy avocado fats

Most of avocado's calories are derived from monounsaturated fat. Monounsaturated fats like oleic oil are one of the main components of the Mediterranean diet, which is known to reduce heart disease, reduce dementia risk and lower cholesterol levels.

An important fat in avocado is called avocadene. Avocadene is actually a fatty alcohol with molecular structure of 16-heptadecene-1,2,4-triol. This particular triol has a number of properties, including being an internal antibacterial agent. Avocadene is also an anti-inflammatory agent. For this reason, it is often recommended as a part of the diet for those with intestinal difficulties and joint inflammation.

In a study of 15 women from Wesley Hospital in Brisbane, Australia (Colquhoun et al. 1992), those eating a monounsaturated oil diet enriched with avocado had a reduction of total cholesterol of 8.2% after only three weeks. LDL cholesterol was also significantly reduced among the avocado group. HDL was unaffected by the avocado-enriched diet.

In another study of 12 women with diabetes (Lerman-Garber et al. 1994), a diet enriched with avocado reduced triglycerides by 20% after only 4 weeks. The avocado diet also increased glycemic control among the patients.

In yet another study (Lopez Ledesma et al. 1996), 67 volunteers (30 of which had high cholesterol) ate either an avocado-enriched diet or control diets. Those eating the avocado diet after only seven days had a reduction in total cholesterol of 16%-17%, a reduction in LDL of 22% and a 22% drop in triglyceride levels. The avocado group also experienced an increase of 11% in HDL (good) cholesterol.

### Avocado does not encourage weight gain

The myth that often circulates among those considering avocados is that avocados are 'fattening.' Yes, this is truly a myth.

To dispel the notion that avocadoes encourage weight gain, South African researchers (Pieterse et al. 2005) gave part of a group of sixty-one obese persons on a weight loss regimen avocado oil to replace their other fat and oil sources. At the end of six weeks, the avocado oil subjects had similar weight loss results as with the other weight loss subjects.

## Anti-inflammatory Foods

A number of foods have been shown in research to decrease inflammation. This relates directly to the food's ability to slow the inflammation cycle which involves the release of pro-inflammatory mediators such as leukotrienes.

As we age, our diet becomes more critical as our body tends to be on an inflammation hair trigger of sorts. This is because our immune system is more sensitive, and weaker at the same time.

Thus the major component of inflammation – after injuries and infections – is our diet. Our diet can stimulate systemic inflammation even if our body is responding to a localized injury or infection.

Red meat, fried foods, refined sugars and simple carbohydrates tend to stimulate inflammation. Red meat, for example, provides the body with too much arachidonic acid – a pro-inflammatory oil. Fried foods present the body with trans and oxidized fats, which tend to damage the arteries and liver, producing inflammation.

Here is a quick list of foods that slow or curb the rate of inflammation within the body:
- Flaxseed
- Fresh pineapple (or bromelain)
- Papaya
- Fresh juices such as carrot, beet, cucumber and beet
- Vegetable broth
- Root foods such as ginger, peanuts, carrots

Most fresh fruits and vegetables are anti-inflammatory. The goal is to alkalize the blood and increase the detoxification capabilities of the liver, to help clear the blood.

Specific fruits and vegetables known to increase detoxification and provide alkalizing effects would include apricots, apples, almonds, artichokes, avocado, banana, lima beans, beets, beet greens, berries, Brussels sprouts, carrots, casaba, cauliflower, celery, coconuts, corn, cranberries, cucumbers, dandelion greens, eggplant, grapes, raw honey, kale, citrus fruits (fresh), lettuce, mango, mushrooms, oats, okra, onions, papaya, parsnips, parsley, peas, pineapple, radishes, raisins, spinach, chard, tomatoes, turnips, walnuts, watermelon, watercress, zucchini.

Fiber can also curb inflammatory response. Increase fiber to 35-45 grams per day. 6-10 servings of raw fruits and vegetables per day to accomplish this.

Garlic, cayenne and onions have quercetin, an inflammatory inhibitor. Also cayenne has been shown to inhibit substance P, one of the cascade elements in migraines. Other anti-inflammatory spices to cook with are turmeric and garlic. Avoid rancid or trans-fat oils. Fresh olive or canola are best cooking oils. A challenge or elimination test to determine any food allergies is suggested. Focus should be on foods that are high in fiber and nutrition, and easy to digest.

## Sterol Foods

Plant sterols, also called phytosterols, are compounds found in most plant foods, including fruits, vegetables, seeds and nuts. There are a variety of different types of sterols, including avenasterol, campesterol and beta sitosterol. These are the lipids that make up the cells membranes of plants. A healthy plant cell membrane made of these phytosterols helps protect the plant's cells from becoming vulnerable to free radicals.

They also help reduce oxidized radicals in human nutrition because they attach and neutralize unstable lipids within the intestines.

Foods high in sterols include fresh corn, with 952 milligrams per 100 grams, rice bran, with 1055 milligrams per 100 grams, wheat germ with 553 milligrams per 100 grams, and flax seed with 338 milligrams per 100 grams. Nuts also have good sterol content. Cashews have 146 milligrams per 100 grams and peanuts have 206 milligrams per 100 grams.

Researchers from Canada's University of Toronto and St Michael's Hospital (Jenkins *et al.* 2011) found that people who ate diets rich in plant-based foods known for lowering LDL-cholesterol, including plant sterols, soy foods, nuts and plant-based fibers showed reductions in LDL-cholesterol by 13% after six months. The average reduction in LDL-cholesterol went from 171 mg/dL on average down 25 mg/dL to 156 mg/dL of LCL-c.

The study was published in the *Journal of the American Medical Association.*

The study followed 345 volunteers who were either instructed to eat a low-saturated fat diet or were given specific dietary advice to eat certain foods known to lower cholesterol during clinic visits. Their LDL-cholesterol levels Those who ate the low-saturated fat diet showed a 3% reduction in LDL-cholesterol levels during the same period. Their levels reduced from the average of 171 mg/dL to 168 mg/dL.

The researchers also divided the specific-foods diet into two additional groups, one that was given two sessions of advice during the six months and the other, given seven clinical dietary sessions during the six months. These two groups showed little difference in their resulting LDL-cholesterol levels. The group given seven advice sessions had 13.8% average reduction in LDL-cholesterol, while the group given two advice sessions showed an average of 13.1% reduction in LDL-cholesterol.

This later result indicates that most people will adhere to diet advice when given occasionally as compared to frequently.

The overall result, however, is consistent with the multitude of research that has shown that plant sterols, cultured soy foods, nuts and high fiber foods specifically reduce LDL-cholesterol.

Higher LDL-cholesterol levels have been associated with higher incidence of heart disease, atherosclerosis (hardening of the arteries), strokes and other cardiovascular issues. This is because LDL-cholesterol is less stable, and readily oxidizes. This oxidation produces free radicals that damage the walls of the blood vessels. This causes scaring, which tends to harden the arteries, as well as releases scar tissue into the blood. This release is what causes thrombosis.

The Canadian researchers concluded that: "Use of a dietary portfolio compared with the low-saturated fat dietary advice resulted in greater LDL-C lowering during 6 months of follow-up." The "dietary portfolio" was the specific foods mentioned, offered within nutrition counseling sessions that taught the volunteers how to incorporate these LDL-cholesterol-lowering foods into their diets.

## The Ancient Grain

Brown rice is an ancient grain that has nourished billions of people for thousands of years. But what about today's rice? Most of it is white. Is there any difference?

Researchers from Japan's University of Tokushima Graduate School of Health Biosciences (Shimabukuro *et al.* 2013) have proven what natural health proponents have been suggesting for decades: Brown rice is superior to white rice, not only nutritionally, but for glucose metabolism and for the prevention of metabolic syndrome.

The researchers ran multiple tests with healthy and obese volunteers, the first to analyze the effect of brown rice consumption on weight management and/or loss, body fat, abdominal fat and glucose metabolism. They also measured the effects of the two types of rice on the health of the arteries (endothelial function and dilation). These effects were also tested in patients who had been diagnosed with metabolic syndrome.

The researchers then randomized 27 male volunteers into groups and for 8 weeks they had the subjects eat various patterns of brown rice or white rice meals. The researchers also mixed the protocols to include a return to white rice consumption for those who ate brown rice for eight weeks.

After the series of tests, the researchers determined that those eating brown rice in their diets had greater weight loss during the eight weeks. Furthermore, most of that weight loss returned after they returned to white rice consumption.

The research also determined that the brown rice consumption resulted in slower glucose metabolism – lower postprandial glucose levels – as compared to white rice consumption.

The researchers also determined that consuming brown rice resulted in a greater dilation of the brachial artery – a measure of the arteries' endothelial health.

The research also found that two months of eating brown rice resulted in lower insulin resistance. Cholesterol levels (LDL-c and total) were also lower after 8 weeks of eating brown rice.

The researchers wrote:

*"In conclusion, consumption of brown rice may be beneficial, partly owing to the lowering of glycemic response, and may protect postprandial endothelial function in subjects with the metabolic syndrome. Long-term beneficial effects of brown rice on metabolic parameters and endothelial function were also observed."*

## Metabolic Syndrome and Whole Grains

Metabolic syndrome is evidenced typically by an overweight status or obesity level of weight, glucose metabolism issues – with either glucose intolerance and/or insulin resistance. Rounding out the effects of these is evidence of coronary artery disease – which typically affects those with glucose metabolism issues due to the formation of free radicals in the blood stream from the greater levels of glucose in the blood.

The research above and others has pointed to the fact that metabolic syndrome is often a factor of eating overly processed foods – and the avoidance of whole foods in general.

The reason for this is that whole foods typically contain greater fibers – in the form of husks, peels, seeds and segment walls. These are typically separated from the food during processing, leaving a mash of starches with limited nutrients. For some foods, a particular nutrient – such as sugar – is extracted from the food and the rest tossed.

The separated, mashed food is then typically heated to high degrees in order to sterilize it – which kills many of the remaining nutrients. This sterilized food is then packaged with preservatives and other chemicals to produce what natural health experts might call "fake food."

In the case of rice, white rice is milled, which means its germ and bran are removed. The remaining kernel is then typically polished and enriched with some of the vitamins it is now missing due to the bran and germ being removed – including folic acid and other important B vitamins.

## Whole Oats and Barley

Oats and barley are also particularly high in soluble fiber, consisting primarily of mixed linkage beta glucans – (1,3)(1,4)-beta-d-glucans. Beta-glucans are unique polysaccharides that have been the focus of much research in recent years. The American Diabetes Association recommends 40 grams of soluble fiber per day to prevent adult-onset diabetes.

Oats and barley also contain considerable amounts of protein. Oats' protein levels are also notable, at 17% – a very high quality protein with a balance of amino acids. And, they are totally free of gluten.

Oats and barley also have a number of important vitamins and minerals. They are also a good source of folate (22% adult DV in a serving for oats), pantothenic acid (21% DV), thiamin (79% DV), calcium (8% DV), iron (41% DV), magnesium (69% DV), potassium (19% DV), zinc (41% DV), copper (49% DV) and manganese (383% DV), along with other nutrients and trace elements.

Oats and barley are also good sources for healthy fats. A serving of oats contains 173 milligrams of omega-3 alpha-linolenic acids, and 3781 mg of omega-6 fatty acids. The fat content of oats – higher than most other grains – is also balanced between monounsaturated and polyunsaturated fats.

Oats also contain a unique combination of glycolipids, diacylglycerols and estolides, and a number of single-, double-, triple- and tetra-bonded diacylglycerols. These unique fatty acids distinguish oats from other grains.

Oats and barley have low glycemic indexes. In oatmeal form, oats have a particularly low glycemic index of 58. Researchers have found that oats provide a 50% reduction in glycemic load or peak, because of the high viscosity of its fiber. The American Diabetes Association recommends 40 grams of soluble fiber per day to prevent adult-onset diabetes. Researchers have found that oats provide a 50% reduction in glycemic load or peak.

Oats reduce cholesterol. In 2007, the UK's University of Teesside's School of Health and Social Care released a Cochrane review study comparing ten different trials reporting on oats' ability to reduce cholesterol.

The study's results concluded that oats lowered total cholesterol and low density lipoproteins an average of 7.7 mg/dL and 7 mg/dL respectively. The mechanism seems to be the beta-glucans' ability to inhibit bile acid absorption.

Oats and barley reduce the risk of artery disease. Oats and barley contain unique alkaloid polyphenols called avenanthramides. Recent research indicates that avenanthramides reduce incidence and complications of atherosclerosis – the scarring and inflammation of the artery walls. Avenanthramides have also shown significant antioxidant capacity.

The best way to eat oats is to cook them lightly. Use either whole rolled or whole groats (also called Irish oats). Whole rolled will require very little cooking. Bring the water to a boil, put in a pinch of whole salt and then the oats at 50/50 water. Cook for less than five minutes, turn off the heat, and add your raisins, cinnamon, raw honey, strawberries, raspberries and other toppings.

For example, cereal grains oats and barley produce a class of compounds called avenanthramides. Avenanthramide content is more than double in whole oat flakes (26-27 mg/kg) than in oat bran (13 mg/kg). Recent research indicates that avenanthramides reduce atherosclerosis – the scarring and inflammation of the artery walls.

Avenanthramides are anti-inflammatory agents. University studies have confirmed that they stimulate immunity by increasing immune cell signaling. A Tufts University study led by Dr. Mohsen Meydani showed that avenanthramides lowered atherosclerosis risk by reducing the growth of vascular smooth muscle cells, while increasing nitric oxide production among artery walls.

In another study led by Dr. Meydani, avenanthramides were shown to increase the stability of the genetic protein p53. The p53 protein regulates tumor necrosis factor, a self-destruct switch that helps the body eliminate cancer-causing cells. Avenanthramides are now thought to be the key constituent giving oats their ability to reduce inflammation around the body.

Avenanthramides are expressed as phytoalexins as part of the oat plant's resistance to disease. The association between crown rust disease on the farm and higher avenanthramides content was established in recent research led by Mitchell Wise, Ph.D. in collaboration with the USDA's Doug Doehlert, Ph.D. and Mike McMullen, Ph.D., a professor at North Dakota State University.

This study tested eighteen grain genotypes in three different growing areas. Crown rust resistance correlated directly with higher avenanthramides levels. As oats resist infections such as crown rust – caused by *Puccinia coronata* – hardy avenanthramide molecules become expressed as part of the plant's immune function. Increases in environmental challenges and infection also translate to increased avenanthramides expression in oat leaves.

Barley, on the other hand, produces the phenolic acids called alk(en)ylresorcinols. This family of compounds produce anti-fungal and antioxidant effects. Barley produces alkylresorcinols for the same purpose that oats produce avenanthramides – as a defense mechanism. In 2004 field testing by scientists from the Agricultural University in Poland, winter barley varieties grown in different regions produced alkylresorcinol content that varied to environmental stress.

## Beta Glucans

Whole cereal grain fiber is rich in beta-D-glucans, which have been shown in university research to maintain healthy cholesterol levels. Researchers from The Netherlands' Maastricht University calculated from multiple studies that healthy cholesterol levels were achieved with every gram of additional beta-glucan soluble fiber added to the diet.

Beta-D-glucans reside in cell walls throughout the bran and endosperm of cereal grains. In 2002, the U.S. Food and Drug Administration, after reviewing scientific evidence from a number of studies, announced that beta-D-glucans soluble fiber had been shown to have significant cardiovascular benefits.

In 2007, the UK's University of Teesside's School of Health and Social Care released a Cochrane review study comparing ten different studies of oats and cholesterol levels. The study's results concluded that oats lowered total cholesterol and low density lipoproteins an average of 7.7 mg/dL and 7 mg/dL respectively. The key mechanism cited was the ability of beta-D-glucans in oats to inhibit bile acid absorption.

Barley beta-D-glucans have illustrated similar results. In a 2007 study at University of Minnesota's Medical School, 155 volunteers were divided into four treatment groups for six weeks of beta-D-glucans consumption or controls.

The beta-D-glucans groups were given either high or low molecular weight barley beta-D-glucans in either 5 gram or 3 gram per day doses. The 5g high molecular weight beta-D-glucan group experienced a 15% reduction of LDL, while the low molecular weight 5g beta-D-glucan group had a 13% reduction of LDL. The 3g groups both experienced 9% LDL reduction, illustrating a dose-relationship between beta-D-glucans consumption and LDL levels.

Beta-D-glucans can also increase high-density lipoprotein levels. In a study at Venezuela's University of Zulia in 2007, 38 volunteers with mild hypercholesterolemia were given either the American Heart Association

Step II diet alone or the AHA Step II diet plus 6 grams of beta-D-glucans per day for eight weeks. HDL levels among the beta-D-glucans group increased by an average of 28% – from 39.4 to 49.5. The beta-D-glucans group also experienced significant decreases in LDL and total cholesterol, and small decreases in VLDL and triglycerides.

## Diabetes Prevention

A number of studies have illustrated that whole cereal grain consumption can significantly decrease the risk of type II diabetes. Mechanisms appear to combine a slower release of glucose into the bloodstream together with improved insulin response.

A study of 18 healthy adult men at New Zealand's University of Auckland in 2007 found that a meal rich in cereal grains significantly reduced the postprandial glycemic and insulin response compared to controls.

A 2005 study in Finland of twelve type II diabetic patients concluded that oat bran flour lowered glucose excursion by 1.6 mmol/l at 30 minutes.

A Swiss study reviewed multiple studies and determined that hyper- and hypoglycemic symptoms are reduced with consumption of cereal grains. The review found a 50% reduction in glycemic peak with the consumption of whole cereal grains. The reviewers proposed that diabetics incorporate these grains into our meals.

Conclusive population studies have found that populations that have transitioning from a traditional grain-based diet to the western red meat-oriented diet are experiencing significant rises in rates of heart disease, cancer and other inflammatory ailments.

(Miyazaki *et al.* 1995; Chihara 1992; Weber *et al.* 1995; Anderson *et al.* 2009; Theuwissen *et al.* 2008; FDA 2002; Kelly *et al.* 2007; Keenan *et al.* 2007; Reyna-Villasmil *et al.* 2007; Muralikrishna and Rao 2007; Poppitt *et al.* 2007; Tapola *et al.* 2005; Würsch and Pi-Sunyer 1997; Murphy *et al.* 2007; Davis *et al.* 2004; Yn *et al.* 1998; Angeli et al 2006; Volman *et al.* 2008; Mattila *et al.* 2005; Bratt *et al.* 2003; Chen *et al.* 2007; Liu *et al.* 2004; Nie *et al.* 2006; Sur *et al.* 2008; Okazaki *et al.* 2004; Zarnowski *et al.* 2002; Zarnowski *et al.* 2004).

## Fiber and The Colon

Without a varied diet of fibrous whole foods, we will not be providing the body with the biochemical structural support that it needs. This is because fiber is a matrix of biochemistry produced through the biological elements of living organisms.

Fiber is either soluble or insoluble. Both soluble and insoluble fibers are not digested. They both move through out intestinal tract, escorting waste, facilitating digestion, and balancing nutrients absorption. They eventually facilitate our bowel movements.

While soluble fiber becomes gelatinous in the presence of liquids, insoluble fiber passes through our small and large intestines without much change. Soluble fiber will bind with fats in the stomach, slowing down the process of absorption. This delays glucose absorption into the bloodstream, which means that it provides an evenly balanced stream of energy to the cells.

For this reason, soluble fiber is good for regulating blood sugar in those who have blood sugar issues – either diabetic (hyper-) or hypoglycemic problems. Soluble fiber also lowers levels of the "bad" forms of LDL cholesterol by rendering LDL particle size at more optimal levels. Soluble fiber is plentiful in oats, flax, vegetables, Psyllium husk, and various other nuts, beans and grains. Apples are a great source as well.

Insoluble fiber facilitates the easier movement of food through our intestines. This means that insoluble fiber helps prevent constipation and helps eliminate toxicity in the colon due to its aiding regular, rhythmic bowel movements. It is like an escort service. Insoluble fiber also helps balance the pH of the intestinal tract.

This of course assists the survival and viability of the important probiotic colonies so important to the immune system. Sources of insoluble fiber include various whole wheats, whole oats, corn, green leafy vegetables (cellulose is an insoluble fiber), and various nuts, seeds, green beans and green peas. Apples are also a great source of insoluble fiber.

A typical adult should have at least 30-40 grams of total fiber in the diet, with about 75% of that fiber being insoluble. By focusing our eating on whole natural foods, we will likely get enough of both fibers. However, should our diet contain a sizeable portion of processed or convenient foods, we might consider taking a count every so often to see what our consumption is. If we have constipation, irritable bowels, or just a lack of regular bowel movements, a lack of insoluble fiber is probably a contributing factor.

Fiber is composed of a number of polysaccharides and oligosaccharides. These are utilized by plants for stability with some flexibility, allowing for circulation and the ability to stand tall against the elements. Plants also use dextrins, inulins, lignans, pectins, chitins, waxy substances, and beta-glucans to create their root, leave and stem structures. All of these bind to toxins in the intestines and lower low density lipoproteins.

The health of the colon is a critical part of the health of the entire body. The colon provides the body with the ability to eliminate waste products. Without good elimination, waste products will putrefy, possibly finding their way back into the bloodstream. Once purification builds within the colon and intestines, the body will attempt to provide a layer of protection to protect the intestinal wall against this mix of bacteria, acidic endotoxins (bacterial poop) and partially digested food.

This self-defensive layer is often referred to as a *mucoid plaque layer*. This layer will build around the inside of the colon, clogging much of the passageway for food and waste to pass. Bacteria and endotoxins will assimilate into the layer, making it all the more unhealthy. This mucoid plaque layer will sometimes be so thick and hard a pencil can hardly fit through the remaining opening. Because pathogenic microorganisms can grow inside the mucoid layer, outside the reach of probiotics, their populations can expand with little hindrance.

There are a number of ailments that have been associated with the build up of mucoid plaque in the intestines and colon. Constipation is obvious, as the opening (or *lumen)* becomes constricted. Other issues not so obvious are sinusitis; allergies; asthma; bronchitis; back pain; liver and gall bladder problems; skin issues like psoriasis and eczema; chronic fatigue and food sensitivities.

Other disorders are worsened by or connected to this build up of mucoid plaque in the colon. Recently there is clinical evidence that the pathogenic bacteria build-up may result in an blood-circulating bacteria, infecting joints and causing rheumatoid arthritis.

Mucin and mucus are the substances providing the layering ability over intestinal walls. As mentioned they are produced by the body to protect the intestinal walls from the acidic environment of the intestine and colon. Much of this mucin and mucus is secreted by *Brunner's glands* located in the duodenum. These glands are stimulated by changes in pH. They harmonically work to balance the pH of the intestinal tract, as an acidic environment will damage the intestinal wall.

Because the stomach produces various acids to break down food and kill microorganisms, the Brunner's glands typically provide just enough mucin and mucous to balance this aspect. However if the food we eat itself has too much acidic quality – such as over-processed foods and meats with their high amino acid content – then these glands will produce more mucus and mucin to provide balance. This extra production provides the glue for the plaque throughout the intestinal and colon walls.

How do we know if we have mucoid plaque? The first symptom is the size of our stool. If the stool is runny and not solid, or perhaps pencil-thin as a norm, then it is likely there is a build up of mucoid plaque preventing our stools from forming correctly. Another giveaway is chronic constipation or irregular bowel movements. Bloating also indicates a strong possibility of mucoid plaque build-up.

Our stools should take place twice or at least once per day – every day. The stool should look solid and husky: Missile-shaped is best and about (depending upon age and size) an inch to two inches in diameter. The longer the stool, the better shape the colon is probably in. Shorter "plops" indicate mucoid plaque build up with small colon lumen.

The easiest solution for mucoid plaque build-up is a combination of fiber, a re-establishment of probiotic colonies and a *colonic*. A colonic is a flushing out of the lower colon utilizing a hydrotherapy colonic machine.

A colonic machine will push water in and out of the colon, washing away the plaque and debris along the colon walls. For difficult cases, this may take 2-3 visits to accomplish. We will typically experience tremendous results after just one treatment though. This treatment has proven very successful among natural therapists.

A number of well-known physicians utilized colonic hydrotherapy in the early to mid twentieth century experienced success treating various illnesses with colon cleansing. Dr. John Kellogg, Dr. William Koch, Dr. Eugene Blass, Dr. J.H. Tilden and Dr. Bernard Jensen and Sir Arbuthnot Lane – King of England's surgeon – all had notable success in treating patients with colon cleansing.

In 1929, Dr. J.F. Burgess, a professor at McGill University and dermatologist at the Montreal General Hospital reported in the *Canadian Journal of Medicine* that his research led him to believe that "alimentary toxins" (build-up of colonic bacteria and plaque) were one of the most important factors in eczema (Burgess 1930).

William Lintz, M.D. successfully treated 472 patients who suffered from allergies with colon cleansing.

Dr. J.H. Tilden successfully treated hundreds of patients with pneumonia during the early 1900s by cleansing their bowels followed by a good diet.

Allan Eustis, M.D., a Tulane University of Medicine professor in 1912, is said to have cured 121 cases of bronchial asthma with colon cleansing.

D. Rochester, M.D. of the University of Buffalo's School of Medicine, made a statement in 1906 saying that after 23 years of observation, he believed that intestinal toxemia is the underlying cause of asthma.

Harvey Kellogg, M.D. once said: *"Of the 22,000 operations that I have personally performed, I have never found a single normal colon, and of the 100,000 that were performed under my jurisdiction, not over 6% were normal."*

## The Need for Seed

Seeds like sunflower, sesame and pumpkin seeds are highly nutritious. In their raw or lightly roasted forms, they supply various omega-3 oils (as we'll discuss later) along with a complete protein foundation of all the essential amino acids.

A number of seeds are helpful for calming inflammation and increasing the body's gentle purification systems. These include Flax, Safflower, Rapeseed, Caraway, Anise, Fennel, Licorice seed, Black seed and others. Seeds contain basic compounds that offer mucilage, saponins and other polysaccharides that contribute to the health of the mucous membranes.

Not surprisingly, combinations or single versions of these seeds have been used in traditional medicine for centuries.

Beans are essentially seeds. The variety of different types of beans are astounding, and most are complete protein foods. These include black beans, soybeans, lima beans, garbanzo beans, pinto beans and many others.

Beans are also are particularly high in a number of phytonutrients, including flavonols like quercetin and kaempferol, and anthocyanins. They also found black beans high in polyphenols like ferulic acid and chlorogenic acid. All of these are potent antioxidants and have been shown to stimulate the immune system (Ranilla et al. 2007).

Flaxseed is also an important seed. A growing cadre of nutritional researchers are beginning to understand that one of key reasons for flax' myriad of health benefits has to do with the fact that those oligosaccharides present in its fiber feeds our probiotic populations.

Other research has shown that supplementing with certain strains of probiotic bacteria also reduces blood pressure.

Research presented at the 2012 American Heart Association scientific session details that a daily dose of flaxseed in breads will decrease blood pressure significantly.

The research comes from the Canadian center for Argi-Food research in health and medicine located in St. Boniface hospital (Leyva et al. 2012). The study followed 110 patients who were over 40 years old who had peripheral arterial disease.

The patients were randomized, and either given 30 grams of milled flaxseed per day within bagels, muffins or buns, or those same breads without flaxseed.

After one year, the patients were retested. The research found that those who consumed the flaxseed within their breads had a reduction of blood pressure by 10 mmHg systolic and 7 mmHg diastolic. Those patients who had high blood pressure prior to the beginning of the study had an even greater reduction in systolic blood pressure – by 15 mm Hg.

Dr. Grant Pierce, the study's lead researcher, stated that the results have surprised many.

> *"The is the largest decrease in blood pressure ever shown by any dietary intervention – including the Mediterranean diet and low-sodium diets."*

Dr. Pierce also indicated that these sort of reductions will reduce heart attack and stroke incidence by as much as 50%.

Flaxseed contains a number of constituents that work synergistically to reduce cholesterol and blood pressure. These include alpha-linolenic acid, linoleic acid, oligosaccharide-rich fiber and various lignans.

Other research has found that flaxseed reduces cholesterol and helps maintain healthy bowel movements.

As we've discussed and will discuss further, seeds and beans also contain various isoflavones and lignans, which balance hormone activity and help produce healthy cholesterol levels.

## Nuts for the Heart

Nuts provide a perfect blend of fats, proteins, isoflavones and minerals. While most of the edible nuts are healthy, some of the best nuts are brazil nuts, almonds, cashews and walnuts (peanuts are not nuts – they are legumes).

Nuts got a bum reputation a few decades ago because of their fairly high fat content. But the type of fats nuts have is the critical point.

A study by researchers from the University of Georgia (Robbins *et al.* 2011) found that tree nuts contain a variety of heart-healthy nutrients.

The researchers studied the nutrient content of ten tree nuts: almonds, black walnuts, Brazil nuts, cashews, English walnuts, hazelnuts, macadamias, pecans, pine nuts, and pistachios. (Peanuts are legumes – not tree nuts).

They found that the percentage of heart-healthy fats to be primarily unsaturated oleic and linoleic fatty acids.

Most of the nuts maintained lower than 10% saturated fats, except for Brazil nuts (24%), cashews (21%), macadamias (17%), and pistachios (13%). These are also known as the more fatty nuts.

The tree nuts also contained heart-healthy tocopherols (natural form of vitamin E), which ranged from 1 to 33 milligrams for every 100 grams of the nut meat.

The researchers also found that six nuts also contained tocotrienols (another type of natural vitamin E): Brazil nuts, cashews, English walnuts, macadamias, pine nuts, and pistachios.

They also found that all the nuts contained significant phytosterol content, and mostly above the levels that have been reported in the USDA National Nutrient Database for Standard Reference.

Heart-healthy phytosterol content was highest in pistachios, containing over 300 milligrams for every 100 grams of the nut meat. Pine nuts came in second, with 272 mg/100 g nutmeat.

While tree nuts are most known for great protein sources – most having all the essential amino acids – a number of studies have confirmed that diets with more nuts provide cardiovascular prevention. The reasons, as this study presents, are their lipid content, phytosterol content, and tocopherol and tocotrienol content.

Walnuts are one of the best nuts. They contain a host of nutrients. A cup of chopped walnuts will contain 18 ounces of protein, or about 15% by weight. Walnuts also contain a host of B vitamins, led by folate at 115 mcg, B6 at 600 mcg and thiamin at 400 mcg. A cup of walnuts also contains 115 milligrams of calcium, 185 milligrams of magnesium and 516 milligrams of potassium. Walnuts are also rich in manganese – with 200% of US Daily Value. Walnuts are also rich in selenium and phytosterols.

But it is walnuts' omega-3 content that blows the doors off of most foods, at 10,623 milligrams of omega-3s per cup. Much of this comes in the form of alpha-linolenic acid (ALA). Healthy livers convert ALA to eicosapentaenoic acid (EPA) and docosahexaenoic acid (DHA) as needed, at a rate of between 7% and 36%.

Studies of men and women conducted at the UK's University of Southampton (Din *et al.* 2011) found an average conversion rate of 36% from ALA to EPA, DHA and other N-3s in women and 16% in men. The liver converts ALA using the delta-6-desaturase and elongase enzymes.

It is not surprising that walnuts have been shown to reduce LDL cholesterol, improve artery health, reduce blood pressure and reduce inflammation. But walnuts also produce vitality in other ways.

In fact, research from the University of California, Los Angeles (Robbins *et al.* 2012) determined that eating 75 grams of walnuts a day for three months increases sperm count and men's fertility in general.

The researchers recruited 117 young men in healthy condition, who consumed a typical Western diet. In this single-blinded, randomized trial, the researchers gave 59 of the men 75 grams of walnuts per day for twelve weeks. The other 58 men avoided tree nuts altogether.

Before and after the twelve weeks the men were tested for sperm parameters and blood parameters. Those who ate the walnuts had a significant improvement in their sperm vitality, their sperm motility and their sperm morphology. Sperm aneuploidy – problems with chromosome quality – was also significantly reduced among the walnut group.

Epidemiological research has estimated that some 70 million couples around the world suffer from infertility issues. From 30% to 50% of infertility issues are due to fertility among men. Between three and five million men seek fertility treatments every year.

The research was led by UCLA Professor Wendie Robbins, Ph.D., R.N. *"The positive finding of walnuts on sperm may be a result of their unique nutrient profile,"* Dr. Robbins stated after the study.

Dr. Catherine Carpenter, an associate professor of medicine at UCLA added:

> *"these findings are not surprising when you look at the nutritious content of walnuts, however the results are amazing considering the impact they might have on men of all ages, including older men, and men with impaired fertility."*

The research findings correlated fertility improvement with the walnuts' alpha-linolenic acid content, along with other nutrients.

Dr. Robbins suggested that the male's diet is rarely considered in modern fertility issues. *"Diet is not just maternal territory anymore,"* she added.

## Hormone-balancing Foods

Foods that may increase and balance hormone levels include complex carbohydrates such as potatoes, yams and hormone regulators that contain isoflavones.

Isoflavones daidzein and genistein are a component of a number of foods, including asparagus; many types of beans including soybeans, fava beans, lupins, mung beans and lentils; seeds such as sesame, linseed and flax; and yams, apples, pomegranates, whole wheat and some others. Isoflavone-rich herbs include black cohosh, licorice root, fennel, anise, hops and chaste berry.

Soy is often made out to be a villain, but the research does not agree (we'll discuss soy in detail later).

As for the isoflavones in soy, an analysis of multiple studies from Sichuan University's Hainan Medical College (Wei *et al.* 2012) confirmed that soy isoflavones effectively increase bone density and reduce bone loss.

The study analyzed multiple published international clinical studies on the application of soy isoflavones to prevent osteoporosis, the central cause of hip fractures and other bone fractures around the world.

In their meta-analysis of the research, the medical researchers found that soy isoflavones increased bone density by 54% while reducing bone loss by 23% as measured by a bone loss marker called deoxypyridinoline, which is found in the urine, especially at higher levels among those women in postmenopause.

The research found that doses above 75 milligrams a day of soy isoflavones had the most effect among postmenopausal women.

Osteoporosis is the leading cause of disability among the elderly. Nearly half of women over 60 will have a hip fracture among industrialized nations.

But remember that the active phytoestrogens within soy isoflavones, genistein and daidzein, are also found among many other isoflavone foods, as listed above.

## Menopause assisting foods

Numerous studies have confirmed that consuming phytoestrogens decreases menopausal symptoms among women, but only among those who maintain particular intestinal probiotics that produce an isoflavone metabolite called S-equol.

Higher circulating levels of S-equol have been linked to decreases in bone loss, reduced prostate cancer and reduced menopausal symptoms, including hot flashes, night sweats and irritability. Some research has also indicated that S-equol reduces the risk of breast cancer and endometrial cancer.

S-equol is produced in the body naturally from isoflavones.

One clinical study (Bicíková *et al.* 2012) tested 28 menopausal women. They were given 80 milligrams of phytoestrogens daily while being tested for S-equol within their urine and bloodstream. Prior to the study, the researchers identified the "S-equol producers" versus "S-equol non-producers."

Among the S-equol producers, their S-equol urine levels went from 0.34 to 10.67 ng/ml after the isoflavone supplementation, while the non-producers' levels went from 0.29 to a scant 0.34.

Meanwhile, Kupperman index ratings decreased substantially, but only for the S-equol producers. In the producers, Kupperman index values went from 23.44 to 14.44, while there was little change among the non-producers.

The Kupperman index measures hot flashes, insomnia, nervousness, melancholia, vertigo, weakness, arthralgia or myalgia (muscle pain), headache, paresthesia (tingling sensations), palpitations (quickening heart beats), and formication (skin sensations). A reduction in the index indicates reduced menopausal symptoms.

Actually, S-equol (4',7-isoflavandiol) – also called 5-hydroxy-equol – is produced by intestinal probiotics after they consume the isoflavones daidzein and genistein we eat. (Some have proposed that S-equol only comes from daidzein but recent research clearly indicates that certain probiotics will produce S-equol from genistein).

Many other studies have shown lower menopausal symptoms among those consuming isoflavones. In one (Jou *et al.* 2008), 96 menopausal Taiwanese women were given 135 milligrams of isoflavones daily for six months. The isoflavone group reported significantly decreased menopausal symptoms. But again, this effect was only among those who were S-equol producers.

This of course points to the health of our intestinal probiotics. Can probiotic supplements help increase S-equol levels? The research has indicated that many of the strains in our probiotic supplements do not increase S-equol production.

This is not to say that just any probiotic supplement will necessarily increase S-equol production. In a 2004 study from the University of Minnesota (Nettleton *et al.* 2004), isoflavone supplementation plus *Lactobacillus acidophilus* DDS+1 and *Bifidobacterium longum* did not generally increase S-equol production among a group of 20 women compared to controls (isoflavones alone). However, S-equol production went up significantly amongst a few of the women. The researchers concluded:

> *"the large differences between plasma and urinary equol in some subjects suggest that equol producer status may be modifiable in some individuals."*

However, in a study from Italy (Benvenuti *et al.* 2011) with twelve menopausal women, *Lactobacillus sporogenes* supplementation resulted in a 24% increase in genistein-related equol, while daidzen metabolite equol production only went up for some of the women but not all.

Another study (Tamura *et al.* 2011) indicated that *Lactobacillus rhamnosus* may increase daidzein S-equol production.

But a study from Germany's Institute of Human Nutrition (Matthies *et al.* 2012) published in the *Journal of Nutrition* has found that the intestinal probiotic bacteria (conveniently) named *Slackia isoflavoniconvertens* will convert both genistein and daidzein to 5-hydroxy-equol.

So while the hunt for the right combination of probiotics to turn "non-equol producers" into "S-equol producers" continues, there is good reason to believe that stronger resident probiotic colonies relate directly to S-equol production. This means the subsequent health benefits related to higher circulating S-equol levels – which include cancer protection, bone health and lower menopausal symptoms – relate directly to healthy intestinal probiotics.

And this relates directly to the Ancestors Diet because this diet is not just about food – it is about cultured food as well. And cultured food, as we'll find, is about consuming the right probiotic bacteria with our diet, just as our ancestors have done for millions of years.

# Chapter Seven

# The Cultured Foods

Our body houses huge populations of living organisms. There are about ten times more probiotic bacteria in our bodies than cells. This means our bodies are more bacterial than cellular. Friendly bacteria make up approximately 70% of our immune system. Scientists are suggesting that the DNA of probiotic bacteria (the microbiome) is more important than our cells' DNA in predicting our vulnerabilities and possible future diseases.

About one hundred trillion bacteria live in the body's digestive system – about 3.5 pounds worth. The digestive tract contains about 400-500 different bacteria species. About twenty species make up about 75% of the population, however. Many of these are our resident strains, which attach to our intestinal walls. Many others are transient. These transient strains will typically stay for no more than about two weeks.

The majority of our probiotics live in the colon, although billions also live in the mouth and small intestines. Other populations of bacteria and yeast can also live within joints, under the armpits, under the toenails, in the vagina; between the toes; and among the body's various other nooks and body cavities.

Microorganisms living within our bodies may be either *pro*biotic, *patho*biotic or *eu*biotic. A probiotic is a microorganism living within the body while contributing positively to the body's health. These friendly bacteria also are also called intestinal *flora* – meaning "healthful." The pathobiotic is a microorganism that harms or impedes the body in one way or another. Eubiotics can be either harmful or helpful to the body, depending upon their colony size and location. A healthy body contains a substantially greater number of probiotics than pathobiotics, while a diseased body likely contains more pathobiotic than probiotic populations.

## Our Cultured Past

Our first major encounter with large populations of bacteria comes when our baby body descends the cervix and emerges from the vagina. During this birthing journey – assuming a healthy mother – we are exposed to numerous species of future resident probiotics. This first inoculation provides an advanced immune shield to keep populations of pathobiotics at bay. The inoculation process does not end here, however.

Because we get much of our bacteria as we pass through the vagina, Caesarean section babies have significantly lower colonies of healthy bacteria. *Bifidobacterium infantis* is considered the healthiest probiotic colonizing infants. Some research has indicated that while 60% of vagina-birth babies have *B. infantis* colonies, only 9% of C-section babies are colonized with probiotics, and only 9% of those are colonized with *B. infantis*. This means that less than one percent of C-section babies are properly colonized with *B. infantis*, while 60% of vagina births are colonized with *B. infantis*.

Our body establishes its resident strains during the first year to eighteen months. Following the inoculation from the vagina, these are accomplished from a combination of breast-feeding and putting everything in our mouth, from our parent's fingers to anything we find as we are crawling around the ground. These activities can provide a host of different bacteria – both pathobiotic and probiotic.

Mother's colostrum (early milk) may contain up to 40% probiotics. This will be abundant in bifidobacteria, assuming the mother is not taking antibiotics. Healthy strains of bifidobacteria typically colonize our body first and set up an environment for other groups of bacteria, such as lactobacilli, to more easily become established.

Picking up a good mix of cooperative probiotic species is a crucial part of the establishment of our body's immune system. Some of the probiotic strains we ingest as infants may become permanent residents. They will continue to line the digestive tract to protect against infection while learning to collaborate with our immune system.

## Cultured Residency

As these early probiotics set up shop within our intestines and other cavities, they become recognized by the body and incubated in parts of the body's lymphatic system. The vermiform appendix, for example, was observed in 2007 by scientists at Duke University as housing resident probiotic strains, and releasing them into the cecum during increased infection. It seems that finally the purpose for the mysterious appendix has been discovered after decades of surgical removal. Other lymph ducts like the tonsils are also suspected to incubate resident probiotic strains as well.

Gaining early probiotic strains from the environment may appear difficult to understand, as we have been taught that dirt is infectious. Rather, natural soils contain huge populations of various bacteria. Many of these are spore-forming *soil-based organisms*. Some soil-based organisms or SBOs can become probiotic populations after early ingestion. Others, which may be less healthy to the body, will allow exposure to probiotic colonies and the immune system to counteract those strains in the future. This training mechanism is critical to the body's future immunity. This means those important infantile occupations – crawling on all fours, eating dirt, making mud pies, having food fights, playing tag and so on – all come together to deliver a stronger immune system later in life.

This has been confirmed by recent research illustrating that infants raised in sterile environments are more likely to suffer from allergies, infections and food sensitivities. Parents should consider living in a natural setting or at least outings to natural environments like pesticide free parks to provide exposure to pathogens and future probiotic colonies.

We can house many transient probiotics, but our resident probiotic bacteria strains do not change through adulthood. Once they take up residence, those strains become part of our body's ecosystem. This does not mean they always remain in strong numbers. Over years of stress, antibiotics and toxin exposure, resident strains may become dramatically reduced.

Supplemented probiotics do not appear to replace these resident strains. Supplemented probiotics typically remain for a couple of weeks, more or less, depending upon the strain and our internal environment. It is believed by some experts that with continued dosing of supplemental strains, resident strains – if they are still present – may increase their colonies.

Illustrating strain-specific survival among children, Polish scientists (Szymański *et al.* 2006) gave *Lactobacillus rhamnosus* to children with diarrhea. The researchers found that some *L. rhamnosus* strains given were found among 80% of patients after 5 days, and among 41.3% after 14 days. One particular strain, *L. rhamnosus* 573L/1, "colonized the G.I. tract more persistently," according to the researchers.

## Cultural Territories

Probiotics line mucosal linings around our oral cavity, gums, teeth, nasal cavity, throat, esophagus, and associated membranes. These probiotics deter the entry of pathogenic bacteria, viruses and fungi through the mouth and nose. Assuming the colonies are strong enough, even if the immune system is not able to properly identify or attack the invader, the oral probiotic system will remove the invader in short order. This will be accomplished by the probiotics producing certain acids and antibiotics that either specifically kill that type of invader or create an environment within which the invader does not feel comfortable.

Oral probiotics, for example, will vigorously defend the areas around the gums and teeth. The problem arises when our diets become overly sugary. As we will discuss later in more detail, probiotics require complex oligosaccharides like inulin, FOS (fructooligosaccharides) and GOS (galactooligosaccharides) for food sources. They do not thrive from simple sugars like glucose and sucrose. Pathogenic bacteria, on the other hand, typically thrive from these simple sugars. In fact, they can grow quite quickly, and may immediately begin to outnumber the probiotic populations, causing caries and gum infections.

Within the intestines, probiotics attach to and dwell in between the villi and microvilli. This allows them to not only keep pathogenic bacteria from infecting those cells: It also allows them to monitor food molecule size of nutrients being presented to the intestinal wall for absorption. This helps prevent the body from absorbing molecules that are too large or not sufficiently broken down. As we will discuss further, large, atypical molecules that have entered the bloodstream will stimulate an inflammatory and allergic response. This is because these larger molecules are not recognized by the immune system.

This is often the case with wheat proteins, milk proteins and nut proteins. For many people, they will be able to drink milk or eat nuts or breads for many years. Then suddenly they become allergic or sensitive to the food. Why? Larger proteins from these foods are being allowed into the bloodstream.

The mouth and intestines are not the only places probiotics guard against invaders. The vagina, urinary tract, belly button and anus are also inhabited by species of probiotics that guard against bacterial intrusion. Healthy colonies of these species protect us against the intrusion of pathogens and toxins into these areas.

Some of our bacteria live peacefully together. Most struggle with other colonies, and mark clearly defined territories with special biochemical secretions. Probiotics within the same colony usually specialize in particular functions. Some work together to help break down foods, and some guard and protect their territory as they consume metabolites. To protect against pathogens, many will produce a number of natural antibiotics designed to reduce the populations of competitors. At the same time, some of their antibiotic secretions aid the body's immune system by stimulating T-cell and B-cell activity.

Many will release antibiotic secretions called bacteriocins that selectively reduce the growth of other pathogens, including yeasts and pathobiotics. In other words, their antibiotic secretions – unlike many pharmaceutical antibiotics – can selectively damage certain strains of pathobiotics and not others. Many probiotics also produce lactic acid, acetic acid, hydrogen peroxide, lactoperoxidase, lipopolysaccharides, and a number of other antibacterial substances. Lactic acid, for example, helps acidify the intestines and prevent harmful bacteria overgrowth.

A study at the Department of Microbiology of the Abaseheb Garware College in India (Watve *et al.* 2001) studied the genus *Steptomyces* since the 1970s, and found that it has been producing new antibiotic substances exponentially over the years. They logistically graphed the count of antimicrobial substances produced over the years, and estimated that the genus is capable of producing more than 100,000 different antibiotic compounds!

Because bacteria are territorial organisms, they will respond to new competition with new antibiotic tools. They will produce different types of biochemicals, and develop different means of attack.

Most bacteria also manufacture waste products. Some of these are toxic and some of them are beneficial. Pathobiotics manufacture substances that increase the risk of disease by raising the body's toxicity level in addition to infecting cells. Various immunological diseases directly or indirectly stem from the waste streams of pathobiotics. Harmful bacteria can overload the liver and lymph systems with toxins. The toxins produced by bacteria are referred to as endotoxins – a technical name for bacteria poop. Bacteria defecate just as any other living organism does. Endotoxins from pathogenic bacteria can contribute to or directly stimulate inflammation and irritation within the intestines, promoting irritable bowel or colitis, Crohn's, polyps, diverticulitis and/or pouchitis. In comparison, probiotic waste is either healthy or inconsequential to the intestines. In other words, probiotic poop can be good for us!

Finnish scientists (Isolauri *et al.* 1994) gave lactobacilli probiotics to 42 children with acute rotavirus diarrhea. They found that the probiotics significantly reduced levels of the bacterial endotoxin urease, and lessened infection duration among the probiotic group compared to the placebo group.

Most bacteria in the digestive tract are anaerobic. This means they live without the need for oxygen. They can thus live in the darkest, bleakest regions of our bodies – including areas with little circulation. Not all biotics are anaerobic however – some are aerobic and some can go either way. These species will live in regions where they can more easily obtain oxygen – including the mouth, the stomach and the vagina. We might compare this to some species on the earth walking on the land and breathing oxygen, while others – like plants – utilize carbon dioxide.

## Cultured Nutrients

Probiotics are called 'friendly' because they boost our immunity and our body's ability to purge toxins and microorganisms from our systems. They make up the strongest part of our living immune system, making up over 70% of our immunity.

Probiotics also help us digest food and they secrete beneficial nutritional products. Unbelievably, probiotics are a good source of a number of essential nutrients. They can manufacture biotin, thiamin (B1), riboflavin (B2), niacin (B3), pantothenic acid (B5), pyridoxine (B6), cobalamin (B12), folic acid, vitamin A and vitamin K. Their lactic acid secretions also increase the assimilation of minerals that require acid for absorption, such as copper, iron, magnesium, chromium, selenium and manganese among many others.

Probiotics are also critical to nutrient absorption. They break away amino acids from complex proteins, and mid-chain fatty acids from complex fats. They help break down bile acids. They help convert polyphenols from plant materials into assimilable biomolecules. They also aid in soluble fiber fermentation, yielding digestible fatty acids and sugars. Among many other nutritive tasks, they also help increase the bioavailability of calcium.

### Nutrients and Probiotic Cultures

| | |
|---|---|
| Biotin | Produced by probiotics |
| Thiamin (B1) | Produced by probiotics |
| Riboflavin (B2) | Produced by probiotics |
| Niacin (B3) | Produced by probiotics |
| Pantothenic Acid (B5) | Produced by probiotics |
| Pyridoxine (B6) | Produced by probiotics |
| Cobalamin (B12) | Produced by probiotics |
| Folic Acid (B9) | Produced by probiotics |
| Vitamin A | Produced by probiotics |
| Vitamin K | Produced by probiotics |
| Copper | Probiotics increase bioavailability |
| Calcium | Probiotics increase bioavailability |
| Magnesium | Probiotics increase bioavailability |
| Iron | Probiotics increase bioavailability |
| Manganese | Probiotics increase bioavailability |
| Selenium | Probiotics increase bioavailability |
| Chromium | Probiotics increase bioavailability |
| Potassium | Probiotics increase bioavailability |
| Zinc | Probiotics increase bioavailability |
| Proteins | Probiotics break down for digestibility |
| Fats | Probiotics break down for digestibility |
| Carbohydrates | Probiotics break down and process |
| Sugars | Probiotics break down and process |
| Milk | Probiotics increase digestibility |
| Phytonutrients | Probiotics increase digestibility |
| Cholesterol | Probiotics bind to + reduce blood levels |

Many of the nutrients found in vitamin supplements and supplemented foods are in fact produced by probiotics. Most commercial forms of vitamin B12, for example, are derived from the probiotics *Propionibacterium shermanii, Pseudomonas denitrificans* or *Streptomyces griseus.*

We should note here that not all probiotics produce the same nutrients. Some, in fact, will consume some nutrients that others manufacture. For example, *Lactobacillus bulgaricus* will produce folic acid in yogurt, and *Lactobacillus acidophilus* will consume folic acid. At the end of the day, a mixture of probiotics will still have a net increase in nutrients, however. For this reason, most cultured dairy products have significantly higher nutrient contents than the milk or cream they were made with.

Probiotics also assist in peristalsis – the rhythmic motion of the digestive tract – by helping move intestinal contents through the system. They also produce antifungal substances such as acidophillin, bifidin and hydrogen peroxide, which counteract the growth of not-so-friendly yeasts. Probiotic hydrogen peroxide secretions are also oxygenating, providing free radical scavenging. In addition, they can manufacture some essential fatty acids, and are the source of 5-10% of all short-chained fatty acids essential for healthy immune system function.

An example of the extent of probiotics' ability to produce antimicrobials is the antibiotic streptomycin. This antibiotic, produced by the probiotic bacteria, *Streptomyces griseus* was discovered in 1943 by Selman Waksman.

Probiotics directly and indirectly break down toxins utilizing biochemical secretions and colonizing activities. Nutrients produced by probiotics have been found to have antitumor and anticancer effects within the body. Some probiotics can prevent assimilation of toxins like mercury and other heavy metals. Others will directly bind these toxins or will facilitate their binding to other molecules in order to remove them.

Probiotic nutrients are instrumental in slowing cellular degeneration and the diseases associated with it. Through their nutritive mechanisms, probiotics help normalize serum levels of cholesterol and triglycerides. Some probiotics even help break down and rebuild hormones.

Probiotic nutrients can also increase the productivity of the spleen and thymus – the key organs of the immune system.

Probiotics are necessary components to healthy digestion. Their populations dwell along and within the intestinal mucosal lining, providing a protective barrier to assist in the process of filtering and digesting toxins and other matter prior to these toxins encountering the intestinal wall cells. This mechanism helps maintain the brush barrier cells and keep the mucosal lining of our intestines from damage caused by foreign molecules coming from our foods and their metabolites. Damage to the brush cells of the intestinal lining is the prime cause for a number of irritable bowel disorders.

Illustrating probiotic production of one critical nutrient, Italian researchers (Strozzi and Mogna 2008) gave 23 healthy volunteers *Bifidobacterium adolescentis* DSM 18350, *B. adolescentis* DSM 18352, or *Bifidobacterium pseudocatenulatum* DSM 18353. Stool samples taken before and 48 hours after administration showed a significant increase of bioavailable folic acid from each of the probiotic strains.

Probiotics will also compete with pathogenic organisms for nutrients. Assuming good numbers, this strategy can check pathobiotic growth substantially. Nutrients produced by probiotics will also help stimulate the immune cell production, and normalize their activity during inflammatory circumstances.

## Foods of Culture

Let's review some of the most available probiotic foods. Most of these are ancient fermented or cultured foods teeming with probiotic bacteria and yeasts. These include yogurt and kefir, but also raw cheeses, traditional cottage cheese, traditional sour cream, traditional buttermilk, traditional sauerkraut, lassi, amasake (Japanese sweet rice drink), traditional miso, traditional tempeh, traditional tamari, traditional shoyu sauce, traditional kombucha tea and others.

Other foods utilize probiotics in their preparation. Traditional sourdough bread and bauerbrot are good examples. Most bread, in fact, uses some sort of (often probiotic) yeast fermentation process to prepare the flour for baking. In these, however, the probiotics are likely all killed during baking.

Some of the foods mentioned here are preceded by the word "traditional" because sadly, many of today's versions are pasteurized or otherwise acidified enough to kill any viable probiotic colonies. Both cottage cheese and butter were originally probiotic foods, for example, when we used to eat dairy products from our local dairies or own farms. Today, these two foods are produced commercially without probiotics. Ironically, even many commercial yogurts are unbelievably pasteurized prior to shipping – killing off most if not all of their viable colonies.

Another example is tamari and soy sauce. Today, most commercial versions are brewed with solvents. Probiotics are no longer part of these processes, as were the traditional versions.

*Here are a few probiotic foods (among many others) to consider adding to our diets:*

### Traditional Yogurt

Good quality yogurt is usually produced using *Lactobacillus bulgaricus, Bifidobacteria bifidus, Streptococcus thermophilus* and sometimes *Lactobacte-*

*ria casei.* Sometimes *Lactobacillus acidophilus* is used, but these will likely be overtaken by the others.

Note that pasteurization kills practically all probiotics. This means that commercial yogurts that pasteurize the yogurt after it has been cultured will have killed most or all of those colonies used to convert the milk to yogurt. Some producers pasteurize the milk first and then make the yogurt.

The best yogurt is made using raw milk. It is quite simple to make yogurt: After heating a pot of milk to 180 degrees F (82 C) momentarily, we can add a half-cup of starter (active yogurt from a previous batch or an active commercial yogurt) into the milk after it cools to about 105 degrees F (40 C). After stirring thoroughly, we can put the container in a warm, clean, dry place, with a clean towel or loose seal over the container. The mixture will sour and gel in about six to ten hours depending upon temperature. Then we can jar and refrigerate.

The ideal blend of probiotic species for a yogurt starter – one that was developed over the centuries by the Bulgarians – is a ratio of seven parts *S. thermophilus* to one part *L. bulgaricus.* This ratio produces the ideal sourness that is tasty yet tart. It also prevents the *L. bulgaricus* from outgrowing and overwhelming the *S. thermophilus.*

This later point is one of the reasons why yogurt starters that include *L. acidophilus* often fail to supply any *L. acidophilus* in the end product. *L. bulgaricus* is a hardy organism that will easily overtake *L. acidophilus* in a culture. The use of *L. acidophilus* in yogurt is not only wasteful, but possibly can result in an overly acidic flavor, as *L. bulgaricus* colonies swell with the lactic acid produced initially by *L. acidophilus.* In addition, it appears that *L. bulgaricus* produce small amounts of hydrogen peroxide – which knocks out the *L. acidophilus* colonies.

The moral of this also is not to expect much in the way of *L. acidophilus* in a commercial yogurt that blends *L. acidophilus* with *L. bulgaricus.*

Yogurt and other fermented dairy foods have little or no lactose. This is because the probiotics convert the lactose to lactic acid. The lactic acid is healthy for the intestinal tract, because it renders a medium that helps promote our own probiotic colonies. Lactic acid also offers a pleasing tart flavor to yogurt and other fermented dairy.

### Traditional Kefir

Kefir is a traditional drink originally developed in the Caucasus region of what is now considered southern Russia, Georgia, Armenia and Azerbaijan. Here Moslem tribe leaders vigorously protected their kefir recipe, as it was considered an esteemed and regal food with healing properties. The secret recipe was eventually ransomed by a young beautiful female Russian emissary who was kidnapped by a local prince. She wrestled a few kefir grains from the secrecy of the prince's family as a settlement for her abduction. She brought kefir into the Moscow market shortly thereafter and it spread as a highly prized healing food all over Russia and Europe. Kefir also became a focus of Soviet research, discovering some of the surprising benefits of probiotics we have outlined in this book.

The basic kefir formula contains *Lactobacillus lactis*, *L. plantarum*, *L. casei*, *L. rhamnosus*, *Bifidobacterium breve*, *Leuconostoc chemoris*, *Streptococcus diacetylactis* and others from the *Streptococcus* and/or *Lactobacillus* families. Secondary bacteria are used to finish and define the surface and flavor. Bulgarian kefir will sometimes often be finished with *Lactobacillus bulgaricus*. It should be noted that some of these bacteria are competitive, and not all will end up in the finished product.

Kefir uses fermented milk mixed with kefir grains that resemble little chunks of cauliflower. One tablespoon of kefir grains can be mixed with whole milk and sealed in a jar at room temperature. The milk is fermented overnight in a warm location with the starter grains. Depending upon the temperature, milk and kefir grains, it will take 1-3 days to completely ferment. The jar should be opened and swirled one to two times a day. The grains are screened or filtered out and utilized for the next batch. Cow's milk is most used, but sheep's milk, goat's milk or deer milk can also be used. It is best to use raw milk for the making of any cultured dairy product. Pasteurized milk is acceptable, but not desired.

## Buttermilk

Buttermilk is a soured beverage that was originally curdled from cream. Traditional buttermilk utilized the acids that probiotic bacteria produce for curdling. Today, forced curdling is done using commercially available acidic products. Cream of tartar, lemon juice or vinegar is added to heated and stirred whole milk at a rate of one tablespoon per cup of milk, until the curdling starts. After standing for 15 minutes and stirring another 15, it is refrigerated. See the butter section for the traditional method.

Buttermilk will usually be finished with *Lactobacillus bulgaricus*, but they can also contain *Bifidobacteria bifidus* and *Streptococcus thermophilus*.

## Traditional Sour Cream

The cream, which rises to the top after churned, can be soured by the use of *Leuconstoc* microflora and *Lactobacillus bulgaricus*. Sometimes *L.*

*acidophilus* and *B. bifidus* are used. Sour cream is a wonderful addition to any meal, as it delivers a rich, creamy consistency and flavor.

### Traditional Butter

Today commercial butter contains no probiotics. Traditionally, butter was made with the cow's natural probiotics. The raw milk sits for a half-day or day depending upon temperature, until the cream rises to the top. The cream is taken from the milk to be churned and aged; letting the probiotics convert lactose to lactic acid. This creates a mix of buttermilk and butter. The buttermilk is strained off, leaving the butter. The butter can be further dried of moisture and mixed with salt for taste. Again, the probiotics from the raw milk will have matured the butter and buttermilk naturally.

*Leuconstoccus cremoris* is the microflora of choice in preparing butter. The characteristic (yummy) flavor or butter is the result of *diacetyl*, a by-product of *Leuconstoc* microflora. *L. acidophilus* and *B. bifidus* are also sometimes used.

### Cheese

For cheeses, more extravagant microflora are used, which include yeasts and molds to culture surfaces along with *Lactobacillus* bacteria. One of the most popular cheese-making probiotic strains is *Lactobacillus helveticus*, because of its smooth flavor. Many other *Lactobacillus* strains produce too much lactic acid, so they aren't that good for cheese-making. Some cheeses also include *Leuconstoccus cremoris and Propionibacterium.*

A good natural cheese without preservatives can be very healthy, but most commercial cheeses are sources of unnatural dairy byproducts of pasteurization as we spoke of earlier. Many commercial cheese cheat by using fermenting enzymes rather than real probiotics. Most commercial cheese should therefore be avoided.

### Traditional Cottage Cheese

Commercial cottage cheese is also now made without probiotics. It was a probiotic process before dairy processors began to pasteurize the product and force the curdling with lactic acids. *L. acidophilus* and *B. bifidus* are sometimes used, but *Leuconstoccus cremoris* and *Lactobacillus bulgaricus* are typical in European versions.

Again, probiotics also produce the lactic acids that were used to curdle the product in traditional cottage cheese making. Skim milk with cream and buttermilk is probably the easiest way to make cottage cheese at home today, using the curds off the cream separation. The probiotics arising from the buttermilk help curdle the thickened milk and cream before separating the curds. Salt is one of the secrets to making a tasty cottage cheese.

## Traditional Kimchi

Kimchi is a fermented cabbage with a wonderful history from Korea. Kimchi was considered a ceremonial food served to emperors and ambassadors. It also was highly regarded as a healing and tonic food. There are a variety of different recipes of kimchi, depending upon the region and occasion.

Kimchi can be made by slicing and mixing cabbage with warm water, salt, ginger, garlic, red pepper, green onions, oil and a crushed apple. It is then put into a sealed jar(s) at room temperature for 24 hours, before putting into the refrigerator to continue the fermenting process (*Lactobacillus kimchii* is a typical colonizer). After several weeks of continued fermentation in the fridge, it is ready for eating.

## Traditional Miso

Miso is an ancient food from Japan. A well-made miso will contain over 160 strains of aerobic probiotic bacteria. This is because the ingredients are perfect prebiotics for these probiotics.

Miso is produced by fermenting beans and grains. Soybeans are often used, but other types of beans are also used. Equal parts soaked and cooked soybeans and rice are mixed. A fungi spore (koji, or *Aspergillus oryzae*) and salt is added to the rice prior to mixing. The mixture is put into a covered container in a dark, dry, room-temperature location and stirred occasionally. It can take up to a year of aging like this for the fermentation to result in a tasty miso.

When other beans other than soy are used, they will produce different varieties of miso. Shiromiso is white miso, kuromiso is black miso, and akamiso is red miso. They are each made with different beans. There are also various other miso recipes, many of which are highly guarded by their makers.

## Traditional Shoyu

Shoyu is a traditional form of soy sauce made by blending a mixture of cooked soybeans and wheat, again with koji, or *Aspergillus oryzae*. The combination is fermented for an extended time. The aging process for shoyu is dependent upon the storage temperature and cooking methods used, and is also guarded.

## Traditional Tempeh

Tempeh is an aged and fermented soybean food. It is extremely healthy and contains a combination of probiotics and naturally metabolized soy. Tempeh is made by first soaking dehulled soybeans for 10-12 hours. The beans are then cooked for 20 minutes and strained. The dry, cooked beans are then mixed with a tempeh starter containing *Rhyzopus oryzae, Rhizopus oligosporus* or both. The mixture is shaped and flattened (about a half-inch high) and put into a warm (room temperature) incubation container for a day or two. The cake will be full with white mycelium (fungal roots) when it is ready. It can then be eaten raw, baked, or toasted.

Other beans other than soy are also sometimes used to make tempeh. The trick is in getting good starter colonies.

## Traditional Kombucha Tea

Kombucha tea is an ancient beverage from the orient. Its use dates back many centuries; and was used by China and Taiwanese emperors. Its use was later popularized in Russia, and then in Eastern Europe, where its reputation grew. A quality kombucha tea will contain a number of probiotics, including *Acetobacter xylinum, Acetobacter xylinoides, Glucobacter bluconicum, Acetobacter aceti, Saccharomycodes Ludwigii, Schizosaccharomyces pombe,* and *Picha fermentans* – and other yeasts in the *Schizosaromyces* genus. The fermenting of these organisms renders a beverage that is full of nutrients and enzymes as well as healthy biotics. Kombucha has enjoyed a reputation of being detoxifying and revitalizing. Many alternative health experts have described it as a tonic.

Kombucha is made by blending a black or green tea with sugar, kombucha starter culture, and sometimes a bit of vinegar to create a slightly acidic environment. It is critical that a healthy starter be used. The mixture is then fermented in a warm, dry environment. It requires oxygen, yet will suffer from any toxins or bacteria from the air. Following a couple of weeks of fermentation, the product should be refrigerated to slow down growth and acidity.

Care should be taken to make sure the yeasts have adequately fermented the ethanols. Otherwise, the kombucha can be as high as 3-5% alcohol, and not healthy. Also be leery of a funky "mother." A kombucha mother might have been passed around for many years amongst those who have brewed their kombucha in their basements or other locales where molds and pathogenic bacteria could have joined and thus contaminated the mother.

## Traditional Lassi

Lassi is a traditional and popular beverage from India – once enjoyed by kings and governors in ancient India. It is quite simple to make, as it is made with kefir or yogurt, with fruit and spices (often mango and cardamom). Lassi can also be cultured with *L. plantarum, l. rhamnosus, Leuconostoc chemoris* and *Streptococcus diacetylactis*. Quite simply, it is a blend of diluted yogurt with fruit pulp – often mango is used in the traditional lassi. A little salt, turmeric and sweetener give it a sweet-n-salty taste. Other spices are also sometimes used. Sugar is often added in today's versions, but honey and/or fruit are preferable.

**Traditional Sauerkraut**

Sauerkraut is a traditional German fermented food. It is made quite simply, by blending shredded cabbage and pickling salt (12:1, or 3 table-spoons of whole sea or rock salt per five pounds of cabbage). Dill can also add flavor The mixture is covered with water and put into a covered bowl or container. It is then stored in the dark in this semi-airtight cover for a few weeks. Then it should be stored in the refrigerator in an en-closed container for a month or two to complete the fermentation of the cabbage. Probiotic bacteria such as *Lactobacillus plantarum* and *Leuconostoc mesenteroides* will typically overtake the early-growth bacteria during fermentation. These bacterial typically live on the surface of cabbage, so they are easily cultured. The salt is essential, as it will prevent the growth of competitive bacteria during the initial stages of the probiotic culture.

The culture can also be encouraged by using a starter brine from a previous batch or a neighbor's brine. A teaspoon of "starter" brine can be used to inoculate the current brine. Culturing can take no more than a few days with this.

A properly fermented sauerkraut can last for years. The probiotics colonize and protect the food from attacking bacteria. Healthy sauerkraut is discernable from the rotten version by the sense of smell. The healthy version will be sour and tangy. The rotten version will smell like rotting cabbage.

**Traditional Kvass**

Here the technique is similar to sauerkraut, except beets, carrots, gin-gers and other root foods can be used. Beets are the most popular, but a blend of these and even fruits can make for a tasty probiotic food. A probiotic starter from a sauerkraut or pickle brine can be used. If you spice with whole salt, garlic, whey and cloves, the *Lactobacillus plantarum* and *Leuconostoc mesenteroides* will likely grow on its own.

**Traditional Pickled Vegetables**

So many different vegetables can be pickled using this same tech-nique, and starter brine. Cucumbers are the most popular, but commercial pickles are pickled using vinegar, which is not a fermented or cultured food (although vinegar-pickled pickles are usually pretty healthy unless they contain a bunch of preservatives. Traditional pickle brine typically contains the *Leuconostoc mesenteroides* and *L. plantarum* bacteria.

Carrots, celery, tomatoes, peppers, onions and other vegetables can be pickled. For a probiotic pickled relish, they can be coarsely grated before adding the salt, spices and brine starter.

Most of these foods are traditional and even ancient foods that have been passed down through generations over thousands of years. This does not mean that we cannot be creative, however.

For example, there is a lot that can be done with yogurt. We've all heard of frozen yogurt, and certainly that is one. But yogurt in some cultures, such as among Indians, is eaten with every meal. It is eaten with and in salads, and rice dishes. Yogurt is creamy and delicious, and can make for an excellent salad dressing with a little oil and vinegar and dill. It can also be added to nearly every sauce to make the sauce creamy and delicious.

Kefir and lassi cultures can be added to nearly every combination of beverage, including smoothies and shakes.

Just about every vegetable can be pickled. Pickles using brine with probiotics is delicious and healthy. We can pickle peppers, olives and so many other foods.

Fermented beverages are now the rage among healthy foods. There are now many fermented beverages, including kombucha and others.

## Milk: Raw vs. Pasteurized

This naturally brings us to the topic of milk, since there are many reports that indicate that dairy may not be so healthy – and not conducive to detoxification processes.

To the contrary, numerous experiments have shown that raw milk, and dairy containing probiotics such as yogurt is not only healthy, but stimulates the immune system and fights off disease.

First let's consider a study by researchers at Switzerland's University of Basel (Waser *et al.* 2007). The researchers studied 14,893 children between the ages of five and 13 from five different European countries, including 2,823 children from farms, and 4,606 children attending a Steiner School (known for its farm-based living and instruction). The researchers found that drinking farm milk was associated with decreased incidence of allergies and asthma. Why?

Raw milk from the cow can contain a host of bacteria, including *Lactobacillus acidophilus, L. casei, L. bulgaricus* and many other healthy probiotics. Cows that feed from primarily grasses will have increased levels of these healthy probiotics. This is because a grass diet provides prebiotics that promote the cow's own probiotic colonies.

219

Should the cow be fed primarily dried grass and dried grains, probiotic counts will be reduced, replaced by more pathogenic bacteria. As a result, most non-grass fed herds must be given lots of antibiotics to help keep their bacteria counts low. Probiotics, on the other hand, naturally keep bacteria counts down.

As a result, the non-grass fed cow's milk will have higher pathogenic bacteria counts than grass-fed cows. This means that the milk itself will also have high counts. When the non-grass-fed cow's milk is pasteurized, the heat kills most of these bacteria. The result is a milk containing dead pathogenic bacteria parts. These are primarily proteins and peptides, which get mixed with the milk and are eventually consumed with the milk.

In other words, pasteurization may kill the living pathogenic bacteria, but it does not get rid of the bacteria proteins. This might be compared to cooking an insect: If an insect landed in our soup, we could surely cook it until it died. But the soup would still contain the insect parts – and proteins.

Now the immune system of most people, and especially infants with their hypersensitive immune system, is trained to attack and discard pathogenic bacteria. And how does the body identify pathogenic bacteria? From their proteins.

In the case of pasteurized commercial milk, our immune systems will readily identify heat-killed microorganism cell parts and proteins and launch an immune response against these proteins as if it were being attacked by the microorganisms directly. This was shown in research from the University of Minnesota two decades ago (Takahashi *et al.* 1992).

It is thus not surprising that weak immune systems readily reject pasteurized cow's milk. In comparison, healthy cow raw milk has fewer pathogenic microorganisms and more probiotic organisms. This has been confirmed by tests done by a California organic milk farm, which compared test results of their raw organic milk against standardized state test results from conventional milk farms.

In addition, pasteurization breaks apart or denatures many of the proteins and sugar molecules. This was illustrated by researchers from Japan's Nagasaki International University (Nodake *et al.* 2010), who found that when beta-lactoglobulin is naturally conjugated with dextranglycylglycine, its allergenicity is decreased. A dextran is a very long chain of glucose molecules – a polysaccharide. The dextran polysaccharide is naturally joined with the amino acid glycine in raw state. When pasteurized, beta-lactoglobulin is separated – where it can become more harmful in the gut.

Raw milk contains many of the nutrients found in mother's milk. These include many vitamins, proteins, nucleotides, minerals, enzymes, immunoglobulins and healthy fatty acids. Raw milk also contains probiotics. These healthy bacteria also lower pathogenic coliform counts—assuming primarily grass-fed cows—as low or lower than some pasteurized milk. Quite simply, raw milk is healthy.

The research supports this. In a study from Switzerland's University of Basel, 14,893 children from five different European countries were tested for asthma and allergy incidence. Those living on family farms or Steiner School farms and drank raw milk had significantly fewer allergies and asthma than other children.

A 2008 study at Spain's Cardenal Herrera University determined that glutathione peroxidase – an important antioxidant contained in milk – was significantly reduced by pasteurization. In 2006, the University also released a study showing that lysine content was significantly decreased by milk pasteurization.

A 2005 study at the Universidade Federal do Rio Grande determined that pasteurizing milk reduced vitamin A (retinol) content from an average of 55 micrograms to an average of 37 micrograms.

A study at North Carolina State University in 2003 determined that HTST pasteurization significantly reduced conjugated linoleic acid (CLA) content – an important fatty acid in milk shown to reduce cancer and encourage good fat metabolism.

Many proteins are denatured or broken down when cooked. In milk, the proteins beta-lactabumin and albumin will denature into peptide combinations—reducing milk's ability to increase our glutathione levels.

### Milk and Constipation

University and Health Department researchers from Australia (Crowley et al. 2013) proved that feeding children homogenized, pasteurized milk produces constipation, and a second recent university study shows that probiotics with milk actually relieves constipation.

The researchers tested 13 children in one trial and 39 children in a second trial. The average age of the children was about 6 and a half year's old. All the children were diagnosed with having chronic constipation (diagnosis = Chronic Functional Constipation).

In the first trial, nine children were given soy milk instead of cow's milk and the others continued the cow's milk. This followed a period where any milk was given (washout period).

All the children given the soymilk all had a resolution of their constipation. This also occurred in the washout period.

These results were confirmed using a crossover design, which allowed each group to reverse their protocol after another washout period.

The second trial also tested for casein type – using A1 milk or A2 milk type casein (more on this later). The results determined that there was little difference between the two milks given – they both showed increased constipation compared to the washout period – when milk was withheld from their diets.

Due to the casein study, the researchers concluded that there was something else other than casein that was causing the constipation. In their conclusion they wrote:

> "The results of Trial 1 demonstrate an association between constipation and cow's milk consumption while trial 2 failed to show an effect from type of casein. Some other component in cow's milk common to both A1 and A2 milk may be causing a problem in these susceptible children. Investigations into the immunological or biochemical mechanism occurring in CFC are required, including investigations of the intolerance reactions and how they affect nerves in the gastrointestinal tract."

Meanwhile, a number of studies have shown that dairy-fermented probiotics actually can relieve constipation.

In one, from Emma Children's Hospital/Academic Medical Center in Amsterdam (Tabbers et al. 2011) twenty children with an average age of a little over seven years old found that a daily dose of dairy-fermented Bifidobacterium breve significantly increased bowel movements and significantly decreased abdominal pain among the children.

Another children's study – this also on twenty constipated children – those given a daily mixture of probiotics including *Bifidobacteria bifidum, B. infantis, B. longum, Lactobacillus casei, L. plantarum* and *L. rhamnosus*, also experienced significantly increased bowel movements (Bekkali et al. 2007).

In addition to this, several studies on adults have found that yogurt or milk fermented with probiotics can significantly reduce constipation (Picard et al. 2005).

Because breast milk and raw milk of various types naturally contain probiotics, and since constipation has been specifically connected with drinking homogenized, pasteurized milk, we must assume that whatever the element is within homogenized, pasteurized milk that is causing the constipation, it is being neutralized by the probiotics within raw milks and yogurt products.

In fact, there is significant evidence to suspect that beta-lactoglobulin may be the culprit from milk that produces the constipation – although we probably still cannot completely eliminate the effects of casein.

And there is clear evidence that both beta-lactoglobulin and casein are neutralized – actually hydrolyzed – by probiotic species (Pescuma et al. 2013).

This means that these two large proteins – not only suspected as culprits in constipation, but also in many food allergies – are largely neutralized by probiotics. This explains why probiotic-supplemented milks or yogurts are curative for constipation.

And this is why raw milk that has been properly tested will likely not have the same effects as homogenized, pasteurized milk.

### Prebiotics in milk

This is not surprising. Natural whole cow's milk also contains special polysaccharides called oligosaccharides. They are largely indigestible polysaccharides that feed our intestinal bacteria. Because of this trait, these indigestible sugars are called prebiotics.

Whole milk contains a number of these oligosaccharides, including oligogalactose, oligolactose, galactooligosaccharides (GOS) and transgalactooligosaccharides (TOS). Galactooligosaccharides are produced by conversion from enzymes in healthy cows and healthy mothers.

These polysaccharides provide a number of benefits. Not only are they some of the more preferred foods for probiotics: Research has also shown that they reduce the ability of pathogenic bacteria like *E. coli* to adhere to our intestinal cells.

The oligosaccharides in milk promote the growth of our probiotics in the intestinal tract. These are referred to as probiotics because they encourage the growth of probiotics, which assist our bodies digest food and fight infection.

These oligosaccharides also provide environments that reduce the availability of separated beta-lactoglobulin. This is accomplished through a combination of probiotic colonization and the availability of the long-chain polysaccharides that keep these complexes stabilized.

This reduced availability of beta-lactoglobulin has been directly observed in humans and animals following consistent supplementation with probiotics (Taylor *et al.* 2006; Adel-Patient *et al.* 2005; Prioult *et al.* 2003). This of course illustrates the fact that raw milk is the only healthy way to drink milk.

It is not surprising, given this information, that people with many conditions have benefited from withdrawing from pasteurized milk and cheese. Raw milk, yogurt, kefir, goat's milk and cheese, along with soy and almond milk, are great alternatives.

Cows and goats produce prolific quantities of these wonderfully healthy foods. Naturally, these animals produce more than their large families supply. The key to obtaining good nutrition from the milk of animals like cows and goats is to treat them with care. Should we torture these poor animals by trapping them into cages while punching them with injections of antibiotics and growth hormones, we will certainly experience the backlash of those acts when we consume the milk.

We might note that the human hands and fingers are perfectly equipped to milk a cow or a goat. Most healthy individuals also produce a prolific amount of enzyme lactase, an enzyme specifically designed to digest lactose – the sugar of cow's milk. Those rare humans who do not produce enough lactase can easily eat naturally cultured milk like cheese and yogurt, because bacteria in these cultured foods produce enough lactase to allow assimilation.

These cultured foods also secret *bacteriocins*, which exhibit otherwise antimicrobial activity. We should also be aware that lactobacilli – the most prevalent probiotics of our intestinal tract – produce lactase as well. As we age, our probiotic colonies should be blossoming with lactase. The antibiotic use of modern society is largely responsible for our lack of healthy probiotics, and the subsequent lack of lactase available.

### What about lactose?

Most healthy individuals also produce a prolific amount of enzyme lactase, an enzyme specifically designed to digest lactose – the sugar of cow's milk. Those rare humans who do not produce enough lactase can easily eat naturally cultured milk like cheese and yogurt, because bacteria in these cultured foods produce enough lactase to allow assimilation.

These cultured foods also secret *bacteriocins*, which exhibit otherwise antimicrobial activity. We should also be aware that lactobacilli – the most prevalent probiotics of our intestinal tract – produce lactase as well. As we age, our probiotic colonies should be blossoming with lactase.

The antibiotic use of modern society is largely responsible for our lack of healthy probiotics, and the subsequent lack of lactase available. And the proliferation of pasteurized dairy has forced our biology to depend upon the production of our own lactase – which is deficient in some people and often slows as we age.

We should note that some ethnicities tend to produce less lactase. This indicates that these cultures relied exclusively on raw milks.

### What About Casein and Beta-lactoglobulin?

In a number of studies, the milk protein casein has been shown to be implicated in a number of conditions, including cancer (Campbell and Campbell 2006).

In addition, beta-lactoglobulin has been implicated in allergies.

For example, Japanese researchers (Nakano *et al.* 2010) found that casein and beta-lactoglobulin were the main allergens in cow's milk – as confirmed by other research. They also found that 97% of 115 milk allergy children had casein-specific IgE antibodies, while 47% had IgE antibodies against beta-lactoglobulin (beta-LG).

However, fermented dairy and probiotic-rich raw dairy presents an altogether different casein and beta-lactoglobulin molecular structure than does pasteurized milk.

When milk is heated to extremely high degrees, the surfaces of casein micelles – minute fat globules about 100 nanometers in diameter – become harder, and more stable. They move within the fluid but remain in a highly rigid state. Other molecules within the milk do not affect these casein micelles. Thus, the consumption of these rigid casein micelles results in a macromolecule – large protein the body does not easily break down.

However, when dairy is fermented, these casein molecules become destabilized by the probiotics. Once a particular acidity is reached in the milk culture, the casein molecules will become sticky, and they will become congealed – observed as "curdling."

As this curdling takes place – driven by the conversion of lactose to lactic acid by probiotic bacteria – an interesting combination occurs. The destabilized casein micelles react with the beta-lactoglobulin whey protein, which produces a *beta-lactoglobulin-kappa-casein complex*. This neutralizes both the effects of separated beta-lactoglobulin molecules and the casein micelles within the body. In other words, both of these proteins – which spawn radicals in the body – become neutralized through the enzymatic processes driven by probiotic bacteria.

As this occurs, another whey protein, called lactoferrin, also undergoes degradation. This process liberates an immune-stimulating derivative called lactoferricin. This lactoferricin released during the degradation of lactoferrins is also produced by probiotic bacteria, most notably *Streptococcus thermophilus* and *Lactobacillus delbrueckii* ssp. *bulgaricus* (Paul and Somkuti 2010).

Thus we find that these whey-casein components and their derivatives create an altogether different combination of elements than pasteurized milk. They also maintain known antimicrobial components such as lactoferricin and other bacteriocins.

### *Organic Milk*

Research has revealed that rBGH – recombinant bovine growth hormones – have negative health effects upon humans. While rBGH is mostly inactive in the human body, rBGH stimulates higher levels of insulin-like *growth factor-1* (IGF-1). Increased absorption of IGF-1 dramatically affects the human body. It is a key biochemical factor stimulating cellular division and growth. Increases in IGF-1 due to rBGH milk has ranged from double its natural value to 360% of natural levels. The ramifications of this absorption has been increasingly seen as hazardous to our health, in the form of increased cancers and endocrine disorders.

The overuse of antibiotics among dairies is also a concern for those drinking the milk or eating the byproducts of these animals. Nearly 25 million pounds of antibiotics are fed to livestock each year – eight times what humans are prescribed. Some of these antibiotics are similar to the antibiotics doctors prescribe to human, except the dosages are much greater and often for a much longer duration. This incredibly large consumption of antibiotics not only reduces our own immune system's strength, but reduces our viable probiotic colonies. It is this level of antibiotic usage, which has helped create antibiotic-resistant strains of bacteria – termed *superbugs – such as MRSA*. We are facing days of stronger bacteria. Our immune systems need all the help they can get, and natural strategies of probiotics and herbal antibiotics should become a greater focus as we face the superbug future.

It cannot be emphasized enough that organic dairy – or at least milk from a dairy that minimizes or declines antibiotic and growth hormone use – is the better health choice for all concerned.

Animals tend to bioaccumulate pollutants in their bodies. Their fatty acids have a tendency of trapping toxic chemicals like polychlorinated biphenyls (PCB). PCBs have been linked to various nerve and brain impairments, as well as infant developmental impairment. PCBs have been showing up more and more in our food supply especially as the move up the food chain.

Certified organic dairies are also required to treat their cows better. Some dairies are better at this than others.

Should we treat animals like the caretakers we are supposed to be, certainly we will reap the benefits of obtaining the best of both worlds when it comes to nutrition.

While nutritionists have noted that there are few nutrients missing from a well-rounded vegetarian diet (most vegetarian diets have more nutrients), the one exception, vitamin B12, is easily gained from through a variety of dairy foods. A couple of cows grazing peacefully in a small pasture could easily supply all of the milk and dairy products for several families.

## Fungal Foods

Baking yeast and brewer's yeast are common yeasts that are primarily derived from an organism called *Saccharomyces cerevisiae*. In most applications, the yeast is not eaten alive, however. It is *heat-killed* prior to eating. This simply means that it is cooked to a temperature that kills off the viable organisms. This doesn't mean that living *S. cerevisiae* organisms are toxic or anything. In reasonable colony sizes, they are perfectly docile, and even healthy to our bodies because they produce nutrients that our bodies use.

For baking, brewing and supplementation, the heat-killed version of this organism can be very healthy, because when it is alive, it produces a variety of nutrients and immune factors that are left behind in whatever food it was used to ferment.

Just before these yeasts die during heating or baking, they will release intense immune factors in an attempt to protect themselves. These immune factors also help protect our bodies, by stimulating our body's detoxification processes and boosting our immune system. In addition, some of their nutrients, such as B-vitamins produced by yeasts, will donate methyl groups to our liver's glutathione radical-neutralizing processes.

Furthermore, because the biofactors that yeasts produce tend to be acidic, they will lend a tart flavor to the food. This of course lends the flavoring that we relish among our traditional probiotic foods such as cottage cheese, pickles, and so many other foods as we discussed above.

This is the case for sourdough bread, for example. Sourdough bread is not only delicious. It is healthy, even if it is made with white flour (for best results, try whole wheat sourdough bread). Fermented brews such as beer and wine Originally, all the fermented brews such as ginger ale and root beer, were all made using probiotic fermentation.

Back to baking, breads, cakes and other recipes made with flour are significantly more healthy when yeast is utilized rather than baking soda or baking powder. This is especially true when aluminum-baking power is considered.

### Yeast Supplements

Baking yeast and Brewer's yeast, Nutritional Yeast and EpiCor®, are all derived from an organism called *Saccharomyces cerevisiae*. This organism is used in brewing and baking. It is thus considered a healthy organism, and acts in a territorial manner to repel organisms and toxins that are seen as foreign to their territories.

For this reason, EpiCor®, Brewer's Yeast or Nutritional Yeast come in dehydrated forms. In other words, the yeast colonies are killed by heat. This heat-killing preserves their nutrients, yet prevents their overgrowth in the body. (However, a person who has mold allergies might still have a reaction to heat-killed yeast because those proteins are still present.)

So what is the difference between EpiCor®, Brewer's Yeast and Nutritional Yeast? The answer lies in their unique processes of fermentation.

**Brewer's Yeast** is a byproduct of the brewing industry, thus it typically does not have the higher levels of nutrients that the other two have. Brewer's yeast still has a variety of nutrients, including many trace elements (such as chromium and selenium), B vitamins (but typically not B12 as many assume), many antioxidants and proteins.

**Nutritional Yeast** will typically produce more of these same nutrients, because it has been prepared in such a way that both stresses the yeasts more, and preserves more of their nutrients. Nutritional yeast will contain chromium and selenium, as well as thiamin, riboflavin, niacin, vitamin B6, folate, vitamin B12, pantothenic acid, magnesium, zinc, and a number of amino acids. It is a great protein source, with 50% protein by weight.

**EpiCor®** is another yeast derivative that is produced using a proprietary method. EpiCor®, however, may have even more enhanced levels of certain nutrients, which include those mentioned above, along with nucleotides and possibly additional antioxidants and immune factors. The reason that EpiCor® may have additional immune factors is because during fermentation, the yeast is *stressed*. Like any organism, when it is stressed, it produces immune factors to protect itself.

After EpiCor® has been stressed, it is then heat-killed, dehydrated and powdered, rendering those immune factors and nutrients.

EpiCor® has been the subject of focused research, which has found that it significantly lowers systemic inflammation.

In one study (Robinson *et al.* 2009), 500 milligrams of EpiCor® or a placebo was given to 80 healthy volunteers with seasonal grass allergies during pollen season. After six and twelve weeks, the EpiCor® group experienced a significant reduction of allergy symptoms compared to the placebo group.

Other EpiCor® studies have shown that it increases salivary IgA (mucosal immunity), and reduces serum IgE (pro-allergy sensitivity).

**Red Yeast Rice:** The yeast *Monascus purpureus,* when fermented with rice, becomes what is known as red yeast rice. Red yeast rice has been shown in research to lower LDL cholesterol (Liu *et al.* 2006). The mechanism renders red yeast the ability to help prevent lipid peroxidation in the body. Red yeast rice has been used in China for over a thousand years.

However, red yeast rice use as a supplement has been questioned by the FDA and pharmaceutical industry. This might have something to do with the fact that correctly fermented red yeast rice can be a significant source of the constituent monacolin K, the primary active ingredient of the statin drug lovastatin.

While there are others, these yeast products have been shown to maximize the body's antioxidant capacities, increase tolerance, and stimulate detoxification processes. They also have considerable research backing up these claims.

Cardiology researchers have now proven in a randomized, double-blinded, placebo-controlled clinical study that red yeast rice combined with lifestyle changes outperforms statins for reducing bad cholesterol and increasing good cholesterol.

Red yeast rice is produced through the fermentation of a yeast, Monascus purpureus, combined with red rice.

Traditional Chinese healers used the red yeast rice to improve digestive conditions along with stimulating circulation of the blood and chi throughout the body.

Interestingly, red yeast rice also contains – among other constituents – phytochemicals called monacolins – whose molecular structure is similar to the molecule used in statin medications. The particular phytochemical in focus as mentioned above is called monacolin K, and it is similar to the drug lovastatin (Mevacor).

The difference is that red yeast rice – like other natural products – contains multiple monacolins along with a variety of other natural constituents which serve to buffer the effects of the monacolins. This does not mean that red yeast rice can render side effects – but its side effects are typically not as serious as statin side effects.

This fact has been confirmed by the fact that two clinical trials have tested patients who could not tolerate statin treatment. These patients did fine with the red yeast rice therapy, and had considerable reductions in bad cholesterol levels and triglyceride levels.

The researchers (Becker *et al.* 2013) conducted their clinical study with 187 patients at Philadelphia's Chestnut Hill Hospital. The patients had high cholesterol and LDL-cholesterol levels – an average of 154 mg/dL of LDL.

The patients were randomly divided into groups and tested for twelve weeks. One group underwent the typical conventional medicine advice – including prescriptive medications – statins. Another group was given 1,800 milligrams of red yeast rice, and another group was given the red yeast rice together with 900 milligrams of phytosterols in addition to making lifestyle changes.

Before and after the twelve weeks, the researchers conducted cholesterol testing and found that the red yeast rice had reduced triglyceride levels in the patients by 24%, reduced total cholesterol by 16%, reduced LDL by 21%, and. increased HDL-cholesterol by 14%.

And compared to the group given statin therapy, the red yeast group given lifestyle changes had 51 mg/dL lower levels of LDL-C compared to 42 mg/dL lower levels from statin therapy, and they were more than twice as likely to have dropped their LDL levels to under 100 mg/dL – often considered the demarcation between healthy and unhealthy levels.

The researchers then followed the patients over a year of the therapy. The group that took the red yeast rice together with lifestyle changes also lost an average of about five pounds, while the typical therapy group lost an average of less than one pound over the course of a year.

This research confirms another study (Becker *et al.* 2009) done with 446 high-cholesterol patients. After eight weeks of red rice yeast therapy, LDL-c levels were reduced by 31%, triglycerides fell by 34% and HDL-c went up by 20%. Other studies have shown similar reductions.

Not that while red yeast rice has far fewer cases of side effects, both statins and red yeast rice can produce headaches, heartburn, gas, bloating, muscle aches, and dizziness. In addition to these, statins can cause rashes, insomnia, diarrhea, and nausea.

## Raw Vinegars

Vinegars are excellent living foods that stimulate the body's living purification systems. Vinegar made from apples, grapes or other fruits also contain a variety of antioxidants, as well as acetic acid, which helps stimulate a good environment for our body's own probiotics, and one that repels pathogenic microorganisms.

There are a variety of different types of vinegars, depending upon the raw material used. In all cases, the raw material of a healthy vinegar will be a plant source, fermented by a healthy yeast culture. The yeast culture will convert the sugars of the plant source (and added sugars if used) to alcohol. As the alcohol is fermented further, it is oxidized by the zymase enzymes in the yeast, which convert to alcohol to carboxylic acetic acids. These acetic acids are the main constituent of vinegar, and what gives vinegar its tartness.

To speed up the process, alcohols are often used commercially to make vinegars. These include cheaper or turned wines, distilled alcohol (from wood or grain) and other spirits. The conversion of alcohol to vinegar is much quicker because the first step (sugar to alcohol) has already been made.

Fresh vinegar is typically made by crushing whole apples, grapes, potatoes, barley or other fruits or grains – even pears, bananas and others –

into a mash. Sugar can be added to speed up the process, typically at a ratio of one-to-four of mash.

Brewer's yeast (*Saccharomyces cerevisiae*) can then be added for fermentation. One-quarter of a yeast cake will typically inoculate a liter of the mash. Alternatively, a "mother" of fresh vinegar that has been retained from a previous vinegar can be used. Such a "mother" will likely contain more yeast species than just the *S. cerevisiae* yeast, and possibly even some probiotic bacteria. The amount needed depends upon the strength of the "mother," but one cup of the mother (from the top center of the previous batch) per liter should probably do it.

The mix is then put aside in a warm place, with the jar covered by a cloth to let in oxygen. The period of fermentation depends upon the sugar content and the temperature stored. The vinegar may be strained or unstrained. Unstrained retains more living yeasts.

Balsamic vinegars will ferment for years in oak barrels, for example. An apple vinegar might take 60 days to nine months. Care should be taken that the alcohol levels are reduced down to well below .5% (legal alcohol limit). Higher acetic acid levels will mean lower alcohol levels. Testing with a round piece of fine marble (5/6 of marble weight reduction equates to acetic acid levels). Look for 30-32 grams reduction per marble piece, after vinegar loses sour taste for a 5% acetic acid vinegar.

Vinegar can be used in salads, for pickling vegetables and other creative recipes. It can also simply be taken by the teaspoon. A traditional raw cider is the Bragg's brand of apple cider vinegars (no financial affiliation).

## Alcoholic Fermentation

A key point to remember regarding fermented beverages is that unless the fermentation process is controls, leaving the product with an alcohol content below .5%, it will be considered an alcoholic beverage.

Alcohol is unhealthy for body. Alcohol is ethanol, which is highly toxic to the liver. Alcohol damages the liver. This means that the liver will produce less enzymes and filter the blood poorly. This leaves the body in a state of increased toxicity. Over time this can produce severe liver disease, which can result in death.

Often people consider that because wines and other spirits are made from natural ingredients, they must be healthy. For example, resveratrol from wine is touted as being healthy. Resveratrol, however, comes from the grapes themselves. While red wine certainly will also contain resveratrol, the alcohol content of the wine can do more damage than the resveratrol can help.

As for those reputed to have been drinking a glass or two of wine every day and remain seemingly healthy, yes, the liver can certainly manage a minimal amount of alcohol every day. This doesn't mean that the alcohol is healthy for the liver. There have been a few studies that have indicated the possibility that a drink or two of wine every day may increase longevity. This type of epidemiological research, however, is highly questionable, notably because those who have a glass or two of wine everyday may also well be doing something else – such as socializing while drinking or reducing stress levels – that might also account for their longevity. Other studies have shown that socializing and reducing stress levels also extend life.

The bottom line is that the research showing that the liver is damaged by alcohol consumption is irrefutable. For example, Canadian scientists (Rehm *et al.* 2010) reviewed seventeen studies that analyzed the relationship between alcohol and cirrhosis of the liver. They found that all of them linked alcohol consumption with liver disease and death from liver disease. They also found that the same amount of alcohol consumption produces a higher incidence of liver disease among women.

Alcohol also damages our probiotic colonies.

## Shrooms

Edible mushrooms are included in the cultured diet because mushrooms, are, in fact, a fungus. Yes, they are a fungus that feeds off of the soil, the bark of a tree or any number of other natural elements. Mushrooms are one of the richest sources of nutrition, and it certain that our ancestors harvested and ate mushrooms, as well as utilized mushrooms for medicinal purposes.

Edible mushrooms offer a significant tool to cleanse out toxins and boost our immunity. We can include delicious mushrooms like Shiitake, Buttons or Chanterelles into our dishes, and we can also take mushroom supplements with Reishi (*Ganderma lucidum*), Hoelen (*Wolfiporia extensas*), Maitake (*Grifola frondosa*), Shiitake (*Lentinula elodes*), Turkey Tails (*Coriolus versicolor or Trametes versicolor*), Agaricus (*Agaricus blazeil*), Cordyceps (*Cordyceps sinensis*) and Lion's Mane (*Hericium erinaceus*). All of these significantly stimulate the immune system, and their constituents bind to toxins within our bodies.

The Agaricus species is the most popular eating mushroom, and this species contains the button mushroom. But there are many, many others. Scientists have cataloged some 50,000 mushrooms, and identified less than 20,000 different mushroom species. Some estimate there may be over 150,000 mushroom species within the Fungi kingdom, which likely encompasses more than 1.5 million total species. Biologists have described less than 5% of Fungi species.

Over 600 mushroom species have been documented to stimulate the immune system. However, the ones mentioned above have received the most attention. Research on these mushrooms have revealed their effects as being antimicrobial, cholesterol-lowering, anti-inflammatory, anti-oxidant, anti-mutagenic, anti-tumor, adaptogenic and immunostimulating.

Cancer has been a significant area of research. A number of these mushrooms have been shown to inhibit cancer cell line growth, for example. American researchers were awakened by Dr. Tetsuro Ikekawa's groundbreaking epidemiological study showing significantly lower cancer rates among Japanese mushroom growers between 1972 and 1986. The research since then has shown significant anticarcinogenic properties among most of the mushrooms mentioned above. While most clinical research to date has been adjunctive to conventional therapies for ethical reasons, human studies have consistently confirmed animal and laboratory models. By August of 2008, there were 4,087 mushroom studies and scientific papers filed with the U.S. National Library of Medicine.

These mushrooms are incredible radical scavengers. For example, lion's mane mushroom has been shown to reduce the risk of Alzheimer's and senility. The mushroom appears to stimulate nerve growth factor, a substance that has can reduce dementia and benefit Alzheimer's patients.

A immune-boosting compound called AHCC – Active Hexose Correlated Compound – has been is derived from shiitake mushroom and their sub-species. This has been shown to stimulate the activity of white blood cells. Further research showed they stimulated interferon (IFN-y) and tumor necrosis factor (TNF-a) as well.

Much of the dramatic immunity effects of mushrooms are due to their polysaccharides and polysaccharide-protein complexes. Laboratory research has isolated multiple polysaccharide types within each species. Twenty-nine unique polysaccharides have been isolated in Maitake, for example.

Mushroom polysaccharides are primarily glucans with different glycosidic linkages, including 1->3 and 1->6 beta glucans, and 1->3 alpha glucans. The complex branching and even helical nature of mushroom glucans appears to be significant. Schizophyllan polysaccharides with (1,3)-b-glucans with 1,3-b-d-linked glucose with 1,6-b-d-glucosyl side groups have been described as "stiff triple-stranded" helices in laboratory research, for example. Schizophyllan (SPG) is an active macrophage stimulator, increasing T cell and NK cell activity and inhibiting various infective agents.

Various immunostimulatory effects have been also attributed to polysaccharide-protein complexes such as PSK (krestin), PSP, lentinan and others. While many varieties contain different levels of the various beta glucans, many researchers believe it is their unique protein sequencing that differentiates effects among species.

Medicinal mushrooms also contain a variety of nutrients. Many mushrooms contain significant amounts of protein. Shiitake can be as much as 17% protein while oyster mushrooms can be 30% protein by weight. Several also contain vitamin B complexes. Most edible mushrooms also contain a variety of macro-minerals and trace elements. Shiitake also can contain as much as 126 mg of calcium, and 247 mg of magnesium per serving, for example. Reishi also contains magnesium, calcium, zinc, iron, copper and trace minerals. Many are good sources of selenium.

Maitake and a number of other mushrooms also contain ergosterols (provitamin D2), along with phosphatidylcholine and phosphatidylserine. Shiitake, Reishi and Maitake have been known to increase from less than 500 IU of D2 in indoor growing conditions to 46,000 IU, 2760 IU, and 31,900 IU respectively, following six to eight hours of sunlight exposure (Stamets 2005).

Various anti-oxidants have been isolated among popular mushroom varieties. Constituents such as ganoderic acid (*G. lucidum*), cordycepic acid (*C. sinensis*), linzhi (*G. frondosa*), agaric acid (several), sizofilan and sizofiran (*S. commune*), galactomannan (*C. sinesis*), and various triterpenoids (several) can actively reduce oxidative radicals and stimulate the immune system.

The density of these in mushrooms is quite incredible. Reishi has over 100 ethanol-soluble triterpenoids. Most of these are antioxidant, and many are anti-inflammatory agents.

Some of the mechanisms of mushrooms to safely stimulate the immune system and produce long-term cleansing benefits are quite complicated. For example, differently branched beta glucans have been observed stimulating immune cells in different ways. For example, certain beta glucans from Maitake will stimulate T-cell production, while differently bonded-chain beta glucans from *Agaricus blazei* stimulate natural killer (NK) cells. Others stimulate B-cells, T-helper cells, lymphokine activated killer cells [LAK], macrophages; and the cytokines interferon gamma, interleukin-2, -12 and tumor necrosis factor [TNF].

Mushrooms significantly detoxify heavy metals inside our bodies, and in their natural environments. Their proteins will bind to certain heavy metals within the soil. These same metabolites become active within the body when eaten, and thus help chelate minerals in our bodies.

For this reason, Cordyceps, Reishi, *Agaricus blazei* and Maitake have been used in China to reduce effects of heavy metal and radiation poisoning.

Mushrooms can be eaten fresh, frozen, drank as teas, cooked with sauces or eaten as supplements. Parts used include the fruiting body (cap and stem) and the mycelia (colonizing rooting network).

234

While each form will stimulate our immune system, fresh or freeze-dried are preferable. Some supplements are hot-water extracted, and some are alcohol extracted. Hot water extracts likely retain more constituents, although alcohol can extract specific medicinal constituents as well.

Even the common recipe mushrooms have medicinal properties. Oyster mushrooms, white button mushrooms, Agaricus mushrooms, and shiitake mushrooms all provide incredible nutrition and healing effects.

## Cultured Soy – The Real Soy Story

Cultured soy is part of many traditional diets for good reason. Soy foods have been shown in numerous studies to reduce breast cancer risk, reduce cholesterol, reduce the risk of heart disease, increase artery health, reduce allergies and reduce the risk of bone fractures (Messina 2010).

In addition, several large epidemiological studies done in the 1990s found that those populations that ate higher levels of tofu in their diets had lower levels of heart disease and many cancers.

Washington state researchers (Lerman *et al.* 2010) found that people with higher LDL cholesterol levels and cardiovascular disease experienced a reduction of LDL cholesterol and smaller particle size, greater HDL cholesterol, lower apolipoprotein levels and lower homocysteine levels. Remember that LDL cholesterol is related to lipoperoxidation, which is what causes artery disease leading to heart attacks and strokes. And lower apolipoprotein levels and lower homocysteine levels mean lower levels of systemic inflammation.

These benefits come from one of soy's isoflavones, genistein. Researchers from Northwestern University's Feinberg School of Medicine, in association with the American Lung Association Asthma Clinical Research Centers (Smith *et al.* 2004) studied asthma severity in 1,033 adolescents and adults. They found that 250 micrograms per 1,000 Kcal per day of the soy isoflavone genistein significantly increased forced expiratory volumes and peak expiratory volumes.

Because some soy nutrients (such as raffinose) can be difficult for some to digest, soy's best antioxidant benefits come when soy is cultured or fermented. Cultured soy foods such as tofu, tempeh, natto, miso and shoyu thus provide easily assimilable sources of soy.

### Is soy really healthy?

Hundreds of studies have illustrated soy's ability to improve or protect against conditions such as postmenopausal symptoms, osteoporosis, hyperlipidemia, prostate enlargement, bladder cancer, hypertension, elevated homocysteine, as well as several types of cancer have been published. Up until about a decade ago, soy had become the ultimate functional food.

The stats support this notion. According to the USDA Nutrient Database for Standard Reference, 100 grams of soybeans supplies 36.5 grams of protein, 277 mg of calcium, 15.7 grams of iron, 280 mg of magnesium, 704 mg of phosphorus, 1797 mg of potassium, 4.9 mg of zinc, as well as vitamins A, E, C, B1, B2, B3, B5, B6 and folic acid. Soybeans also contain bioactive constituents such as polyphenolic isoflavones (200mg/100g – primarily genistein and daidzein) and various saponins known for their chemoprotective and antimutagenic effects.(1,2) A half-cup of tofu provides 40% DV of protein, 25% DV of calcium and 87% of women's and 130% of men's DV in iron.

These facts didn't seem to prevent a flurry of anti-soy sentiment from flooding the press over the past few years. An American Heart Association 22-study review resulted in about a 3% LDL reduction, which translates to a 6% reduction of heart disease risk.

Another meta-analysis of 23 studies published in the *American Journal of Clinical Nutrition* on 1381 subjects, showed a 3.7% reduction in total cholesterol, 5.25% reduction in LDL cholesterol, and 7.27% reduction of triglycerides. Additionally, HDL cholesterol increased on an average of 3.03% (Zhan *et al.* 2005).

Outside of the AHA statement, much of the anti-soy press has seemed to be driven by statements stemming from a rather small group of focused individuals gathering under a pro-animal diet organization, an organization which will go unnamed in this text. The organization has put out a flurry of pro-animal products books, along with websites promoting the benefits of meat consumption while ignoring the proven risks.

Some of their literature strenuously promote soy as a dangerous food, accusing it of disrupting endocrine glands, affecting fertility, containing pro-clotting lectins while robbing the body of nutrients through trypsin inhibition.

Meanwhile, many esteemed health experts have defended soy's positive benefits and accused the literature of exaggerating and sensationalizing soy's negative effects. Statements by leading heart-healthy advocates Dean Ornish, M.D. and James McDougall, M.D. provided balance to the issue by reminding readers of the large library of research data confirming soy's many health benefits.

Meanwhile the science has been reviewed by leading health experts such as Andrew Weil, M.D., Michael Murray, N.D. and Joseph Pizzorno, N.D. who have cited soy's therapeutic uses in prostate enlargement, breast cancer, menopause, male infertility, osteoporosis and premenstrual syndrome.(Murray and Pizzorno 1998; Weil 2004).

Interestingly most soy scientists accept, even some of the anti-soyists, that heat and processing – especially fermentation – rids soy of much of its protease trypsin-inhibitor effects.

It should also be pointed out that a large array of other healthy foods like grains, legumes and vegetables like spinach also contain varying amounts of trypsin inhibitors.

In a review of some of this anti-soy literature by the Tufts University Department of Nutritional Science for scientific website accuracy, the main website of the organization was given an *"unacceptable"* rating in 2003.

In its review of the website, Tufts scientists stated:

*"they appear to select obscure studies, take study results out of context and use undocumented 'facts' from their own publications to forward their agenda."*

The lectin/hemagglutin position, though seemingly sensational, may well have been challenged by research illustrating soy isoflavones' ability to reduce platelet aggregation and blood clotting related to stroke and heart attack. A 2006 double-blind, randomized placebo-controlled study from the Universidad de Chile on 29 post-menopausal women with an average age of 53.5 concluded that soy isoflavones daidzein and genistein decreased TxA2 receptor density, which *"reduce the risk of thrombogenesis,"* according to lead researcher Professor Argelia Garrido (**Garrido** *et al.* **2006**).

Warnings by several government agencies regarding soy-based infant formula have attracted anti-soy comments. The United Kingdom, New Zealand, Australian, French, Israeli and Swiss governments have all made statements warning mothers against soy-based infant formulae, some recommending doctor's advice prior to its use. Anti-soy advocates have heralded these announcements as confirming the legitimacy of their position on infantile endocrine disruption.

However, this is specific to the issue of replacing breast milk with soymilk – which we are not advising in the Ancestors Diet. Breast milk is the intended food for infants, and this is confirmed by hundreds of studies.

Rather, the Ancestors Diet advocates soy as a nutritional food best eaten in its fermented forms, including tofu, tempeh and natto.

The reality that soy is a highly nutritional food has been proven in the research. A review of 11 studies in *Menopause – The Journal of the North American Menopause Society* – concluded that there was consistent relief from hot flush number and frequency with dosages of at least 15 mg of genistein per day (Williamson-Huges *et al.* 2006).

And a meta-analysis done by the Griffith University School of Medicine (Howes *et al.* 206) reviewed data from 17 randomized and controlled studies of four weeks or more. The researchers commented:

> *"The results of the study tend to support the recommendation of the North American Menopause Society that "... for women with frequent hot flashes, clinicians may consider recommending soy foods or soy isoflavone supplements.""*

This research confirms multiple epidemiological studies of soy-eating Asian women reporting a fraction of the hot flashes North American and European women have. Protective effects for postmenopausal osteoporosis (Arjamdi *et al.* 1998, Scheiber *et al.* 2001; Picherit *et al.* 2001) and increased frontal lobe cognitive function (File *et al.* 2005) have also been reported.

We've discussed some of the other fermented soy products earlier. Let's now cover a new one.

### Natto

An enzyme-extracted from natto, nattokinase has been proven to be a significant nutraceutical. Natto is a traditional fermented soy dish of Japan and Thailand. The fermenting process utilizes a strain of *Bacillus subtilis* to produce the enzyme. Recent studies confirm profibronolytic (clot-dissolving) effects of natto and its extract, (Suzuki *et al.* 2003; Peng *et al.* 2005). making nattokinase useful for stroke prevention. One study showed a 12% reduction in airline venous thrombosis during long airline flights (Cesarone *et al.* 2003).

## The Prebiotic Diet

One of the most important factors in establishing a healthy environment for our probiotic colonies is making sure they have the right mix of nutrients available. The nutrients our probiotic families favor are called prebiotics. In other words, some foods are particularly beneficial for *bifidobacteria, lactobacilli* and other probiotic populations. These are the oligosaccharides, fructooligosaccharides, galactooligosaccharides, and transgalactooligosaccharides – also referred to as inulin, FOS, GOS and TOS. Even two or three grams of one of these prebiotics will dramatically increase probiotic populations assuming healthy colonies. Inulin, FOS, GOS and TOS are also antagonistic to toxic microorganism genera such as *Salmonella, Listeria, Campylobacter, Shigella* and *Vibrio.* These and other pathogenic bacteria tend to thrive from refined sugars as opposed to the complex saccharides of inulin, FOS, GOS and TOS.

Oligosaccharides are short stacks of simple yet mostly indigestible sugars (from the Greek *oligos*, meaning "few"). If the sugar molecule is fructose, the stacked molecule is called a fructooligosaccharide. If the sugar molecule is galactose, the stacked molecule is called a galactooligosaccharide. These molecules are very useful for human cells and probiotics because they can be processed directly for energy as well as be combined with fatty acids to create cell wall structures and cellular communication molecules. These nutrients also provide energy and nourishment to our probiotic colonies.

The oligosaccharides inulin and oligofructose are probably the most recognized prebiotics. Inulin is a naturally occurring carbohydrate used by plants for storage. It has been estimated that more than 36,000 plant species contain inulin in varying degrees (Carpita *et al.* 1989). The roots often contain the greatest amounts of inulin.

Commercial sources of inulin include Jerusalem artichoke, agave cactus and chicory. Chicory, the root of the Belgian endive, is known to contain some of the highest levels of both inulin at 15-20%, and oligofructose at 5-10%. Inulin from agave has been described as highly branched. This gives it a higher solubility and digestibility than inulin derived from Jerusalem artichoke or chicory.

Notable prebiotic FOS-containing foods include beets, leeks, bananas, tree fruits, soybeans, burdock root, asparagus, maple sugar, whole rye and whole wheat among many others. Bananas contain one of the highest levels of FOS. Bananas are thus a favorite food for both humans and probiotics.

GOS and TOS are natural byproducts of milk. They are produced as lactose is enzymatically converted or hydrolyzed within the digestive tract. This process can also be done commercially. Before much of the recent research on prebiotics was performed, nutritionists simply thought of GOS and TOS as indigestible byproducts of milk.

A lesser known yet important prebiotic is the polysaccharide arabinoxylan-oligosaccharide. This is a component of wheat bran. We will discuss this further in our chapter on grains.

It is the longer-chain polysaccharides that provide the most benefit to our probiotics. These are contained in whole, plant fiber foods.

On the other hand, foods that have been stripped of these important plant fibers, creating refined simpler sugars, feed the more aggressive disease-causing bacteria and yeasts such as Staphylococcus and Candida.

Another element in plant foods providing prebiotic nutrition for probiotics is the polyphenol group. Polyphenols are groups of biochemicals produced in plants such as lignans, tannins, resveratrol, and flavonoids.

There is some uncertainty as to which of these are most helpful to probiotic populations.

Some prebiotics have interesting side effects. For example, there seems to be a relationship between oligofructose inulin and calcium absorption. Inulin has been shown to improve calcium absorption by 20%, and yogurt supplemented with TOS has increased calcium absorption by 16% (van den Heuvel *et al.* 2000)

Galactooligosaccharides have another side effect that is important to note. Dr. Kari Shoaf and fellow researchers at the University of Nebraska (Shoaf *et al.* 2006) found in laboratory tests that galactooligosaccharides reduce the ability of *E. coli* to attach to human cells within tissue cultures. This effect was isolated from GOS' ability to nourish probiotics. This means that GOS provides more than nutrition to our probiotic colonies. This once considered useless indigestible nutrient also helps keep *E. coli* and other pathogenic bacteria from attaching to our cells. A nice package deal indeed.

FOS and GOS have been known to cause digestive disturbance in rare cases. Such a digestive disturbance is likely caused by dysbiosis, however.

Conclusively, a preponderance of scientific literature indicates that probiotics thrive from a diet of plant-based natural foods with plenty of phytonutrients, while overly processed, sugary and meat diets tend to promote pathogenic bacteria and their disease-causing endotoxins.

## Cultures and Digestion

Dysbiosis is a state where the body has an imbalance between probiotic populations and pathogenic bacteria populations. In other words, the system is being overrun by the pathogenic bacteria and there are not enough probiotics in place to control their populations. When the body is lacking probiotics, or is overgrown with pathobiotic populations, there is typically an intestinal infection of some type. The extent of the infection, of course, depends upon the type of pathogenic bacteria present, and their populations in proportion to probiotic populations.

Many disorders can be traced back to dysbiosis. Some are direct and obvious, and some are not so obvious, and often appear as other disorders. In general, most digestive disorders are either caused by or accompanied by a lack of balanced intestinal probiotic populations. There are several types of dysbiosis.

We can usually detect *putrefaction dysbiosis* from the incidence of slow bowel movement. Symptoms of putrefaction dysbiosis include depression, diarrhea, fatigue, memory loss, numbing of hands and feet, sleep disturbances, joint pain and muscle weakness. Many of these disorders and others are often due directly to the overgrowth of pathobiotics. The bacteria are burdening the blood stream with endotoxin waste products and neurotoxins; infecting cells, joints, nerves, brain tissues and other regions of the body.

Another overgrowth issue is *fermentation dysbiosis*. This is often evidenced by bloating, constipation, diarrhea, fatigue, and gas; and the faulty digestion of carbohydrates, grains, proteins and fiber. This is also a result of pathobiotic overgrowth, but in this type of dysbiosis, yeasts are prevalent among the overgrowth populations. As we know from baking bread, yeast will ferment quickly in warm, humid environments.

Either type of dysbiosis can result in an acute case of watery diarrhea. While diarrhea in itself may not sound that dangerous, the critical loss of body water will result in dehydration, which can be lethal. This is because the body's water is being purged faster than our ability to replace it.

A few years ago, researchers (Allen *et al.* 2004) published a review of twenty-three studies that trialed probiotics on patients with acute diarrhea. These twenty-three studies were randomized and controlled, and carefully chosen to meet stringent control criteria. Together the review gathered data on 1,917 patients in countries with low infant mortality rates. The overall conclusion of this review was that probiotics reduced the risk of infection substantially, and the duration of diarrhea episodes by an average of 30.48 hours.

For example, German scientists (Rosenfeldt, *et al.* 2002) gave sixty-nine children hospitalized with rotavirus enteritis a placebo or the probiotics *Lactobacillus rhamnosus* or *Lactobacillus reuteri* twice per day for five days. The probiotic treatment group had a significantly reduced period of rotavirus excretion, reduced hospital stays and duration of episodes. Studying another group of forty-three children with mild gastroenteritis recruited from day care centers, the researchers found that probiotic treatment resulted in average diarrhea episode lengths of 76 hours – versus 116 hours among the non-probiotic group.

A body with low probiotic populations will create havoc for the immune system. *Deficiency dysbiosis* is related to an absence of probiotics, leading to damaged intestinal mucosa. This can lead to irritable bowel syndrome, food sensitivities, and intestinal permeability. The lack of probiotics allows the intestinal wall to come into contact with foreign molecules. This can open up the junctions between the intestinal brush barrier cells. This can in turn lead to the entry of these toxins along with larger more complex food particles into the bloodstream – such as larger peptides and protein molecules – as we have discussed. Because these molecules are not normally found in the blood stream, the immune system identifies them as foreigners. The body then launches an inflammatory immune response, leading to *sensitization dysbiosis*. Linked to probiotic deficiency, sensitization dysbiosis causes food intolerances, food allergies, chemical and food sensitivities, acne, connective tissue disease and psoriasis. Intestinal permeability has also been suspected in a variety of lung and joint infections.

The obvious signs of dysbiosis include hormonal imbalances and mood swings, high cholesterol, vitamin B deficiencies, frequent gas and bloating, indigestion, irritable bowels, easy bruising of the skin, constipation, diarrhea, vaginal infections, reduced sex drive, prostate enlargement, food sensitivities, chemical sensitivities, bladder infections, allergies, rhinovirus and rotavirus infections, influenza, and various histamine-related inflammatory syndromes such as rashes, asthma and skin irritation.

Furthermore, the infection of various parts of the body – either from pathogenic bacteria or their endotoxins – can cause various ailments typically associated with autoimmune or degenerative etiologies. Autoimmune type diseases of the liver, the urinary tract, the joints, gums and ears, heart and lungs can directly result from any one of the above forms of dysbiosis. An example of this is Grave's disease – considered a classic autoimmune disorder caused seemingly by the immune system attacking healthy cells of the thyroid gland. Tests have shown that some 80% of Grave's sufferers test positive for *Yersinia enterocolitica* antibodies. Dysbiosis is often accompanied by an overgrowth of the bacteria, *Yersinia enterocolitica*. Yersina endotoxins can attach to thyroid cells, stimulating the overproduction of thyroid hormone – one of the symptoms of Grave's disease.

## Health Benefits of Cultures

The following chart summarizes some of the research findings of what probiotics do within the body. Each of these have been specifically detailed and reviewed in the author's book, *Probiotics: Protection Against Infection*. Please consult this book for references and further information about probiotics in general.

| Allergies | reduce Th1/ Th2 ratio; decrease Th2 levels; lower TGF-beta2; increase IgE |
| Anorexia nervosa | increase appetite; increase assimilation; increase lymphocytes |
| Antibiotics | produce antibiotic and antifungal substances (such as acidophillin and bifidin) that repel or kill pathogenic bacteria, adjusting to pathogen and resistance |
| B-cells | modulate and redirect B-cell activity |
| Bile | break down bile acids |

| Biochemicals | secrete lactic acids, lactoperoxidases, formic acids, lipopolysaccharides, peptidoglycans, superantigens and others to manage pH and repel pathogens. |
|---|---|
| Bladder cancer | reduce recurrent bladder cancer incidence and inhibit new tumors |
| Blood pressure | reduce hypertension; inhibit ACE |
| Calcium | increase serum calcium; decrease parathyroid hormone |
| Cancer (general) | reduce mutagenicity; increase natural killer tumoricidal activity; increase survival rates |
| Candida overgrowth | control populations; reduce overgrowths |
| CD cell orientation | modulate and direct particular CD cells depending upon condition, including CD56, CD8, CD4, CD25, CD69, CD2, others |
| Cell degeneration | slow cellular degeneration and associated diseases among elderly persons |
| Colds and Influenza | reduce infection frequency; reduce infection duration; reduce symptoms; prevent complications; decrease worker sick days |
| Colic | reduce crying time; decrease infection; increase stool frequency; decrease bloating and indigestion |
| Colon cancer | reduce recurrence; increase survival rates; reduce beta-glucosidase; inhibit cell abnormality and mutation; increase IL-2 |
| Constipation | increase bowel movement frequency; ease colon and impacted feces |
| Control pathogens | compete with pathogenic organisms for nutrients, thus checking their growth |
| C-reactive protein | reduce levels in blood |
| Cytokines | stimulate the body's production of various cytokines, including IL-6, IL-3, IL-5, TNF alpha, and interferon |
| Dental caries | reduce and control cavity-causing bacteria |
| Digestion | reduce gas, nausea and stress-related gastrointestinal digestive difficulty |
| Digestive difficulty | secrete digestive enzymes; help break down nutrients from fats; proteins and other foods |
| Diverticulosis | reduce polyps and strengthen intestinal wall mucosa |
| Ear infections | hasten otitis media healing response; prevent infections |
| EFAs | manufacture essential fatty acids, including important short-chained FAs, and help body assimilate EFAs |
| Fiber digestion | aid in soluble fiber fermentation, yielding fatty acids |

| | and energy |
|---|---|
| Food poisoning | increase resistance to food poisoning; battle and remove pathogenic organisms; reduce diarrhea and other symptoms |
| Glucose metabolism | improve glucose control |
| Gum disease | reduce gum infections; deplete gingivitis |
| *H. pylori* | reduce *H. pylori* infections; reduce ulcers |
| HIV/AIDS | stimulate immune system; reduce symptoms; reduce co-infections; increase survival rates |
| Hormones | balance and stimulate hormone production |
| Hydrogen peroxide | manufacture H2O2 – oxygenating/antiseptic |
| IBS | decrease bloating, pain, cramping |
| Immunoglobulins | modulate IgA, IgG, IgE, IgM to weakness |
| Inflammation | modify prostaglandins (E1, E2), IFN-gamma, reduce CRP; modulate TNF-alpha; increase IgA; slow inflammatory response as needed |
| Intestinal Permeability | protect against IIPS; block penetration of toxins; work cooperatively with villi and microvilli; attach to mucosa; improve barrier function |
| Intestine walls | protect walls of intestines against toxin exposure and colonization of pathogens |
| Iron absorption | increase iron assimilation; increase hemoglobin count |
| Keratoconjunctivitis | decrease burning, itching and dry eyes |
| Kidney stones | reduce urine oxalates; reduce blood oxalates |
| Lipids/Cholesterol | reduce LDL, triglycerides and total cholesterol; increase HDL |
| Liver | stimulate liver cells (hepatocytes); stimulate liver function; reduce cirrhosis symptoms; reduce liver enzymes |
| Liver cancer | stimulate immune response; decrease infection and complications after surgery |
| Lung cancer | increase survival rates; reduce chest pain and other symptoms |
| Mental state | improve mood; stimulate positive mood hormones like serotonin and tryptophan |
| Milk digestion | aid dairy digestion for lactose-intolerant people; produce lactase |
| Monocytes | increase oxidative burst capacity |
| Mucosa | coat intestines, stomach, oral, nasal and vagina mucosa, providing protective barrier |
| NF-kappaB | modulate activity to condition |
| NK-cells | stimulate natural killer cell activity |
| Nutrition | manufacture biotin, thiamin (B1), riboflavin (B2), niacin (B3), pantothenic acid (B5), pyridoxine (B6), |

| | cobalamine (B12), folic acid, vitamin A and/or vitamin K; aid in assimilation of proteins, fats and minerals |
|---|---|
| Pancreatitis | reduce pancreas infection (sepsis); reduce necrosis; speed healing |
| pH control | produce a number of other acids and biochemicals, modulating pH (see biochemicals) |
| Phagocytes | increase phagocytic activity as needed |
| Phytonutrients | convert to bioavailable nutrient forms |
| Premature births and Low birth weights | speed growth; reduce infection; improve immune response; increase nutrition |
| Protein assimilation | break down amino acid content; inhibit assimilation of allergic polypeptides |
| Respiratory infections | inhibit pneumonia; reduce duration of infection; inhibit bronchitis; inhibit tonsillitis |
| Rotavirus infections | speed healing times; prevent infection; ease abdominal pain; eradicate infective agents |
| Spleen | stimulate spleen activity |
| Stomach cancer | inhibit tumors; reduce H. pylori overgrowths |
| T-cells | modulate T-cell activity to condition |
| Th1 - Th2 | decrease Th2 activity; increase Th1 (increases healing and decreases allergic response) |
| Thymus | increase thymus size and activity |
| Toxins | break down toxins; inhibit assimilation of heavy metals, chemicals, and endotoxins |
| Ulcers | control H. pylori; speed healing; improve mucusa; moderate acids; reduce pain |
| Vaccination | increase vaccine effectiveness |
| Vaginosis/Vaginitis | reduce infection; re-establish healthy pH; reduce odor |

## Cultural Supplementation

Eating plenty of cultured and prebiotic foods may not be enough during times of dysbiosis or other inflammatory issues related to an overgrowth of toxic pathogens.

For those who are trying to revitalize their digestive tracts to enable the proper digestion or sensitivity to certain foods such as grains and fibers, for example, supplementing probiotics daily is a good idea.

The supplementation of probiotics to discourage food sensitivities must be done with the science in mind. This is vital, because not every species, every strain and every dose has been shown to be useful for food sensitivities. Rather, research has shown that specific species and strains,

245

used in specific doses alongside prebiotic-rich diets are most beneficial, as we've illustrated in this book.

First we should know which species aid in food sensitivities. After reviewing hundreds of clinical studies, some quoted in this book and many more discussed in the author's *Probiotics – Protection Against Infection* (2009), we summarize here the probiotics that have been shown useful for food sensitivities, together with a selection of research findings related to digestive issues:

### Lactobacillus acidophilus

*Lactobacillus acidophilus* is by far the most familiar probiotic to most of us, and is also by far the most-studied probiotic species to date. They are one of the main residents of the human gut, although supplemented strains may still be transient. In addition to helping digest lactose, probably the most important benefit of *L. acidophilus* is their ability to inhibit the growth of pathogenic intestinal microorganisms such as *Candida albicans, Escherichia coli, Helicobacter pylori, Salmonella, Shigella* and *Staphylococcus* species.

The research has found that L. acidophilus help digest milk, reduce stress-induced GI problems; inhibit *E. coli*, reduce various intestinal infections, reduce intestinal permeability, control *H. pylori*, reduce inflammation, reduce dyspepsia, help relieve IBS and colitis, inhibit and control Clostridium spp., inhibit Bacteroides spp., and inhibit Candida spp. overgrowths.

### Lactobacillus helveticus

*L. helveticus* was made popular by cheese-makers from Switzerland. The Latin word *Helvetia* refers to Switzerland. *L. helveticus* is used to make Swiss cheese and other varietals, as it produces lactic acid but not other probiotic metabolites that can often make cheese taste bitter or sour.

### Lactobacillus salivarius

*L. salivarius* are residents of most humans. They are found in the mouth, small intestines, colon, and vagina. They are hardy bacteria that can live in both oxygen and oxygen-free environments. *L. salivarius* is one of the few bacteria species that can also thrive in salty environments. *L. salivarius* produce prolific amounts of lactic acid, which makes them hardy defenders of the teeth and gums. They also produce a number of antibiotics, and are speedy colonizers.

### Lactobacillus casei

*L. casei* are transient bacteria within the human body, but are residents of cow intestines. Thus they are readily found in naturally raw milk and colostrum. *L. casei* have been reported to reduce allergy symptoms and increase immune response. This is accomplished by their regulating the immune system's CHS, CD8 and T-cell responsiveness – an effect seen among immunosuppressed patients. *L. casei* are also competitive bacteria that will overtake other probiotics in a combined supplement. So it is best to supplement *L. casei* individually.

### Lactobacillus rhamnosus

Much of the research on this species has been done on a particular strain, *L. rhamnosus* GG. *L. rhamnosus* GG have been shown in numerous studies to significantly stimulate the immune system and inhibit allergic inflammatory response as noted earlier. This is not to say, however, that non-GG strains will not perform similarly. In fact, studies with *L. rhamnosus* GR-1, *L. rhamnosus* 573/L, and *L. rhamnosus* LC705 strains have also showed positive results. The GG strain is trademarked by the Valio Ltd. Company in Finland and patented in 1985 by two scientists, Dr. Sherwood Gorbach and Dr. Barry Goldin, who also led most of the exhaustive research on this strain.

### Lactobacillus reuteri

*L. reuteri* is a species found residing permanently in humans. As a result, most supplemented strains attach fairly well, though temporarily, and stimulate colony growth for resident *L. reuteri* strains. *L. reuteri* will colonize in the stomach, duodenum and ileum regions. *L. reuteri* will also significantly modulate the immune response of the gastrointestinal mucosal membranes. This means that *L. reuteri* are useful for many of the same digestive ailments that *L. acidophilus* are also effective for. *L. reuteri* also have several other effects, including the restoration of our oral cavity bacteria. They also produce a significant amount of antibiotics.

### Lactobacillus plantarum

*L. plantarum* has been part of the human diet for thousands of years. They are used in numerous fermented foods, including sauerkraut, gherkins, olive brines, sourdough bread, Nigerian ogi and fufu, kocha from Ethiopia, sour mifen noodles from China, Korean kimchi and other traditional foods. *L. plantarum* are also found in dairy and cow dung.

*L. plantarum* is a hardy strain. The bacteria have been shown to survive all the way through the intestinal tract. Temperature for optimal growth is 86-95 degrees F. *L. plantarum* are not permanent residents, however. When supplemented, they vigorously attack pathogenic bacteria, and create an environment hospitable for incubated resident strains to expand before departing. *L. plantarum* also produce lysine, and a number of antibiotics including lactolin. They also strengthen the mucosal membrane and reduce intestinal permeability.

### Lactobacillus bulgaricus

We owe the *bulgaricus* name to Ilya Mechnikov, who named it after the Bulgarians – who used the bacteria to make the fermented milks that produced the original kefirs apparently related to their extreme longevity. In the 1960s and 1970s Russian researchers, notably Dr. Ivan Bogdanov and others, began focused research on *L. bulgaricus*. Early studies indicated antitumor effects. As the research progressed into Russian clinical research and commercialization, it became obvious that even heat-killed *L. bulgaricus* cell fragments have immune system stimulating benefits.

*L. bulgaricus* bacteria are transients that assist in *bifidobacteria* colony growth. They significantly stimulate the immune system and have antitumor effects. They also produce antibiotic and antiviral substances such as bulgarican and others. *L. bulgaricus* bacteria have also been reported to have anti-herpes properties. *L. bulgaricus* require more heat to colonize than many probiotics – at 104-109 degrees F.

The research has shown that L. bulgaricus will help increase absorption of dairy (lactose).

### Bifidobacterium bifidum

These are normal residents in the human intestines, and by far the largest residents in terms of colonies. Their greatest populations occur in the colon, but also inhabit the lower small intestines. Breast milk typically contains large populations of *B. bifidum* along with other bifidobacteria. *B. bifidum* are highly competitive with yeasts such as *Candida albicans*. As a result, their populations may be decimated by large yeast overgrowths. This will also result in a number of endotoxins, including ammonia, being leached out of the colon into the bloodstream. As a result, *B. bifidum* populations are extremely important to the health of the liver, as has been illustrated in the research. They produce an array of antibiotics such as bifidin and various antimicrobial biochemicals such as formic acid. *B. bifidus* populations can also be severely damaged by the use of pharmaceutical antibiotics.

### Bifidobacterium infantis

*B. infantis* are also normal residents of the human intestines – primarily among children. As implicated in the name, infants colonize a significant number of *B. infantis* in their early years. They will also colonize in the vagina, leading to the newborn's first exposure to protective probiotic bacteria. For this reason, it is important that pregnant mothers consider probiotic supplementation with *B. infantis*. *B. infantis* are largely anaerobic, and thrive within the darkest regions, where they can produce profuse quantities of acetic acid, lactic acid and formic acid to acidify the intestinal tract.

### Bifidobacterium longum

*B. longum* are also normal inhabitants of the human digestive tract. They predominate the colon but also live in the small intestines. They are one of our top four bifidobacteria inhabitants. Like *B. infantis,* they produce acetic, lactic and formic acid. Like other bifidobacteria, they resist the growth of pathogenic bacteria, and thus reduce the production of harmful nitrites and ammonia. *B. longum* also produce B vitamins. Healthy breast milk contains significant *B. longum.*

### Bifidobacterium animalis/B. lactis

*B. animalis* was previously thought to be distinct from *B. lactis,* but today they are considered the same species with *B. lactis* being a subspecies of *B. animalis*. *B. lactis* has also been described as *Streptococcus lactis.* They are transient bacteria typically present in raw milk. They are also used as starters for traditional cheeses, cottage cheeses and buttermilks. They are also found among certain plants.

### Bifidobacterium breve

*B. breve* are also normal inhabitants of the human digestive tract – living mostly within the colon. They produce prolific acids, and also B vitamins. Like the other bifidobacteria, they also reduce ammonia-producing bacteria in the colon, aiding the health of the liver. Latin *brevis* means short.

### Streptococcus thermophilus

*Streptococcus thermophilus* are common participants in yogurt making. They are also used in cheese making, and are even sometimes found in pasteurized milk. They will colonize at higher temperatures, from 104-113 degrees F. This is significant because this bacterium readily produces lactase, which breaks down lactose. (This is the only streptococci known to do this.) Like many other supplemented probiotics, *S. thermophilus* are temporary microorganisms in the human body. Their colonies will typically inhabit the system for a week or two before exiting (unless consistently consumed). During that time, however, they will help set up a healthy environment to support resident colony growth. Like other probiotics, *S. thermophilus* also produce a number of different antibiotic substances, including acids that deter the growth of pathogenic bacteria.

### *Saccharomyces boulardii*

*S. boulardii* are yeasts (fungi). They render a variety of preventative and therapeutic benefits to the body. Yet should this or another yeast colony grow too large, they can quickly become a burden to the body due to their dietary needs (primarily refined sugars) and waste products. *S. boulardii* are known to enhance IgA – which, as we've discussed, will typically reduce IgE atopic sensitivities. This is likely why this probiotic helps clear skin disorders. *S. boulardii* also help control diarrhea, and have been shown to be helpful in Crohn's disease and irritable bowel issues. *S. boulardii* have also been shown to be useful in combating cholera bacteria (*Vibrio cholerae*).

## Probiotic Supplement Considerations

The main consideration in probiotic supplementation is consuming live organisms. These are typically labeled as "CFU" which stands for *colony forming units*. In other words, live probiotics will produce new colonies once inside the intestines. Dead ones will not. So the key is keeping the probiotics alive while in the capsule and supplement bottle, until we are ready to consume them. Here are a few considerations about probiotic supplements:

## Capsules

Vegetable capsules contain less moisture than gelatin or enteric-coated capsules. Even a little moisture in the capsule can increase the possibility of waking up the probiotics while in the bottle. Once woken up, they will starve and die. Enteric coating can minimally protect the probiotics within the stomach, assuming they have survived in the bottle. Some manufactures use oils to help protect the probiotics in the stomach. In all cases, encapsulated freeze-dried probiotics should be refrigerated (no matter what the label says) at all times during shipping, at the store, and at home. Dark containers also better protect the probiotics from light exposure, which can kill them.

## Powders

Powders of freeze-dried probiotics are subject to deterioration due to increased exposure to oxygen and light. Powders should be refrigerated in dark containers and sealed tightly to be kept viable. They should also be consumed with liquids or food, preferably dairy or fermented dairy. If used as to insert into the vagina, a douche mixture with water and a little yogurt is preferable.

### Caplets/Tablets

Some tablet/caplets have special coatings that provide viability through to the intestines without refrigeration. If not, those tablets would likely be in the same category as encapsulated products, in terms of requiring refrigeration.

### Shells or Beads

These can provide longer shelf viability without refrigeration and better survive the stomach. However, because of the size of the shell, these typically come with less CFU quantity, increasing the cost of a therapeutic dose. Another drawback may be that the intestines must dissolve this thick shell. An easy test is to examine the stool to be sure that the beads or shells aren't coming out the other end whole.

### Lozenges

These are new and exciting ways to supplement with probiotics. A correctly formulated chewable or lozenge can inoculate the mouth, nose and throat with beneficial bacteria to compete with and fight off pathogenic bacteria as they enter or reside in our nose, throat, mouth and even lungs. However, the probiotics in a lozenge will not likely survive the stomach acids and penetrate the intestines.

Still, lozenges are an excellent way to protect against new infections and prevent sore throats when we are traveling or working in enclosed spaces. The bacteria in a lozenge or chewable ease out as we are sucking or chewing, leaving probiotics dispersed throughout our gums and throat, rendering increased immunity. This type of supplement should still be kept sealed, airtight and cool. Refer to the author's book *Oral Probiotics* (2010) for detailed information regarding species and strategies for oral probiotic lozenges.

### Liquid Supplements

There are several probiotic supplements in small liquid form. One brand has a long tradition and a hardy, well-researched strain. A liquid probiotic should be in a light-sealed, refrigerated container. It should also contain some dairy or other probiotic-friendly culture, giving the probiotics some food while they are waiting for delivery.

### Probiotic Dosage

A good dosage for intestinal probiotics for prevention and maintenance can be ten to fifteen billion CFU (*colony forming units*) per day. Total intake during an illness or therapeutic period, however, will often double or triple that dosage. Much of the research shown in this text utilized 20 billion to 40 billion CFU per day, about a third of that dose for children and a quarter of that dose for infants. (*B. infantis* is often the supplement of choice for babies.)

Supplemental oral probiotic dosages can be far less (100 million to two billion), especially when the formula contains the hardy *L. reuteri*.

People who must take antibiotics for life-threatening reasons can alternate doses of probiotics between their antibiotic dosing. The probiotic dose can be at least two hours before or after the antibiotic dose. (Always consult with the prescribing doctor first.)

Remember that these dosages depend upon delivery to the intestines. Therefore, a product that passes into the stomach with little protection would likely not deliver well to the intestines. Such a supplement would likely require higher dosage to achieve the desired effects.

# Chapter Eight

# Sweets, Fats and Salts

These three foods are critical foods, simply because they direct taste and smell, and drive us towards eating certain foods. The reason being, that these three types of foods are critical to the body's health.

Sweeteners are critical to our health because our body is driven by the conversion of glucose and oxygen to energy and heat. This means that glucose is our central fuel.

Fats are our body's secondary source of fuel, and a form of fuel storage. In addition, fats – also called lipids – make up many of our body's primary structures, most importantly, our cell membranes.

Salts are also critical to our body because they provide essential ions – also called minerals and trace elements – that give our body structure and provide the means for energy conductance. This means that without salts, we could not fire nervous responses between nerves and cells, and we could not maintain an electrolyte balance in our body's tissues.

## Sugar: The Good and the Bad

Sugar has gotten a bad rap. Some say sugar is the cause for many of the diseases of modern society. These include dental decay, type 2 diabetes, obesity, metabolic syndrome, yeast infections and a host of others. Why is sugar so bad for you? And are all sugars bad?

Researchers from the University of California at San Francisco (Lustig et al. 2012) concluded that sugar is not simply empty calories – sugar, they find, is the cause of chronic disease and early death.

The paper, written by Dr. Robert Lustig, Dr. Laura Schmidt and Dr. Claire Brindis, was published in the scientific journal, Nature last week. They submitted:

*"A growing body of scientific evidence shows that fructose can trigger processes that lead to liver toxicity and a host of other chronic diseases. A little is not a problem, but a lot kills — slowly."*

All three authors are professors at the University of California. Dr. Lustig is a medical doctor and professor of Clinical Pediatrics. He is one of the foremost experts on the central nervous system and childhood obesity.

White sugar is composed of primarily sucrose, while corn syrup is more than a third fructose, about a third glucose and the rest in maltose, depending upon how highly refined the corn syrup is. The more refined corn syrups, such as high fructose corn syrup or HFCS, can have up to 38% fructose.

Refined sugars such as HFCS and table sugar have been stripped away from the nutrients and fiber of the original food source – cane, beets or corn – and thus subject the blood stream to immediate hikes in blood sugar levels. This overloading puts pressure on the liver and pancreas, and is linked to insulin insensitivity – eventually leading to diabetes and inflammatory conditions.

The paper illustrated research that shows that refined sugars and corn syrups are one of the primary causes for obesity, heart disease, diabetes and other metabolic-oriented diseases. This, they point out, is cause to regulate sugar products, just as tobacco and alcohol are regulated. They state:

> *"If international authorities are truly concerned about public health, they must consider limiting fructose — and its main delivery vehicles, the added sugars HCFS (high fructose corn syrup) and sucrose — which pose dangers to individuals and to society as a whole."*

Today, refined sugar consumption has skyrocketed in the United States, going up with rates of obesity, high blood pressure, heart disease, cancer and diabetes over the decades. Over the past three decades, our sugar intake has tripled. The average American now consumes about 22 teaspoons of sugar a day – or more than 75 pounds of sugar a year. This is well over the 6 and 9 teaspoons suggested for women and men respectively by the American Heart Association.

Most packaged foods now contain either sugar and/or HFCS as ingredients. Sodas and sports drinks supply the bulk of Americans' sugar intake, at 36%. Desserts are second at 19%. Fruit drinks and packaged foods follow.

The authors also underscored the addictive quality of sugar. *"Sugar promotes the same phenomena in the brain that addictive substances do,"* Dr. Lustig told NBC in a recent interview.

The most controversial point of the paper published in Nature was the proposal that sugary foods and beverages be taxed to limit their consumption. The paper states:

> *"If international authorities are truly concerned about public health, they must consider limiting fructose — and its main delivery vehicles, the added sugars HCFS (high fructose corn syrup) and sucrose — which pose dangers to individuals and to society as a whole."*

Though controversial, this is not a new concept. Dr. Kelly Brownell and Thomas Frieden, M.D., Ph.D. have argued for taxing sugar. They co-authored such a proposal in a paper published in the New England Journal of Medicine in 2009. Dr. Frieden is the Director for the U.S. Centers for Disease Control and Prevention, and Dr. Brownell is the Director of Yale's Rudd Center for Food Policy and Obesity.

Research supports this. A study published in the *Archives of Internal Medicine* (Duffey et al. 2010) followed 5,115 young adults for 21 years. They found that taxing soda 10% reduced caloric consumption by 7%. The study calculated that an 18% tax would reduce caloric intake by 56 calories for each person, equating to five pounds of weight loss per year.

These researchers concluded:

> *"In conclusion, our findings suggest that national, state or local policies to alter the price of less healthful foods and beverages may be one possible mechanism for steering U.S. adults toward a more healthful diet. While such policies will not solve the obesity epidemic in its entirety and may face considerable opposition from food manufacturers and sellers, they could prove an important strategy to address overconsumption, help reduce energy intake and potentially aid in weight loss and reduced rates of diabetes among U.S. adults."*

### The main reason most people think sugar is bad

Sugar has been demonized because it can be immediately absorbed into the blood. This stimulates the pancreas to produce and release insulin into the bloodstream. Insulin escorts glucose into the cells and the mitochondria in the cells use it for making energy (e.g., the Krebs cycle).

Afterward, blood sugar levels can drop, leaving the body in a state of "sugar blues." In other words, the initial "sugar high" from mitochondrial energy production is followed by that sinking "sugar low."

This gyration of highs and lows theoretically stresses the pancreas and somehow causes the cells to become insensitive to insulin and glucose.

What's wrong with this overly simplified explanation? The main problem is that sugars are contained in practically every meal, and they are necessary for life. Most foods, especially carbohydrates, will raise blood sugar levels.

### Will the real culprit please stand up?

The problem with this explanation is that there is no reason why the body should not be able to handle sugar loading. After all, many other loading events take place around the body, including the beating of the heart and the gasping of the lungs. The body was designed for periodic loading.

Plus, we need glucose to feed our cells. Besides, leftover glycogen stored in the liver should be able to bridge the sugar highs and lows. Put it this way: Our bodies are energy machines. Why can't they handle a few candy bars now and again?

255

In other words, this "sugar rush" explanation just doesn't cut it alone. It doesn't fully explain type 2 diabetes, metabolic syndrome, yeast infections, obesity, dental decay and many other problems now connected to refined sugar loading.

In fact, even though about every child in America gorges on candy bars, ice cream and other sugary foods, only a few percent will contract type 2 diabetes or metabolic syndrome.

The biggest problem with sugar is that it is *bacteria food*. Pathogenic bacteria love simple, refined sugars.

Speaking of gorging: Pathogenic bacteria within the mouth and intestines gorge on certain refined sugars. Refined sugars help them grow exponentially (called colonization). As they grow in numbers, they begin to wreak havoc on our entire physiology.

In the mouth, they produce acids that wear away the dentin and enamel of our teeth. Eventually the bacteria climb inside and domesticate our gums. Once inside the gums, they leak their acids and other endotoxins (their poop) into the bloodstream.

They can also and swarm to other body cavities such as the ears, throat, nose and lungs. As these infections grow, they can cause COPD, allergies, sinusitis, throat infections, ulcers (*H. pylori* bacteria) and a variety of intestinal infections.

These infective bacteria poison the body. In some cases, they can leak into the bloodstream and colonize regions of the body not readily reachable by the immune system. These areas include the joint capsules and pleural cavity. The endotoxins they propel into the bloodstream act as free radicals. Free radicals eat away at veins and artery walls, the heart, the joints and many other tissue systems around the body. They will also damage the liver and the pancreas.

And when these wretched radicals reach the cells, they can infiltrate and damage cell membranes – and the ATP-potassium ion channels that transport glucose into the cell. They can also damage the mitochondria within the cell. This can contribute to cells becoming less sensitive to glucose and insulin.

When the heart, blood vessels, liver, pancreas, cells and mitochondria all become damaged by pathogenic microorganism endotoxins, they function poorly. Even a little sugar can pose a threat, as a damaged pancreas cannot produce the insulin needed, and damaged cell membranes cannot adequately absorb glucose.

When the liver is damaged by endotoxins, glycogen deficiencies result. All of this throws off the balance between blood glucose levels, glycogen levels, insulin and fat storage. The result is the body-wide inflammatory state called metabolic syndrome.

### This is supported by the research

The research supports a conclusion that microorganisms at least contribute to glucose and fat metabolism disorders. Studies have confirmed that probiotic yogurts change propionate and butyrate levels within the blood. Increased hydrogen produced in breath tests is caused by the consumption of the simple sugars by pathogenic bacteria in the gut.

Diabetics also happen to experience more fungal infections and bacterial infections. The outcomes and complications associated with infections of *Staphylococcus aureus* are worse in diabetics. Long-term high-fiber, no-refined sugar diets have proven in many cases to slow and even reverse glycemia problems. This is all proven research.

Let's not forget yeast infections. Yes, simple sugars are also great food for yeasts. As yeast populations grow, they migrate to different regions of the body.

The bottom line is that the buildup of pathogenic yeast and bacteria within the body is stimulated by the excessive refined sugars. This is the biggest problem with refined sugar.

### Which sugars are the worst?

You mean what are the best foods for bacteria and yeast? Refined simple sugars that produce the most fructose and glucose – stripped of all the plant fiber and phytonutrients from the plant – are by far the best bacteria foods.

This means that foods with refined sucrose (breaks down to 50/50 glucose and fructose), high-fructose corn syrup (can range from 40 percent fructose and 60 percent glucose to 90 percent fructose), evaporated cane juice (99 percent sucrose), brown sugar (83 percent sucrose) and organic sugar (99.7 percent sucrose) are the worst foods, because they contain more of the refined sugars pathogenic bacteria love.

Processed, refined versions of honey, agave and refined fruit juices are almost as bad. These are altogether different from raw honey, whole fruit juices and maple syrup, however. These latter sweeteners are better because they are not refined. Their sugars are still complexed within plant nutrients and polysaccharides.

Of the refined sweeteners, brown rice syrup, malt syrup, wheat syrup and molasses are better, because they contain more maltose – a more complex and nutritious sugar.

Plant-based beneficial sugars like mannose, xylitose and galactose are particularly healthy. Mannose and xylitol are in fact antibacterial. Mannose and xylitol have both been shown in numerous studies to reduce bacteria adhesion. They have thus been used for urinary tract infections and for reducing dental cavities. Stevia is also a great sweetener that has proven to be healthy to the body and oblivious to pathogenic bacteria.

Once we strip away the plant's own antibacterial ingredients, leaving the sugar molecules naked and ready for gorging, we are giving pathogenic bacteria a ticket to ride. Polysaccharides complexed in foods, including lactose, galactose, fructooliglycerides (fibrous plant sugars) and galactooligosaccharides (contained in milk), nourish our probiotics. Pathogenic bacteria don't like these so much.

The solution is to not let pathogenic bacteria and yeast rise to such great numbers in the first place. This means sticking to the types of whole food and nutritive sweeteners mentioned above, and eating probiotic foods and taking supplements on a consistent basis.

After all, one bug's poison can be another bug's medicine.

## The Problems with Refined Sugars

Naturally, our bodies and minds are attracted to sweetness. Sweetness occurs at a number of levels. The two that stand out for most of us are nutritional sweetness and mental sweetness. Frankly, the inner self is attracted to sweetness because the spiritual dimension is full of sweetness. We come from sweetness.

For this reason, we seek the various pleasures associated with the physical world. We therefore consider physical pleasures 'sweet.' We might call an attractive person of the opposite sex "sweet." We might also call an appealing performance "sweet." We also might refer to a situation where we are enjoying our senses as "sweet." These sub-conscious referrals reflect the fact that we crave sweetness.

When the physical body achieves sweetness, either with sweet foods or with obtaining other "sweet" perceptions; dopamine, sometimes serotonin and sometimes endorphins are secreted into the bloodstream and limbic system. These neurotransmitter secretions indicate positive feedback to the limbic system, which flashes onto the screen of the mind. These sweet reactions cause the inner self to become enraptured with sweetness. As a result, we find ourselves perpetually seeking sweetness.

The taste of almost any sort of saccharide – whether glucose, fructose, lactose (from milk) or maltose (from grains) – will stimulate an impulse through the tongue's receptors to the lower brain and limbic system. This is then translated through the cerebral cortex, where its biochemical structure is compared with the cell's needs for energy. For this reason, the simpler sugars yield a more positive the physical response.

The sugar molecule itself must be absorbed through the digestive tract to have its physical impact upon the cells. The affect upon the limbic system is stimulated through the biochemical fingerprint of the molecule. We might compare this to watching a movie preview versus watching the movie. The preview is a virtual impression of the movie.

It is for this very reason that the Romans developed the method of regurgitation, allowing them to taste the sweetness of their food in excess of their capacity to digest it. They would eat sumptuously, then exit for a regurgitation in a nearby vomitorium. This would allow them to regurgitate and return for more good-tasting food.

Following an effective screening by the mind, the quality of the sugar's sweetness is recorded for future use. This is confirmed by its energizing effects on our cells – as they cascade from a euphoric sugar-high to the sugar-low. The only problem is, we tend to be very optimistic when it comes to negative feedback: We tend to remember the high and forget the low. This cascading sensual flash with an energy rush bonus precipitates the addiction to sugar.

This is not to say that eating sweet foods are not good for the body. Assuming the sugar molecules are bound within their natural environment, sugar is a balanced form of energy. Wholesome sweet foods like fresh fruits, raw honey, raw milk and sweet grains are perfectly healthy. Also many vegetables are sweet: carrots and beets are not only sweet but have lots of phytonutrients – as long as they are eaten whole (steamed beats are delectably super-sweet for example).

When we refine and isolate the sugars, making corn, cane or beet syrup, we strip away the various fibers and nutrient complexes that balance and slow down the sugar absorption. This leaves the purified sweeteners ready for immediate presentation to the bloodstream and liver. In this state, they are immediately converted to glycogen to be absorbed immediately and all at once into the bloodstream, starting the sugar blues cascade of elevated blood sugar followed by a hypoglycemic state – or a sugar low.

We can certainly gain energy from refined sugar isolated from beets or cane. However, our bodies will quickly become out of balance, due to the spiking of blood sugar levels. This results in the spiking of insulin, glucose absorption and resulting sugar low characteristic of refined sugar foods. Some call this the *sugar-high-rebound* effect.

## Sweeteners and Triglycerides

A new study from the Department of Internal Medicine at Eberhard-Karls University in Germany has confirmed that high fructose corn syrup significantly raises triglyceride levels.

The research was performed on twenty healthy volunteers with an average age of 30 years old. They were given 150 grams of very high fructose or glucose for four weeks. Both the fructose and the glucose groups experienced decreased insulin sensitivity, but only the fructose group experienced higher triglyceride levels.

Triglycerides are associated with very low density lipoproteins. VLDL is associated with artery disease due to the peroxidation of lipids. This produces free radicals which damage the arteries and tissues of the body, producing cardiovascular disease.

This study confirms a twenty-four hour metabolic study that was done at the University of California-Davis in 2008. This study gave 24 human subjects either sucrose or high-fructose corn syrup, and measured metabolic levels over a 24-hour period. While triglyceride levels changed little just following the meal, levels changed significantly the next morning, over the baseline prior to sucrose or HFCS consumption. The resulting triglyceride levels among the sucrose group increased by 28 mg/dl while the triglyceride levels increased by 19 mg/dl among the high fructose corn syrup group. The increased levels of triglycerides were significantly higher among those men and women with higher body fat. Women over 32% body fat increased by 29 mg/dl for sucrose and 16 for HFCS, while men over 22% body fat increased by 48 mg/dl for sucrose and 22 for HFCS.

In this study, the researchers also found that leptin levels were significantly raised by both sucrose and HFCS. However, the raised levels of leptin were about the same between sucrose and HFCS. Raised leptin levels are associated with overeating.

This research illustrates that both refined sugars and refined fructose are damaging to our health, because they both raise triglyceride levels, insulin levels and leptin levels. However, the German study showed that glucose alone did not raise triglycerides.

## Synthetic Sweeteners

The modern multinational corporate food industrial complex has decided that profits are more important than the health of consumers. This is indeed short-sighted as sick or dead customers aren't repeat customers.

In fact, corporate market studies have found that sugar-laced foods achieve better resale performance because of the addictive quality of sugar. For this reason, these companies mass produce foods formulated with refined simple sugars, knowing that we will often forego our own health in favor of gaining a little sweetness.

Over the past few decades, consumers have demanded foods with less added sugar due to the proven link between refined sugars and obesity and diabetes. In a twisted, profit-only move, corporate food has developed several sugar-analogues with varying degrees of success. In some cases, it has lead to disastrous health effects as we will see in the following discussion of synthetic sweeteners.

## Aspartame

Despite the fact that aspartame is touted as a safe food by the FDA, research continues to reveal various risks associated with its use. Two hundred times sweeter than sugar, aspartame is now used in many "low-sugar" or "sugar-free" or "diet" products. It is now present in sugar-free gums; diet soft drinks of all sorts; coffee sweetener packets; topping mixes; desserts and laxatives. Aspartame is far from a real food. It has three main components: *phenylalanine, aspartic acid* and *methanol.*

Methanol is also known as methyl alcohol or wood alcohol. It is known to convert to formaldehyde, formic acid and diketopiperazine in metabolic reductions. Methanol is poisonous when consumed in small doses. Toxic levels of methanol can cause blindness. Methanol can cause inflammation of pancreas and heart. It can also cause the brain to swell.

In the body, phenylalaline will utilize phenylalanine hydroxylase to convert to tyrosine. Tyrosine is used by the body to convert to dopamine and nor-epinephrine. Assuming there is enough of the hydroxylase enzyme available; the tyrosine may be useable by the body. However, if the body is lacking in phenylalanine hydroxylase for any reason, a dangerous build-up of phenylalanine can accumulate in the brain. Accumulations in brain cells can cause brain damage and nervous conditions. People with *phenylketonuria*, or the inability to produce the required enzyme (common among those with kidney disease or iron deficiencies) will be subject to this dangerous and sometimes lethal disorder. A buildup of phenylalanine has been known to cause mental retardation and other mental disorders.

Aspartic acid or aspartate has been referred to as neurotoxic, or destructive to brain cells. It has been known to destroy cells in the hypothalamus as well. It has been linked, along with MSG, to fibromyalgia. Aspartame consumption has also been linked to vision defects, mood disorders, migraine headaches, nausea, diarrhea, sleep disorders, memory loss, confusion, convulsions, magnesium deficiency and imbalance, Graves disease, Parkinson's disease, fibromyalgia and others. Aspartame may be more dangerous for children and those more chemically sensitive.

## Sucralose

Sucralose, trademarked Splenda™ was developed in 1976 by researchers working for Tate & Lyle, Ltd, a British sugar conglomerate, who teamed with Johnson & Johnson to market the product under the umbrella of the McNeil Specialty Products Company. There are few human studies on sucralose, and reliance has been primarily on studies of rats, mice and rabbits. Sucralose was approved by the FDA in 1998 for consumption using only studies on rats and rabbits and one study of human metabolic rates. It was approved by Canada in 1991, but not yet approved in most European countries.

Sucralose's chemical structure is 1,6-dichloro-1,6-dideoxy-beta-D fructofuranosyl-4-cloro-4-deoxy-alpha-D-glactopyranoside. It is manufactured via a multiple step process whereby three hydroxyl groups are replaced by three chlorine atoms. It registers on the mind as about 600 times sweeter than sugar.

One of the main arguments is how much sucralose is actually absorbed into the bloodstream. This is of critical concern because the molecule is so damaging upon the body's various organs and will build up in the tissues. Chlorine ions can also form some pretty toxic bonding formations. Sucralose is said to be absorbed and metabolized by the human body at rates of 11-27%, though the Japanese government says as much as 40% is absorbed by the body. Once in the body, sucralose will break down into small amounts of 1,6-dichlorofructose. Other chlorinated toxic metabolites are also suspected to form as well. The half-life of sucralose has been documented to range from 2-36 hours by animal studies. While the manufacturer says it passes through the body unabsorbed in that time, a study on dogs noted 20% non-recovered after four days and 4-7% non-recovered after five days on humans. This means the non-recovered portion was still in the body.

The chlorinates used to manufacture sucralose are similar compounds utilized by pesticides and other chlorinated toxins. Metabolites can include trace amounts of arsenic, heavy metals and methanol due to toxins introduced during manufacturing. There is concern of liver toxicity, as sucralose has been associated with enlargement of the liver and kidneys. One study of rats showed higher incidences of pelvic mineralization and epithelial hyperplasia, notably in high-dose females. Rats studied with sucralose also showed decreased thymus and spleen weights, lymphocytopenia and cortical hypoplasia of the spleen and thymus. One study of sucralose in diabetics showed glycosylated hemoglobin increase, indicating possible future diabetic control complications.

Other effects associated with sucralose, mostly anecdotal, include lymph follicle atrophy, growth reduction, red blood cell count decrease, pelvic hyperplasia, pregnancy complications, and diarrhea. Many people have complained of stomach cramping, depression and anxiety because of sucralose consumption.

## Saccharin

Saccharin was discovered by I. Remsen and C. Fahlberg from Johns Hopkins University in 1879 as a derivative of coal tar. It has been made popular by Sweet-n-low™. In 1971, the FDA proclaimed that saccharin was a carcinogen and a warning label was required to be put on all labels containing it. In 1998 the National Toxicology Program removed saccharin from the carcinogen list, and in 2000, Bill Clinton signed an act removing saccharin's warning label requirement. The controversy surrounding saccharin's carcinogenic risks are based on a lack of human evidence and the high dosage levels with different metabolisms. This controversy of its potential as a carcinogen has overshadowed other potential risks of saccharin consumption in humans.

Saccharin's molecular structure is o-sulfobenzimide; 2,3-dihydro-3-oxobenzisosulfonazole. It is a white aromatic chemical, 300-500 times sweeter than sugar. As saccharin itself is not water-soluble, its sodium salt is used as the sweetener replacement. Saccharin is a sulfimide, and readily forms acids. Saccharin is highly polar and a strong organic acid, with a pKa of approx 2.0.

Saccharin is almost completely ionized in the acid or salt form, unionized portions forming in the stomach. Absorption occurs in the small intestines, where about 95% is absorbed. Metabolism and biotransformation of saccharin in the body has yet to be established. Saccharin is known to accumulate in plasma and in the tissues. Accumulated saccharin will transfer to the fetus and to the baby through breast milk in ionized form.

Most assume that there is no toxicity, because much of saccharin passes through the kidneys unmetabolized. However, others have disputed this assumption. Sodium saccharin altered the intestinal microflora content in rat testing. Saccharin and saccharin-containing drugs have been shown to be toxic to the liver in some cases. Hamster studies have shown clastogenicity in lung cells and chromosomal aberrations and sister chromatid exchanges in the hamsters' ovaries. Sodium saccharin has induced DNA damage in the stomach and colon in mice studies and *in vitro* studies.

In a study comparing memory and recovery among the elderly, saccharin-dosed patients scored substantially below those consuming glucose. Although interestingly the study was focused on the effects of glucose on brain function and saccharin was used as the control substance, the results infer that either saccharin's plasma binding slowed brain function; or glucose improved function. Since saccharin is a glucose-replacement and normally in the diet, it is assumed that saccharin replacement has negative effects on memory and brain function.

Since most of the research on saccharin has focused on whether it is a carcinogen, despite thousands of studies, very few have studied other possible negative effects on humans.

In a group of 42 patients with adverse effects resulting from consumption of saccharin in pharmaceutical agents, pruritus and urticaria were the most common reactions, followed by eczema, photosensitivity, and prurigo. Other reactions include wheezing, nausea, diarrhea, tongue blisters, tachycardia, fixed eruptions, headache, diuresis, and sensory neuropathy. In one study, ingestion of saccharin-adulterated milk formula by infants was associated with irritability, hypertonia, insomnia, opisthotonos, and strabismus. Two reports of adult saccharin overdose resulted in edema, oliguria and persistent albuminuria. As a result, the AMA has recommended limits for saccharin use among children and pregnant or nursing women

## Xylitol

Xylitol is actually a naturally occurring sweetener. In the late nineteenth century, German chemists discovered xylitol from birch tree bark. Xylitol also appears in a wide variety of other plants and fruits. Berries, corn, lettuce, and mushrooms are sources of xylitol. Xylitol is also manufactured in the human body. While xylitol has the same sweetness as sugar, it is not a sugar. It is a 5-carbon sugar alcohol – a phenol. Because it is short of the 6th carbon atom which makes up carbohydrates, it is absorbed slowly and only partly utilized by the body. Xylitol contains 40% less calories than sugar. It is extensively used in products in Europe and is considered safe for human consumption up to about 90 grams per day. However, beyond about 20 grams, it can result in diarrhea.

Xylitol has been shown to reduce dental caries when consumed regularly, thus it being used as a commercial dentifrice.

While considered a naturally occurring element, out of its natural complex of phytonutrients it can potentially have metabolic effects. Since xylitol has been used for many years in Europe without toxicity reported in humans, most feel that there is little or no risk, especially at moderate dosages.

One study showed possibility of benign thymus tumors in rats because of large doses of xylitol. However this study has not since been duplicated. Another study showed potential for alteration of calcium ions, causing secondary pheochromocytomas (adrenal medulla hyperplasia) in rats. Xylitol has been shown to be diuretic. It can increase levels of organic acid excretion, possibly reflecting impaired mitochondrial oxidation. Xylitol can also alter the mucosal intestinal lining, resulting in mucosal hyperplasia as a result of partial absorption

## Mannitol

Mannitol is another natural botanical derivative. It can be extracted with ethanol from plants like celery, or it can be produced using yeasts or probiotics. This it is considered a natural sweetener, and healthy as long as it has not been isolated and refined. Mannitol is a polyol – an alcohol and sugar. It is similar to xylitol and sorbitol. However, it will oxidize in aqueous solution (lose hydrogen ions), causing the solution to become acidic.

In therapeutic intravenous doses, mannitol has been shown to shrink coupled endothelial cells, thereby opening the blood brain barrier. It is recognized as a vasodilator and has been used to reduce cranial pressure. It has also been used to treat patients with oliguric renal (kidney) failure, and can be administered intravenously. Mannitol is laxative in doses over 20 grams. It can also alter the mucosal intestinal lining, resulting in mucosal hyperplasia.

## Sorbitol

Sorbitol is a white crystalline powder with a melting point of 95C. It is a sugar alcohol, with the same sweetness as sugar. It is classified as an artificial sweetener. It has four calories in every gram, same as table sugar. It is used as a sugar-replacer in many commercial foods such as gums, ice cream, etc.

Although sorbitol is produced by the body, too much has been known to cause damage to cells. Excessive sorbitol has been linked to diabetic retinopathy and neuropathy. Short of a sixth carbon atom (carbohydrate), it is absorbed slowly and only partly utilized by the body. This results in its laxative effects.

Studies have shown that sorbitol and mannitol can cause gastrointestinal discomfort or even severe diarrhea at 10-50 grams consumed. In 1999, The Center for Science in the Public Interest petitioned the FDA to add a warning to sorbitol labels regarding possible GI problems. Like xylitol, it has been shown to reduce dental caries when consumed regularly, and is thus used in commercial dentifrices. Sorbitol along with xylitol has been shown to be diuretic and to increase levels of organic acid excretion in rats, possibly reflecting impaired mitochondrial oxidation. Like xylitol and mannitol, sorbitol can alter the mucosal intestinal lining, resulting in mucosal hyperplasia because of their partial absorption.

# Nature's Sweeteners

The over-consumption of quickly-absorbing simple sugars such as white sugar and corn syrup have been associated with type II diabetes and obesity. Other complications of simple sugars in the diet include mineral leaching, mental imbalances, nervous disorders, hypoglycemia, hepatic disorders, adrenal and thyroid disorders and a host of other ailments.

Natural plant-based sweeteners that have been minimally processed, leaving more natural constituents that slow and balance absorption provide nutrition and complexity that slow absorption and conversion to blood glucose

Natural, less processed sweeteners that have natural mineral content and micronutrients left from the natural source to balance glycemic reaction in the bloodstream, thus have lower glycemic indexes and glycemic loads.

Natural, minimally-processed sweeteners have more complex sweetener molecular components and more complex long-chain sugars as well as simple sugars, for example honey has fructose, glucose and maltose, rice syrup has glucose and maltose, barley malt extract has fructose, maltose and glucose. These combinations and complexities slow and balance glucose absorption because the conversion to blood glucose is slower. Let's review some of the natural sweetener choices

> **Agave** is one of the lowest glycemic index and load sweeteners. This sweetener is extracted from the Agave cactus plant, and contains naturally-occurring fructose, dextrose, maltotriose and maltose. Currently most agave is produced in Mexico where the plant is indigenous. Agave has small levels of calcium, potassium and magnesium and a number of other micronutrients.

> **Raw honey** contains naturally-occurring fructose, glucose and maltose. In its raw form honey can have up to 35% protein with half of all the amino acids, a number of micronutrients and minerals, B vitamins and vitamins C, D and E. Honey is categorized by the flowers that the bees draw from. Manuka honey, for example, is from bees that harvest the Manuka tree in New Zealand and Australia, and is known for its many health benefits due to beneficial enzymes and micronutrients.

> **Brown rice syrup** is made from sprouted brown rice, and composed of glucose and maltose, and is thus slowly digesting. It also is a source of niacin, calcium and potassium. Brown rice has one of the lower glycemic loads.

> **Wheat and barley malt syrups** are primarily composed of maltose and glucose. These syrups are slower in conversion to blood glucose because of their complexity and long sugars, as well as composition with other nutrients in the syrup which creates further complexity. Wheat syrup is a good source of calcium, magnesium, phosphorus, potassium and sodium. Maltose and maltotriose have been shown to be absorbed more slowly than glucose or sucrose in the body. Thus sweeteners with these components have a slower, more time-released effect upon the bloodstream.

➢ **Organic cane juice or organic evaporated cane juice** is processed more minimally than conventional white sugar, without the second-cycle bleaching and further chemical extraction and screening that takes place in conventional white sugar, which removes virtually all nutrients and isolates the glucose content without fiber. Thus organic sugar has more nutritional content, more minerals and thus is absorbed somewhat slower than white sugar. Organic cane juice and organic evaporated cane juice have about 11 mg of calcium and 6 mg of potassium per 100 grams. Organic sucanat is sugar without the molasses removed. Thus it has 150 mg of calcium, 440 mg of potassium and 5.2 mg of iron per 100 grams.

➢ **Molasses** is made from cane juice crushing without extracting, refining and bleaching steps. It has more complexity, and is a good source of calcium (550mg per 100 grams!), iron and potassium.

➢ **Oat syrup** contains maltose, glucose and fructose but is mostly maltose. It is a good source of iron, magnesium, B vitamins, phosphorous, zinc, copper and calcium at 170 mg and potassium at 1143 mg per 100 grams.

➢ **Maple syrup** contains mostly sucrose, and is a good source of calcium, potassium and iron with a healthy dose of phenolic compounds other healthy enzymes and micronutrients. It is made from the sap of the maple tree, with minimal processing to concentrate the sap down to the syrup.

➢ **Stevia**: Concentrated powder from the *Stevia rebaudiana* plant is 300 times sweeter than sugar. This is truly a natural and healthy sweetener. It is a native to Paraguay and used for hundreds of years as a leaf for wound healing. It also has been used as a digestive aid. No adverse side effects have been reported in its use. It can leave a bitter taste if excessive amounts eaten at a sitting however. Studies on rats have shown stevia extract increases glucose tolerance, and lower doses significantly increase glucose transport and insulin stimulation – almost the opposite effect refined sugar has. Meanwhile larger doses have been shown to increase whole-body insulin sensitivity. It has been concluded that stevia should have potential therapeutic effects on at type 2 diabetes patients. Stevia has also been shown to lower blood pressure in rat experiments. It has been proposed that stevia may improve nutrient-sensing mechanisms and increase cystolic acyl-coenzyme activity. In an acidic environment, stevia was shown to inhibit intestinal *E. coli* growth as well. Once again, nature produces the best option.

## Oils and Fats

Fats are oils with unique biochemical structures required by the body for energy and structure. Lipids (fats) and phospholipids (phosphorus molecules connected to fatty acids) are essential to the health and maintenance of the body's cellular structures, organs, immunity, nervous system, cardiovascular system, pulmonary system and endocrine system. They make up the cell membranes: in side by side "stacks," permitting osmosis in between. Phospholipids will work together with the cell to repair and maintain the membrane and certain organelles.

Lipids are the building block molecules in the production of prostaglandins, which manage most of the body's functions, including as clotting activation; blood pressure regulation; heart rate regulation; thyroid hormone regulation; adrenal hormone production; and digestive processes. Lipids attach, help assimilate and process fat-soluble vitamins like B-vitamins, vitamin A, D and E. They deliver amino acids to the liver and other cells for protein synthesis.

Lipoproteins are lipids attached to protein molecules. They make up the structure of many proteins and enzymes. Lipoproteins deliver cholesterol to cells to make up tissue and fibrin, for example. In damaged and inflammatory environments, low-density lipoproteins can also deliver cholesterol to the artery walls, clogging arteries, causing atherosclerosis and heart disease.

Generally, fats are known by their bonding types, as either monounsaturated, polyunsaturated or saturated. Most are a combination of two or three types – and those with the most of one type of bond are referred to as that type of fat. Fats (or lipids) contain special molecules called fatty acids. Fatty acids are prevalent in seeds, grains, vegetables, nuts and beans. *Essential Fatty Acids*, or EFA's are defined as lipids necessary (i.e., the body does not manufacture enough) for adequate health.

EFA's are usually considered long-chain polyunsaturated fatty acids derived from shorter-chain linolenic, linoleic and oleic acids. The main EFAs are omega-3s – primarily *alpha linolenic acid* (ALA), *docosahexanoic acid* (DHA) and *eicosapentaenoic acid* (EPA); omega-6s – primarily *linoleic acid;* and omega 9s – primarily *oleic acid*. These all can be considered essential in some sense. A healthy human body will produce DHA from ALA, and EPA is a derivative of DHA. Many health researchers consider only omega-3s as essential, because the body produces small quantities of omega 9; and omega-6 is readily available in most plant foods. The real issue becomes getting the right mix and balance of these critical fatty acids.

Monounsaturated oils are typically considered to be high in omega 9 fatty acids like oleic acid. A monounsaturated fatty acid has one double carbon-hydrogen bonding chain. Oils from seeds, nuts and other plant-based sources have the largest quantities of monounsaturates. Oils that have large proportions of monounsaturates such as olive oil are known to lower heart disease when replacing saturated fat in diets. Monounsaturates also aid in skin cell maintenance; improve glycemic tolerance by increasing glucagon-like peptide – GLP-1; and increase insulin levels when needed.

Polyunsaturated fats, which contain a higher proportion of polyun-saturated fatty acids have at least two double carbon-hydrogen bonding chains. They typically come from plant and marine sources.

DHA and EPA are long-chained polyunsaturated oils. They are known to lower heart disease and increase artery-wall health. However, a typical polyunsaturated fatty acid is more prone to alteration by heat, which can change the fatty acid to a trans fat or other mutated vibration. Linoleic and linolenic acids (omega-6 and omega-3) are likely the more prevalent polyunsaturates.

Saturated fats, or fats with high levels of fatty acids without double bonds (the hydrogens "saturate" the carbons), are typically highest in animal fats and tropical oils such as coconut and palm. Milk products such as butter and whole milk contain saturated fats, along with a special type of fatty acid called CLA or *conjugated linoleic acid*. Most experts agree that a maximum of about 10% of one's oil consumption should be saturated.

*Trans-fats* are oils that have either been overheated or have undergone hydrogenation, which is heating while bubbling hydrogen ions through the oil. The "trans" refers to the positioning of part of the molecule, as opposed to "cis" positioning. The cis positioning is the orientation the body works best with. Trans-fats have been known to be a cause for in-creased free radicals in the system; damaging artery walls; contributing to heart disease, high LDL levels, liver damage, diabetes; and other metabolic dysfunction. It should be noted that CLA is also a trans-fat, but this is a healthy trans-fat, produced by cows.

The omega-3 fatty acids have a orientation that is extremely stable. *Alpha linolenic acid* (ALA) is the primary omega-3 fatty acid the body can most easily assimilate. Once assimilated, the healthy body will convert ALA to eicosapentaenoic acid (EPA) and docosahexaenoic acid (DHA) at a rate of about 7-15%, depending upon the health of the liver.

Docosahexaenoic acid and eicosapentaenoic acid act together within the brain and nervous system. EPA and GLA (see below) will be converted to eicosanoids. Eicosanoids are the building blocks to hormones and phosopholipids which make up cell membranes. Excellent sources of omega-3 oils are flaxseeds, walnuts, pumpkin seeds, Brazil nuts, sesame seeds, many green leafy vegetables, spirulina, avocados, hempseed oil, flaxseed oil, pumpkin oil, walnut oil, canola oil.

Some people – especially those who are immune-suppressed or burdened with toxicity such as cigarette smoke, may not convert ALA to DHA well. Researchers suspect that gamma linolenic acid consumption is also necessary for conversion of ALA to DHA. For those with low levels of DHA, or have problems converting ALA and DHA, a natural algae from the Pacific called Golden Algae produces a pure form of DHA.

This type of DHA is preferable to fish oil, which also typically accompanies saturated fats as well as toxins such as mercury and PCBs coming from the fish. We propose it is best to obtain DHA from as low on the food chain as possible – both harmonically and for pure health reasons.

DHA is important for the central nervous system. It increases brain cell functionality, aids in nerve cell maintenance and development, balances good (HDL) cholesterol while limiting LDL (LDL is considered "bad" cholesterol, though recent studies have confirmed it is really the size of the LDL particle). DHA also aids in the flexibility of blood vessel walls and assists in blood vessel wall health in general. Deficiencies in DHA can cause decreased memory and mental cognition, tingling sensations, decreased immunity, hypertension, heart dysfunction, menopausal disorders and blood clots. It is widely accepted that omega-3 deficiency in the US is widespread.

One of the culprits is the abundance of meat-eating and high proportions of polyunsaturated oil consumption, while ignoring important the essential fatty acids like ALA and GLA required to convert to DHA. ALA comes from flaxseeds, canola, perilla seed, purslane, walnuts, pumpkin seeds and soybeans.

Omega-6 fatty acids are the most available form of fat in the plant kingdom. Linoleic acid is the primary omega-6 fatty acid and it is found in most grains and oilseeds. A healthy body will convert linoleic acid into GLA readily, utilizing the same delta-6 desaturase enzyme used for ALA to DHA conversion. (Many think the ALA to DHA and the LA to GLA conversion as stepped and related). From GLA the body produces di-homo-gamma linoleic acid, which cycles through the body as an eicosinoid.

GLA aids in skin health, assists in joint movement and healthy synovial fluid, and is critically important to nerve conduction. Limited conversion of both LA to GLA and ALA to DHA is thought to be related to trans-fat consumption, smoking, pollution, stress, infections, and various other metabolic agents that effect the liver.

For those who may not convert easily, GLA is also obtained from the oils of borage seeds, evening primrose, hemp seed and also from spirulina. Excellent food sources of LA include flaxseed, hempseed, grapeseed, pumpkin seeds, sunflower seeds, safflower seeds, soybeans, olives, pine nuts, pistachio nuts, peanuts, almonds, cashews, chestnuts, and their respective oils.

Omega-9 fatty acids are technically not "essential" as the body manufactures a limited amount. However, monounsaturated fatty acids like oleic acid has been shown in studies to lower heart attack risk, aids in blood vessel health, and are suspected as anti-carcinogenic. The best sources of omega-9s are olives, sesame seeds, avocados, almonds, peanuts, pecans, pistachio nuts, cashews, hazelnuts, macadamia nuts, several other nuts and their respective oils.

Recent research has shown that the right balance of oil consumption is about 30-40% omega 6s, 30-40% omega 3s, 10% saturated fats, and about 10% GLA. The American diet has been estimated at about a 20-1 proportion between omega-6 to omega-3. This imbalance of omega-6 has been associated with heart disease, obesity, various autoimmune diseases, diabetes, arteriosclerosis/atherosclerosis, high cholesterol, and other cardiovascular dysfunction. When oil consumption is out of balance, the body will have trend towards an environment of inflammation and autoimmune response.

From a biochemical viewpoint, this is because omega 6 oils convert more easily to arachidonic acid. AA seems to push the body toward the processes of inflammation. While this is often portrayed somewhat virtually in the literature, there is a practical reason for this tendency towards inflammation.

The cascading conversion of fatty acids toward their intentional use as phospholipids, lipoproteins, energy fats and storage fats is a cycle. Just as any biological cycle, balance between all the components is necessary. Should an imbalance exist, the process will create a balance through an increase in certain byproducts. In the case of the fatty acid cascade, healthy fatty acids convert to the very phospholipid membranes lining our body's cell network. Too much consumption of the wrong fatty acids leave these membranes inadequately structured, leaving the cell contents vulnerable to the infusion of undesirable chemistry.

Too little EFAs will also leave nerve cells with inadequate sheathing. This leaves the nerve vulnerable to misfiring, causing numbness and pain. The wrong cell membrane chemistry also opens the artery wall cells up to damage. In addition, the incorrect fatty acid consumption can affects the body's lipoprotein contents. Examples of lipoproteins are cholesterol, hormones and neurotransmitters.

Having the wrong mix of biochemistry effects the balance among these important messenger biochemicals. The net result of these various imbalances is, of course, inflammation. They body begins to slowly incinerate because of a lack of appropriate structure. The immune system begins attacking its own cells because these cells either become damaged, or are simply inadequate due to their lack of the right chemistry.

It is the long-chain PUFAs (polyunsaturated fatty acids) like ALA, DHA and GLA provide the balance for these components. While many doctors are now prescribing a regular diet of salmon or other fatty fish, it should be cautioned that these fatty fish also contain saturated fats, and many types of toxins – depending upon where they are caught or farmed. Farmed fish now dominate the market. While we might think farmed fish are safer because they are in a controlled (and seemingly clean) environment, this is not confirmed by the research.

In one study, a team of researchers from Indiana University (Carlson and Hites 2005) analyzed salmon from over 700 fish farms, supermarkets and wild salmon catches to test dioxin, PCBs and other carcinogenics. They compared the levels with the Environmental Protection Agency's standards, and determined that a fish meal eaten more than once or twice a month (San Francisco area=twice/Los Angeles area=once) would exceed the EPA's safe levels of these toxins in the diet.

Other areas, such as European cities, had even higher levels of toxins in their fish. This is not to mention the biochemical and environmental issues related to the imbalances created within our oceans; and the pain fish feel. While many claimed several years ago that fish farming was the answer to environmental concerns, this has backfired.

We are now finding new and dangerous strains of diseases and genetic mutation incubating in these fish farms. The diseases are now leaking into the wild habitat and threatening the populations of wild fish. Vegetarianism and algae-derived DHA certainly appears to be less risky to our health and the health of the planet.

## Oil Pressing

It is important to select expeller pressed oils versus solvent extracted. Most commercial oils are solvent extracted. Most natural food oils or organic oils are expeller pressed. Solvent extraction is when chemical solvents are added to either a mechanical extraction or a slurry of the oil-seed, to extract a larger percentage of the oils from the seeds or plant.

These solvents can include a mixture of ethanol and other chemicals. Solvent extraction typically leaves chemical residues in the oil. Expeller pressed is the preferred process. In expeller pressing, the seeds are mechanically crushed with large presses.

The weight of the press is the only action upon the seed or plant material. The pressure behind the press can produce heat in the resulting oil. To prevent the oil from being damaged, the pressure is carefully measured. Always insist upon expeller-pressed oils! It is easy to tell the difference between expeller-pressed and solvent-extracted.

The solvent-extracted oil is typically water-white and very clear. Sometimes clarity can be quite high in expeller-pressed oil, especially if it goes through additional refining after pressing – which is also not good because this over-refining will create more heat in the oil. The best oils look, smell and taste as though they come from food. They will typically have a browner color, sometimes cloudy. They will also have a distinctive "nose" or smell that smells like the seed or plant they were crushed from. When smelling, we should also note whether there is any rancidity, which would indicate that the oil is too old.

The color of an oil should also tell us whether the oil is refined, partially-refined or is a virgin oil. Refining is a process of filtering and screening oil to purify it. Organic refining is usually done without chemicals. Instead, *diatemacous earth* is used to attract residues. Conventional refining can contain various bleaching chemicals, which will whiten and clarify the oil. Refining removes many of the natural sterols, polyphenols and other phytonutrients (plant origin nutrients) left in the oil after crushing.

Oil refining will sometimes extend the shelf life and decrease the likelihood of rancidity, but can also oxidize more easily, creating free radicals and trans-fats among the oil. This is because those polyphenols and other phytonutrients provide biochemical stability to the oil molecules – much the same as fiber provides stability to polysaccharides. While chemically refined oils may be more "stable" as far as rancidity, they are not as "stable" once we consume them.

Many commercial oils are very stable when left crude or virgin. Such is the case of olive oil, which can last for many months without refrigeration. Still any crude or virgin oil should be packed in a dark bottle to delay the break down of the phytonutrients sensitive to light and refrigerated to preserve its phytonutrients.

Noting these points, we might want to avoid eating fried foods, as high-heating oils creates trans-fats and other byproducts. If we do fry we can use the lowest-heat possible and not use older oil to fry with. Good cooking oils include canola, which is a balanced omega-3 and omega-6 oil. Olive oil is also good to cook with and is a good monounsaturated with numerous health benefits, but it does not supply any omega-3s.

We might want to avoid all hydrogenated or partially hydrogenated (worse) oils or foods made with vegetable shortening. We can replace vegetable shortening with unrefined oils from coconut, palm or even olive oil. We can also eat raw nuts and seeds when possible, replacing chips and oil-cooked snacks. Raw or even mildly roasted nuts and seeds will supply a good mix of healthy oils without the potential problems associated with crushing, heating and extracting. We can also eat baked chips and crackers rather than fried chips and crackers. We can buy unrefined oils when possible, or if refined, buy organically refined oils. Trans-fat labels are now required by the FDA. Its probably best to reach for zero trans-fats.

Milk and cheese, especially from organic cows, have a fatty acid called conjugated linoleic acid, a polyunsaturated fatty acid that has been shown to be anti-carcinogenic, anti-inflammatory agent, has been known to increase immunity and brain function.

Peanuts and peanut oils have been shown to have a number of benefits. A 1999 study at Penn State University (Kris-Etherton, PM *et al.* 1999) showed that a diet of peanuts, peanut oil and peanut butter were superior than a low-fat diet. The peanut diet reduced heart disease by 21% while low-fat diet reduced it by 12% Several large long-term population studies have shown that eating one serving of nuts or peanut butter five or more times a week can reduce heart disease by 50%. Peanut oil is also a good massage oil, helping to sooth and relax stressed muscle fibers.

## Our Ancestors' Fats

The types of fats we eat relate directly to detoxification because some fats result in more radicals and other fats result in fewer radicals. As a result, some fats are pro-inflammatory while others are anti-inflammatory.

Here we refer to the anti-inflammatory fats as being *living food fats,* because these come from low-processed plant-sources that maintain high levels of what the plant utilized for its own development and procreation (as most healthy plant fats come from the seeds of plants). A few of the healthy fats come from algae sources, as we'll discuss.

The fat balance of our diet is critical to cleansing because our cell membranes are made of different lipids and lipid-derivatives like phospholipids and glycolipids. An imbalanced fat diet therefore can lead to weak cell membranes, which leads to cells that have restricted or inconsistent pores. The cell membrane pores allow nutrients in to the cells and waste out of the cells. Unhealthy fats also lead to weaker cell membranes that are more prone to damage by oxidative radicals – producing more cell damage and more toxicity in the body.

An example of this is the International Study of Asthma and Allergies in Childhood (ISAAC) conducted among eight Pacific countries, which included Samoa, Fiji, Tokelau, French Polynesia and New Caledonia. The research found that margarine consumption was one of the leading predicating factors in current asthma and wheezing among children.

Furthermore, they found that the risk factors for increased rhinoconjunctivitis included the regular consumption of meat products, butter and margarine among others. Allergic eczema was also associated with regular meat consumption and butter consumption among others.

Here is a quick review of the major fatty acids and the foods they come from:

## Major Omega-3 Fatty Acids (EFAs)

| Acronym | Fatty Acid Name | Major Dietary Sources |
|---------|-----------------|-----------------------|
| ALA | Alpha-linolenic acid | Walnuts, soybeans, flax, canola, pumpkin seeds, chia seeds |
| SDA | Stearidonic acid | hemp, spirulina, blackcurrant |
| DHA | Docosahexaenoic acid | Body converts from ALA; also obtained from certain algae, krill and fish oils |
| EPA | Eicosapentaenoic acid | Converts in the body from DHA |

## Major Omega-6 Fatty Acids (EFAs)

| Acronym | Fatty Acid Name | Major Dietary Sources |
|---------|-----------------|-----------------------|
| LA | Linoleic acid | Many plants, safflower, sunflower, sesame, soy, almond especially |
| ARA | Arachidonic acid | Meats, salmon |
| PA | Palmitoleic acid | Macadamia, palm kernel, coconut |
| GLA | Gamma-linolenic acid | Borage, primrose oil, spirulina |

## Major Omega-9 Fatty Acids

| Acronym | Fatty Acid Name | Major Dietary Sources |
|---------|-----------------|-----------------------|
| EA | Eucic acid | Canola, mustard seed, wallflower |
| OA | Oleic acid | Sunflower, olive, safflower |
| PA | Palmitoleic acid | Macadamia, palm kernel, coconut |

## Major Saturated Fatty Acids

| Acronym | Fatty Acid Name | Major Dietary Sources |
|---------|-----------------|-----------------------|
| Lauric | Lauric acid | Coconut, dairy, nuts |
| Myristic | Myristic acid | Coconut, butter |
| Palmitic | Palmitic acid | Macadamia, palm kernel, coconut, butter, beef, eggs |
| Stearic | Stearic acid | Macadamia, palm kernel, coconut, eggs |

***Essential fatty acids (EFAs)*** are fats the body does not form. Eaten in the right proportion, they can also lower inflammation and speed healing. EFAs include the long-chain polyunsaturated fatty acids – and the shorter chain linolenic, linoleic and oleic polyunsaturates. EFAs include omega-3s and omega-6s. The omega-3s include alpha linolenic acid (ALA), docosahexaenoic acid (DHA) and eicosapentaenoic acid (EPA). EPA and DHA are found in algae, mackerel, salmon, herring, sardines, sablefish (black cod). The omega-6s include linoleic acid, (LA), palmitoleic acid (PA), gamma-linoleic acid (GLA) and arachidonic acid (ARA). The term *essential* was originally given with the assumption that these types of fats could not be assembled or produced by the body – they must be taken directly from our food supply.

This assumption, however, is not fully correct. While it is true that we need *some* of these from our diet, our bodies can readily convert LA to ARA, and ALA to DHA and EPA as needed. Therefore, these fats can be considered essential in the sense that they are not generated by the body, but we do not necessarily have to consume each one of them.

**Monounsaturated fats** are high in omega-9 fatty acids like oleic acid. A monounsaturated fatty acid has one double carbon-hydrogen bonding chain. Oils from seeds, nuts and other plant-based sources have the largest quantities of monounsaturates. Oils that have large proportions of monounsaturates such as olive oil are known to lower inflammation when replacing high saturated fat in diets. Monounsaturates also aid in skin cell health and reduce atopic skin responses.

Monounsaturated fatty acids like oleic acid have been shown in studies to lower heart attack risk, aid blood vessel health, and offer anti-carcinogenic potential. They are typical among Mediterranean diets, which have been shown to reduce heart disease risk and cancer risk – related to their lower levels of lipid peroxidative radicals. The best sources of omega-9s are olives, sesame seeds, avocados, almonds, peanuts, pecans, pistachio nuts, cashews, hazelnuts, macadamia nuts, several other nuts and their respective oils.

**Polyunsaturated fats** have at least two double carbon-hydrogen bonds. They come from a variety of plant and marine sources. Omega-3s ALA, DHA and EPA simply have longer chains with more double carbon-hydrogen bonds. ALA, DHA and EPA are known to lower inflammation and increase artery-wall health. These *long-chain* omega-3 polyunsaturates are also considered critical for intestinal health.

The omega-6 fatty acids are the most available form of fat in the plant kingdom. Linoleic acid is the primary omega-6 fatty acid and it is found in most grains and seeds.

**Saturated fats** have multiple fatty acids without double bonds (the hydrogens "saturate" the carbons). They are found among animal fats, and tropical oils such as coconut and palm. Milk products such as butter and whole milk contain saturated fats, along with a special type of healthy linoleic fatty acid called CLA or *conjugated linoleic acid.*

The saturated fats from coconuts and palm differ from animal saturates in that they have shorter chains. This actually gives them – unlike animal saturates – an antimicrobial quality.

Medium chain fatty acids like coconut and palm oils have been shown in human studies to lower lipoprotein-A concentrations in the blood while having fibrinolytic (plaque and clot reduction) effects (Muller *et al.* 2003).

***Trans fats*** are oils that either have been overheated or have undergone hydrogenation. Hydrogenation is produced by heating while bubbling hydrogen ions through the oil. This adds hydrogen and repositions some of the bonds. The "trans" refers to the positioning of part of the molecule in reverse – as opposed to "cis" positioning. The cis positioning is the bonding orientation the body's cell membranes work best with. Trans fats have been known to be a cause for increased radical species in the system; damaging artery walls; contributing to inflammation, heart disease, high LDL levels, liver damage, diabetes, and other metabolic dysfunction (Mozaffarian *et al.* 2009). Trans fat overconsumption slows the conversion of LA to GLA.

***Conjugated linolenic acid (CLA)*** is a healthy fat that comes from primarily from dairy products. CLA is also a trans fat, but this is a trans fat the body works well with – it is considered a healthy trans fat.

Researchers from St Paul's Hospital and the University of British Columbia (MacRedmond *et al.* 2010) gave 28 overweight adults 4.5 g/day of CLA or a placebo for 12 weeks in addition to their medications. After the twelve weeks, those in the CLA group experienced significantly better lung function compared to the placebo group. The CLA group also experienced a significant reduction of weight and BMI compared with the control group. The CLA group also had lower leptin/adiponectin ratios – associated with balanced metabolism.

Other research has also found that CLA can to reduce lipid peroxidation and provide better balance among lipids (Noone *et al.* 2002).

***Arachidonic acid (ARA):*** ARA is considered an essential fatty acid, and research has shown that it is vital for infants while they are building their intestinal barriers. However, ARA is pro-inflammatory and stimulates pro-inflammatory mediators like leukotrienes. Too much of it as we age thus burdens our immune systems, pushing our bodies towards systemic inflammation and slower detoxification.

Red meats provide the highest levels of arachidonic acid. Because arachidonic acid stimulates the production of pro-inflammatory prostaglandins and leukotrienes in an enzyme conversion process, too much ARA leads to a greater level of toxicity, producing more inflammation.

Interestingly, carnivorous animals cannot or do not readily convert linoleic acid (found in many common plants) to arachidonic acid, but herbivore animals do convert linoleic acid to arachidonic acid, as do humans. This conversion – on top of a red meat-heavy diet – produces high arachidonic acid levels. In contrast, a diet that is balanced between plant-based monounsaturates, polyunsaturates and some saturates (such as the Mediterranean diet) will balance arachidonic acids with the other fatty acids.

**Gamma linoleic acid (GLA):** A wealth of studies have confirmed that GLA reduces or inhibits the inflammatory response. Leukotrienes produced by arachidonic acid stimulate inflammation, while leukotrienes produced by GLA block the conversion of polyunsaturated fatty acids to arachidonic acid. This means that GLA lowers inflammation, and promotes a healthy immune system.

A healthy body will convert linoleic acid into GLA readily, utilizing the same delta-6 desaturase enzyme used for ALA to DHA conversion. From GLA, the body produces *dihomo-gamma linoleic acid,* which cycles through the body as an eicosinoid. This aids in skin health, healthy mucosal membranes, and down-regulates inflammatory hypersensitivity.

In addition to conversion from LA, GLA can also be obtained from the oils of borage seeds, evening primrose seed, hemp seed, and from spirulina. Excellent food sources of LA include chia seeds, seed, hempseed, grapeseed, pumpkin seeds, sunflower seeds, safflower seeds, soybeans, olives, pine nuts, pistachio nuts, peanuts, almonds, cashews, chestnuts, and their respective oils.

The conversion of LA to GLA (and ALA to DHA) is reduced by trans fat consumption, smoking, pollution, stress, infections, and various chemicals that affect the liver.

**Docosahexaenoic acid (DHA)** obtained from algae, fish and krill, has significant therapeutic and anti-inflammatory effects according to the research. DHA is also associated with stronger cell membranes, and lower levels of lipid peroxidation.

It appears that the anti-inflammatory effects of DHA in particular relate to a modulation of a gene factor called NF-kappaB. The NF-kappaB is involved in signaling among cytokine receptors. With more DHA consumption, the transcription of the NF-kappaB gene sequence is reduced. This appears to reduce inflammatory signaling (Singer *et al.* 2008).

DHA readily converts to EPA by the body. EPA degrades quickly if unused in the body. It is easily converted from DHA as needed. Our bodies store DHA and not EPA.

Because much of the early research on the link between fatty acids and inflammatory disease was performed using fish oil, it was assumed that both EPA and DHA fatty acids reduced inflammation. Recent research from the University of Texas' Department of Medicine/Division of Clinical Immunology and Rheumatology (Rahman *et al.* 2008) has clarified that DHA is primarily implicated in reducing inflammation. DHA was shown to inhibit RANKL-induced pro-inflammatory cytokines, and a number of inflammation steps, while EPA did not.

The process of converting ALA to DHA and other omega-3s requires an enzyme produced in the liver called delta-6 desaturase. Some people – especially those who have a poor diet, are immune-suppressed, or burdened with toxicity such as cigarette smoke – may not produce this enzyme very well. As a result, they may not convert as much ALA to DHA and EPA.

For those with low levels of DHA – or for those with problems converting ALA and DHA – low-environmental impact and low toxin content DHA from microalgae can be supplemented. Certain algae produce significant amounts of DHA. They are the foundation for the DHA molecule all the way up the food chain, including fish. This is how fish get their DHA, in other words. Three algae species – *Crypthecodinium cohnii*, *Nitzschia laevis* and *Schizochytrium spp.* – are in commercial production and available in oil and capsule form.

Microalgae-derived DHA is preferable to fish or fish oils because fish oils typically contain saturated fats and may also – depending upon their origin – contain toxins such as mercury and PCBs (though to their credit, many producers also carefully distill their fish oil). However, we should note that salmon contain a considerable amount of arachidonic acid as well (Chilton 2006).

Thus, the DHA derived from fish sources, because it requires increased levels of filtering and processing to remove PCBs and mercury, would not be considered a living source of DHA, as it is too far removed from the living source. Algae-derived DHA is a wholesome source, as it is derived directly from living algae. Algae-derived DHA also does not strain sensitive fishery populations.

Algal-DHA also decreases pro-inflammatory arachidonic acid levels. One study (Arterburn *et al.* 2007) measured pro-inflammatory arachidonic acid levels within the body before and after supplementation with algal DHA. It was found that arachidonic acid levels decreased by 20% following just one dose of 100 milligrams of algal DHA.

For those who consider fish the superior source of DHA: In a study by researchers from The Netherlands' Wageningen University Toxicology Research Center (van Beelen *et al.* 2007), all three species of commercially produced algal oil showed equivalency with fish oil in their inhibition of cancer cell growth. Another study (Lloyd-Still *et al.* 2007) of twenty cystic fibrosis patients concluded that 50 milligrams of algal DHA was readily absorbed, maintained DHA bioavailability immediately, and increased circulating DHA levels by four to five times.

In terms of DHA availability, algal-DHA is just as good as fish. In a randomized open-label study (Arterburn *et al.* 2008), researchers gave 32 healthy men and women either algal DHA oil or cooked salmon for two weeks. After the two weeks, plasma levels of circulating DHA were bioequivalent.

***Alpha-linolenic acid (ALA)*** is the primary omega-3 fatty acid the body can most easily assimilate. Once assimilated, the healthy body will convert ALA to omega-3s, primarily DHA, at a range of about 7-40%, depending upon the health of the liver. One study of six women performed at England's University of Southampton (Burdge *et al.* 2002) showed a conversion rate of 36% from ALA to DHA and other omega-3s. A follow-up study of men showed ALA conversion to the omega-3s occurred at an average of 16%.

We should include that ALA, which comes from plants, has been shown to halt or slow inflammation processes, similar to DHA. In studies at Wake Forest University (Chilton *et al.* 2008), for example, flaxseed oil produced anti-inflammatory effects, along with borage oil and echium oil (the latter two also containing GLA).

Furthermore, flaxseed has been recommended specifically for toxicity and inflammation for centuries. This is not only because of its omega-3 levels: it is also because flaxseed contains mucilage, which helps strengthen our mucosal membranes.

***The healthy fat balance:*** In a meta-study by researchers from the University of Crete's School of Medicine (Margioris 2009), numerous studies showed that long-chain polyunsaturated omega-3s tend to be anti-inflammatory while omega-6 oils tend to be pro-inflammatory.

This, however, simplifies the equation too much. Most of the research on fats has also shown that most omega-6s are healthy oils. Balance is the key.

Research has illustrated that reducing animal-derived saturated fats reduces inflammation, cardiovascular disease, high cholesterol and diabetes (Ros and Mataix 2008). All of these relate to toxicity, because as we've discussed, lipid peroxidation lies at the root of these conditions.

The relationships became clearer from a study performed at Sydney's Heart Research Institute (Nicholls *et al.* 2008). Here fourteen adults consumed meals either rich in saturated fats or omega-6 polyunsaturated fats. They were tested following each meal for various inflammation and cholesterol markers. The results showed that the high saturated fat meals increased inflammatory activities and decreased the liver's production of

HDL cholesterol; whereas (good) HDL levels and the liver's anti-inflammatory capacity were increased after the omega-6 meals.

What this tells us is that the omega-3/omega-6 story is complicated by the saturated fat content of the diet and subsequent liver function. High saturated fat diets increase (bad) LDL (lipid peroxidation) content and reduce the anti-inflammatory and antioxidant capacities of the liver. Diets lower in saturated fat and higher in omega-6 and omega-3 fats encourage antioxidant and anti-inflammatory activity.

We also know that diets high in monounsaturated fats – such as the Mediterranean diet – are also associated with significant anti-inflammatory effects. Mediterranean diets contain higher levels of monounsaturated fats like oleic acids (omega-9) from foods like olives and avocados (and their oils); as well as higher proportions of fruits and vegetables, and lower proportions of saturated fats.

High saturated fat diets are also associated with increased obesity, and a number of studies have shown that obesity is directly related to inflammatory diseases – including allergies as we've discussed. High saturated fat diets and diets high in trans fatty acids have also been clearly shown to accompany higher levels of inflammation – illustrated by increases in inflammatory factors such as IL-6 and CRP (Basu *et al.* 2006).

To maximize anti-inflammatory factors, the ideal proportion of omega-6s to omega-3s is recommended at about two to one (2:1). The Western diet has been estimated by researchers to up to thirty to one (30:1) of omega-6s to omega-3s. This large imbalance (of too much omega-6s and too little omega-3s) has also been associated with inflammatory diseases, including asthma, arthritis, heart disease, ulcerative colitis, Crohn's disease, and others. When fat consumption is out of balance, the body's metabolism will trend towards inflammation. This is because in the absence of omega-3s and GLA, omega-6 oils convert more easily to arachidonic acid. And remember, ARA is pro-inflammatory (Simopoulos 1999).

Noting the research showing the relationships between the different fatty acids and inflammation, and the condition of the liver (which can be burdened by too much saturated fat), scientists have logically arrived at a model for dietary fat consumption for a person who is either dealing with or wants to prevent inflammation-oriented conditions and toxicity:

| Omega-3 | 20%-25% of dietary fats |
|---|---|
| Omega-6+Omega-9 | 40%-50% of dietary fats |
| Saturated | 5%-10% of dietary fats |
| GLA | 10%-20% of dietary fats |
| Trans fats | 0% of dietary fats |

Nuts, seeds, grains, beans, olives and avocados can provide the bulk of these healthy fats in balanced combinations. Walnuts, pumpkin seeds, flax, chia, soy, canola and algal-DHA can fill in the omega 3s. Healthy saturated fats can be found in coconuts, palm and dairy products.

### What about fish oil? And heart disease?

Yes, fish contains long-chain DHA and EPA, and these are known to curb inflammation, help brain health and reduce heart disease.

Unfortunately, fish today also come with baggage in the form of mercury, dioxin, and other pollutants. Why? Because fish are higher in the food chain and they bioaccumulate the toxins that are floating around in our waters. And yes, our bodies of water around the earth have become our dumping zone. So when we eat fish, we are in effect eating the fat-soluble toxin that our society is dumping into our waters.

Some fish also contain significant amounts of saturated fats, and fatty fish have high amounts of arachidonic acid – as we discussed earlier.

Plant-based fats also deliver these long-chain PUFAs in healthy forms without these bioaccumulated (up the food chain) toxins. Many plants deliver ALA which converts to DHA and EPA in the body in healthy individuals. For those whose livers are not so healthy, algal-DHA is the best, safest option in terms of less risk of mercury and other toxins.

And plant-based fats deliver on the heart health issue – surprisingly, even better than fish fats.

In fact, two large research reviews by medical scientists have determined that omega-3 fatty acids from plants reduce the incidence of heart disease and heart attacks while fish oil has only a slight ("insignificant") effect.

The most recent study focusing on the omega-3 fatty acid alpha-linolenic acid (ALA) comes from researchers at Harvard Medical School (Pan et al. 2012) along with several other prestigious universities. The researchers analyzed 27 clinical trials that studied 251,049 human subjects. The studies included over 15,000 heart attacks and other cardiovascular events.

The cardiovascular events were cross-referenced against either supplementation or blood levels of ALA. In total, increased consumption of alpha-linolenic acid omega-3 fatty acids resulted in a 14% total reduction of heart attacks and associated cardiovascular events. And as trends were pooled and examined with ALA blood biomarkers, the reduction in cardiovascular events was as high as 20%.

Another large review of research, published in September's *Journal of the American Medical Association*. The research comes from medical researchers from Greece's Ioannina University Medical School and Hospital

(Rizos *et al.* 2012). In this study, researchers utilized the Cochrane Central Register of Controlled Trials of research for fish oil and cardiovascular events research through August of 2012.

The researchers analyzed 20 studies involving 68,680 human subjects. Among these, there were 3,993 deaths from heart attacks and cardiovascular events, 1,150 sudden deaths, 1,837 heart attacks and 1,490 strokes. Against these were cross-referenced marine-sourced (fish) omega-3 fatty acids, which include DHA and EPA, along with saturated fats (yes, fish oil typically contains saturated fats).

The research found that fish oil supplementation did slightly reduce the incidence of heart attacks by 11% and heart attack deaths by 9%. However, given the scale of the margin of error, the researchers concluded that fish oil supplementation, *"was not associated with a lower risk of all-cause mortality, cardiac death, sudden death, myocardial infarction, or stroke based on relative and absolute measures of association."* In other words, there wasn't enough of a difference from the margin of error to claim fish oil reduces heart attacks or cardiovascular events.

Supporting the conflicting evidence, the researchers also stated:
> *"Treatment with marine-derived omega-3 polyunsaturated fatty acids (PUFAs) for the prevention of major cardiovascular adverse outcomes has been supported by a number of randomized clinical trials (RCTs) and refuted by others."*

The research on plant-based alpha-linolenic acid omega-3s has not been so controversial because research over the years has consistently shown ALA's ability to help prevent cardiovascular events and cardiovascular disease. And this is illustrated with the size of the study analysis (totaling 251,049 humans).

Alpha-linolenic acid is one of the primary fatty acids found in various seeds, nuts and grains. Some of the highest levels are found in chia seeds (64%), kiwi fruit seeds (62%), flax seeds (55%) and hemp seeds (20%). Other good sources include walnuts, pumpkin seeds, sesame seeds, olives, canola, kale, spirulina, spinach and others.

In addition to being well utilized by the body, alpha-linolenic acid (ALA) is also converted to docosahexaenoic acid (DHA), eicosapentaenoic acid (EPA) and other important omega-3s within the body. The primary liver enzyme used in the conversion of ALA to DHA is delta-6 desaturase. DHA converts to EPA in the body as needed. A healthy person will convert ALA to DHA at a rate of from 7% to 15% according to research.

For those who convert ALA to DHA at a slower rate, algal DHA provides the purest form of DHA. DHA is produced by algae and travels up the marine food chain. Algal DHA does not contain saturated fats as many fish do. DHA-producing algae is farmed in tanks in the absence of mercury, PCBs and dioxins that have been known to bioaccumulate within fish.

DHA and EPA are the central fatty acids in fish oil besides saturated fat. It also should be noted that fatty fish such as salmon also contain a considerable amount of arachidonic acid. Foods rich in arachidonic acids have been shown to increase inflammation in the body.

### Algal DHA and heart disease

Let's discuss algal DHA oil a little further.

Remember that DHA stands for docosahexaenoic acid, an omega-3 fatty acid. Microalgae species *Crypthecodinium cohnii*, *Nitzschia laevis* and *Schizochytrium* spp. all produce algal DHA.

Research from New York's Rockefeller University (Bernstein *et al.* 2012) determined that DHA sourced from microalgae lowers serum triglycerides and Low-density lipoprotein (LDL) in overweight adults, and reduces VLDL particle size.

This conclusion was confirmed by a new meta-study from the Cleveland Clinic's Wellness Institute (Neff *et al.* 2011), which found that algae-derived DHA lowers serum triglycerides in healthy persons.

In the Rockefeller University study, 35 overweight or obese adult volunteers took either two grams of algal DHA per day or a placebo. The DHA group had significantly lower triglyceride levels, and lower levels of VLDL (very low density lipoprotein) cholesterol.

Furthermore, the particle sizes of all the cholesterol types within the DHA group were greater, including their HDL, LDL and VLDL cholesterol. Other research has found that smaller sized cholesterol particles are associated with cardiovascular disease and atherosclerosis – the hardening of the arteries.

The newer meta-study from the Cleveland Clinic analyzed the results of eleven clinical studies that included 485 healthy volunteers. In these studies, triglyceride levels were significantly lower in the algal-DHA groups, and HDL/LDL levels were higher among healthy persons.

Other research has established that the DHA derived from algae has the same beneficial effects and safety as DHA derived from fish oil. The body stores this long-chain fatty acid in the form of DHA, and converts DHA to EPA as needed.

### Algal DHA and the brain

Omega-3 fatty acids, and especially docosahexaenoic acid (DHA), are critical for the functioning of nerve and brain cells. They aid in nerve cell maintenance and development. Alpha linolenic acid (ALA) is the most available omega-3 fatty acid – available from whole grains, seeds, beans and other foods. Once assimilated, a healthy body will convert ALA to eicosapentaenoic acid (EPA) and docosahexaenoic acid (DHA) at a rate of about 7-15%, depending upon the health of the liver.

However, those who eat a poor diet, who are immune-suppressed, or burdened with toxins such as cigarette smoke or various chemicals may not convert ALA to DHA optimally. Researchers suspect that gamma linolenic acid (GLA) consumption is also necessary for conversion of ALA to DHA.

For those with low levels of DHA, or have problems converting ALA and DHA, the natural algae derived from the Pacific Ocean called Golden Algae produces a pure form of DHA. Many health experts feel that this type of DHA is preferable to fish oil that typically contains saturated fats and a greater risk of mercury and PCBs coming from the fish (depending upon the producer). Algal DHA is produced from algae from controlled tanks as opposed to potentially polluted ocean or fish farm habitats.

Oxford University researchers (Richardson *et al.* 2012) determined that DHA derived from algae increases reading performance, memory and behavior in children who are underperforming or have attention-deficit disorders.

The researchers conducted a double-blind, placebo-controlled study of 362 healthy children who were seven to nine years old. The children attended school among 74 schools in Oxfordshire, U.K.

The researchers gave the children either 600 milligrams of algal DHA daily for 16 weeks or soybean oil capsules that matched the color and taste of the algal DHA supplement. The children were given the supplements either by parents or schools alternatively.

The research found that those children who were underperforming in reading skills and had behavioral issues such as ADHD symptoms had noticeable improvement in these areas, including cognition, memory, behavior and reading performance, as tested by teachers and reported by parents.

The improvement in reading among the DHA group averaged either 20% more or 50% more among the subgroups of children who were underperforming.

This improvement led to an average of nearly two months of increased reading levels among the poorest reading group.

Among those children with ADHD symptoms, parents of the algal-DHA group reported significant behavior improvement using a 14-point symptom grading scale.

The researchers concluded:

*"DHA supplementation appears to offer a safe and effective way to improve reading and behavior in healthy but underperforming children from mainstream schools."*

## Our Ancestors' Salt

Salt is one of those elements the body needs in nature's doses, and within a matrix of its natural structure. Once again, we have abandoned the natural version, opting for the white refined version.

Is sodium bad for you and how much is bad?

Well for starters, research from University of California (McCarron et al. 2013) has determined that conventional medicine's assumption of salt intake outside a certain range being a cause of hypertension and heart disease has been wrong.

The new research, a compilation of clinical studies that piggybacked onto a 2009 study done at UC-Davis, which accumulated numerous studies including 19,151 human subjects who were tested for their 24-hour urinary sodium excretion rates.

This new study accumulated an additional 129 studies, which included 50,060 human subjects, again being tested for their 24-hour sodium excretion rates. The research also gauged sodium intake together with excretion rates.

The researchers also analyzed the various studies regarding salt intake and hypertension, along with heart conditions in general, along with the salt intakes over the decades around the world.

This international focus has now produced evidence showing that the assumptions of conventional western medicine that sodium intake at certain levels is associated with a greater risk of hypertension – with safe levels being defined as 1,500 to 2,500 milligrams of sodium (salt) per day.

One of the main assumptions of conventional medicine is that sodium levels within the blood that lead to hypertension are produced by higher intakes of sodium in the diet.

This was disproven by the research, which found that the body self-adjusts and regulates the sodium intake within the body, yielding healthy levels. This regulation takes place through the discharge of sodium outside of healthy levels.

The research also determined that around the world, the consumption of sodium by healthy humans tends to range from 2,622 to 4,840 milligrams per day. The upper level of this range is nearly twice the range given by conventional medical institutions regarding maximum sodium intakes.

The researchers identified several other falsehoods regarding the assumptions between salt intake and heart disease/hypertension, as stated in the *American Journal of Hypertension:*

*"No consistent data had appeared in the scientific literature specifically demonstrating that lower sodium intake was associated with a reduction in either all-cause or CVD mortality."*

They also stated that even though it was assumed that because many consumer products had reformulated with lower salt levels,

*"There was no evidence that sodium intake was declining in the United States."*

This meant that the assumptions that hypertension rates were slowing because of changes in sodium assumption were wrong. The researchers went on to describe how studies that were supposed to have shown how reducing sodium intake reduces the risk of hypertension and heart disease actually did not result in sodium intakes at the targeted levels.

This is because the body maintains its internal sodium levels by increasing what the researchers call "sodium appetite." When the body senses its sodium levels are too low, it will engage the person to seek foods with higher sodium levels in order to accomplish enough sodium.

Then, if too much sodium is consumed, the body will automatically adjust its internal sodium levels by excreting sodium in the urine. The mechanism the body uses is the renin-angiotensin-aldosterone system to balance sodium levels.

Decades of research proved this was true for animals. Western medicine thought humans were an exception to this principle.

In fact, recent studies, such as one from Albert Einstein School of Medicine (Alderman et al. 2012) of more than 360,000 human subjects, and another from Canada's McMaster University (O'Donnell et al. 2011) of 4,729 human subjects – have determined that sodium levels less than 2,500 milligrams per day and 3,000 milligrams per day (respectively) actually increased the rate of cardiovascular disease.

And the upper levels of these studies – levels above which increased the rate of heart disease – were above 6,000 and 7,000 milligrams a day respectively.

The bottom line of this research is that the study of salt and cardiovascular disease has been wrought with assumption and miscalculation. This has actually resulted in endangering the lives of those who have taken the recommendations to cut salt out of the diet.

### *What about mineral balance?*

The reality is, modern salt is not a healthy dietary agent. Modern vacuum-evaporated salt contains numerous chemical additives such as tricalcium phosphate, silica dioxide, sodium ferrocyanide, ferric ammonium citrate and/or sodium silico-aluminate.

Worse, modern salt (even many "sea salts") have been "purified" through separation, resulting in the removal of nature's balance of minerals that are important co-factors for sodium consumption. These include potassium, calcium, magnesium and many trace elements that are naturally present in salt extracted from mines or even sea water, and necessary in our diet.

The most dangerous thing about this modern salt is the imbalance that it can create among our other minerals: Consuming too much of one mineral and not enough of others creates imbalances throughout our tissues.

And this research illustrates that while the body may adjust for the over-consumption of sodium, the under-consumption of important minerals like sodium, potassium, magnesium and many others is more lethal to our heart, blood vessels and other tissues.

### Refined Salts versus Whole Salts

Refined table salts start innocently enough: they are collected from seawater (much of America's salt comes from the not-so-pristine waters of the South San Francisco Bay – noted as one of the most polluted bays in America, for example) or harvested from underground salt mines. After water flushing, table salt manufacturers will typically treat and precipitate out unwanted elements using chemical agents such as barium, sulfuric acid and chlorine.

The resulting brine is vacuum-evaporated, and anti-caking chemicals such as tricalcium phosphate, silica dioxide, sodium ferrocyanide, ferric ammonium citrate and/or sodium silico-aluminate may be added, depending upon the manufacturer. Many manufacturers also add iodine and dextrose; and many foreign manufacturers add fluoride. The result is 'purified' salt – around 99% sodium chloride: A miracle of industrial modification.

Humans have treasured unrefined whole salts for their health-giving, anti-microbial, and culinary properties for thousands of years. And for good reason. Natural whole salt chipped from mines or solar-evaporated from water is not simply sodium chloride.

Whole salt may contain up to 80 minerals and trace elements: Important minerals such as potassium, which primarily resides inside the cell membrane to balance sodium levels on the outside of the cell membrane;

as well as boron, silica and zinc — all essential to healthy bones, muscles, nerves and enzyme metabolism. Even healthy traces of mercury, arsenic, and cadmium are found in real whole salt. Over the past few years research has begun to link mineral and trace element deficiencies to a host of ailments, including arthritis, cardiovascular disease, asthma, and a number of autoimmune disorders.

While whole salt's levels of macro minerals like calcium, magnesium, potassium may not reach daily recommended allowance levels, whole salt contains a balanced spectrum of the trace elements missing from many modern diets. Whole salt is also alkalizing; helping provide a neutralizing environment. Many holistic practitioners believe the crystalline structure of whole salt also renders its mineral ions more easily and energetically absorbed. Whole salt's potential ability to assist in detoxification is also gaining attention. Some holistic doctors are reporting success with whole salts used adjunctively as anti-microbial/anti-parasitic agents. Some have noted that whole salts help improve immunity and metabolism among their patients.

A 1998 study led by Michael Alderman, M.D. awakened us to this possibility when it showed a greater mortality rate among lower sodium users within a population of 11,348 participants. As a result, many physicians now concede that both too much and too little sodium may stress the body. Although peer-reviewed research is lacking on whole salts, holistic doctors have observed reductions in blood pressure among patients using whole salts. Customer testimonials from whole salt companies also appear to be consistent with these observations.

How about iodine? Is not white salt our primary source of iodine? It should not be and does not have to be. For a narrow diet devoid in dairy, berries like strawberries, sea vegetables and land vegetables, there may be a risk of low-iodine levels. Although many studies have related regional goiter levels to low-iodine levels, other studies — like a 35,999-person study (Trowbridge *et al.* 1975) done among 10 states in the U.S. — found no relationship between goiter and low-iodine consumption. In fact, this study showed higher goiter levels among higher iodine excretion levels.

Higher goiter levels have also been seen amongst adequate iodine diets, and some research has related mal-absorption to be the causal issue. As such, it appears that both low- and high-iodine consumption can be problematic.

In a low-iodine diet, white iodized salt may be a reasonable source, however as in any isolated supplement program, we should point out that iodine absorption and utilization is dependent upon full-spectrum nutrition.

For example, the body requires minerals like selenium to properly process iodine into T3 and T4, and selenium is typically present in whole salts. It should also be noted that a mere 1.6g of iodized salt will result in approximately 122µg of iodine, while absorbing diets under 100µg of iodine appear to be adequate for goiter prevention, while excess iodine diets have been linked to chronic high volume thyroid disorders. Most dieticians agree that there is enough iodized salts available in our diet anyway, should we eat out or buy prepared or canned foods.

While the term 'sea salt' conjures the ocean, experts agree that all salt is 'sea salt' – even salt mines are just ancient seabeds. Meanwhile the *term* 'sea salt,' whole salt manufacturers complain, is also a source of confusion to consumers looking for whole salt. Be aware of salts labeled "sea salt" or "natural sea salt," they say. Even the most refined salt can be called "sea salt."

Traditionally seashore-evaporated whole salts are different. They contain the full spectrum of minerals from their environment – assuming their environment is clean. There are traditional, hand-harvested whole sea salts from the French coast of Brittany, for example. This artisan salt is unique because the natural evaporation clay-base is thought to add beneficial elements while absorbing toxins. Boasting a mere 82% sodium chloride level (with 12%+ moisture), this salt contains a number of macro and trace minerals, based on independent analysis.

Although a traditional source of salt for thousands of years, mined whole salt has recently been gaining attention in the natural health community. These ancient underground whole salts are pressurized into complex crystalline form over millions of years of volcanic and tectonic plate movement.

One such cache lies within the famous Pakistan salt range – the oldest working salt mine in Asia – said to be 200-250 million years old. Still harvested by local traditional miners, its crystallized rock salt is labeled and distributed after importation into the U.S.

An independent lab assay of one of these whole mineral salts examined by the author showed over 80 elements – albeit many in trace quantities – with sodium chloride levels over 97%. The larger, pinkish salt crystal rocks are also sold as negative ion lamps, which are said to remove impurities from the air and energize indoor space.

This mineral-rich pink rock salt is also found in the United States. A 155-million-year old volcanic ash-covered salt mine near Redmond, Utah is the site of some of the earth's purest salt crystals. We have seen company assay reports showing around 97% sodium chloride with up to 74 minerals and trace elements within the remaining 3% from this salt.

As almost every chef worth his/her spatula agrees, whole salts add exquisite taste to any meal due to their mineral content – each whole salt lending its own unique flavor. Some of these salts have won culinary awards for their distinct taste. While whole salts can provide a great source of trace minerals to our diet, they can also provide better-tasting meals.

Bottom line: use whole salts instead of refined salts, but eat enough iodized salt to retain healthy iodine levels. These can be consumed with kelps as well. A few whole salts are now iodized.

# Chapter Nine

# The Fallacy of Gluten-Free

Without a varied diet of fibrous whole foods, including grains produced by mother nature, we will be robbing the body of some of nature's best resources for a healthy body. The humble grain produces seeds for procreation, but from this process sprouts essential nutrients that benefit every cell, organ and metabolism within our bodies. These include an array of vitamins, minerals, essential oils, and complex phytocompounds – some of which are only available in grains.

Yet we find online and among some books the pitch that grains containing gluten are hazardous to our health. Are they really?

Certainly this negates decades of scientific research and thousands of years of healthy traditional diets eaten by billions of people around the world.

This anti-gluten postulation opposes decades of scientific research that shows precisely the opposite: Whole grain plant foods contain important nutrients, fibers and phytocompounds that extend our lives.

Those who have bought into this anti-gluten postulation also end up turning their diets upside down as they seek alternatives to healthy whole grains. They also find themselves on the wrong side of the fiber equation, because most grains that supply important soluble and insoluble fibers also happen to contain gluten. We've discussed fiber and intestinal health at length earlier.

As the theory goes, lectins and gliadins within grains cause inflammation, and phytic acid from grains (and nuts) blocks mineral absorption. They also make a claim that wheat germ – a healthy food rich source of B-vitamins and other nutrients – is supposedly a cause for "leaky gut syndrome" because it contains wheat germ agglutinin.

Anti-gluten pundits also claim that whole cereal grains – which have been proven by scientific research published in peer-reviewed medical supposedly harm the heart and brain. Is this proven among the large studies that have shown that whole grains reduce the risk of disease and inflammation? No.

Sure, some obscure and inconclusive sterile laboratory tests may show that these compounds could enable conditions which might possibly produce inflammation if the body was like the sterile laboratory.

But the body is not like a sterile laboratory. As we will show throughout this book, the body is alive with not only living cells and organs, but over 500 trillion different bacteria and yeasts, all of which consume various components of our foods and produce a myriad of enzymes that help digest our foods and provide nutrition.

The anti-gluten position ignores the conclusive research that has studied the health effects of whole grain consumption throughout the world, not only from an epidemiological (large human populations) approach, but also from a double-blind, placebo-controlled clinical research perspective.

The anti-gluten position also attempts to support the opinion that the "paleo diet" – a diet that emphasizes eating mostly red meat and other animal products – is the healthiest diet.

Yet this opinion ignores the massive and conclusive scientific research showing that diets rich in red meat increase the risk of several types of cancer, heart disease and other inflammatory conditions. This conclusion has been supported by the American Heart Association, the American Cancer Society and other research groups, because it is backed by peer-reviewed medical research. These studies illustrate that the Mediterranean diet and similar diets rich in fresh fruits, vegetables and whole grains provide the best protection against inflammatory diseases such as heart disease, cancer and others.

## Confusing the Issue: Refined Flour Foods

Part of the misunderstanding about gluten grain comes from the fact that much of the grain we are consuming in the Western diet is overly processed and lacks the essential nutrients our ancestors ate. Let's review the problems with modern overly-processed grain and flour foods.

Let's start with the humble wheat berry, put forth by the wheat grass for procreation purposes. Today's commercial farmer begins by turning over the rich layers of soil to expose its nutrients and denitrifying bacteria to the sun. Chemical fertilizers are then spread over the soil. Then he plants wheat berry seeds treated with fungicides for bunt, smut and other potential diseases. Chemical pesticides sprayed on and around the crop as it sprouts and grows.

Wheat typically grows with very little other attendance. A couple of waterings during the summer will usually suffice in dryer areas. Once the mature wheat is ready for harvest, the commercial farmer drives large combine harvesters through the field and cuts the wheat. The combine is equipped with blades that cut the wheat and threshers, which strip the chaffs off the stalks and separate the wheat berries off the chaff.

Before the combine – named because it combined the process of cutting and threshing the wheat – farmers cut wheat by hand. Farmers used scythes to cut the wheat, and hand-threshed the wheat with flails on a wheat threshing floor – basically by whacking it against a rock or threshing floor to knock out the wheat berries.

Once the commercial farmer's wheat berries are separated, they are typically brought to a grain elevator, where they are stored until needed for milling. Once the mill is ready, truckloads of grain will be delivered from the elevators. The mill is equipped with various roller-grinding machines called millstands, which grind up the grain to the specifications needed in the flour.

In today's large industrial mills, the bran (the outer part) and the germ (the next layer in) are typically separated from the endosperm (the inner part) using large steel rollers. Some of the rollers are serrated while some are smoother, and the grain is conveyed from one roller to another and ground at different rates to achieve various flour consistencies. The endosperm is eventually milled into white flour. Depending upon the mill, the germ and the bran are typically sold for animal feed. Sometimes it is just spread out onto a dormant field.

Increasingly, this bran is being retained and used for adding fiber to food as a food additive. Wheat germ is now sold for use in various food applications by some mills. This has a degree of difficulty, however, because the germ must be refrigerated. It has lost its natural protective covering in the milling process.

In some mills, the bran and part of the germ is milled into whole-wheat flour. This is becoming increasingly popular as modern nutritionists have only recently discovered the need for fiber in the diet.

The wheat mill evolved from using a stone to grind the wheat berry against another stone to produce flour. Human ingenuity produced the gristmill, a stone-grinding apparatus developed to grind larger quantities at once. In both of these, however, there was no separation of the bran and germ from the endosperm. Flour was ground-up wheat berries, and that's what our ancestors baked and ate for thousands, even millions, of years.

Today, after the commercial white flour has been ground, it is sent off to a bakery. Today's industrialized bakeries are set up with automated baking and mixing equipment. The flour is dumped into large vats where it is typically mixed with water, blended with aluminum baking powder and/or dried yeast, sugar, refined salt and other chemicals as preservatives and flavor enhancers. The result: white bread, donuts, coffee cakes, and *ad nauseam*.

These of course are the fuel for most of our western society. These fuel our taste buds along with our significant obesity rates. In the U.S., for example, over 60% of us are overweight and more than a third of us are obese. So much for the romantic wheat berry.

Most of us know when we strip the bran and the germ off the berry, we end up with a product that has little or no fiber. Do we realize that the bran and germ also contain many valuable nutrients? Some might have heard that wheat bran and wheat germ contains B vitamins like thiamin and riboflavin. Do we understand the entire nutritional and energetic content of whole-wheat berries outside of a few vitamins?

In reality, whole grains have micronutrients and phytochemicals critical to our health. Grains contain a host of phytosterols, lignans, fatty acids and amino acids. They also contain various levels of thiamin, riboflavin, niacin, vitamin E, potassium, iron, magnesium, zinc, selenium, copper, chromium, manganese, molybdenum, selenium and iodine, among others.

Meanwhile, our white breads and coffee cakes are so depleted of these nutrients that federal law now requires they are enriched with some synthetic B vitamins and iron to give them some semblance of food.

And yes, eating these types of gluten-containing overly-processed foods can certainly produce inflammatory conditions. This has been shown in the research. These overly-processed foods have been robbed of the balance of nutrients delivered by whole grain. They are foods gone awry.

But let's not throw out the baby with the bath water.

## Whole Grains Provide Many Health Benefits

Whole grains are rich in anti-inflammatory components and healthy fiber. Peer-reviewed research over the past two decades has confirmed that insoluble and soluble dietary fibers in whole grains provide a variety of health benefits.

These include lowering the risks of heart disease, diabetes, asthma, obesity, stroke, ulcer, acid reflex, diverticulitis, hemorrhoids and others. While the balance of water insoluble and soluble fibers appears to be necessary, soluble fibers specifically have been shown to help lower blood pressure, reduce glycemic and insulin response, lower colon cancer risk, and lower LDL cholesterol.

As mentioned earlier, health researchers have determined that at least 25 grams of total fiber should be in the diet, optimally 30-40 grams. Whole grains provide both soluble and insoluble fiber. They contain arabinoxylans, oligosaccharides, beta-glucans and other polysaccharides that help balance our cholesterol levels and our blood glucose levels.

The health of our colon and intestines is improved by consuming whole grains. This is the conclusion of a significant amount of research, much of which we have discussed. Cereal grasses are one of the most nutritious plants because they mine nutrients from deep within the soil. The grain contains more than just what is in the stalk. Grains also contain hormone-balancing phyto-estrogens, as we discussed earlier. Some of the research supporting these points are contained in the sections entitled "Fiber and the Colon," "Sterol Foods," and "Hormone-balancing Foods."

## Gluten and Gliadins: The Real Story

In a study that analyzed treatment alternatives for celiac disease from George Washington University School of Medicine (Bakshi *et al.* 2012), the researchers found that probiotics provide a viable solution for gluten digestion and intestinal health – and likely their absence provides the smoking gun for the cause of gluten sensitivities.

Celiac disease – an inflammatory immune response to the gliadin protein in gluten – has been increasing over the past few years, and research is illustrating that celiac disease is more prevalent than previously considered.

Gluten sensitivities also appear to be increasing, with more and more people in western countries – especially in the U.S. – opting for gluten-free diets. This typically comes from a sense many have had that the gluten foods in their diet produce intestinal irritations, including bloating and indigestion. For this reason, the term "gluten-free" has become ubiquitous among health food stores and consumers.

Meanwhile, we find that grain-based foods have been part of the human diet for thousands of years, and some of the healthiest diets – including the Mediterranean Diet – contain gracious quantities of wheat and other whole grains. This is not to mention of course the fiber content among whole grains and the research that has shown foods rich in fiber reduce heart disease and other metabolic disorders.

And many traditional societies – producing the diets of a majority of the world's population, many of which are known for long lifespan – have grains as the cornerstone of their diet. These cultures also come with an absence of a history of intestinal problems.

This leads to the logical question: Has humanity really been poisoning itself with wheat and other gluten-containing grains (including barley, rye and others)? In a word, no.

The fact is, humanity has been eating these grains for thousands of years, and it has genetically, biologically and probiotically adapted to eating these foods.

Significant research focus and several teams of investigators have confirmed that the inflammatory response to gliadin – initiated with an interleukin-15 mediated response – is inhibited by healthy intestinal probiotics.

In fact, intestinal probiotics break down gliadin into healthy, non-inflammatory components.

A 2012 paper by three medical school professors studied the various means by which the effects of celiac disease may be mitigated – by inhibiting the inflammatory response. The paper's authors include two professors who are gastroenterology professors at George Washington

University School of Medicine, Anita Bakshi, M.D. and Sindu Stephen, M.D. Two other clinical M.D.s co-authored the research.

The researchers focused first upon the mechanisms of wheat gliadin protein upon the intestinal cells – which produce inflammation and intestinal permeability. These include the activation of a CD4+ T-cell response among the intestinal cells – which induces the secretion of a protein called zonulin. Zonulin then stimulates an increase in the spaces in the tight junctions between the intestinal cells, creating gut permeability.

This opening between intestinal cells is accompanied by an even greater inflammatory response as the immune system responds to larger proteins having potential contact with the bloodstream.

While there are a number of studies that have shown these effects, the researchers singled out a few studies that clearly and specifically illustrated how intestinal probiotics in a healthy body will inhibit this process by breaking down gluten through protease (enzyme) activity.

In one of these, Irish researchers found that two enzymes produced from probiotic bacteria – prolyl endopeptidase and endoprotease B – were able to break down gluten into non-reactive elements, completely sidestepping the possible intestinal response.

This research was confirmed in a clinical setting by scientists at the Celiac Sprue Research Foundation in Palo Alto, California. Here 20 celiac patients were given small doses of gluten with and without (double-blind, randomized, cross-over) being pretreated with one of these probiotic-produced enzymes – prolyl endopeptidase. The cross-over study utilized two 14-day treatment periods in total, in a staged format.

The pretreatment with the enzyme allowed a majority of the celiac patients to avoid malabsorption of carbohydrates and fats – a typical symptom of celiac sprue response.

The researchers concluded that:

> "Pretreatment of gluten with prolyl endopeptidase avoided the development of fat or carbohydrate malabsorption in the majority of those patients who developed fat or carbohydrate malabsorption after a 2-week gluten challenge."

In a series of studies from Finland's University of Tampere Medical School, researchers tested the probiotics strains *Lactobacillus fermentum* and *Bifidobacterium lactis* with gluten digestion and the inflammatory effects of gliadin.

They found these live probiotics were both able to inhibit the inflammation response among sensitive intestinal (Caco-2) cells. In both instances the probiotics prevented the inflammatory response as well as prevented the formation of "membrane ruffles."

The researchers stated:

> "B. lactis inhibited the gliadin-induced increase dose-dependently in epithelial permeability, higher concentrations completely abolishing the gliadin-induced decrease in transepithelial resistance."

This of course means the probiotics reduced the amount of intestinal damage caused by the inflammatory response related to the gluten ingestion.

And in their conclusion, the researchers stated:

> "We conclude thus that live B. lactis bacteria can counteract directly the harmful effects exerted by coeliac-toxic gliadin and would clearly warrant further studies of its potential as a novel dietary supplement in the treatment of coeliac disease."

While the inflammatory response in celiac sprue is typically described as being the result of a genetic abnormality, intestinal irritation and indigestion to gluten in non-celiac people provokes similar mechanisms of inflammation – though not as vigorous – and not linked with genetic abnormality (yet).

The UGW researchers concluded after reviewing the research that: "Inclusion of probiotics appears to be able to reduce the damage caused by eating gluten-contaminated foods and may even accelerate mucosal healing after the initiation of a gluten-free diet."

These results have been confirmed by other research. In a 2013 study from Argentina's University of Buenos Aires tested a probiotic supplement with 22 adults with celiac disease. The patients were given either capsules with the probiotic *Bifidobacterium infantis* or a placebo for 3 weeks.

Those taking the probiotic supplement had significantly lower levels of indigestion, constipation and other intestinal symptoms as gauged by the Gastrointestinal Symptom Rating Scale. Levels of IgA antibodies to gluten were also lower among the probiotic group.

The researchers stated:

> "The study suggests that B. infantis may alleviate symptoms in untreated celiac disease."

Certainly adult celiac patients are dealing with a dramatically heightened genetic response to the gluten protein, which is significantly greater than what is experienced by those even with some gluten sensitivity. And we cannot necessarily suggest that the inflammatory immune response of a celiac sprue patient can be completely eliminated by gliadin enzymes released by probiotics, which break down those gliadin proteins. This is because the gliadin genetic imprint may still be recognized by the immune system – producing the antibody-driven inflammatory response.

However, the non-genetic immune response that produces some bloating and/or indigestion for non-celiac people sensitive to gluten has many of the same mechanisms – especially when it comes to creating intestinal permeability. And the research is showing that even among celiac patients, symptoms of gluten intolerance are reduced. So it would only be logical to conclude – as have many researchers – that gluten sensitivities outside of celiac disease may be alleviated with healthy intestinal flora.

We also have only been looking through a narrow beam of research investigating only a few enzymes and probiotics. A healthy human intestine is a microcosm of thousands of strains of probiotic bacteria which produce a myriad of enzymes that assist our body with the digestion of nature's foods. So we are merely scratching the surface, yet the surface truly reveals the culprits involved.

After reviewing the research (before this last study), the GW medical professors supported this conclusion by stating:

*"Supplementation with a variety of bacterial strains can help inhibit gluten/gliadin-induced damage in the small intestine."*

The research clearly identifies the smoking gun for the growth of intestinal irritability and gluten insensitivity: The steady and growing destruction of healthy probiotics within our intestines through an unbridled use of antibiotics and antiseptics. This lack of probiotics exposes the intestines to large unbroken gliadin molecules the intestines are not intended to contend with. Healthy probiotic colonies would otherwise break these gliadins down into components our intestines were designed to deal with.

When we examine the evidence: The fact that gluten sensitivities have been growing as the use of antibiotics and antiseptics have become increasingly utilized together with the findings that enzymes produced by probiotics break down gluten and gliadin into non-toxic constituents, we can only arrive at the conclusion that our gut microflora has everything to do with wheat and other gluten sensitivities.

And with this conclusion, avoiding all forms of gluten in our diets can not only be an arduous and close to impossible task – but it may become unnecessary if we learn how to maintain healthy intestinal probiotics.

## Grains Feed Our Probiotics

In fact, research from UK researchers has determined that gluten grains – and wheat in particular – also provide critical nourishment (prebiotics) for our intestinal probiotics. This has now been established in a number of laboratory and human clinical studies over the past couple of years.

For example, in research led by Professor of Food Microbial Sciences at the UK's University of Reading, Dr. Glenn Gibson, 55 healthy men and women were given different doses of a wheat bran for three weeks. Those eating more wheat bran showed an increase in healthy probiotic bifidobacteria in their intestines and colons.

Another study led by Dr. Gibson tested 40 adults, and found the same conclusion: A polysaccharide named arabino-xylan-oligosaccharide – a component of wheat bran – was found to be the prebiotic. After many additional studies, it has been confirmed that arabino-xylan-oligosaccharide is critical for the health of our intestinal probiotics – and this nutrient is now considered a prebiotic. We'll discuss the importance of probiotics later on.

And as far as the agglutinin in wheat germ – it has been shown in several human clinical studies that wheat germ reduces intestinal inflammation, help the liver, stimulate immunity and help normalize cholesterol levels.

(Bakshi *et al.* 2012; Pyle *et al.* 2005; Lindfors *et al.* 2008; Stenman *et al.* 2009; Smecuol *et al.* 2013; Maki *et al.* 2012; Walton *et al.* 2012; Grant *et al.* 2001; Farkas 2005; Ostlund 2003; Cara *et al.* 1992; Demidov *et al.* 2008).

## What About Phytic Acid?

Anti-wheat proponents also contend that gluten grain's phytic acid content is too high. Yet phytic acid is not only within gluten-containing grains. It is found in a large range of foods. In fact, some of the highest amounts of phytic acid are contained among some of the healthiest nuts such as Brazil nuts and almonds, as well as sesame seeds and other healthful foods. These mentioned nuts can have as much as twice the phytate levels as many gluten-containing grains.

Yes, research has found that many unprocessed nuts and grains contain phytic acid. Phytic acid has been shown in multiple laboratory studies to potentially decrease the absorption of certain minerals, including calcium, iron and zinc.

However, it is not as simple as that. Phytic acid – also called inositol hexakisphosphate as well as phytate – is broken down into its soluble components (hydrolyzed) during soaking, cooking, fermentation and germination processes.

301

Phytates are also hydrolyzed by enzymes called phytases – which become available during the processes just mentioned. In the presence of a phytase, phytates are converted to inositolphosphates such as myo-inositol triphosphate, which do not block mineral absorption.

Phytases are available throughout nature. Upon germination, most grains will produce phytases to neutralize phytates. (Yes, nature is intelligent.)

And many bacteria also produce phytase – including intestinal bifidobacteria such as *Bifidobacterium infantis* – a bifidobacterium passed from mother to infant during birth and within breastmilk – and lactobacilli such as *L. acidophilus*, *L. plantarum* and *L. paracasei* – which are present in the guts of healthy persons. These and many other probiotic strains produce phytase, which in turn hydrolyze any remaining phytic acids not hydrolyzed during soaking, cooking, fermentation and/or germination (Sandberg 1991; Famularo *et al.* 2005).

Multiple studies have successfully tested the ability of these and other probiotic strains to hydrolyze phytic acid by producing phytase content. The probiotics that have been found to produce phytase include *Bifidobacterium bifidum* (Nalepa *et al.* 2012); *Bifidobacterium pseudocatenulatum, Bifidobacterium longum* (Tamayo-Ramos *et al.* 2012); and other bifidobacteria (Sanz-Penella *et al.* 2012). This adds to other Lactobacillus strains that have also been shown to produce the phytase enzymes (Tang *et al.* 2010; Lavilla-Lerma *et al.* 2013).

And it is for this reason that the Ancestors Diet promotes the consumption of cultured foods and supplements.

Grains have nourished billions of people for thousands of years. The ancient Ayurvedic formula for consuming grains with meals is to include yogurt with the meal. Though the soaking and longer cooking style of Ayurvedic rice and other grains (curried with turmeric and other spices) naturally reduces its phytic acid content, the accompanying yogurt helps immediately jump start the fermentation process.

This is followed up by the phytase produced by the intestines probiotics – leaving little if any phytic acid hydrolyzed.

The bottom line: If we care for our microbiome – our gut's probiotics – we shouldn't have to worry much about gluten sensitivity. Unless of course we are celiac – which very few of us are.

For the rest of us – our bodies and our gut's probiotics were designed to digest gluten-containing grains, along with so many other plant-based and cultured foods.

# Chapter Ten

# To Supplement or Not?

As we've discussed, antioxidant nutrition can significantly lighten our body's inflammatory load, and stimulate our detoxification processes. But do we need to supplement the Ancestors Diet?

For example, researchers from the Human Nutrition Research Center on Aging at Tufts University (Tucker *et al.* 2004) studied the relationships between homocysteine and B vitamins. They studied 189 healthy volunteers between 50 and 85 years old.

They gave the subjects either one cup daily of fortified cereal (with 440 micrograms of folic acid, 1.8 milligrams of vitamin B-6, and 4.8 micrograms of vitamin B-12) or an unfortified cereal (placebo). After twelve weeks, the fortified cereal eaters had significantly less homocysteine levels than did the placebo cereal.

A diet with a variety of plant-based fresh foods of sufficient quantity should require little if any supplementation, assuming an array of organically-grown foods and/or foods grown in healthy soils is eaten.

This said, there is also a likelihood that our diets may be lacking in some nutrients, especially if we live stressful lives and/or suffer from any sort of systemic inflammation.

In the latter condition, we are likely eating a narrow range of foods and/or exposed to a significant amount of toxins or infections. In other words, because toxins and infections 'burn up' nutrients – as the body requires these to neutralize radicals and produce enzymes – a person with systemic inflammation living in a toxic environment will likely require more nutrients than a healthy person living in a natural environment.

There are a number of isolated nutrients that have been shown to help reduce toxins. A few, like antioxidant vitamins C, A, D, and E and others have been shown to reduce inflammation by modulating inflammatory mediators and balancing Th1 and Th2 (Mainardi *et al.* 2009). Others, such as selenium, directly relate to the liver's glutathione processes for reducing toxins and radicals.

When a person's diet is lacking in an important nutrient, the body sometimes responds with critical weaknesses in immunity and inflammation. This can produce a greater tendency for toxin accumulation, simply because the body's supply of radical-neutralizing nutrients is decreased.

## Will the Ancestors' Diet Deliver on Nutrition?

We might entertain the argument that eating red meat is required for nutrition. Yet numerous studies have shown that vegetarian adults and children and those on the Mediterranean diet receive adequate nutrition on almost every aspect, and experience fewer deficiencies (Janelle and Barr 1995). A diet with cultured dairy, probiotic yeast foods and a broad range of nuts, grains, seeds and greenfoods (including, if needed, DHA-producing microalgae) will supply all the nutrients needed for health, including vitamin B12, as we'll expand upon.

## Nutrient Savvy

Many people are deficient in some or many nutrients, depending upon their diet. Even people who regularly take multi-vitamins become deficient in some nutrients. Why is this? This is an extremely complicated subject – one that could take an entire book to fully explore. To summarize, there are a number of reasons why people don't get the nutrients their body needs. These range from the more obvious – of poor diet choices – to the less obvious – of not being able to absorb certain nutrients due to enzyme issues, probiotic deficiencies and/or intestinal defects.

As has been shown in a number of studies, especially regarding B vitamins, a person may take a good multivitamin yet still be deficient because they lack the intrinsic factors that help assimilate those nutrients. In other cases, there is a chelation problem, where the nutrient is not absorbed because it doesn't have the right intestinal biofactors available within either the diet or the intestines. In still other cases, a nutrient may not be in a form that the body recognizes. This is often the case with synthetic multivitamins. In some cases, the body might treat the particular nutrient as a foreign molecule, and decide to break it down and expel it!

For those who are deficient in one or more nutrients, a good food-source supplement or change in the diet can immediately help their inflammatory hypersensitivity. Yet for another person, who may not be deficient in that nutrient, the nutrient supplement may not offer a significant change in toxicity and/or inflammation.

If a person is not deficient in the nutrient, taking more of the nutrient may not help them at all. Furthermore, overloading on isolated nutrients that have been shown to help those who are deficient can lead to a worsening of inflammation. This is due to the fact that synthesized, isolated nutrients can overload the liver and detoxification systems, as they have to be broken down. Some vitamins, such as vitamin A, can be toxic if over-supplemented. The bottom line is that for the most part, more is not necessarily better when it comes to nutrients.

So it is essential that we engage in a supplement strategy very logically. First, we need to have a healthy amount of plant-based foods in our diet, with raw, fresh foods with plenty of fiber and phytonutrients. This will create a solid foundation.

Secondly, we can add a food-based multivitamin as a sort of insurance policy to make sure we get enough of the most important nutrients. A food-based multivitamin is one where the nutrients are sourced directly from foods, or grown on food substrates such as spirulina. These sorts of multivitamins are more recognized by the body.

Thirdly, we can pay closer attention to certain nutrients that have been shown in some research to decrease inflammation. For these nutrients, we may decide to take a focused combination or isolated nutrient. But here we need to understand that many isolated nutrients can imbalance our body and create other deficiencies. Therefore, we need to approach isolated nutrient supplementation with caution. Best to err on the side of nature's balance of whole food sources, in other words.

For example, if we are taking more vitamin C, we can use a food-based or mineral ascorbate vitamin C supplement that offers chelated versions, and bioflavonoids that help the body assimilate and utilize the vitamin C.

If we are taking a mineral supplement like magnesium, we can take one that offers a chelated version together with calcium and trace minerals – offered by coral or mined sources, for example. The point here is that taking excess magnesium without the supporting and balancing minerals can exhaust the body of calcium, zinc and other essential, supporting elements.

We can also consult with a nutritionally-oriented health professional who can test our body's nutrient levels. Tests range from urine tests to blood tests and hair analyses – the latter of which may be appropriate to establish cellular mineral levels (Wilson 1998). This can be very helpful when trying to determine if we have a particular nutrient deficiency.

## Food-based Supplements

A food-source supplement is one where the nutrients have been produced by a living organism. The three key sources of natural nutrients are those produced by plants, those produced by probiotics, those produced by yeasts or those produced by the earth. These are nature's nutrients. Living organisms produce nutrients to protect themselves from the environment or other species. Thus, the nutrients they produce stimulate our immune system.

Our immune system also readily recognizes the nutrients, and our body and liver can readily metabolize these nutrients. They can be easily broken down and utilized, in other words.

Nutrients that are produced in a lab or manufacturing facility using synthesized substrates and catalysts can be recognized as a nutrient by the body, but many may not, especially if the immune system is already subject to inflammation. Such an immune system may not tolerate many synthetic nutrients.

As a result, the best nutrients on the market are:
> Nutrients that have been grown by yeasts or probiotics
> Nutrients that have utilized natural substrates (many use spirulina)
> Nutrients that have been derived directly from plant sources (vitamin C from acerola, for example)
> Nutrients that have been gathered from mines or dead coral (magnesium and calcium carbonate, for example)

Because these types of nutrients are produced by living organisms, they are well-recognized by the body, and well-utilized by the body.

## Nutrients Not to Isolate

With that said, we should know that nearly every nutrient has a role in the body's immune system and/or the liver's detoxification process. Thus we can really list practically every nutrient here. Instead, we'll just list a few "heavy-hitters" that are known to significantly stimulate cleansing. Remember, however, that the body needs a balance of nutrients. Therefore, it is advisable to not focus on isolated nutrients, but rather on living nutrients combined (chelated) within natural supplement substrates.

**Quercetin:** We also discussed quercetin foods previously. Quercetin supplements may be appropriate if the diet is lacking in plant-based foods. As mentioned earlier, this flavonoid inhibits histamine and leukotrienes – inflammatory mediators – in the body.

**Vitamin C** is considered by researchers as one of the "first line of defense" antioxidants, because it is readily available to neutralize free radicals at mucosal membranes and tissue fluids. A number of studies have shown that vitamin C can reduce inflammation.

Vitamin C supplement doses aimed at reducing inflammation typically range from one to three grams per day. As mentioned, chelated versions and versions with bioflavonoids help the potency of vitamin C. Some health researchers have also noted that vitamin C and quercetin tend to work well together. This is why apples and onions are so healthy. While fruits and many vegetables offer readily-assimilable doses of vitamin C with bioflavonoids, vitamin C drink powders with chelated ascorbates also provide a good way to supplement extra vitamin C.

**Lycopene:** This phytonutrient, usually isolated from tomatoes, has been shown in some research to reduce inflammation. Best approach here is to consume tomatoes, which have been found to contain about 10,000 different nutrients.

*Beta-carotene and other Carotenoids:* These vitamin A precursors are essential antioxidants often lacking in many diets. Some research has shown that carotenoids can reduce radical damage to the eyes and other organs.

*Vitamin E:* Vitamin E supplementation has been shown to provide significant antioxidant benefits. As a result, studies have shown that vitamin E can help prevent cardiovascular disease, respiratory diseases and cognitive impairment.

A few recent studies on vitamin E have shown inconclusive findings, however. What is going on here?

Most people consider vitamin E a single nutrient. But there are actually at least eight forms of vitamin E. Four of them are tocopherols, which include alpha-tocopherol, beta-tocopherol, gamma-tocopherol, and delta-tocopherol. There are also four tocotrienol forms of vitamin E. This includes alpha-tocotrienol, beta-tocotrienol, gamma-tocotrienol, and delta-tocotrienol. The primary vitamin E form in most supplements is alpha-tocopherol.

Most of the research on vitamin E has utilized only alpha-tocopherols. Ongoing research has established that alpha-tocopherols do provide some benefits, but a mix of tocotrienols provide more benefit – especially with regard to cardiovascular health.

Diets can vary in terms of their vitamin E forms. Western diets are typically restricted to alpha-tocopherols and gamma-tocopherols. However, a mixed plant-based diet that includes coconut and palm foods, whole grain rice and other whole grains will render more of the tocotrienol forms.

The bottom line is that the E vitamins are essential antioxidants that help prevent lipid peroxidation – as discussed earlier.

*Vitamin Bs:* All the vitamin Bs are important to the body's detoxification systems. They are most known for donating methyl groups, used by the liver and glutathione to scavenge free radicals. We should also note that toxins and pharmaceuticals will reduce our stores of Bs. Also, many people lack the intrinsic factor that allows for B vitamin – especially B12 – assimilation. For these people, many doctors have advised B12 shots.

Research has recently illustrated, however, that sublingual (under the tongue) B12 is absorbed just as readily into the blood as a B12 shot. There are several sublingual B vitamin supplements on the market today.

## Superfoods for Vitality

Isolated nutrients in large doses can also throw off the body's balance of other nutrients, as we've discussed. Many nutrients are called cofactors because their effectiveness requires the presence of other nutrients. This sort of cooperative character of nutrients is simply because the body's processes are heavily related to each other. As opposed to a lot of research, very little occurs in the body within a vacuum.

Superfood supplements are quite simply, extremely nutritious foods. Many – such as wheatgrass, spirulina, chlorella, barley grass and others – also typically contain generous levels of chlorophyll – which alkalizes the blood, stimulates more red blood cells, and helps neutralize radicals.

Many of these are available as supplements, as they may be dehydrated and encapsulated or pressed into tablets – or simply taken as a powder. Many superfood supplements – primarily nutritious fruits and vegetables such as noni, mangosteen and wheat grass – may also be eaten raw as we've discussed. We've covered some of these as greenfoods earlier, but we'll summarize some of them again just to underscore their importance to cleansing and reducing inflammation. We'll also introduce some new superfoods as well:

**Cereal Grasses**
Wheat grass is the young grass of the wheat species, *Triticum aestivum*. In addition to a plethora of vitamins, minerals, amino acids, phytonutrients, metabolic enzymes – including superoxide dismutase and cytochrome oxidase.

Early research by Dr. Charles Schnabel, Dr. George Kohler and Dr. A.I. Virtanen in the 1925-1950 era found that cereal grasses like wheatgrass achieved their highest nutrient content at around 18 days – right before the first jointing.

Wheat grass can increase blood hemoglobin levels. Wheat grass tablets decreased blood transfusion needs by 25% among 20 children requiring frequent blood transfusions in a recent study.

Barley grass maintains similar properties. Research has found that barley grass is a potent free radical scavenger; significantly reduces total cholesterol and LDL-cholesterol; and inhibits LDL oxidation. Barley grass juice powder can have 14 vitamins, 18 amino acids, 15 enzymes, 10 antioxidants, 18 minerals and 75 trace elements.

Another cereal grass is Kamut grass. The khorasan wheat has higher protein levels than most wheat varieties, and contains higher zinc, selenium and magnesium content. Selenium is known for stimulating glutathione activity as we've discussed.

Cereal grasses will contain up to 70% chlorophyll. Chlorophyll has been shown by laboratory and clinical studies to be antiseptic and bacteriostatic. In other words, chlorophyll kills or repels various types of bacteria, making it useful for various internal infections.

Chlorophyll has also been shown to increase hemoglobin levels in cases of anemia, especially in combination with supplemental iron. For this reason, because the grasses contain iron, they make great blood content builders. For this very reason, many athletes have found that eating cereal grasses gives them a competitive edge when it comes to endurance and speed.

Wheat grass, barley grass and kamut grass have been used with success for various healing and detoxification purposes. Nutritionists and alternative health professionals have recommended cereal grasses to alkalize the body--increasing the blood's ability to detoxify while boosting the productivity of the immune system. The combination of chlorophyll and antioxidant nutrients makes it the perfect way to protect the body against the stresses of our toxic world.

Cereal grasses have been shown to reduce inflammation and have beneficial effects upon the cardiovascular system as well. As the inflammation cascade is central to many disorders, cereal grasses are a great way to help deter or reduce the incidences of autoimmunity, allergies, and heavy metal toxicity.

Making cereal grasses part of our everyday diet is not hard. There are various juice grass powders available on the market. Look for dehydrated juice powder instead of simply dehydrated grass. To avoid the grassy taste simply blend the powder into a whole fruit smoothie. One to two teaspoons per day is enough to provide a wealth of health and energy.

For the quintessential wheat grass connoisseur, wheat grass can be easily grown in the kitchen or pantry. There are many small kitchen wheat grass kits available. One small tray of wheat grass can last for weeks, as the grass can be harvested (clipped with scissors) multiple times. Wheat grass is very sweet when fresh. It can be juiced or added to salads or sandwiches.

## Aloe

*Aloe vera* has been used traditionally for inflammation, constipation, wound healing, skin issues, ulcers and intestinal issues for at least five thousand years. Aloe's constituents include anthraquinones and mucopolysaccharides, which help replenish the mucosal membranes.

## Mushrooms

We discussed Reishi mushroom and Hoelen mushroom (*Wolfiporia extensas*) in the Chinese herbal medicine section earlier. Other mushrooms, such as Maitake (*Grifola frondosa*), Shiitake (*Lentinula elodes*), Turkey Tails (*Coriolus versicolor or Trametes versicolor*), Agaricus (*Agaricus blazeil*), Cordyceps (*Cordyceps sinensis)* and Lion's Mane (*Hericium erina-*

*ceus*) all have the distinction of stimulating the immune system and increasing tolerance. Blends of mushrooms are readily available in encapsulated supplement form.

## Lecithin

This is derived primarily from brewer's yeast and soy, and is known to contain choline and inositol – two nutrients beneficial for cell membranes and nerve cells. Lecithin has been shown to relax nerves and help smooth muscle function.

## Green Papaya

This superfood has been used to help rebuild weakened mucosal membranes. It contains a special enzyme called papain, as well as vitamins A, C, E and Bs. In fact, it contains more vitamin A than carrots and more vitamin C than oranges on a per-content basis.

## Bee Products

**Bee Pollen** has been recommended by traditional practitioners for inflammatory conditions because it contains a variety of antioxidant nutrients, enzymes, and proteins – many of which are derived from pollen. Clinicians have documented observing that bee pollen can increase tolerance and immunity in many of their patients. Bee pollen is best used from hives and honeybees harvesting pollens from the local plants if possible.

**Bee Propolis** is a resin collected from the conifer tree buds. Honeybees use it to plaster to their hives for stability and protection. Lab research has found more than 300 active constituents in propolis. These include aromatic oils, polyphenols, phenolic aldehydes, sequiterpene quinines, coumarins, flavonoids, esters, terpenes, lectins, cinnamic acids amino acids, minerals, vitamins to name a few. These appear to work synergistically to give bee propolis its reputation as antimicrobial and anti-inflammatory. Propolis extracts have been reported to increase healing rates, and have illustrated anti-tumor effects in a number of laboratory protocols. Free radical reduction and bone healing effects have also been observed in the research on propolis. In vitro lab studies show propolis appears to improve liver cell function.

**Royal Jelly:** This superfood, made by the Queen, supplies similar nutrients as bee pollen, along with others. Royal jelly supplies vitamins A, C, D, E, Bs, enzymes, steroid hormones, trace minerals and all the essential amino acids. Royal jelly is also a rare source for natural acetylcholine. Royal jelly has been recommended for inflammatory conditions for many centuries. It is also reputed to stimulate the adrenal and thyroid glands.

***Manuka Honey:*** Raw honey in general has been shown to be anti-microbial and soothing to the mucosal membranes. Thus, it is often used in cough syrups and sore throat remedies as we've described. Manuka honey is a special honey that comes from honeybees that harvest from the flowers of the Manuka bush (*Leptospermum scoparium*). This particular honey is thought to exert stronger health properties than normal raw honey. It is also reputed to be a remedy for ulcers, sinus infections and irritable bowels. Most of the world's supply comes from New Zealand, where the Manuka tree flourishes. This honey is also typically treated very gently to preserve its antioxidant and antimicrobial properties.

## Super Brans, Fibers and Seed Supplements

These include psyllium seed, oat bran, rice bran, fennel seed, flax seed, sesame seed, sunflower seeds and others. These supply mucilage, lignans and important plant fibers that stimulate mucosal membrane health and decrease levels of lipid peroxidation-sensitive LDL cholesterol.

## Plant Gums

These include guar gum and glucomannan. Most gums derived from plants provide mucilage and glucuronolactone, and other special polysaccharides. These constituents help maintain the health of our mucosal membranes. They also bind to toxins. Glucuronolactone is also a key component in many of the body's flexible connective tissues, which include the lungs.

## Sea Grasses and Algaes

(*Some duplication here with previous discussion of this topic. These are foods that can also be supplemented.*) Kelps might be called seaweeds, but these phyto-nutrient powerhouses are anything but weeds. About 1,500 species of sea kelps flourish, many in the North Pacific and North Atlantic oceans.

Most kelps are stationary, and sustainably harvested in the wild. This means they must be allowed to regrow to guarantee future harvests. *Asco-phyllum nodosum* kelp contains an impressive array of vitamins – more than many vegetables. They include over 60 essential minerals, amino acids and vitamins. They also contain growth promoters, according to kelp researchers.

Most kelps also contain fucoidan, a sulfated polysaccharide. Laboratory studies have indicated fucoidan has anti-tumor, anticoagulant and anti-angiogenic effects. It down-regulates Th2 (inhibiting allergic response), inhibits beta-amyloid formation (implicated in Alzheimer's), inhibits proteinuria in Heymann nephritis and decreases artery platelet deposits.

Other kelps include dulse, sargassi seaweed, *Undaria pinnatifida*, sea palm and others.

### Spirulina

Spirulina use dates back to the Aztecs. A good source of carotenoids, vitamins (including vegan B12 according to independent laboratory tests) and minerals, spirulina contains all essential and most non-essential amino acids, with up to 65% protein by weight. It also contains antioxidant phytonutrients such as zeaxanthin, myxoxanthophyll and lutein. It also will contain antioxidant carotenoids, vitamins and minerals.

Spirulina also contains phycobiliprotein, a unique blue pigment anti-inflammatory and antioxidant. Research has showed that phycobiliproteins can protect the liver and kidney from toxins. They are also anti-viral, and stimulate the immune system.

In one study from the University of California-Davis, 12 weeks of 3000 milligrams of Hawaiian spirulina per day significantly increased hemoglobin concentration and mean corpuscular hemoglobin among 30 adults over the age of 50. IDO (indoleamine 2,3-dioxygenase) enzyme activity – a sign of increased immune function – was also higher among the subjects.

### Chlorella

More than 800 published studies have verified the safety and efficacy of *Chlorella pyrenoidosa*. Chlorella's reputation of drawing out heavy metals and other toxins make it a favorite among health practitioners.

Chlorella maintains considerable vitamins minerals, and phytonutrients – including chlorella growth factor (CGF), known to stimulate cell growth. It is also a complete protein, with about 60% protein by weight and every essential and non-essential amino acid. Clinical studies have shown that chlorella stimulates T-cell and B-cell activity and contributes to the improvement of fibromyalgia, ulcerative colitis and hypertension. Another study showed that chlorella increases IgA levels and lowers dioxin levels in breast milk.

Chlorella's tough cell wall must be broken down mechanically to allow these nutrients' bioavailability. Our digestive enzymes cannot digest these outer cell walls. For this reason, quality chlorella growers will pulverize this tough outer cell wall.

### Haematococcus and Astaxanthin

Another greenfood algae is *Haematococcus pluvialis*, known for its high astaxanthin content. Astaxanthin is a strong carotenoid similar to beta-carotene. For this reason, astaxanthin is one of the most powerful natural antioxidants known. It also has anti-inflammatory effects, and has been used for eye health, joint healthy, muscle soreness, cardiovascular health, and skin health. It can also protect against damage from UV radiation.

### Blue-Green Algae from Klamath Lake

(*Some duplication here with previous. Left in for emphasis!*) *Aphanizomenon flos-aquae* or AFA, grows on the pristine waters of Klamath Lake in Oregon. Commercial AFA harvesting began in the early 1980s. This rich volcanic Klamath Lake gives AFA a good source of protein and all the essential and non-essential amino acids. It also has many vitamins, minerals and phytonutrients. AFA contains about 60% protein by weight, and at least 58 minerals at ppm levels, along with significant chlorophyll content.

One of the more exciting phytonutrient compounds discovered in AFA is phenylethylamine (PEA). PEA has been called the 'love molecule,' as it serves to increase positive moods. PEA is also found in chocolate. AFA has significantly more PEA, however.

### Red Algae

Red algae – from the *Rhodophyta* family – have been used for thousands of years for inflammation-oriented conditions.

Researchers from the National Taiwan Ocean University (Kazłowska *et al.* 2010) studied the ability of the red seaweed *Porphyra dentata*, to halt allergic responses. The researchers found that a *Porphyra dentata* phenolic extract suppressed nitric oxide production among macrophages using a NF-kappa-Beta gene transcription process. This modulated the hypersensitivity immune response on a systemic level. The phenolic compounds within the Red algae have been identified as catechol, rutin and hesperidin.

### Aloe Vera

While aloe has long been known for its skin irritation and wound healing abilities, science on its internal use is still emerging.

Aloe is now used for gastrointestinal health, immune support and cardiovascular health, as well as the health of the skin and mucosal membranes.

Aloe may also help prevent kidney stones. A study published in the *Journal of the Thailand Medical Association* found that 200 grams of fresh aloe gel a day significantly decreased urinary oxalate excretion.

In addition, a study from London's Queen Mary School of Medicine on 44 active ulcerated colitis patients found that internal aloe use resulted in clinical improvement. And double-blind, randomized research using Aloecorp's Qmatrix processed aloe has shown that it reduces oxidative stress markers and stimulates the immune system.

Aloe can be taken as a juice or a gel.

### Pine Bark Extract

Traditional herbalists have used pine bark extracts for respiratory conditions for centuries. The process of extraction is complex, however. Pine bark contains numerous constituents that yield health benefits, but also contains a high-density tannin complex requiring careful purification.

Today's standard for pine bark extracts is an extract of French Maritime Pine (*Pinus pinaster*) called Pycnogenol®. This extract is produced using a process patented by the Swiss company Horphag Research, Ltd. The process renders a number of bioavailable procyanidolic oligomers (PCOs), including catechin and taxifolin, as well as several phenolic acids.

Pycnogenol® has undergone extensive clinical study and laboratory research. Today, Pycnogenol® has been the subject of nearly 100 human clinical studies, testing over 7,000 patients with a variety of conditions. This extract's unique layered proanthocyanidin content has been shown, among other things, to significantly reduce systemic inflammation.

For example, in a German study (Belcaro *et al.* 2008), Pycnogenol® lowered C-reactive protein levels – known to increase during systemic inflammation and allergies – after 156 patients were given 100 milligrams of Pycnogenol® or placebo for three months. The average CRP decrease went from 3.9 to 1.1 following the treatment period. This is a 354% reduction in this important systemic inflammation marker after only three months of use.

In a study from the National Research Institute for Food and Nutrition in Rome, Italy (Canali *et al.* 2009), 150 milligrams of Pycnogenol® were given to six healthy adults for five days. After the five days, blood tests showed that Pycnogenol® interrupted the genetic expression of 5-lipoxygenase (5-LOX) and cyclooxygenase-2 (COX-2). It also inhibited phospholipase A2 (PLA2) activity. The Pycnogenol® supplementation program also reduced leukotriene production and altered prostaglandin levels. As discussed earlier, COX-2 and 5-LOX production is tied to inflammation processes.

Pycnogenol® also reduces histamine, another critical systemic inflammatory mediator as we've discussed. Researchers from Ireland's Trinity College (Sharma *et al.* 2003) found that Pycnogenol® inhibited the release of histamine from mast cells. The researchers commented that this effect appeared to be the result of the significant bioflavonoid content of Pycnogenol®.

Pycnogenol® has also been shown to reduce and inhibit NF-kB by an average of 15%. NF-kB is involved in the expression of inflammatory leukotrienes, as well as adhesion molecules. The matrix metalloproteinase 9 (MMP-9) enzymes known as conducive to inflammatory responses, is also reduced by Pycnogenol® (Grimm *et al.* 2006).

The bottom line is that Pycnogenol®, an extract bark of the French maritime pine tree, has been shown not only to reduce systemic inflammation in general through the radical scavenging abilities of procyanidolic oligomers.

## Living Minerals

Calcium research and media regarding calcium intake has been highly suggestive and to some degree mis-informative. The media and medical community has suggested that a person with a typical diet, especially as they age, is deficient in calcium. While it may be true that such a person, eating a western-modern diet of processed foods and meat may be experiencing a bone-calcium loss, the solution is not as easy as adding more calcium to the diet. Firstly, calcium is critical to numerous biochemical and metabolic activities within the body. While most of it is contained in the bones and teeth, it is also prevalent in nerve cells, artery wall cells, muscle tissues and many organs. It is necessary for muscle contraction, and is critical to the flexibility of the blood vessel walls.

It is also a vital part of the messaging systems of the nerves. We have discussed the calcium ion channels. These are key signally devices, passing intention throughout the body. Calcium is also a key component used in the expression of various hormones and enzymatic processes. These of course are signaling systems as well. We might conclude that while calcium gives our bodies structure, it is also a key element providing the key physical processes of communication through the body.

While we might think bones are fairly stable and permanent, they actually undergo a constant recycling process of remodeling. This is actually a biochemical process – a slow-moving oscillation between the deposit of minerals like calcium, boron and strontium into bone; and *resorption* – or a breakdown of these elements. While the body is young, there is more formation than resorption, yet the process is ongoing. The younger body's bones develop and grow: As the body ages, the bones resorb more than they form. They begin to grow more porous and even shrink and fuse in places. As a result, the recommended consumption of calcium grows as our body ages, as we attempt to replace the calcium we lose. Recommended allowances for a three year old are 500 milligrams a day, while those for a person over the age of 51 are 1200 milligrams a day.

It should be noted that these recommendations were made in consideration of the modern Western diet. This means the meat eater's diet. Countries with less meat eaters experience far less osteoporosis than those who eat higher quantities of meat or otherwise eat higher levels of protein. This is because the excess amino acid content in the bloodstream of a meat eater draws calcium from bones to become neutralized.

It should also be noted that calcium alone will not cause more bond formation. Boron, strontium, selenium, zinc and vitamin D are all elements necessary for good bone formation. Therefore, it is important we have balanced calcium supplementation. This means eating calcium from natural sources, which also have a balance of the other elements needed – along with good sunlight so we produce enough vitamin D.

Coral calcium is a good natural source of not only calcium, but various other trace elements. Despite the controversial history of coral calcium, interest and consumption of this supplement appears to be steadily growing. With over 70 ionic trace minerals and copious amounts of assimilable calcium carbonate, coral calcium is now a serious marine nutraceutical, and supply appears more sustainable than other marine calcium sources such as oyster shells.

Some debate now focuses on whether coral calcium is detrimental to living reef systems. Most agree that harvesting live coral is not sustainable, as world coral populations are on the decline. Many also have an issue with dry-land mining of dead coral from islands like Okinawa, which analyses show significantly reduced mineral content with increased heavy metal content. One company we noticed has a unique process of gathering the dead coral sediment from the ocean floor, which the company says sweeping it out provides for a healthier growing environment for the live coral around it. We have seen assays showing this coral powder with an almost ideal 2:1 calcium-to-magnesium ratio to add to a generous mineral content of more than 60 trace elements.

There is a great interest in bone mass maintenance today. Bone is actually an organ. It has a scaffolding-type matrix that distributes calcium bonded with a number of different ions. The bones do change dramatically with diet and activity, and without a healthy diet of various minerals as well as calcium and vitamin D, we can easily lose our body's bone mass prematurely (it is normal to lose bone mass very late in life as the body begins to die).

One of the key minerals that works conjunctively with calcium is strontium. Because it has been eclipsed in news reports by calcium and magnesium, strontium is not that well known. The reality is that strontium is a component of bone, and without it, calcium cannot properly build bone mass. Recent research using a pharmaceutical combination of strontium and renelic acid (called strontium renelate) has determined that strontium together with calcium and vitamin D aids bone mass building better than calcium and vitamin D alone (Marie 2006).

## Magnesium, Sulfur, Zinc and Other Minerals

Minerals are critical to our detoxification and cleansing processes because they donate ions that neutralize radicals, and are part of key en-

316

zymes. Without enough of these important minerals, the body's metabolic systems slow down, due to the lack of enzymes.

*Magnesium* deficiency has been found to be at the root of a number of conditions, especially those related to anxiety, spasms and muscle cramping. Not surprisingly, inflammation can be significantly reduced with magnesium supplementation.

Magnesium, along with calcium, is critical for smooth muscle tone and nerve conduction. Magnesium is part of the calcium ion channel system. Magnesium regulates calcium infusion into the nerves, which helps keep them stabilized and balanced. This is why magnesium deficiencies within the calcium ion channel system causes overstrain among muscles. This translates to spasms, cramping and muscle fatigue.

If magnesium levels are low, the ion channels will be unstable, stimulating nerve hyperactivity. This nerve hyperactivity can cause changes in the flow of nutrients into cells and toxins out of cells. In other words, magnesium deficiency can result in toxemia.

Magnesium is also a critical element used by the immune system. A body deficient in magnesium will likely be immunosuppressed. Animal studies have illustrated that magnesium deficiency leads to increased IgE counts, and increased levels of inflammation-specific cytokines. Magnesium deficiency is also associated with increased degranulation among mast/basophil/neutrophil cells, which stimulates the allergic response.

Dr. Jabar from the State University of New York Hospital and Medical Center, notes the blood magnesium levels can help determine if magnesium supplements can help. Magnesium levels among red blood cells indicate whether magnesium will likely have any effects.

It is no surprise that magnesium has also been shown to benefit anxiety, as it helps balance nerve firing. Magnesium has also been shown to have anti-inflammatory effects when combined with dosing with larger (one gram or more) doses of vitamin C.

Foods high in magnesium include soybeans, kidney beans, lima beans, bananas, broccoli, Brussels sprouts, carrots, cauliflower, celery, cherries, corn, dates, bran, blackberries, green beans, pumpkin seeds, spinach, chard, tofu, sunflower seeds, sesame seeds, black beans and navy beans, mineral water and beets.

*Calcium* is also critical for the functioning of nerves and muscles. Every cell utilizes calcium, evidenced by calcium ion channels present in every cell membrane. Therefore, calcium is necessary for healthy lungs and airways. Thus, calcium deficiency results in more than bone problems. Muscle cramping and airway constriction are also side effects of calcium deficiency. Low calcium levels also result in deranged nerve firing, which can produce anxiety and depression. Supplementing calcium should also be accompanied by magnesium supplementing. For example, a supplement with 1,000 mg of calcium can be balanced by 600 mg of magnesium along with trace minerals.

Good calcium foods include dairy, bok choy, collards, okra, soy, beans, broccoli, kale, mustard greens and others.

**Zinc** is another important mineral for toxemia. Researchers from Italy's INRAN National Research Institute on Food and Nutrition (Devirgiliis *et al.* 2007) have investigated the relationship between zinc and chronic diseases. Their research determined that an "imbalance in zinc homeostasis" can impair protein synthesis, cell membrane transport and gene expression. These factors, they explained, stimulate imbalances among hormones and tissue systems, producing inappropriate inflammation.

As zinc ions pass through the cell membrane, they assist the cell in the uptake of nutrients. Zinc transporters interact with genes to regulate the transmission of nutrients within the cell, and the pathways in and out of the cell. Zinc concentration within the cell is balanced by proteins called metallothioneins. These proteins require copper and selenium in addition to zinc. Metallothioneins are critical to the cell's ability to scavenge various radicals and heavy metals that can damage the cells. Deficiencies in metallothioneins have been seen among chronic inflammatory conditions, and even fatal diseases such as cancer.

Not surprisingly, research has also shown that zinc modulates T-cell activities (Hönscheid *et al.* 2009).

Good zinc foods include cowpeas, beans, lima beans, milk, brown rice, yogurt, oats, cottage cheese, bran, lentils, wheat and others.

**Selenium:** Research has shown that greater levels of lipid peroxidation (due to greater consumption of poor fats and fatty foods) decrease our body's levels of selenium. This is because selenium is a critical component of , glutathione peroxidase – which reduces lipid peroxidation. Those with higher levels of lipid peroxidation tend to require more selenium because they exhaust this nutrient more readily, as we discussed earlier. While selenium supplements might offer generous amounts of selenium, one brazil nut will supply about 120 micrograms of selenium. This is 170% of the recommended daily value.

**Sulfur:** Research has also confirmed that dietary sulfur can significantly relieve inflammation and hypersensitivity. In a multi-center open label study by researchers from Washington state (Barrager *et al.* 2002), 55 patients with allergic rhinitis were given 2,600 mg of methylsulfonylmethane (MSM) – a significant source of sulfur derived from plants – for 30 days. Weekly reviews of the patients reported significant improvements in allergic respiratory symptoms, along with increased energy. Other research has suggested that sulfur blocks the binding of histamine among receptors.

Another study (Kim *et al.* 2006) of 50 patients with knee osteoarthritis given either 6 grams per day of MSM) or a placebo for 12 weeks found that after 12 weeks, the MSM group had significantly less pain and significantly more mobility than the placebo group.

Supplemental MSM is typically derived from plant sources. Good food sources of sulfur include avocado, asparagus, barley, beans, broccoli, cabbage, carob, carrots, Brussels sprouts, chives, coconuts, corn, garlic, leafy green vegetables, leeks, lentils, onions, parsley, peas, radishes, red peppers, soybeans, shallots, Swiss chard and watercress.

***Potassium*** is lowered by many pharmaceutical medications, toxins and sweating. Low potassium levels will contribute to imbalances in blood pressure and the kidneys. These issues reduce our ability to cleanse toxins.

Good potassium foods include bananas, spinach, sunflower seeds, tomatoes, pomegranates, turnips, lima beans, navy beans, squash, broccoli and others.

***Trace minerals:*** These should not be ignored in this discussion. Trace elements are important to nearly every enzymatic reaction in the body.

While minerals have been shown to provide therapeutic results, we must be careful about mineral supplements, especially those that provide single or a few minerals. Minerals co-exist in the body, and a dramatic increase in one can exhaust others as the body depletes the oversupply. Thus, an isolated macro-mineral supplement can easily produce a mineral imbalance in the body, which can produce a variety of hypersensitivity issues.

Better to utilize natural sources of minerals. These include, first and foremost, mineral-intensive vegetables. Nearly all vegetables contain generous mineral content in the combinations designed by nature. Best to eat a mixed combination of vegetables to achieve a healthy array of trace minerals.

Whole food mineral sources also contain many trace minerals in their more-digestible *chelated* forms. Chelation is when a mineral ion bonds with another nutrient, providing a ready ion as the body needs it.

Most organically-grown plant-based foods provide a rich supply of trace minerals, assuming we are eating enough of them. Other good sources of full spectrum trace minerals include natural mineral water, whole (unprocessed) rock salt, coral calcium, spirulina, AFA, kelp and chlorella. These sources will typically have from 60 to 80 trace elements, all of which are necessary for the body's various enzymatic functions. See the author's book, *Pure Water.*

We should also note that research by David Brownstein, M.D. (2006) has illustrated that whole unprocessed salt does not affect the body – high blood pressure, cardiovascular disease, diabetes and so on – as do refined salts (often called sodium).

These naturally-chelated mineral sources also prevent the side effects known for mineral supplements. For example, magnesium can easily produce diarrhea in the 2,000-5,000 milligram level. While this might be considered a minor side effect, diarrhea can also produce dehydration.

Numerous holistic doctors now prescribe full-spectrum mineral combinations for inflammatory conditions. Many have attested to their clinical successes in recommending minerals to balance the inflammatory response and stimulate healthy mucosal membranes. Full range supplements that have RDA levels of the macrominerals combined with trace levels of the other minerals can provide a good foundation. Eating more than 5-6 servings a day of fruits and vegetables can provide the rest.

## Vitamin B12 Solved

We might entertain the argument that eating red meat is required for nutrition because it supplies vitamin B12.

Yet numerous studies have shown that vegetarian adults and children and those on the Mediterranean diet receive adequate nutrition on almost every aspect, and experience fewer deficiencies (Janelle and Barr 1995). A diet with cultured dairy, probiotic yeast foods and a broad range of nuts, grains, seeds and greenfoods (including, if needed, DHA-producing microalgae) will supply all the nutrients needed for health, including vitamin B12.

Recent studies out of India have indicated that as the country has become more developed, rates of coronary artery disease and heart disease in general have increased.

Some have erroneously applied the cause to vegetarianism. As the theory goes, vegetarians do not get enough B12, and this has caused the increase in heart disease.

The study (Kumar et al. 2009) that is being quoted tested 386 coronary artery disease patients and 448 control subjects for vitamin B12 deficiency, homocysteine and cysteine levels. In this test, the heart disease patients had lower levels of vitamin B12 and higher levels of cysteine. The researchers were puzzled by this, because they expected higher levels of homocysteine, not cysteine.

The researchers assumed that vegetarianism caused the B12 deficiency because most of the B12 deficient people were vegetarian (but so are a lot of people in India), so vegetarianism must be at the root of the coronary artery disease. Right?

Wrong.

Numerous studies over the past four decades have illustrated that vegetarians have lower rates of heart disease worldwide, and meat-eating increases the rate of heart disease. We've documented only a few of these in this book. Countries with the highest meat diets have the highest rates of heart disease (Jolliffe and Archer 1959).

Just to name a few recent studies, researchers from Harvard's Department of Nutrition (Bernstein et al. 2010) followed 84,136 women between 30-55 years old for 26 years. Those who ate the most red meat had the highest rates of heart attack.

In a study by Spain's University of Madrid School of Medicine researchers (Guallar-Castillón et al. 2010), 40,757 people between the age of 29 and 69 years old were followed for eleven years. They found that the Mediterranean diet was associated with significantly lower risks of coronary heart disease.

The Physicians Health Study by researchers at Boston University's School of Public Health (Ashaya et al. 2010) followed 21,120 men with an average age of 55 years old from 1982 to 2008. They found that red meat consumption was associated with higher risks of heart failure. Furthermore, they found that the more red meat consumed, the higher the risk.

The assumption that vegetarian diets lead to B12 deficiencies is also a false one. Among developing countries vitamin B12 deficiency is increasing across the board, especially so amongst countries known for their meat diets.

In a review of B12 deficiency around the world by University of Colorado researchers (Stabler and Allen 2004), Europeans have one of the highest levels of B12 deficiency in the world, along with South Americans, Central Americans, Africans and Mexicans. These are not countries known for being vegetarian. In fact, these countries have some of the highest meat-eating rates.

Furthermore, most of the vegetarians of India consume cow's milk, a rich source of vitamin B12 (however, many in the poor regions may not have adequate dairy availability).

The fact is, B12 deficiency, or pernicious anemia – an inability to absorb vitamin B12 is a complex disorder that may involve the loss of intrinsic factor, a lack of intestinal receptor sites, sprue, gluten allergy, ileitis, or even parasites. A lack of probiotics, or other intestinal problems may also be at issue (another topic altogether).

In fact, some of the same regions mentioned above these are also areas known for higher levels of *H. pylori* infections. In a study from researchers from Turkey's Gülhane Military Medical Academy (Kaptan et al. 2000), 77 of 138 patients suffering from vitamin B12 deficiency were infected by *H. pylori*. Eradication of H. pylori led to healthy levels of B12 absorption and a reversal of B12 deficiency symptoms in 40% of the patients. Others likely had other absorption problems.

In a study from Sweden's University of Gothenburg (Lewerin et al. 2008), elderly subjects with B12 deficiencies also had higher levels of gastritis and *H. pylori* antibodies.

Furthermore, among Americans, where a meat diet is widespread, 10-15% of people over the age of 60 has B12 deficiency according to research from the USDA's Human Nutrition Research Center on Aging at Tufts University (Baik and Russell 1999).

In other words, it is no surprise that coronary artery disease patients in an Indian Hospital are low in vitamin B12, and not surprising that most were also vegetarian, because most people in India are vegetarian. This select study was focused upon heart disease patients, most of whom also have problems with B12 absorption.

Like many other developing countries, India is experiencing more heart disease because of its increase in refined, foods, processed foods and fried foods. These foods damage intestinal health, promote free radicals, and are nutrient-poor. Frying foods also produces acrylamide (Ehling et al. 2005). Acrylamide (as we've discussed) can lower the body's levels of glutathione, which may well be why the Indian patients in the Kumar study mysteriously had high levels of cysteine (a component of metabolized glutathione.) And it is also interesting that countries with higher levels of B12 deficiency also happen to be developing countries known for diets high in fried foods.

Furthermore, why would heart disease be growing in India only recently? Indians have been primarily vegetarian for thousands of years.

Assuming healthy B12 digestive absorption, the Ancestors Diet delivers plenty of B12 from cultured milk, yogurt, whey, nutritional yeast, malts and probiotic (cultured) foods. Vegans may have to look to nutritional yeast, cultured foods, fortified foods and supplements for their B12.

## Getting D

Multiple studies have found that inflammatory diseases are significantly greater among regions further from the equator and those with less sunlight exposure. In both Europe and the U.S. – with the exception of urban areas with greater air pollution – those living in Southern regions have shown significantly lower incidence of many degenerative diseases, along with fewer hospital visits.

Vitamin D induces cathelicidin production (Grant 2008). Cathelicidins are proteins found within the lysosomes of macrophages and polymorphonuclear cells (PMNs). These immune cells are intensely antiviral and antibacterial in nature. They are also stimulated and regulated by vitamin D within the body.

Many conditions have been shown to be improved or prevented by therapeutic sunlight and/or vitamin D.

These include, lupus vulgaris, small pox, Pick's disease, tuberculosis, asthma, nervous diseases, adrenal insufficiency, hormone imbalances, congestive heart failure, cardiovascular disease, multiple sclerosis, rheumatoid arthritis, Crohn's disease, irritable bowel syndrome, acne, psoriasis, jaundice, depression, eczema, high blood pressure, heart disease, diabetes, hypothyroidism, angina, prostate cancer, lung cancer, colon cancer, ovary cancer, kidney disease, hyperparathyroidism, uterine cancer, stomach cancer, kidney cancer, lymphoma, pancreatic cancer, ovarian cancer, tooth loss, bone loss, obesity, joint inflammation, insomnia, Parkinson's disease, fibromyalgia and a variety of immune- and autoimmune-related diseases.

In all, research over the past ten years has found that sunlight and/or vitamin D deficiency is implicated in over 70 disease conditions.

The sun's ultraviolet-B rays stimulate our bodies to synthesize vitamin $D_3$. Vitamin D is more of a hormone than a vitamin. It is a critical biochemical for the body. The cholesterol derivative *7-dehydrocholesterol* undergoes a *conrotatory electrocyclic reaction* to produce a pre-vitamin D. The pre-vitamin D molecule undergoes hydroxylation in the liver and kidneys to convert to the final $D_3$ structure – 1,25 dihydroxyvitamin D (or 25-OHD).

Within a 7-dehydrocholesterol-saturated biomolecular environment of the epidermis, specialized cells called *melanocytes* produce a protective biochemical called *melanin*. Skin melanocytes are primarily located at the lower strata of the epidermis. Other melanocytes located around the body produce specialized forms of melanin. Melanocytes within the uvea, which contains the iris, produce the melanin that gives the color to our irises. Melanocytes around our hair follicles give color to our hair. Melanocytes within the leptomeninges residing within our brain and spinal cord produce a type of melanin thought to support cerebrospinal fluid circulation.

Once produced in skin melanocytes, melanin is transferred to the keratinocytes, which lie on the external skin barrier. Melanin is the biochemical pigment that makes the skin turn brown. Melanin also provides a natural sunscreen for the skin: The greater the melanin level, the fewer ultraviolet-B rays reach the 7-dehydrocholesterol molecules, and the less vitamin $D_3$ is produced. Vitamin D is used in thousands of metabolic processes around the body. What is not used is stored within fat cells for later use.

Vitamin D is considered a cell membrane antioxidant. It specifically inhibits the lipid peroxidation process. Research has found that vitamin D inhibits lipid peroxidation better than cholesterol – a typical inhibitor. One study found its lipid peroxidation properties have anti-cancer benefits (Wiseman 1993).

While some mushrooms and some seafood can be good sources of vitamin D, the best source is the sun. Additional effects and mechanisms of sunlight and vitamin D are discussed in my book, *Healthy Sun.*

# Chapter Eleven

# Preparing the Ancestors Diet

## The Art of Eating

In our modern world, food preparation has nearly become a lost art. Our ancestors respected and revered the eating ceremony as a nutritional necessity. We appreciated the magical flavors and colors of food with thankfulness and spiritual ceremony.

In drastic contrast, modern western society has turned the eating function into a wolf-down race of convenience and haste.

As we race through our stressful modern technologies, we grab overly processed convenience meals, sacrificing nutrition for a full belly.

The result of this process is not only indigestion, but a lack of harmony with our diet. In our haste we have truly missed the essence of the food our bodies need for nourishment. And we have missed the conscious aspect completely.

This is not just mumbo-jumbo. Researchers from the UK's University of Southampton Medical College (Grimshaw *et al.* 2013) determined that an infant fed an early diet incorporating more homemade foods and more fruits and vegetables is significantly less likely to have food allergies.

The researchers tested 41 infants who had been diagnosed with food allergies along with 82 other infants who did not have food allergies. Food allergies were determined with food challenges.

The researchers collected food diaries from the mothers for all of the children through their first two years of life. They then analyzed the food diaries for eating patterns, including their intake of fruits and vegetables, processed foods, homemade foods and so on.

The researchers found that the children who ate more homemade foods with fruits and vegetables and fewer processed foods during their first year of life were significantly less likely to have food allergies by the age of two.

The researchers concluded:

> *"An infant diet consisting of high levels of fruits, vegetables, and home-prepared foods is associated with less food allergy by the age of 2 years."*

In an interview with Reuters Health, Dr. Kate Grimshaw – lead author of the study – gave some background on the possible relationship between early diet and food allergies:

*"We know that there are nutrients in the diet that educate the immune system. And one could argue that if they're not there in adequate amounts when the child's immune system is developing, that may be one way that this is working."*

This relationship between foods and our immune system doesn't end during childhood.

From a purely chemical level, when we eat a gigantic bite and wash it down with liquids, we completely bypass the all-important functions of chewing and oral enzymes. In order to properly digest our food, we must thoroughly masticate it.

If our bodies didn't have such a narrow, long windy digestive tract, mastication wouldn't be so important. Most of us have seen how snakes can swallow a mouse whole. This is because their digestive tracts are radically different from ours – they are wide and short, with powerful enzymes.

A masticated food mass mixed with chyme is called the *bolus*. As the bolus reaches our stomach, it should be more fluid than solid. This allows for the stomach's gastrin and pepsinogen to reach most of the molecular matter to begin breaking it down and preparing it for its path through the small intestines.

The right bolus is accomplished by chewing intently until the food can slide down the esophagus without the necessity of fluids. The bolus should have the consistency of a smoothie.

The salivary glands aid this process by infusing amylase into the food. Amylase is a potent enzyme that breaks down complex carbohydrates and fibers into more simple carbohydrates. We might say the mouth is the first stomach.

While we are chewing, we can calmly breathe. Breathing while eating calms the body and slows the rush to swallow. It also gives the body a good dose of oxygen – a necessary element to aid digestion. And by oxidizing the bloodstream, which in turn supplies energy via the gastric arteries to the fundus glands, the pyloric glands and the cardiac glands lying within the stomach are nourished. These glands produce the various digestive juices such as pyloric acid, gastric acid, pepsin converted from pepsinogen, and other stomach enzymes. Balancing these acids are various hormones secreted by the cells of the mucosal membrane of the stomach. Hormones such as *gastrin, somatostatin, enteroglucagon* and *inhibitory peptide* (or GIP) all work to balance the acidic content of the stomach. Without a balanced secretion of these hormones the stomach is faced with the prospect of peptic ulcers and GERD – commonly known as *acid reflux*. A good supply of oxygen also helps relax the vagus nerve, which is involved in the stimulation and release of the various stomach enzymes and hormones from the stomach's glands, the liver and the gall bladder.

The digestive tract was designed for small, frequent meals. If we can imagine foraging around the forest, eating fruits, nuts, leaves and berries as we find them, and then having a periodic group or family meal, this would probably best describe how our digestive tracts work. Most of our diet research has supported this fact as well. People who eat 4-6 smaller meals a day tend to keep the weight off more easily. This is primarily because the carbohydrate and fat parts of our meals are more thoroughly assimilated and more efficiently used, as opposed to converted to fatty acid molecules and stored into adipose cells for later use.

On the other hand, should we breathlessly stuff our food down, not only will we lack the oxygen to feed these glands and cells, but our mental intensity resonates through the limbic system to the vagus nerve. This biochemical cascade stops the flow of digestive enzymes. This physiological response is rooted in the survival situation. If a tiger started running towards us while we were eating our bodies would respond by halting all digestive activities and redirecting that blood flow and nervous energy towards our muscles, eyes and other regions to escape the tiger. This might cause a bit of ingestion but it might save our body.

Preventing our body from responding to our anxieties means we have to put our anxieties away while we're eating. This means relaxing and breathing while we're eating. We might also consider meditative thinking or engaging in relaxing and pleasing discussions with other members at the table. Laughing is also good for digestion. We may have to try to stagger the laughter between bites a bit, but laughter both soothes the vagus nerve and relaxes the diaphragm and chest for easier breathing. Breathing easy with a lack of tension while chewing slowly and thoroughly will create the foundation of good nutrient absorption. After all, why eat if we are not absorbing our food and just getting indigestion?

Research over the past decade has indicated that over half of ulcer cases are accompanied by a bacterial infection of *Helicobacter pylori*. This bacteria species has been observed colonizing sections of the stomach damaged with ulcers. While the research is compelling, to make the assumption that ulcers are caused by an infection of *H. pylori* appears a bit hasty. The question is how, in the presence of tremendous acidity within the stomach (with pH levels from four to five), such a bacteria could survive. The question also becomes how this infection became rooted in the first place. The facts lend themselves to the reality that the environment of the infected person was somehow compromised.

In addition to this reality, the "hole" of the peptic ulcer – *H. pylori* infection or not – is a wearing away of the mucosal membrane that protects gastric cells from the acids secreted into the stomach. Should this membrane become weakened the stomach acids will begin destroying the gastric cells, producing the ulcer. Something has weakened this mucous membrane protecting the stomach. When this mucous membrane – made up of some of the secretions mentioned above – becomes thinner or changes chemistry, this compromised environment leaves our bodies open to both infection and damage from the acidic secretions.

The key here is a balanced diet of phytonutrients and a good supply of oxidized blood while we're eating. This means breathing during eating. If we are shoveling food in while talking, we're not getting much in the way of oxidized blood to the glands mentioned above. An excess of fatty and overcooked foods will render the stomach open to the effects of free radicals. These radicals can begin their damage of the mucosal lining, just as they damage the blood vessel walls. A balance of phytonutrients with each meal will go far to provide antioxidant and neutralizing effects. Phytonutrients will also supply the nutrients needed for the body to protect the wall of the stomach. This is accomplished by the production of an alkalinic mucosal membrane lining within the walls of the stomach and esophagus.

This brings us to the topic of antacids and acid-blockers. Many who have experienced GERD or indications of pre-ulceration either reach for over the counter antacids or acid-blockers. Often a doctor will prescribe these as medications.

While a temporary blocking of stomach acid may be necessary to heal an ulcer after surgery or while undergoing therapy, the use of these medications comes with dangerous implications, which may well be connected to the *H. pylori* epidemic. Antacids include aluminum-based magnesium hydroxide (Maalox® and Mylanta® for example); aluminum carbonate (Basajek®); aluminum hydroxide (AlternaGEL®); calcium carbonate (Rolaids®, Tums®); or magnesium hydroxide (Milk of Magnesia®). Obviously, many of these mineralized chemicals, especially the aluminum-bases, offer us a dangerous build up of undesired metal ions. Antacids work by neutralizing our acids. This is dangerous because with our acids neutralized, our stomachs are open to allowing foodborne bacteria into the body. The hydrochloric acid content of the stomach is part of our immune system. It prevents infection. Antacids have also been shown to inhibit absorption of phosphorus, calcium, folic acid and citrate. (Gaby 1997; McHardy 1978; Spencer and Kramer 1983; Nolan *et al.* 1990; Russell *et al.* 1988).

Histamine (H-2) blockers such as Tagamet®; Pepcid®, and Zantac® block the production of stomach acids. This opens the stomach not only to infection as mentioned above, but also prevents the assimilation of various nutrients required by the body. These include vitamin B12, magnesium and iron. In addition, these H-2 blockers also appear to reduce vitamin D activation. (Threlkeld 1998; Aymard *et al.* 1988; Salom *et al.* 1982; Bachmann *et al.* 1994; Anonymous 1985; Threlkeld 1994).

Another way to block stomach acid production is with proton pump inhibitor medications. These drugs have been shown to cause an almost complete loss of stomach acid, causing a reduction of assimilation of beta-carotene, vitamin B12 and folic acid. Again this strategy also opens the stomach and the rest of the body to bacterial infections.

Could the combination of *H. pylori* infection observed in over fifty percent of ulcer patients be caused by their prior use of these types of medications? Have the studies screened the patients for use of these to eliminate that possibility? Hardly. As most of these studies are led by researchers or institutions funded by or connected to the pharmaceutical companies, that screen would be risky. (Tang *et al.* 1996; Koop and Bachem 1992; Schenk *et al.* 1996; Russel *et al.* 1988; Marcuard *et al.* 1994; Brummer *et al.* 1997; Threlkeld 1998).

Nature provides a range of solutions to GERD and ulcerative conditions. These include various botanicals called *demulcents,* such as slippery elm, licorice, marshmallow root, and ginger. These botanicals stimulate the action of the various gastric glands. They also promote the production of the mucosal lining of the stomach, along with the various hormones and enzymes that protect the gastric cells from being damaged by stomach acids. These herbs, along with the proper amount of water consumption (as a healthy stomach lining requires good water intake), healthy probiotic colonies, and a balanced botanical diet will ensure a strong and healthy gut.

The above discussion indicates the extent of the biological qualities of digestion. Our entire digestive tract moves within the undulations of peristalsis. As we discussed previously, peristalsis is the rhythmic contraction of the smooth muscles governing the stomach, intestines, and colon, but also connecting the digestive operations of mouth, esophagus, liver, and rectum. The contraction of the muscles around these regions encourages the various secretions of the liver, gall bladder, stomach glands, and intestinal cells. While muscles in each region contract slightly differently and to different rhythms, they all synchronize to complete overall rhythms. While three to eight cycles per minute are seen around the stomach, ten to twenty cycles per minute are seen in the intestines. The colon's rhythm tends to mirror the pacing of the stomach. These slow oscillations vibrate at frequencies reflecting the 'grounded' plane of survival. For this reason we often feel comforted by food. We will connect food with our anxieties related to family, loneliness, and acceptance.

This is a good practical example of how rhythms can be transmuted from the external environment to ones internal physical processes. At the biochemical level, the bio-voltaic balance of acids, enzymes, hormones and mucosal lining all work to keep the system acidic enough to sterilize and break down food, yet alkaline enough to create a chyme ready to enter the sensitive intestinal tract. A disruption of the delicate balance is quite easy, as we are faced with a hostile or uncomfortable situation. Anxiousness or fear initiate autonomic responses, immediately altering the rhythms associated with our breathing rate, our peristalsis rate and the various enzyme and hormone secretions required for proper digestion.

The art of delivering the correct food into our body brings together a number of skills. These skills include selection of the proper food. The food should have the right color, aroma, ripeness, cleanliness, texture, nutrition, and timing. A view towards the conscious elements of the food will limit the impact we have upon other creatures. The food we choose must then be prepared for eating. A humble respect towards the raw food and its completeness during preparation can render a dish rich in phyto-nutrients. A more conservative preparation will usually result in a more nourishing meal. Giving a spiritual context to our meal and sharing food with the people we hold dear helps facilitate relaxation while digesting. We might want to avoid eating during any traumatic or stressful circumstances. This way, our meal can be eaten with respect and calmness. We can chew slowly and breath a little while chewing.

Following a graceful and appropriate conclusion to the meal – without getting too full – we can take a nice walk or another calm activity. This will help to escort the food through the system with a minimum of regurgitation, heartburn, indigestion, or bloating. Most nutritionists agree that eating too late or plunking down on the couch after a big meal is not that good of an idea. Our digestive processes all work better if we follow our meal with a gentle walk or other movement. A soft and gentle self-massage in the abdominal region in a clockwise fashion can be added help stimulate the digestive processes.

Ron Rosedale, M.D., and author of the bestseller *The Rosedale Diet*, has done extensive research on the physiological characteristics common among longer-living organisms. Dr. Rosedale has compiled research performed since the 1930s on various species of organisms – including humans. This research has studied rodents, worms, monkeys, and humans. After analyzing these various studies, Dr. Rosedale has concluded a number of commonalities between longer-living organisms, in contrast with their shorter-living counterparts:

Longer living organisms tend to have lower fasting insulin levels. They tend to have lower fasting glucose. They tend to have lower body temperatures. They tend to have lower body fat levels. They tend to have reduced thyroid hormone levels. They tend to have lower levels of triglycerides. Some have also shown lower fasting leptin levels (because leptin levels have only recently begun to be measured).

Taken as a whole, this means those who live longer are those who eat less; eat less sugary and fatty foods; relax more; have lower levels of metabolism; have lower levels of body fat; and have lower blood-based triglyceride levels.

What does this mean for a healthy diet? We should probably eat only as much as we need to sustain health. We should probably eat healthy foods with lower levels of processed fats and processed sugars. We should probably try to maintain our balance, and take things with 'a grain of salt.' We should exercise regularly.

## Local, Organic, Rotated

Over the past 20 years, the organic movement has grown from a whisper to a roar. In the early years of organic farming and distribution, the thought of growing foods without the use of dangerous pesticides and herbicides was considered radical. Let's restate this another way: The methods of growing foods humankind has been using for thousands of years – without the use of chemicals – was considered radical.

When we consider that today millions of tons of chemicals are being dumped onto our mother earth not intended to be there in the name of greater food production and profits, it is not hard to understand that food was not meant to grow this way. The entire picture of chemical farming is one of imbalance. Organic food producers have proven that food can be grown without dangerous chemicals. The original intent of chemicals was to preserve and protect crops from the ravages of various insects and disease which destroy crops from time to time. This seemingly positive intent has gone awry due to humankind's arrogance that nature cannot provide its own mechanisms to achieve these results.

Consider for a minute that most diseases and pest issues are caused by an imbalance between humankind's activities and nature's rhythms. For example, instead of growing crops indigenous to that particular locality and environment, we choose to mix and match regions with various seed varieties. Instead of farming while adapting to the particular biodiversity of the property, we prefer to clear the land and grow row crops. Instead of each of us growing our own food, or supporting local farmers in growing our foods, we prefer to ship unripe food thousands and thousands of miles from where it is grown.

In nature, there is a balance to all things on both gross and subtle levels. We can see this balance existing in all actions. There is a reaction for every action. For every act made without respect, sensitivity, and humility, a resulting reaction serves to remind us that there is a superior design engaging a greater intelligence and consciousness among nature.

Not so long ago a family farm produced a myriad of crops the family and children ate, including vegetables, corn, squash, cabbage and others. Today's farms are a different animal altogether, and monoculture food production is not only proving to be hard on the land, but it is also increasingly causing allergies in our children.

Allergy specialists from France's Nancy University and the Allergy Vigilance Network (Moneret-Vautrin *et al.* 2012) conducted a large-scale study of children and adults with regard to their sensitivity to the monoculture crops of corn and rapeseed – grown on giant farms in the midst of small towns scattered throughout Europe.

The sixty-nine allergy researchers, members of the Allergy Vigilance Network, included 2,515 children and 2,857 adults in the study. The subjects were tested for either having an allergy or sensitivity to these crops – or having an immune sensitivity that would likely to develop into an allergy.

The research found that among the 5,372 total people tested, 62% suffered from some sort of allergy with symptoms, while 10% had an allergy but no symptoms, and 27% had no allergies. Of those who had allergies, 26% were allergic to maize/corn pollen while nearly 12% were allergic to rapeseed pollen. And over 8% were allergic to corn seed.

But among those who lived closer to monoculture farms that planted and harvested these crops, the allergy rates to those crops were much higher. Of the allergic individuals, nearly 14% of those living near rapeseed crops were allergic to rapeseed, while over 21% of the asymptomatic allergic people were sensitive to rapeseed (compared to 8% among the study population).

Of those asymptomatic allergy sufferers who lived closer to farms, over 30% were allergic to corn/maize pollen (compared to 19% among the study population).

These statistics reveal not only a growing trend of allergies related to monoculture crops, but the closer we live to the farms, the more likely their allergies to these crops are.

The researchers concluded:

> *"The incidence of sensitization to rapeseed and maize pollen is positively correlated to the level of exposure.... The frequency of sensitization confirms the allergenicity of these plants destined for food supply and demonstrates the importance of monitoring for respiratory allergies to these pollens, not only in workers exposed to these types of crops, but*

*also in atopic patients living in regions that contain a high density of rapeseed and maize fields."*

The researchers also correlated other studies that have shown that pollen sensitivities can lead to certain food allergies:

*"Cross-reactivities between pollens and seeds could potentially elicit cross-reacting food allergies."*

In the last fifty years, families throughout the world have increasingly given up the production of food for their families and communities. Huge populations of people who once homesteaded their land to produce food have moved to the cities, where population density and pollution is making us sicker and our environment more polluted.

This trend is spawning the growth of giant monoculture farming companies that typically do not replenish the soil, but use chemical fertilizers and monoculture crops. This depletes precious soil nutrients – causing massive soil erosion. And the widespread use of chemical fertilizers is wrecking havoc in our oceans and waterways – producing "dead zones" throughout the world with massive sealife die-offs.

Monoculture has also resulted in the loss of nearly three-quarters of the plant varieties that once gave us nutrition.

Should we continue along this path, the future will no only bear us more limited varieties of food that tastes the same where ever we go: It may also result in us becoming allergic to many of our own foods.

Though we have the power of choice, we certainly do not have the power of control (otherwise, we could control the reaction). Should we act as though we have the power of control, we are served up with an education process. This education illustrates that we should be acting within the physical environment with humility, respect, and sensitivity. This means respecting and utilizing nature's design.

Should we continue to act as if in control (and thus out of balance) even through we have been served with education, the natural reaction can become more traumatic. This is what is occurring around the process of global warming. Global warming is nature's response for our arrogant abuse of natural resources.

Rather than organic farming being radical, it should be considered balanced and respectful. We can understand it is balanced as we review the research indicating that organically grown foods contain higher levels of nutrients and lower levels of pesticide residue. We can understand that organic food has greater balance when our research tells us that the soils used in organic cultivation are healthier, contain more nutrients, and do not erode as fast. We can understand organic production is harmonically correct when we observe that organically grown grain has a greater tolerance for drought and a greater resistance to pests.

One of the central reasons that organic farming is a balanced form of agriculture is because it requires that crops are rotated. Rather than re-tilling and chemically-fertilizing, followed by planting the same crop – which can lead to erosion and soil deprivation – organic farmers must plant cover crops and alternative crops between repeating crops. This follows nature's biochemical patterns, as each type of crop adds back different features to the soil, depending upon the time of year.

We can see, taste, and smell this balance when we compare organic fruit with fruit grown with pesticides. While the organic fruit may not look as "perfect" as the conventional fruit, the taste and nutrition reveal the inner balance. All of these biological attributes – nutrition, taste, smell and sustainability – all illustrate that organic food production is quite simply the better way to eat and produce food.

There are also other considerations to make when we select our foods – some of which may require us to compromise on organic. We should know where the product was grown.

Long-distance shipping of foods is problematic for several reasons:

The most obvious being the amount of carbon dioxide created. The second is the effect this transportation has upon the food itself. Shipping and storing food requires extra preservation techniques. Preservation requires either refrigeration, freezing or cooking and jarring/canning in order to travel the journey. Other techniques include using outright preservatives, nitrogen flushing, and/or various grades of plastic containers. Preservation techniques can have damaging effects upon the food to one degree or another – especially those involving chemicals that can leach into the foods to produce radicals and toxins.

While shipping may be necessary to gain access to fresh foods for some areas; if the food is also grown locally, why should we buy the shipped-in version?

## Organic Foods Proven More Nutritious

Several studies have illustrated that organic foods not only have less pesticide residue, but they are more nutritious as well.

A study from French and Brazilian researchers (Oliveira *et al.* 2013) affiliated with France's University of Avignon and Brazil's Federal University Ceara compared organic tomatoes grown in the Northeast region of Brazil with conventionally-grown tomatoes grown in the same region under similar conditions.

The researchers then took numerous samples through the growing season, and compared various nutritional components, including brix levels (natural sucrose), pH, antioxidant activity, phenolic content, anthocyanin content and yellow flavonoid content, vitamin C content, enzyme content, fatty acid content, chlorophyll content and lipid peroxidation levels.

At the ripe stage, the organic tomatoes had significantly higher levels of many of these nutrients and medicinal benefits. The organic tomatoes at the ripe stage had:

- *139% higher levels of total phenolics — more than double*
- *140% higher phenylalanine ammonia lyase levels — a measure of enzyme activity*
- *90% higher antioxidant potency — measured by superoxide dismutase levels — a measure of free radical scavenging potential*
- *72% higher yellow flavonoid content*
- *57% higher levels of vitamin C*
- *28% higher levels of acidity — % of citric acid*
- *57% higher brix levels, which influence taste — sweetness*

At the same time, the organic tomatoes were 40% smaller when mature compared to the conventionally grown tomatoes.

The researchers also found evidence that the organic tomato plants produced more nutrients as a result of being stressed more than the conventional tomatoes. The primary elements related to the comparative increases in both phenolics (or polyphenols) and enzyme levels. Because stress tends to increase enzyme activity, this likely resulted in the higher phenolic content.

In their conclusion the researchers stated:

> *"Our work clearly demonstrates that tomato fruits from organic farming have indeed a smaller size and mass than fruits from conventional growing systems, but also a substantially better quality in terms of concentrations in soluble solids and phytochemicals such as vitamin C and total phenolic compounds. Until recently, the focus has been mainly on yield rather than on gustative and micronutritional quality of fresh plant products. This might be all right for staple food, but, as far as fruits and vegetables are concerned, it may be argued that gustative and micronutritional quality matter more than energy supply."*

As we have mentioned earlier, polyphenols are plant compounds that have been linked with preventing heart disease, dementia and cancer.

Furthermore, the researchers found that the "gustative" levels — a quality of taste — of the organic tomatoes were significantly higher than the conventional tomatoes. In other words, the organic tomatoes quite simply tasted better.

This new finding confirms previous research that also showed that organic fruits tend to contain higher levels of certain nutrients such as lycopene, vitamin C and phenolic content.

For example, researchers from Warsaw University of Life Science's Faculty of Human Nutrition and Consumer Sciences (Hallmann *et al.* 2012) have determined that organically grown sweet bell peppers contain more antioxidants than conventionally grown sweet bell peppers.

The research, led by Professor Ewa Rembialkowska and Dr. Ewelina Hallmann, performed a side-by-side comparison of organic sweet bell peppers and conventional sweet bell peppers (*Capsicum annuum* L.).

The researchers found that the level of carotenoids and polyphenols were significantly higher among the organic bell peppers. Levels of vitamin C, total carotenoids, beta-carotene, alpha-carotene, total phenolic acids, gallic acid, chlorogenic acids, quercetin D-glucoside and kaempferol were all higher in the organic bell peppers compared to conventional bell peppers. These phytonutrients are all key antioxidant compounds that have been independently confirmed as being able to neutralize free radicals in the body, stimulate the immune system, and deter infections by bacteria, viruses and fungi.

This is not the first study that has shown that organic foods maintain higher levels of nutrients.

Other research (Mohammed *et al.* 2011) has illustrated that organic tomatoes contain more vitamin C, quercetin, kaempferol and other phenolic acids than conventionally grown tomatoes.

Other studies comparing organic grains, vegetables and fruits have all resulted in similar conclusions.

The central reason that organic foods typically contain more nutrients is because organic farmers utilize natural forms of fertilizers. These natural fertilizers provide the soil with a host of soil nutrients not supplied by conventional fertilizers. Conventional fertilizers, typically chemical-based, will spike up levels of a limited range of nutrients. This might include, for example, nitrogen and phosphorus and a few others.

An organic fertilizer will also contain these, plus up to 70 different trace elements and many other soil nutrients. Organic fertilizers also supply soil with humus and organic matter that adds soil fertility and beneficial organisms. These include nitrogen-fixing bacteria and worms that keep the soil loose and rich.

Continual use of synthetic fertilizers, on the other hand, can produce soil erosion. The lack of beneficial organisms and a broad range of nutrients causes the soil to become malnourished, producing weaker plants. In this state, the soil results in reduced nutrient content among the plants.

Organic growers also typically rotate their crops. This means they might grow a vegetable crop one year, followed by a grain crop or a cover crop the next year. This alternating of crops allows the soils to replenish their nutrient content, especially when cover crops are plowed back into the soil.

Organic certification agencies require this sort of soil stewardship by organic growers. Organic means the soil is being nurtured, allowing for sustainable crop production. This contrasts greatly to conventional crop production, where there is no oversight, causing widespread soil erosion.

Organic farming is also better for our environment because it does not utilize pesticides and herbicides that damage our environment. These toxic chemicals are now are seeping into our drinking waters where they are polluting our bodies. As this website has reported, the use of certain types of pesticides has also been linked to the bee colony collapse, which is decimating our bee populations throughout the U.S. Bees are necessary to pollinate crops.

The easiest way to support organic growing methods is to buy organic foods. We'll be healthier, and we'll make the world more sustainable.

In other words, we can change the world with our wallets.

Economically, organic tomatoes provide more bang for the buck, so to speak — at least when it comes to taste and nutrition. Thus in most cases, organic is well worth the slightly higher price — especially when we consider the disastrous effects pesticides, herbicides and chemical fertilizers are having on our environment.

A farmer's market question to ponder is whether organic food trumps locally grown. The answer is unclear, and we will each probably need to decide this for ourselves depending upon the situation. For some foods, we can easily find locally produced organic alternatives. No brainer. For others, we cannot find anything locally that comes close. How important is the imported food to our health?

Of course there needs to be some criteria set forth to make a decision between distant organic or locally grown conventional foods. At some point the distance organic might add more negative health consequences to our environment than a locally grown food that sprayed once or used some nitrogen fertilizer. Most likely the organic food will still be healthier, but at some distance away for the organic food, the conventional local food might. Anyway, this will be a personal decision.

Buying locally-grown foods also synchronizes our bodies with the seasonal and genetic nature of our local growing region. Eating foods with the season harmonizes nature's output with our needs. For example, nature will produce more vitamin-C rich fruits such as citrus and apples during the fall and winter season. This is also the time of year when our bodies require more vitamin C, as they face the additional stresses of changing weather and colder temperatures – and additional indoor time. Increasing our apple and citrus intake during the winter months will naturally increase our immunity. Just as nature intended.

At the end of the day, it is probably wise to utilize locally grown foods as much as possible, while seeking out or suggesting our local growers either convert to organic or reduce their spraying habits.

If most of us were to have our own private or local gardens, and eat locally as a community, we would find the need for storage and freight would be minimized. There would be less need for refrigeration because much of the food is kept fresh on the vine until it is ready to be eaten. Food may be dried, frozen, or even canned for use in the winter. Compare this to gigantic industrial farms, where large harvesting machines gobble up huge quantities of petroleum to operate, then requiring gigantic storage facilities to store the foods. This requires some foods to be fumigated for preservation and to prevent insect damage. Some foods will require massive refrigeration units. Then the food will usually require packaging in plastic containers to be shipped to the markets. One of the more interesting phenomena regarding this process is that the local communities where these massive farms and processing facilities are located do not experience lower costs than the markets located thousands of miles away for those goods grown in the community. What is wrong with this picture?

All of this extra processing creates an increased amount of complexity to a process largely solved with local community farms. The various processing manipulations required for this massive enterprise applies increasing negative biochemical interference to the food. The food is picked early, stored, chilled, warmed, rechilled, pasteurized, put in plastic and then sealed under nitrogen. By the time it gets to our table, it has probably lost much of its nutrition and health-giving properties.

This is especially the case when the food is altered structurally and repackaged.

## Risks of Pesticides

Today over five billion pounds of pesticides are applied to our crops, households and other areas we share with insects. Many of these pesticides have been shown to be neurotoxic – they damage nerves and nerve transmission. Three-quarters of the twelve most dangerous chemicals (aka the "dirty dozen") used by man are pesticides according to the Stockholm Convention on Persistent Organic Pollutants.

Many of these pesticides have been proven to be neurotoxins. Organochlorine hydrocarbons are one of the most widely used types of pesticides in commercial farming enterprises. These include DDT (dichlorodiphenyltrichloroethane), which is banned in the U.S. but not in many other countries where lots of our food is grown. DDT's analogs such as dicofol and methoxychlor are also in use. Other neurotoxic organochlorine hydrocarbons include hexachlorocyclohexane, lindane, gamma-hexachlorocyclohexane, endosulfan, chlordane, heptachlor, aldrin, dieldrin, endrin, kelevan, mirex, chlordecone, toxaphene and isobenzan. Most of these will cause changes to the central nervous system by altering potassium, sodium or calcium ion channels.

Today many of the organochlorines have been replaced by organophosphates, but these will alter neurons by blocking acetylcholinesterase enzymes. Cholinesterase enzymes are acetylcholine inhibitors. Increased acetylcholine availability leads to excessive to neuron firing, resulting in nerve excitability, long term nervousness, nerve weakness and even paralysis.

We have heard about the toxicity of pesticides. Let's look at an example of just how real this toxicity is.

A review of research from Belgium's Catholic University of Louvain (Van Maele-Fabry *et al.* 2012) found that Parkinson's disease is linked to occupational exposure to pesticides.

The researchers, working with the Louvain Center for Toxicology and Applied Pharmacology, analyzed studies between 1985 and 2011 that looked at pesticide exposure by workers who handled pesticides. These included farm workers who sprayed pesticides.

The research found that those who handled pesticides were significantly more likely to contract Parkinson's disease. In four studies, where the Parkinson's diagnoses were confirmed by neurologists, those handling pesticides had an average of over two-and-a-half times the risk of contracting Parkinson's disease. The increased risk ranged from 46% higher to almost four-and-a-half times higher among the workers.

Three cohort studies, which followed larger populations and compared them to the general population, concluded that workers handling pesticides had close to twice the risk of contracting Parkinson's disease than the rest of the population. (It should also be noted that the general population typically also has constant contact with pesticide residue in the form of foods and household pesticides.)

One of these cohort studies showed workers handling pesticides had almost three times the rate of contracting Parkinson's disease.

The researchers found significant rates of increased Parkinson's disease risk among workers in banana plantations, sugarcane fields and pineapple farms.

Another study, this from the University of California (Gonzalez *et al.* 2012), tested Mexican-American mothers and their children living in agricultural regions with higher pesticide exposure. The researchers monitored 202 mother-and-daughter pairs for relative levels of paraoxonase, acetylcholinesterase, and butyrylcholinesterase enzymes and their respective activity among neurons. The researchers confirmed that pesticide exposures not only affect adult acetylcholinesterase levels, but also affect children under the age of nine years old more than adults. They also concluded that children born of pesticide-exposed parents have even lower levels of acetylcholinesterase – relating to the higher risks of nerve disorders.

Other pesticides, such as imidacloprid and related neonicotinoids are neurotoxins in turn bind to nicotinic acetylcholine receptors – important to healthy nerve firing. These pesticides are also suspected in bee colony collapse disorder.

Manufacturers of neonicotinoid pesticides have claimed that the chemicals will not affect human acetylcholine receptors. However, a study by researchers from the Tokyo Metropolitan Institute of Medical Science (Kimura-Kuroda *et al.* 2012) found that the neonicotinoids imidacloprid and acetamiprid "had greater effects on mammalian neurons than those previously reported in binding assay studies."

As for those of us not handling pesticides on the job or at home, pesticide residues are found on a majority of commercially grown foods. In a review of the research by Cornell University's Dr. David Pimentel (2005), 73% to 90% of conventional fruits and vegetables contain pesticide residues, with at least 5% of those pesticide levels above FDA tolerance amounts.

While the cost of organic foods might be a tad higher in the store, the price paid in the long run for pesticides in terms of liver disorders and nervous disorders such as Parkinson's – as well as environmental damage to our bees, waterways and soils – makes the real price for organic foods cheap in comparison.

## Cooking for Health

Hopefully this book has clarified that cooking should be done minimally. How do we minimally cook our foods?

First, some foods are best eaten cooked. This is especially true for practically every grain, as cooking softens the bran and fibers, depletes phytates and in general, makes the grain tastier and easier to eat.

First start with whole grains or beans. Brown rice, whole grain couscous, whole lentils, whole peas, whole grain pasta and so forth.

Cooking grain is typically done with boiling water, but it can also be done with soaking. In fact, if we prefer, we can soak the grain – assuming it is vital – until it sprouts, and just heat it.

However, this will not taste so good, as the polysaccharides will be consumed during sprouting, making the dish a little sour.

Some profess doing these to completely deplete the phytates, but as we discussed in the gluten chapter, healthy intestinal bacteria produce phytases that break down phytates.

Bringing the water to a boil first is preferred but not necessary to cook grains or pasta. Salt is helpful for flavor, but utilize one of the natural salts discussed in the salt section.

Then it is about not overcooking. This is accomplished by testing. The grain or bean should be just soft but not mushy. The grain should be easily crushed between the fingers but not mashable.

When it comes to pasta, we're talking al dente: This is when the pasta is soft enough to be minimally sticky. The famous test is to through it against the wall, but just between the fingers is fine. It should just barely be sticky, but again soft enough to be crushed between the fingers.

As for other foods, vegetables and roots should be either eaten fresh or steamed. Broccoli, squash, carrots, beets, spinach, bok choy, even celery can be steamed.

Pass on the butter (unless it is unpasteurized) and go straight for the raw coconut oil to "butter" up the vegetables. Delicious!

Steaming is also great for potatoes instead of boiling or baking. While baked potatoes are delicious, pass on the aluminum foil or over an open flame. These all overcook the potato, leaving a once-nutritious food a mashable lump of starchy carbohydrates. Steamed potato can be eaten whole or cut up and mashed, and "buttered" with coconut oil. Yum.

Another option to baking is a convection oven. These circulate the heat to create a more evenly-baked food, possibly using less overall heat.

At issue, as we've discussed, is destroying precious phytonutrients. Minimally cooking means getting the food into tasty, delicious form but not mushy and overcooked.

When it comes to baking breads, rolls or any other flour-based food, best to start with a whole wheat flour and then use yeast or sourdough mix rather than baking powder – which can contain aluminum or similar metals.

Yeast and sourdough are best because they help break down phytates, gliadins and other grain components. Cooking the bread will also help break these down as well, but baker's yeast is a digestive aid. A good baker's yeast is also a source of B vitamins and other nutrients.

In general, baking is better than frying, boiling is better than baking and steaming is better than boiling. Raw beat all of these in the case of most fruits and veggies.

Steaming is second best because it retains the most because the food is buffered from the highest temperatures by the water moisture. This helps preserve more of the precious phytonutrients.

The reason boiling is better than baking is that the water will help retain nutrients, plus some phytonutrients will end up in the water and soak back into the food. For this reason, when boiling roots or vegetables, it is better to just bring the heat to a boil and then turn the heat off, and let the food stand in the water until it cools enough to serve and eat. This will preserve more nutrients.

This can also be done with cooking grains, beans and legumes. Instead of cooking to the end, put a little less water in, and cook to the point where there is still some water left at the bottom (maybe a ¼ inch) and then cover the pan and let the grain steam cook for the remainder.

Frying should be done sparingly if at all. Frying overheats the food and chars it. This will produce HCAs and PAHs as we've discussed earlier.

This also goes for open-flame cooking. If you must use an open flame, put a pan over the fire and steam or boil the food instead of grilling it. Grilling is one of the worst things we can do to our body, even if the food is vegetarian.

## Microwave or Not?

We are increasingly preparing our foods in microwaves. Is this smart? Let's take a closer look.

Microwaves produce two different forms of radiation: High frequency radiowaves producing an electromagnetic frequency in the range of 2450 megahertz, together with 60 hertz magnetic fields. This bombardment of combined electronic pulse and magnetic fields polarize the molecules of the water or food. It is thought this electromagnetic combination will rotate food molecules at speeds approaching the 2450 million cycles per second.

This tremendous kinetic movement translates to heated water or food. The problem is, along with this heat, other electromagnetic effects upon the food are observed. The thin rays can break and damage the biochemical bonds between food molecules and atoms. It is the breaking of the bonds releases energy in the form of heat. These are the nutrient bonds in the food. Because the biochemical bonds have been altered and rearranged by the sporadic pulses of radiation, we cannot be convinced the nutritional aspects will remain the same. Certainly simple observation confirms dramatic effects not seen when we cook food otherwise. A well-cooked microwave dinner reveals dry and rubbery textures not seen in real food.

Studies (Knize *et al.* 2007) at the University of California Lawrence Livermore Laboratory concluded that microwaves produced *heterocyclic aromatic amines* and *polycyclic aromatic hydrocarbons*. Both are suspected carcinogens. Frying forms primarily the polycyclic aromatic hydrocarbons.

Dr. Lita Lee's 1989 *Microwaves and Microwave Ovens* report reveals a number of interesting facts regarding the history, use and research on microwaves: Microwave ovens were developed by the Nazis for the war operations. After the war, the research the Germans performed on microwaves were classified by the U.S. War Department. The Soviets also obtained some of this information after the war. The Soviet Union shortly thereafter banned the use of microwaves. They issued an international warning on the health hazards of microwaved foods. Other Eastern European researchers reported the microwave's harmful effects as well.

*The Atlantis Rising Educational Center* in Oregon determined that a number of carcinogens form during microwaving in nearly all types of foods. Microwaving meats caused formation of the carcinogen *d-nitrosodiethanolamine*. Microwaving milk and grains converted amino acids into carcinogenic compounds. Thawing frozen fruit by microwave converted glucosides and galactyosides into carcinogenic chemicals. Short-term microwaving converted alkaloids from plant foods into carcinogenic compounds. Carcinogenic radicals formed from microwaving root vegetables.

In December of 1989, British Medical Journal *Lancet* reported that microwaves converted trans-amino acids to cis-isomers in baby formulas. Another amino acid, L-proline, converted to a d-isomer version. This version has been classified as a *neurotoxin* (toxic to the nerves) and *nephrotoxin* (toxic to the kidneys).

Research from Russia indicated nutritional reductions of sixty to ninety percent in microwave tests. Decreases in bioavailable vitamin Bs, vitamin C, vitamin E, minerals, and oil nutrients were observed. Confirming the Oregon research, alkaloids, glucosides, galactosides and nitrilosides – all phytonutrients – were found damaged by microwaving. Other proteins were degraded as well.

The leakage of various toxins from packaging during microwaving has also been documented. A 1990 *Nutrition Action Newsletter* reported various toxins leaked onto microwaved foods from food containers. Suspected carcinogens benzene, toluene and xylene were among chemicals released into food. Also found was polyethylene terphtalate (PET). Various plasticizers are almost certainly to be included in this list, as they will quite easily out-gas when heated.

Dr. Lee also reported pathogenic changes observed among micro-waved food consumers. They include increased lymphatic disorders, increased cancer cell formation rates, increased rates of stomach and intestinal cancers, and a higher rate of digestive disorders.

Dr. Becker's *The Body Electric* reported various disorders such as cardiovascular difficulties, stress, headaches, dizziness, anxiety, irritability, insomnia, reproductive disorders, and cancer in the Soviet Union among microwave-exposed workers when the Soviets were developing radar during the 1950s.

One issue to realize is that microwaving – -unless done for extended periods – rarely completely sterilizes a food. This should be a warning for all those who pack leftovers into the fridge – which attracts bacteria – and think two minutes in the microwave will kill all those buggers.

Well, sorry. There may be some die-off in the localized areas where the wave pulses cause higher-energy heat releases. For the most part, there are still bacteria remaining in that food. The longer the food was kept after its original cooking, the more bacteria it will probably be infested with – refrigeration or not. (Yes, bacteria do live in the fridge. Bacteria will also live in the freezer as well. We can wipe them down with vinegar and baking soda periodically to help control their populations.)

If the microwave is not avoidable there are a few things we can do to slow down the bond-mutating process. One is to apply a teaspoon or two of water around the food being cooked. We can sprinkle the top of the food with water as well. This way the water bonds are broken by the radiation, providing heat to the food hopefully before too many of the food's own bonds are broken. This should help preserve some of the nutritive energy of the food, while at the same time providing a better foundation for sterilization of the food.

The controversy over microwaves can be solved personally by this one experiment. While there are a number of experiments that have shown the negative effects of microwaved food and water, they have been refuted by a number of well-respected researchers and governmental agencies who do not want to see any difference in the health effects of microwaved water and food. Most researchers do agree however, that microwaves do not sterilize food as cooking does. This fact has been un-avoidable by the *Salmonella* outbreaks among those who took food home in doggie bags to microwave later.

This bombardment of food molecules is not the intended use for microwaves. We can however, cook food with natural microwaves. Natural microwaves traveling from the sun and other radiating sources are based upon direct current, while microwaves utilize an alternating current of up to 1000 watts. This alternating current creates an additional polarized oscillation exerting a different set of waveform influences.

These polarizing frequencies can reverse molecular and atomic polarity at speeds in the billions of times per second, as mentioned earlier. This action creates the friction that heats the surrounding molecules. As this takes place, a process called *structural isomerism* takes place. This is the damaging and deforming of molecular structure. This can also cause the decay of some of the molecules – a *radiolytic* effect.

This polarity reversal effect has been observed on amino acids of microwave-cooked foods. Swiss food scientist Dr. Hans Ulrich Hertel and Dr. Bernard Blanc of the Swiss Federal Institute of Technology reported in a 1991 paper that microwave food created cancerous effects within the bloodstream.

The small but controlled study had eight volunteers consume either raw milk; conventionally-cooked milk, pasteurized milk; microwave-cooked milk; organic raw vegetables; conventionally-cooked vegetables; the same vegetables frozen and warmed in a microwave; or the same vegetables cooked in the microwave oven. Blood tests were taken before and after eating.

Subjects who ate microwaved milk or vegetables had decreased hemoglobin levels, increased cholesterol levels and decreased lymphocyte levels. Interestingly, the Swiss Association of Dealers for Electro-apparati for Households and Industry brought charges of "interfering with commerce" against Dr. Hertal and Dr. Blanc. They were convicted and issued a "gag order." Five years later the European Court of Human Rights reversed this decision.

The increase in leucocytes concerned Dr. Hertel the most. Increased leukocyte levels in the bloodstream are generally connected with infection or tissue damage. As this element is combined with the molecular damage and polarity reversals, it is logical to assume that microwaves create an increase in radicals damaging to tissues and cells.

Ever wonder why the microwave door is grated and heavily paneled to keep microwaves from leaking out? While many focus their concern on the damage that might be done to our bodies should their be a leak, we might want to focus a bit more on what is happening to the food being put in our bodies after being pummeled with alternating-current microwaves.

We can do a simple test to determine whether we want this type of electromagnetically radiated water in or around our body. Start with two plants of the same kind and age. Water one with tap water that has been microwaved and cooled to room temperature, and water the other with the same tap water but without microwaving. After a short period we will see that one of the plants is not healthy. That will be the one watered with microwaved water.

In 2006, Marshall Dudley's granddaughter completed a science fair project that did just that: She compared plant feeding between stove-boiled filtered water and the same filtered water source but microwaved. She took several genetically identical, same-aged potted and pruned young plants of identical health. She fed one group of plants filtered water boiled in a pan and cooled.

She fed another group the same filtered water, but microwaved until boiling and cooled. The 'watering study' went on for a period of nine days, and pictures of each plant were taken each day. Then method allowed for a simple assessment of each plant's health through the photographs; allowing the monitoring simply by observing the color, shape and texture of their leaves and their rate of growth through the study period.

Each day the effect of microwave water between the two groups become increasingly apparent: The plants being fed the microwave water were dying. The boiled water group kept growing taller, with greater foliage. The microwave-water fed group became increasingly withered and slumped over in obvious stress. By the ninth day, the microwave-watered plant had lost most of its leaves while the boiled-watered plant stood tall with crisp green leaves.

Nothing is more emphatic than pictures. In this case, it was extremely clear that microwaves damage the molecular structure of not only water, but also as Drs. Hertel and Blanc revealed through their research, that food has no place being irradiated through microwaving.

## About Juicing

Juicing has been advocated for many years by a number of health experts and nutritionists. Many have promoted juicing for detoxification and cleansing. This is not the case here.

However, juicing is a suboptimal way to glean the benefits of fruits and vegetables. This is because while juicing definitely retains many of the water-soluble phytonutrients, it leaves behind this phytonutrients that are not water-soluble. Many phytonutrients are complexed within the plant fibers of fruits and vegetables. And most juicing machines separate out the fiber, where they'll end up in the trash or compost. What a crime against nutrition!

The moral here is that plant fibers together with water-soluble phytonutrients will render more nutritional benefits than the water-soluble phytonutrients will alone. While many water-soluble phytonutrients are antioxidants that bind to toxins and neutralize radicals such as lipid peroxides, fiber attaches to LDL cholesterol in the intestines, which prevents them from becoming lipid peroxides in the first place. Fibers also attach to numerous other radicals and toxins within the intestines, flushing them out through the colon. *This prevents their entry into the bloodstream.*

While juicing is may be practical for a few hard fiber vegetables like carrots, the best strategy for most other fruits and vegetables is to make smoothies.

A smoothie is made by putting the whole fruit or vegetable into a blender (after peeling in the case of oranges and the like, although orange peels are also a great cleansing nutrient). To the fruit we can add some water, a greenfood powder, and perhaps some kefir or yogurt, and don't forget some form of fiber – either flaxseeds, wheat germ or chia seeds.

Kiwis with the skins on are also great sources of fiber and antioxidants. For thinner consistency, simply add more water, and for thicker consistency, less water. Some incredible frozen fruits are available at most stores – including berries, mango, pineapple and so on. Add bananas for prebiotic sweetness.

While juice can also be added to our smoothies, juices are not recommended in the living cleanse diet. This is because juices have been separated from their fibers, and this makes the juice not wholesome. Furthermore, many commercial juices are pasteurized or flash-pasteurized, rendering many of the enzymes and antioxidants useless, and often denatured.

Furthermore, the sugars in pasteurized juices can turn to more simplified versions, rendering them unstable and acidic upon consumption and subject to becoming radicals within the body.

This denaturing can easily be observed. Simply pour some pasteurized filtered orange juice into a glass. Now peel an orange and put into the blender. Pour that into a glass next to the juice glass. Now take a gulp of the juice, and then take a gulp of the orange smoothie.

You will taste the difference. As you let the juice slide past your throat, take an extra swallow and see if you do not sense the acidification of the juice on the epithelia of the throat/esophagus. Now do the same with the smoothie. The smoothie will go down, uh, okay, *smooth.*

## Antioxidant Food Remedies

Okay, so I couldn't help myself but to add a few – but just a few – recipes. These are not just typical recipes though. They provide superior antioxidant power. They are remedies that help stimulate detoxification and immunity:

- *Super salsa:* This Mexican dish provides cilantro, garlic, cayenne peppers and tomatoes to stimulate blood purification. Chop and mix to taste. Fresh diced tomatoes are best.

- *Honion syrup:* Equal parts chopped onions and raw honey provides constituents to stimulate the immune system. Heat on low for 5 minutes, then cool.

- *Horseradish syrup:* Equal parts grated horseradish and honey will clear the sinuses and open the airways, while providing an alkalizing effect.

- *Lemon and honey:* This remedy is often blended with an herbal tea such as peppermint or chamomile. The combination of lemon juice and honey provide an alkalizing and cleansing effect. Add honey and lemon together after tea is finished seeping, just before drinking.

- *Garlic syrup:* Garlic and raw honey combine two antimicrobials and immune-system boosters. Crush a bulb of garlic and add one tablespoon of raw honey.

- *Super pickles:* Jerusalem Artichokes, celery and carrot, pickled in apple cider vinegar provide a great alkalizer and blood purifier. Cut the vegetables in large pieces, soak in the vinegar for a day or two.

- *Raw vegetable juices:* Juiced endive, celery and carrots. These feed us with immediate nutrients that stimulate our immune system and alkalize our blood. Better with a blender.

- *Super soup:* Barley, celery, carrots, beets and ginger. These also provide significant blood alkalizing effects, liver cleansing and stimulate the immune system. Mix together into boiling water. Simmer on low heat. When vegetables are soft, serve.

- *Super fruits:* Raw apricots, blueberries, blackberries, strawberries. These provide significant levels of antioxidants. Cut and blend into a bowl. Add plain yogurt.

- *Miso soup:* Miso provides a fermented form of soybeans that stimulates immunity. This remedy has been a long-time favorite among Asian countries.

- *Turmeric curry dishes:* Ayurvedic cooking provides many traditional dishes steeped in spices that stimulate the immune system and provide antioxidants. Turmeric is a favorite that has shown to reduce cancer risk. This is only one type of spiced dish that Ayurvedic cooking provides. Add a teaspoon of turmeric to cooked rice and stir. Consult Ayurvedic cookbook for great recipes.

## Raw and Fresh

Most nutrients are heat-sensitive. Vitamin C, fat-soluble vitamins A, E and B vitamins are reduced during pasteurization. Many fatty acids are transformed by high heat to unhealthy fats. Important plant nutrients, such as anthocyanins and polyphenols, are also reduced during pasteurization, along with various enzymes. Proteins are denatured or broken down when heated for long. While this can aid in amino acid absorption, it can also form unrecognized peptide combinations. In milk, for example, some of the nutritious whey protein, or lactabumin, will denature into a number of peptide combinations that are not readily absorbed.

A 2008 study on strawberry puree from the University of Applied Sciences in Switzerland showed a 37% reduction in vitamin C and a significant loss in antioxidant potency after pasteurization. A 1998 study from Brazil's Universidade Estadual de Maringa determined that Barbados cherries lost about 14% of their vitamin C content after pasteurization. During heat treatment, vitamin C will also convert to dehydroascorbic acid together with a loss of bioflavonoids.

A 2006 study on bayberries at the Southern Yangtze University determined that plant antioxidants such as anthocyanins and polyphenolics were reduced from 12-32% following UHT pasteurization. Polyphenols, remember, are the primary nutrients in fruits and vegetables that render anti-carcinogenic and antioxidant effects.

One of the most important losses from pasteurization is its enzyme content. Diary and plant foods contain a variety of enzymes that aid in the assimilation or catalyzing of nutrients and antioxidants. These include xanthenes, lysozymes, lipases, oxidases, amylases, lactoferrins and many others contained in raw foods.

The body uses food enzymes in various ways. Some enzymes, such as papain from papaya and bromelain from pineapples, dissolve artery plaque and reduce inflammation. While the body makes many of its own enzymes, it also absorbs many food enzymes or uses their components to make new ones.

Pasteurization also typically leaves the food or beverage with a residual caramelized flavor due to the conversation of the enzymes, flavonoids and sugars to other compounds. In milk, for example, there is a substantial conversion from lactose to lactulose (and caramelization) after UHT pasteurization. Lactulose can cause intestinal cramping, nausea and vomiting.

In the case of pasteurized juices, pasteurization can leave the beverage in a highly acidic state, which can irritate our mucous membranes and intestines.

As for irradiation, there is little research on the resulting nutrient content outside of a few microwave studies (which showed decreased nutrient content and the formation of undesirable metabolites). There is good reason to believe that irradiation may thus denature some nutrients.

Whole foods in nature's packages are significantly different from pasteurized processed foods. Fresh whole foods produced by plants contain various antioxidants and enzymes that reduce the ability of microorganisms to grow.

The Creator also provided whole foods with peels and shells that protect nutrients and keep most microorganisms out. Microorganisms may invade the outer shell or peel somewhat, but the peel's pH, dryness and density – together with the pH of the inner fruit – provide extremely effective barriers to microorganisms and oxidation.

For this reason, most fruits and nuts can be easily stored for days and even weeks without having significant nutrient reduction. Once the peel or shell is removed, the inner fruit, juice or nut must be consumed to prevent oxidation and contamination – depending upon its pH and sugar content.

Whole natural foods also contain polysaccharides and oligosaccharides that combine nutrients and sugar within complex fibers. These combinations also help prevent oxidation and pathogenic bacteria colonization. With heat processing, however, the sugars are broken down into more simplified, refined form, which allows microbial growth and oxidation. Why?

Because simple sugars provide convenient energy sources for aggressive bacteria and fungi colonies. By contrast, our probiotics are used to eating the complexed oligosaccharides in fibrous foods. In other words, heat-processing produces the perfect foods for pathogenic microorganism colonization.

As we discussed in the last chapter, pathogenic microorganisms provide the fuel for systemic inflammation. They can infect the body's (and airways') tissues directly, and/or their endotoxins – waste products – stream into our bloodstream to max out our immune system and detoxification processes. This causes systemic inflammation, and toxicity.

### Whole is better than cut and packaged

Nowadays, prepackaged salads are big business. But there is a reason lettuce is best harvested whole.

Research from the University of Illinois and the U.S. Department of Agriculture's Agricultural Research Service (Yang *et al.* 2012; Bezanson *et al.* 2012) determined that field coring lettuce – the practice of removing the lettuce core in the field – dramatically increases the risk of the lettuce harboring *E. coli* contamination.

Many prepackaged salad producers core lettuce in the field as it is being picked by farm workers. The two 2012 studies found that because the workers maintain contact with the soil while picking and coring, both the coring knives and the coring ring can maintain and transfer Escherichia coli microorganisms from the soil onto the leaves of lettuce after coring. Once there, the hardy bacteria can continue to grow, even sometimes surviving the washing process.

Removing the core from lettuce allows the leaves to be easily packaged. Coring is typically done in the field for prepared salad mixes packaged into plastic bags. The coring is done in the field because it increases the efficiency of the process that takes the lettuce off the farm. At the plant, the loose leaves are then cut, washed and packaged into bags.

The University of Illinois at Urbana-Champaign research found that frequently washing the coring rings and knives with chlorine during the coring process reduces the risk of contamination. They also developed a new coring device that also cuts down *E. coli* contamination.

Over the past decade a number of *E. coli* outbreaks have resulted from cored and bagged lettuce or spinach packaged into plastic bags. Theories ranged from the farms being too close to dairy farms to organic farming methods – both of which have since been debunked.

Buying whole heads of lettuce uncored not only reduces the risk of contamination. It also reduces carbon emissions used for the extra manufacturing processes.

Coring lettuce at home is simple and fun. Iceberg lettuce can be decored simply by smashing the head core-first onto a cutting board. Romaine and other lettuces can be decored by simply pulling off the leaves.

Refrigeration is vital for storing lettuce whether cored or not. Another study – this from Korea's Chung-Ang University (Tian *et al.* 2012) – found that maintaining temperatures below 5 degrees C (41 degrees F) deters the growth or kills off *Salmonella enterica serovar Typhimurium, Staphylococcus aureus, Listeria monocytogenes,* and *E. coli.* Temperatures above 15 degrees C (60 degrees F) allowed most of these microorganisms to grow.

Because a plant's immune system typically defends against *E. coli* contamination when growing, maintaining the core and the lettuce head through to the time of salad preparation in the kitchen is an easy and less expensive way to reduce the risk of contamination. And under no conditions should a bagged packaged lettuce or even a fresh head of lettuce be left out of the refrigerator for very long.

# Spicing Up Our Diet

There are numerous herbs and spices that have been utilized in traditional medicine to modulate the immune system and stimulate the body's purification processes. Many of these also so happen to be delicious spices that we can add to practically any dish.

The incorporation of these culinary spices and herbs have a gradual and gentle effect upon the body. Their effects are seen by the stimulation of the strength of those organs and tissue systems that drive our body's purification programs. They can:

- ➢ Strengthen the immune system
- ➢ Increase tolerance
- ➢ Stimulate detoxification processes
- ➢ Donate key nutrients
- ➢ Balance and strengthen the adrenal glands
- ➢ Subdue anxious nervous response
- ➢ Strengthen mucous membranes
- ➢ Feed probiotics
- ➢ Reverse systemic inflammation
- ➢ Alkalize the bloodstream
- ➢ Rebuild the airways
- ➢ Relax smooth muscles
- ➢ Neutralize free radicals
- ➢ Strengthen the adrenal glands

Those common herbs are easily accessible in western society. They can easily be grown in our gardens and purchased at most stores. We can blend into our food recipes, and steep them into herbal teas.

These uses are by far the most sustainable means to use these herbs, and they are also the safest. This is because nature provides a full spectrum of nutrients among an herb's active ingredients among the natural parts of the plant. The roots, stems, leaves and flowers of one of these herbal plants typically provide a safe means of consumption – assuming we are selecting one of these herbs and not some poisonous plant we have never seen.

On the contrary, an herbal formulation that has undergone extraction or refining can eliminate some of these natural buffers – such as fibers, polysaccharides and mucilages. Cooking these away can result in side effects and pronounced effects that might not be expected. Following are a few culinary spices that can be added to our meals.

## Black Pepper

In Ayurveda, *Piper nigrum* is considered medicinal. Yet it is probably one of the most common spices used in Western foods. In fact, the world probably owes its use of Black pepper in foods to Ayurveda.

Black pepper is used in a variety of Ayurvedic formulations because of its anti-inflammatory action. Ayurvedic doctors describe Black pepper as a stimulant, expectorant, carminative (expulsing gas), anti-inflammatory and analgesic. It has been used traditionally for rheumatism, arthritis, bronchitis, coughs, asthma, sinusitis, gastritis and other histamine-related conditions. It is also thought to stimulate a healthy mucosal membrane among the stomach and intestines.

Black pepper used as a spice to increase taste is certainly not un-healthy, but it takes a significantly greater and consistent dose to produce its anti-inflammatory effects.

A traditional Ayurvedic prescription for gastroesophageal reflux or GERD, for example, is to take Black pepper in a warm glass of water on an empty stomach first thing in the morning over a period of time. This dose of Black pepper, according to Ayurveda, stimulates mucosal secre-tion, and purifies the mucosal membranes of the stomach and intestines.

Researchers from South Korea's Wonkwang University (Bae *et al.* 2010) found that the *Piper nigrum* extract piperine significantly inhibited inflammatory responses, including leukocytes and TNF-alpha.

## Long Pepper

The related Ayurvedic herb, *Piper longum,* has similar properties and constituents as Black pepper. It is often used in Indian recipes. It is used to inhibit the inflammation and histamine activity that results in lung and sinus congestion. Like Black pepper, Long pepper is also known to strengthen digestion by stimulating the secretion of the mucosal mem-branes within the stomach and intestines. It is also said to stimulate en-zyme activity and bile production. One study by researchers from India's Markandeshwar University (Kumar *et al.* 2009) found that the oil of Long pepper fruit significantly reduced inflammation.

## Turmeric

*Curcuma longa* has been extensively used as a medicinal herb for many centuries, and this predicated its use as a curry food spice – as Ayurveda has long incorporated healing herbs with meals. The roots or rhizomes of Turmeric are used. It is a relative of Ginger in the *Zingiberaceae* family.

Just as we might expect from a medicinal botanical, Turmeric has a large number of active constituents. The most well known of those are the curcuminoids, which include curcumin (diferuloylmethane, demeth-oxycurcumin, and bisdemethoxycurcumin). Others include volatile oils

353

such as tumerone, atlantone, and zingiberene; as well as polysaccharides and a number of resins.

As stated in a recent review of research from the Cytokine Research Laboratory at the University of Texas (Anand 2008), multiple studies have linked Turmeric with *"suppression of inflammation; angiogenesis; tumor genesis; diabetes; diseases of the cardiovascular, pulmonary, and neurological systems, of skin, and of liver; loss of bone and muscle; depression; chronic fatigue; and neuropathic pain."*

Indeed, Turmeric has been used for centuries for arthritis, asthma, inflammation, gallbladder problems, diabetes, wound-healing, liver issues, hepatitis, respiratory disease, menstrual pain, anemia, and gout. It is described as alterative, antibacterial, carminative and stimulating. It is also known for its wound-healing, blood-purifying and circulatory powers. Studies have illustrated that curcumin has about 50% of the effectiveness of cortisone, without its damaging side effects (Jurenka 2009).

A number of studies have proved over the past decade that Turmeric and/or its key constituents such as curcumin halt or inhibit both inflammatory COX and LOX enzymes. Curcumin has specifically been shown to inhibit IgE signaling processes, and slow mast cell activation (Aggarwal and Sung 2009; Thampithak *et al.* 2009; Sompamit *et al.* 2009; Kulka 2009).

## Coriander/Cilantro/Parsley

*Coriandrum sativum* has documented throughout traditional medicines as an anti-allergy and antioxidant herb. The seeds are called Coriander, and the leaves are called Cilantro. Cilantro has been popularly used throughout Central America, Italy, and also Asia – where it is sometimes called Chinese parsley. Cilantro is the backbone ingredient – together with tomatoes and garlic – of salsa. It is related to Italian parsley, with many of the same constituents. Coriander is taken as fresh or juiced fresh, and it has been used by Ayurvedic practitioners primarily for allergic skin rashes and hay fever.

Fresh Italian parsley can readily be found in supermarkets and farmers' markets. While often used as a garnish (for looks and/or to clean the breath), a therapeutic quantity of parsley is about a *bunch*. A bunch of parsley is about two ounces or about ten stalks together with their branches and leaves. A *bunch* can be added to a salad or put into a soup. Parsley can be delicious with tomatoes, vinegar and olive oil. And of course, it can also freshen the breath.

## Szechwan Pepper

This is the fruit from *Zanthoxylum simulans* which is also sometimes referred to as *Fructus Zanthoxyli Bungeani* or *Pericarpium zanthoxyli bungeani* in traditional Chinese medicine. More precisely, this herb is also referred to as Sichuan pepper. The tree is also called Prickly ash, and is grown around the world. The small peppers that come from the Prickly ash tree can be dried and ground or used fresh.

Chuan Jiao is also referred to as Fagara, Sansho, Nepal pepper or Szechwan pepper.

Because it is very spicy and hot, it is often used in Sichuan dishes – known for their spiciness. Chuan Jiao contains limonene, geraniol and cumic alcohol, among with a number of other medicinal constituents.

In traditional Chinese medicine, Chuan Jiao is known to remove abdominal pain, vomiting, nausea and parasites – especially roundworm. It is also used as a skin wash for eczema, and has a mild diuretic effect.

## Licorice and Gan Cao (Chinese Licorice)

*Glycyrrhiza uralensis* is also called Chinese Licorice. It is not the common Licorice (*Glycyrrhiza glabra*) known in Western and Ayurvedic herbalism. However, the two plants have nearly identical uses and constituents. So this discussion also serves *Glycyrrhiza glabra*.

Chinese licorice is known in Chinese medicine as giving moisture and balancing heat to the lungs. It has thus been extensively used to stop coughs and wheezing. It is also known to clear fevers. Taken either internally or topically, it is known to ease carbuncles and skin lesions. It is also soothing to the throat and eases muscle spasms. The root is thus described as antispasmodic.

Researchers from New York's Mount Sinai School of Medicine (Jayaprakasam *et al.* 2009) extensively investigated *Glycyrrhiza uralensis*. They found that *G. uralensis* had five major flavonoids: liquiritin, liquiritigenin, isoliquiritigenin, dihydroxyflavone, and isoononin. Liquiritigenin, isoliquiritigenin, and dihydroxyflavone were found to suppress inflammation via inhibiting eotaxin. Eotaxin stimulates the release of eosinophils during inflammation.

Licorice also contains glactomannan, triterpene saponins, glycerol, glycyrrhisoflavone, glycybenzofuran, cyclolicocoumarone, glycybenzofuran, cyclolicocoumarone, licocoumarone, glisoflavone, cycloglycyrrhisoflavone, licoflavone, apigenin, isokaempferide, glycycoumarin, isoglycycoumarin, glycyrrhizin and glycyrrhetinic acid (Li *et al.* 2010; Huang *et al.* 2010).

One of its main active constituents, isoliquiritigenin, has been shown to be a H2 histamine antagonist (Stahl 2008). Chinese Licorice has been shown to prevent the IgE binding that signals the release of histamine. This essentially disrupts the histamine inflammatory process while modulating immune system responses (Kim *et al.* 2006).

Another important constituent, glycyrrhizin, is a potent anti-inflammatory biochemical. It has also been shown to halt the breakdown of cortisol produced by the body. Let's consider this carefully. Like cortisone, cortisol inhibits the inflammatory process by interrupting interleukin cytokine transmission. If cortisol is prevented from breaking down, more remains available in the bloodstream to keep a lid on inflammation.

This combination of constituents gives Licorice aldosterone-like effects. This means that the root stimulates the production and maintenance of steroidal corticoids. Animal research has confirmed that Licorice is anti-allergic, and decreases anaphylactic response. It also balances electrolytes and inflammatory edema (Lee *et al.* 2010; Gao *et al.* 2009).

### Ginger

This is *Zingiberis officinalis,* also called *Rhizoma zingiberis officinalis* in traditional Chinese medicine. It is quite simply common Ginger root.

Ginger is extensively used in both Chinese and Ayurvedic medicine. It is also commonly used in Western herbalism and a number of other traditional medicines around the world.

Ginger is one of the most versatile food-spice-herbs known to humanity. In Ayurveda – the oldest medical practice still in use – Ginger is the most recommended botanical medicine. Ginger is referred to as *vishwabhesaj* – meaning "universal medicine" – by Ayurvedic physicians.

An accumulation of studies and chemical analyses has determined that Ginger has at least 477 active constituents. As in all botanicals, each constituent will stimulate a slightly different mechanism – often moderating the mechanisms of other constituents. Many of Ginger's active constituents have anti-inflammatory and/or pain-reducing effects. These include a number of gingerols and shogaols.

Clinical evaluation has documented that Ginger blocks inflammation by inhibiting lipoxygenase and prostaglandins in a balanced manner. This allows for a gradual reduction of inflammation and pain without the negative GI side effects that accompany NSAIDs. Ginger also stimulates circulation, inhibits various infections, and strengthens the liver.

Properties of Ginger supported by traditional clinical use include being analgesic, anthelmintic, anticathartic, antiemetic, antifungal, antihepatotoxic, antipyretic, antitussive, antiulcer, cardiotonic, gastrointestinal motility, hypotensive, thermoregulatory, analgesic, tonic, expectorant, carminative, antiemetic, stimulant, anti-inflammatory, antimicrobial and more.

Ginger has therefore been used as a traditional treatment for bronchitis, rheumatism, asthma, colic, nervous disorders, colds, coughs, migraines, pneumonia, indigestion, respiratory ailments, fevers, nausea, colds, flu, ulcers, hepatitis, liver disease, colitis, tuberculosis and many digestive ailments to name a few.

## Cinnamon

This is *Cinnamomum cassia*, also referred to as *Ramulus cinnamomi cassiae* in traditional Chinese medicine. It is commonly called cinnamon – a delicious culinary spice present in most kitchens.

Cinnamon is used in just about every traditional medicine. The bark is often used, although the twigs are also utilized. Its constituents include limonene, camphor, cineole, cinnamic aldehyde, gums, mannitol, safrole, tannins and oils.

According to Western herbalism, Ayurvedic medicine and traditional Chinese medicine, it is useful for colds, sinusitis, bronchitis, dyspepsia, asthma, muscle tension, toothaches, the heart, the kidneys, and digestion. It is also thought to strengthen circulation in general. Its properties are described as expectorant, diuretic, stimulating, analgesic and alterative. In other words, it is an immune-system modulator. It is also thought to dilate the blood vessels and warm the body according to these traditional disciplines.

## Jujube

The *Ziziphus zizyphus* plant produces a delicious sweet date that tastes very much like a sweet apple. The fruit has many different properties in traditional medicine. It has been used to stimulate the immune system. It has been used to reduce stress, reduce inflammation, sooth indigestion, and repeal GERD.

Jujube contains a variety of constituents, including mucilage, ceanothic acid, alphitolic acid, zizyberanal acid, zizyberanalic acid, zizyberanone, epiceanothic acid, ceanothenic acid, betulinic acid, oleanolic acid, ursolic acid, zizyberenalic acid, maslinic acid, tetracosanoic acid, kaempferol, rutin, quercetin and others.

## Panex Ginseng

*Panex ginseng* is an immune stimulant with thousands of years of use. Panax ginseng will come in white forms and red forms. The color depends upon the aging or drying technique used.

When Ginseng is cultivated and steamed, it is called 'red root' or Hong Shen. Ginseng root will turn red when it is oxidized or processed with steaming. Some feel that red root is better than white, but this really depends upon its intended use, the age of the root, and how it was processed. Soaking Ginseng in rock candy produces a white Ginseng that is called Bai shen. This soaking seems odd, but this has been known to increase some of its constituent levels such as superoxide and nitric oxide. When the root is simply dried, it is called 'dry root' or Sheng shaii shen. Korean Red Ginseng is soaked in a special herbal broth and then dried.

There are a number of species within the *Panax* genus, most of which also contain most of the same adaptogens, referred to as gensenosides. Most notable in the *Panex* genus is American Ginseng, *Panax quinquefolius.*

Ginseng contains camphor, mucilage, panaxosides, resins, saponins, gensenosides, arabinose and polysaccharides, among others.

*Eleutherococcus senticosus,* often called Siberian Ginseng, is actually not Ginseng. While it also contains adaptogens (eleutherosides), these are not the gensenoside adaptogens within Ginseng that have been observed for their ability to relieve hypersensitivity.

Researchers from Italy's Ambientale Medical Institute (Caruso *et al.* 2008) tested an herbal extract formula consisting of *Capparis spinosa, Olea europaea, Panax ginseng* and *Ribes nigrum* (Pantescal) on allergic patients. They found that allergic biomarkers, including basophil degranulation CD63 and sulphidoleukotriene (SLT) levels were significantly lower after 10 days. They theorized that these biomarkers explain the herbal formulation's *"protective effects."*

Researchers from Japan's Ehime University Graduate School of Medicine (Sumiyoshi *et al.* 2010) tested *Panax ginseng* on mice sensitized to hen's eggs. After the oral feedings, they found that the Ginseng significantly reduced allergen-specific IgG Th2 levels. It also increased IL-12 production, and increased the ratio of Th1 to Th2 among spleen cells. In addition, it enhanced intestinal CD8, IFN-gamma, and IgA-positive counts. The researchers concluded that, *"Red Ginseng roots may be a natural preventative of food allergies."*

Ginseng has been found to stimulate circulation and improve cognition. It is also known to reduce fatigue, and stress. Herbalists also use it to improve appetite, and as a mild stimulant and potent antioxidant.

## Cumin Seed

*Cuminum cyminum* has a long history of use among European and Asian herbalists. It is described as antispasmodic and carminative, so it tends to soothe inflammatory responses. Like Fennel, Cumin has been used traditionally to ease abdominal cramping and gas.

Cumin seed contains mucilage, gums and resins. Traditional herbalists consider these constituents primarily responsible for Cumin's ability to help strengthen the mucosal membranes. This makes Cumin part of a strategy to rebuild the mucosal membranes of the airways.

## Fennel

*Foeniculum vulgare* contains anetholes, caffeoyl quinic acids, carotenoids, vitamin C, iron, B vitamins, and rutins. Ayurvedic and traditional herbalists from many cultures have used Fennel to relieve digestive discomfort, gas, abdominal cramping, bloating and irritable bowels; and to treat inflammation. Fennel stimulates bile production. Bile digests fats and other nutrients, increasing their bioavailability.

One of Fennel's constituents, called anethole, is known to suppress pro-inflammatory tumor necrosis factor alpha (TNF-a). This inhibition slows excessive immune response. The combination of anethole and antioxidant nutrients such as rutin and carotenoids in Fennel also strengthen immune response while increasing tolerance.

Fennel is not appropriate for pregnant moms, because it has been known to promote uterine contractions. As with any herbal supplement, Fennel should be used under the supervision of a health professional. Those with birch allergies should also be aware that they may also be sensitive to Fennel. (The same goes for Cumin, Caraway, Carrot seed and a few others).

## Mints and Menthol

The plants of the mint family include Peppermint (*Mentha piperita*), Watermint (*Mentha aquatica*), Spearmint (*Mentha spicata*), Pennyroyal (*Mentha pulegium*) and several others. They have a variety of common constituents, of which menthol is the most applicable to respiratory issues. Other active constituents of many mints will include menthylacetate, menthone, mentofuran, limonene, cineole, isomenthol, neomenthol, azulenes and rosmarinic acid.

Mint is well-known for its ability to settle digestion and ease flatulence. These effects are due to azulene's ability to relax the smooth muscles around the intestines. Azulene also relaxes the smooth muscles around the airways as well. Note that Chamomile also contains azulene.

Menthol is most known for its ability to clear congestion and expand the airways. It is the expectorant property of menthol that produces this effect. Menthol reduced coughing in a study from Britain's Leicester University Hospitals (Kenia *et al.* 2008) of 42 children.

All the mints make delicious herbal teas, a great addition to any breakfast or after-dinner beverage.

## Basil

*Osimum basilicum* contains ursolic acid and oleanolic acid, both shown in laboratory studies to inhibit inflammatory COX-2 enzymes. Basil is also calming and refreshing. It makes a great Italian food spice.

## Garlic

*Allium sativum* probably deserves a larger section, but that information could easily encompass a book in itself – as was well documented by Paul Bergner: *The Healing Power of Garlic* (1996). Garlic is an ancient medicinal plant with a wealth of characteristics and constituents that stimulate the immune system, protect the liver, purify the bloodstream, reduce oxidative species, reduce LDL lipid peroxidation, reduce inflammation, and stimulate detoxification systems throughout the body. This is supported by a substantial amount of rigorous scientific research.

Garlic is also one of the most powerful antimicrobial plants known. A fresh garlic bulb has at least five different constituents known to inhibit bacteria, fungi and viruses. Much of this antimicrobial capability, however, is destroyed by heat and oxygen. Therefore, eating freshly peeled bulbs are the most assured way to retain these antimicrobial potencies.

Cooked, aged or dehydrated garlic powder also has a variety of powerful antioxidants, but little of its raw antibiotic abilities. Garlic is also a tremendous sulfur donor as well. The combination of garlic's antibiotic, antioxidant, anti-inflammatory and immune-building characteristics make it a *must* spice-herb-food for any inflammatory condition.

## Oregano

*Origanum vulgare* contains at least thirty-one anti-inflammatory constituents, twenty-eight antioxidants, and four significant COX-2 inhibitors (apigenin, kaempherol, ursolic acid and oleanolic acid).

## Rosemary

*Rosmarinus officinalis* contains ursolic acid, oleanolic acid and apigenin – a few of the many constituents in this important botanical – shown to inhibit inflammatory enzymes in laboratory studies. Research has also shown that rosemary's volatile oils can halt airway constriction by inhibiting mast cell degranulation.

## Other Great Spices

The list does not end here. Still other spice herbs have been used among traditional medicines throughout the world to reverse the toxic, inflammatory metabolism. Many of these are not direct pulmonary herbs, but rather, serve to purify the blood, strengthen the liver, strengthen the adrenals, strengthen the immune system and inhibit inflammation. Here is a short list:

> ➤ Aloe (*Aloe vera*)
> ➤ Anise (*Pimpinella anisum*)
> ➤ Cayenne (*Capsicum* spp.)
> ➤ Chamomile (*Matricaria chamomilla*)
> ➤ Comfrey (*Symphytum officinale*)
> ➤ Green Tea (*Camellia sinensis*)
> ➤ Lemongrass (*Cymbopogon citratus*)
> ➤ Nutmeg (*Myristica fragrans*)
> ➤ Thyme (*Thymus serphyllum*)
> ➤ Tulsi (*Ocimum gratissimum*)
> ➤ Wild onion (*Hymenocallis tubiflora*)

There are certainly many more gentle herbs we can to this collection. But these are certainly good candidates to consider for one's garden, tea or spice cupboard.

### Adding Anti-inflammatory Spices to Our Meals

The sign of a therapeutic dose of these spices within a dish is when the spice can be readily tasted. That is, the pungent flavor of the spice stands out in the food. If the amount of spice simply flavors the food a little, then it will probably not be enough to stimulate any immune response. If the spice can be specifically tasted (for example, *"that dish tastes garlicy"* or *"tastes peppery"*) then the spice will likely be enough to stimulate a therapeutic response.

That said, if multiple spices are used, the dose of each spice can be smaller. After all, the meal should also taste good. This, however, is why traditional Chinese and Indian food is so spicy. The recipes come from therapeutic traditions.

Another element of the therapeutic dose is consistency. It is not enough to have one or more of these spices once a week with a particular dish. The spice(s) should be added to at least one meal every day.

In addition, care must be taken to protect therapeutic spices from degradation. This can occur when spices are left in the light or sun for an extended period, or when spices are left open to oxygen. Often spices are left in kitchen racks exposed to the lights of the kitchen and window, or left in unsealed containers or shakers. Oxygen and light degrade the biochemical constituents that give these spices their therapeutic properties.

This latter point is likely one of the main reasons our culinary spices cannot be considered therapeutic. Leaving the spice exposed can take place during processing, packaging and shipping; as well as in the kitchen. Therefore, we should consider purchasing our therapeutic spices from a bulk herb store, or from suppliers or brands that respect their therapeutic nature.

By far the best way to consume or add these foods to our diet is in their fresh form. Many of these herbs can be grown in our garden or purchased from a local farmers' market or grocery store as fresh. As discussed earlier, fresh foods maintain more bioactive nutrients. This is because their beneficial constituents are naturally sealed within the food's peel, shell or cell walls.

Note also that these anti-inflammatory herbal spices (and most of the other natural products contained in this chapter) will typically not stimulate a therapeutic response immediately. Depending upon the status of our immune system, it may take weeks or months before the daily dosing of these natural elements is seen in the form of strengthening our immunity and reducing our toxin levels.

## Food Selection

There have been some radical diets out that maintain regimented and complex ways to select our foods. Some call for our blood type. Others call for our race or gender. Others use body type.

The bottom line in choosing our foods is that first they are as whole and unprocessed as possible. And secondly, they should appeal to our senses. Thirdly and not to be forgotten, we should be able to readily digest them without any cramping, constipation or other intestinal discomfort.

When a physician visits with a patient, he or she typically reviews the body's symptoms together with the patient's history. The physician will look at the vital signs; the heart beat, the blood pressure, and so on. He or she might also look at the sclera of the eyes, perhaps the tongue, and then begin to review specific parts of the body for pain, range or motion or function.

We should perform this same analysis for food, using our senses.

### The Olfactory Sense

Because the olfactory nerve endings and olfactory bulb process nerve impulses, allowing us to be able to assess many aspects of the food before we eat it. We can validate its nutritive qualities and revealing its potential to stress our bodies. This takes what many call a keen sense of smell, yet most everyone possesses this ability. We simply have to be aware we have it, and then use it.

Frankly, nutritious food should appeal to our sense of smell. However, we need to distinguish this from a conditioned response to those unhealthy foods of our past. Odors given off by frying any food, for example, are particularly deceptive, because our olfactory senses are made up of nerve cells that are surrounded by lipid (fat) membranes. Thus, we should disregard the olfactory sense related to fried foods.

This can easily be distinguished if our intent is to eat healthy.

We need to carefully smell a food before we purchase it or eat it. It should appeal to the olfactory senses. If a food smells bitter, fermented or overly pungent, we need to further investigate the food for consumption, and possibly reject it. If the characteristic is not typical for that food we should probably not eat it until we know what has changed it. A fermented food will likely contain a range of bacteria. If the food is not specifically cultured with probiotics or using vinegar or lemon juice (faux fermentation), then the food is likely infected with pathogenic bacteria.

If a food smells burnt or rotten, we should probably reject it. If a food has a chemical smell it should be rejected. If the food smells caramel-sweet it is likely overcooked. The caramelization is produced by the glycation of protein with sugar, and this is not healthy.

**Our Visual Sense**

A food should also appeal to us visually. This is tested by our initial reaction when we first look at the food. Did the initial glance make us look twice at it or did we look on to the next thing without a second thought?

Again we must distinguish between something naturally visually attractive, and a past memory. For example, donuts sprinkled with colored dots might remind us of eating donuts as children, and they might look pretty attractive. But their attractiveness is derived from their artificial colors combined with our recollection of sweetness.

If a food has lost its natural color and structure, we should be cautious. A healthy food will have the color of the ripened fruits, vegetables, nuts, or grains it was made with. A healthy cooked meal should retain considerable color. When the colors are gone, much of the nutrition will also be gone. Natural browns, greens, yellows, oranges and even reds and blues will indicate that the food still retains some kind of functional nutrition. This can of course be deceived by chemically altered foods with food dyes. This is usually revealed by the food color being unrealistically bright for a prepared food, or even an unnatural shade of the color.

Food should also appear to maintain its natural texture as much as possible. While it may be mashed, grated, blended, or chopped, a real food will retain a fibrous appearance regardless of what condition it is in. A mushy, slimy texture would indicate that the fiber has been removed. Typically, fiber renders a grainy, fibrous texture to the food. A food without this appearance should be immediately suspect.

## Touching Our Foods

Foods should be touched. Today we use forks and knives to stab and cut our food. Why do we avoid touching our food? It is completely understandable if we do not have clean hands. It is far better to give our hands a good washing and eat as much of our food with our natural forks – our fingers. Touching our food as we eat it loses our tactile sense of it.

Using our tactile senses while eating provides sensory protection, preventing us from eating a food that is too hot, too cold, too hard and stale, or otherwise not appropriate to eat. By "escorting" the food into our mouths with our hands, we also prepare the mouth and stomach for the incoming food. Whether it is hot, cold, hard, soft, crunchy, sticky or fibrous, our mouth will be prepared for its entry.

This might be comparing handing a person a gift rather than mailing it to them. As we hand someone the gift we are able to exchange a full range of communications and reactions.

As we touch a food, we test its structure. A food that has lost its structure will likely be over-processed and lacking fiber. This is a sign that the food no longer retains the nutritional effects of real food. If the product is hard and brittle, we might consider that food suspicious and find out why it became so hard. It may have been left outside and become rancid, bug-eaten or otherwise degraded by oxygen and light.

If the food is slimy or sticky, we might want to smell and look at it more carefully. In general, a food should have structure and firmness, unless of course it is a sauce or extract. If it is cooked or mashed it should still have resistance when it is pushed on or touched.

## Tasting Our Foods

The tongue contains thousands of tiny taste receptors called taste buds on its surface. These receptors are receivers – comparable to tiny antennas. The locations of the taste buds have been arranged in such a way that similar types of receivers are in common proximity. This creates specific taste regions. For example, bitter taste buds are located at the back of the tongue. Sour taste buds are located at either side of the tongue towards the back. Salty taste buds are located on the sides closer to the lips. The tip of the tongue contains primarily sweet taste buds.

The molecular elements of a particular food render its fingerprint, which translates into brain waveforms perceived as particular tastes and odors. These impulses are translated through the glosopharyngeal cranial nerves, where they converted into feedback in the gustatory center of the lower brain.

Taste is critical to understanding the nature of the food and what effect it will have in the body.

According to Ayurvedic food science there are six types of tastes or *rasas: sweet, salty, bitter, pungent, astringent, and sour.* Because each produces a different neurological response, each has a different physiological effect and an effect upon our moods.

Healthy food should not have an extreme flavor in any single category. The most balanced foods have a combination of at least two of these flavors. Sweet foods should also have a bit of sourness. That might be categorized as tangy. A tree-ripened fruit may be described as sweet, but most fruit are also tangy. While the middle of some fruits are quite sweet, the outer parts like the rind will likely balance the sweet with sour to get to tangy. For most fruit, we might try eating the rind or at least the inner layer of it, as the rind will carry many nutrients not found in the inner part. The perfect example is citrus, which we discussed earlier.

This kind of balance exists within nature. As soon as we disrupt this balance by – for example, trying to juice the fruit while screening out the pulp and the rind, we will be removing the molecular balance from the food. This is expressed by its lack of fiber, overly sweet flavor, and missing nutrients. For this reason, filtered (and especially pasteurized) fruit juice is almost as rough on the body's metabolism as refined sugar. It spikes our blood sugar and insulin levels, and will stimulate the sugar high and low. If the fruit is eaten whole, the sweetness will be balanced by its fiber and oil content – which slow absorption.

We might compare this situation to a person extracting a statement out of context from a speech or story. The statement is not balanced by the words occurring around it. In the same way, nature has provided us with a balance of molecules within living foods for a good reason: to keep us healthy.

## Hydration Strategies

We will likely die of starvation if we don't eat in a month or two. But we'll die within days without water.

The fact that dehydration (lack of sufficient fluid intake) can contribute to systemic inflammation and toxicity has been confirmed by research.

In a dehydrated state, our mucosal membranes and tissues weaken. Every cell is stressed. It is for this reason that other research has found that many ulcerated conditions can be cured simply by drinking adequate water (Batmanghelidj 1997).

Water is directly involved in inflammatory metabolism. Research has revealed that increased levels of inflammatory mediators such as histamine are released during periods of dehydration in order to help balance fluid levels within the bloodstream, tissues, kidneys and other organs.

Research by Dr. Batmanghelidj (1987; 1990) led to the realization that the blood becomes more concentrated during dehydration. As this concentrated blood enters the capillaries of the respiratory system, histamine is released in an attempt to balance the blood dilution.

The immune system is also irrevocably aligned with the body's water availability. The immune system utilizes water to produce lymph fluid. Lymph fluid circulates immune cells throughout the body, enabling them to target specific intruders. The lymph is also used to escort toxins out of the body.

Intracellular and intercellular fluids are necessary for the removal of nearly all toxins – and pretty much every metabolic function of every cell, every organ and every tissue system.

Water also increases the availability of oxygen to cells. Water balances the level of free radicals. Water flushes and replenishes the digestive tract. Thus, water is necessary for the proper digestion of food, as well as nutrition utilization. The gastric cells of the stomach and the intestinal wall cells require water for proper digestive function. The health of every cell depends upon water.

There is certainly reason to believe that dehydration is a key factor for toxicity and inflammation.

As Dr. Jethro Kloss pointed out decades ago (1939), the average person loses about 550 cubic centimeters of water through the skin, 440 cc through the lungs, 1550 cc through the urine, and another 150 cc through the stool. This adds up to 2650 cc per day, equivalent to a little over 2-½ quarts (about 85 fluid ounces).

Meanwhile many have suggested drinking eight 8-oz glasses per day. This 64 ounces would result in a state of dehydration. In 2004, the National Academy of Sciences released a study indicating that women typically meet their hydration needs with approximately 91 ounces of water per day, while men meet their needs with about 125 ounces per day. This study also indicated that approximately 80% of water intake comes from water/beverages and 20% comes from food. Therefore, we can assume a minimum of 73 ounces of fresh water for the average adult woman and 100 ounces of fresh water for the average adult man should cover our hydration needs. That is significantly more water than the standard eight glasses per day – especially for men.

The data suggests that 50-75% of Americans have chronic dehydration. Fereydoon Batmanghelidj, M.D., probably the world's foremost researcher on water, suggests a ½ ounce of water per pound of body weight. Drinking an additional 16-32 ounces for each 45 minutes to an hour of strenuous activity is also a good idea, with some before and some after exercising. More water should accompany temperature and elevation extremes, and extra sweating or fevers. Note also that alcohol is dehydrating.

A glass of room-temperature water first thing in the morning on an empty stomach can significantly help our mucosal membranes. Then we should be drinking water throughout the day. Our evening should accompany reduced water consumption, so our sleep is not disrupted by urination.

There are easy ways to tell whether we are dehydrated. A sensation of being thirsty indicates that we are already dehydrated. A person with toxicity and/or inflammation should thus be drinking enough water to not ever feel thirsty. Dark yellow urine also indicates dehydration. Our urine color should be either clear, or bright yellow if after taking multivitamins.

Drinking just any water is not advised. Municipal water and even bottled water can contain many contaminants that can burden the immune system, and trigger inflammation. Care must be taken to drink water that has been filtered of most toxins yet is naturally mineralized. Research has confirmed that distilled water and soft water are not advisable. Natural mineral water is best. Please refer to the author's book, *Pure Water* for more information on water content, filters and water therapy.

# Chapter Twelve

# Essential Considerations

## A Practical Choice

This text does not assume that every reader is prepared to completely give up eating red meat. We are simply laying out the facts showing the connection between the Western diet and greater levels of inflammation and toxicity, together with the evidence that a diet with more plant-based foods will present less toxicity and systemic inflammation.

A diet with more plant-based foods and less red meat will enable a stronger immune system and faster detoxification.

We can each make our own decisions with regard to how to incorporate this information into our diet. For some, it will simply mean eating less red meat, which will have the effect of decreasing our disease potential. For others, it might mean adopting the Mediterranean diet. For still others, it might mean a full commitment to the wisdom of our ancestors.

## Eating Environmentally

There are also many environmental and ecological reasons the Ancestors Diet is correct. Meat eating is a terrible use of our dwindling world's resources. 18% of our carbon input into greenhouse gases and 22% percent of our methane pollution is caused by animal husbandry and slaughter operations. The cattle and hog industry is one of humanity's most polluting industries – infecting our waterways with bioactive manure, antibiotics and other pollutants.

Because of massive over-fishing, our oceans are now depleted of 90 percent of the largest predatory species compared to only fifty years ago. A typical meat-based diet requires over five times the resources a plant-based diet requires. It takes about 5.86 plant protein pounds to produce one animal protein pound. In addition, one pound of animal protein requires about one hundred times the water a pound of plant protein requires. One steer's lifetime water intake could float a battleship. In a world of dwindling resources, it truly becomes an ethical choice.

The earth is bursting with an excessive population of cattle due to the meat industry. While over 1.2 billion domesticated cattle populate the planet – rivaling human population – cattle disrupt more than half the world's land. In the past fifty years, about sixty percent of the world's rangelands have been damaged from overgrazing.

In addition to these destructive practices, overcrowded commercial egg and poultry farming operations provide a potent incubation location for various diseases, including the bird flu. The flu pandemic of 1918 was a bird flu virus. It killed between 50 million and 100 million people around the world. Today we are faced with another growing virus, the H5N1 flu strain, which has already killed about 200 people worldwide. While early blame was made upon migrating wild birds, it is now increasingly evident that cramped and overcrowded commercial poultry and egg operations are the likely vectors for the virus.

In 2006, research presented at an international veterinary and agricultural science conference concluded that commercial poultry operations were the likely vectors for the H5N1 virus outbreak. In these operations, living beings with feelings and emotions – are caged and camped by the hundreds of thousands in indoor facilities. In these operations viruses can easily become rampant. Many infections have hit poultry operations over the years, forcing hundreds of thousands of sick birds to be immediately slaughtered (Greger 2007).

There is clear scientific research gathered over the past thirty years proving that eating meat wastes the world's food resources. Should a majority of western populations assume a plant-based diet, we would easily free up enough food to generate a world-wide surplus of food.

Meat eating is also one of the larger contributors of atmospheric carbon levels. Meat production contributes an astonishing 18% of the carbon pollution. Cattle and other animal ranching also contributes dramatically to the deforestation of the world's rainforests.

There is yet another dimension of the Ancestors Diet to consider. There is a deeper, conscious result of slaughtering animals and eating them unnecessarily. Yes, we now know our bodies are not designed for eating meat. Indeed, our bodies are designed for living peacefully and using our higher intellects to aspire for spiritual growth. In fact, our useful position as the planet's most intelligent organism puts us in the position of being a caretaker of the animal kingdom. To provide nurturing for animals allows us to shepherd these souls as they progress into higher states of consciousness.

By "unnecessarily," it means we do not need meat for our survival. Not only is the diet described here substantial enough to satisfy the nutritional needs of the human organism, but it provides an increased level of health and increased survival. During situations where there is not the plant life to sustain health, this may become a different matter. To eat meat as a matter of survival in the absence of options – just as some colder-weather populations have done for thousands of years during icebound winters – does not have the same biological impact.

370

Certainly, this is not the case for most populations of the world, especially today with a healthy business of food trade to draw from. Most of the first and second world countries now have plenty of wholesome plant-based and dairy foods to utilize. Most of the third world does too, though there are pockets of isolated and poor populations without adequate resources.

With the advent of farming methods and food distribution transportation, our abilities to access nourishing non-violent foods are overwhelming. Today we add to our outdoor farming methods the ability to grow many foods in greenhouses during the winter time. This together with local dairies and the storage of summer fruit production, we can sustain our health quite fabulously without killing animals in most northern latitude locations.

There are many who propose that animals are not conscious living creatures. This is refuted by simple observation as well as scientific research. A simple observation of our pets should give us the immediate understanding that animals truly experience pain, experience pleasure, and seek loving relationships. If we consider how far a dog will go to please his or her master, and how a cat will pine to be petted, we can see that animals seek love and attention just as we do. We can hear animals of every kind cry when they are in pain. Some animals such as the elephant even produce tears when they are in pain.

Researchers have been observing and experimenting on rats, monkeys and so many other animals for years. Here they not only observe various social and conscious activities amongst these animals, but use these findings to associate with human behavior. Recently one study (Rutte and Taborsky 2007) determined that Norway rats, a common subject for inflicting all sorts of experiments, were able to reciprocate with other rats, understanding exchange, relationships, and justice. They were able to understand that an action could be exchanged for another, and they were able to judge a fair exchange between them – an understanding of justice. The textbooks and journals are full of evidence that animals experience love and respect between other animals and even humans.

With these points in mind, with permission from EarthSave (1989), we quote some revealing statistics, though there may be some variances relating to today's population and currency:

> *Human population of United States: 243,000,000*
> *Number of Human beings who could be fed by the grain and soybeans eaten by U.S. livestock: 1,300,000,000*
> *Sacred food of Native Americans: Corn*
> *Percentage of corn grown in United States eaten by human beings: 20*

➤ *Percentage of corn grown in United States eaten by livestock: 80*

➤ *Percentage of oats grown in United States eaten by livestock: 95*

➤ *Percentage of protein wasted by cycling grain through livestock: 90*

➤ *Percentage of carbohydrate wasted by cycling grain through livestock: 99*

➤ *Percentage of dietary fibre wasted by cycling grain through livestock: 100*

➤ *How frequently a child dies of starvation: Every 2 seconds*

➤ *Pounds of potatoes that can be grown on 1 acre of land: 20,000*

➤ *Pounds of beef that can be produced on 1 acre of land: 165*

➤ *Percentage of U.S. agricultural land used to produce beef: 56*

➤ *Pounds of grain and soybeans needed to produce 1 pound of feedlot beef: 16*

➤ *Pounds of protein fed to chickens to produce 1 pound of protein as chicken flesh: 5 pounds*

➤ *Pounds of protein fed to hogs to produce 1 pound of protein as hog flesh: 7.5 pounds*

➤ *Number of children who starve to death every day: 40,000*

➤ *Number of pure vegetarians who can be fed on the amount of land needed to feed 1 person consuming meat-based diet: 20*

➤ *Number of people who will starve to death this year: 60,000,000*

➤ *Number of people who could be adequately fed by the grain saved if Americans reduced their intake of meat by 10%: 60,000,000*

➤ *Historic cause of demise of many great civilisations: Topsoil depletion*

➤ *Percentage of original U.S. topsoil lost to date: 75*

➤ *Amount of U.S. cropland lost each year to soil erosion: 4,000,000 acres (size of Connecticut)*

➤ *Percentage of U.S. topsoil loss directly associated with livestock raising: 85*

➤ *Number of acres of U.S. forest which have been cleared to create cropland to produce a meat-centred diet: 260,000,000*

➤ *How often an acre of U.S. trees disappears: Every 8 seconds*

➤ *Amount of trees spared per year by each individual who switches to a pure vegetarian diet: 1 acre*

➢ *A driving force behind the destruction of the tropical rainforests: American meat habit*

➢ *Amount of meat imported annually by U.S. from Costa Rica, El Salvador, Guatemala, Nicaragua, Honduras and Panama: Less than the average American housecat*

➢ *Current rate of species extinction due to destruction of tropical rainforests and related habitats: 1000/year*

➢ *User of more than half of all water used for all purposes in the United States: Livestock production*

➢ *Quantity of water used in the production of the average cow sufficient to: float a destroyer*

➢ *Water needed to produce 1 pound of wheat: 25 gallons*

➢ *Water needed to produce 1 pound of meat: 2,500 gallons*

➢ *Cost of common hamburger meat if water used by meat industry was not subsidised by U.S. taxpayers: $35/pound*

➢ *Current cost for pound of protein from wheat: $1.50*

➢ *Current cost for pound of protein from beefsteak: $15.40*

➢ *Cost for pound of protein from beefsteak if U.S. taxpayers ceased subsidising meat industry's use of water: $89*

➢ *Length of time world's petroleum reserves would last if all human beings ate meat-centred diet: 13 years*

➢ *Length of time world's petroleum reserves would last if all human beings ate vegetarian diet: 260 years*

➢ *Principal reason for U.S. military intervention in Persian Gulf:*

➢ *Dependence on foreign oil: Barrels of oil imported daily by U.S.: 6,800,000*

➢ *Percentage of energy return (as food energy per fossil energy expended) of most energy efficient farming of meat: 34.5%*

➢ *Percentage of energy return (as food energy per fossil energy expended) of least energy efficient plant food: 328%*

➢ *Pounds of soybeans produced by the amount of fossil fuel needed to produce 1 pound of feedlot beef: 40*

➢ *Percentage of raw materials consumed in U.S. for all purposes presently consumed to produce current meat-centred diet: 33*

➢ *Percentage of raw materials consumed in U.S. for all purposes needed to produce fully vegetarian diet: 2*

➢ *Production of excrement by total U.S. human population: 12,000 lbs./sec*

➢ *Production of excrement by U.S. Livestock: 250,000 pounds/second*

➢ *Sewage systems in U.S. cities: Common*

➤ *Sewage systems in U.S. feedlots: Nil*
➤ *Amount of waste produced annually by U.S. livestock in confinement operations which is not recycled: 1 billion tons*
➤ *Relative concentration of feedlot wastes compared to raw domestic sewage: Ten to several hundred times more highly concentrated*
➤ *Where feedlot waste often ends up: In our water*
➤ *Number of U.S. medical schools: 125*
➤ *Number of U.S. medical schools with a required course in nutrition: 30*
➤ *Training in nutrition received during 4 years of medical school by average U.S. physician: 2.5 hours*
➤ *How frequently a heart attack strikes in U.S.: Every 25 seconds*
➤ *How frequently a heart attack kills in U.S.: Every 45 seconds*
➤ *Most common cause of death in U.S.: Heart attack*
➤ *Risk of death from heart attack by average American man: 50%*
➤ *Risk of death from heart attack by average American vegetarian man: 15%*
➤ *Risk of death from heart attack by average American purely vegetarian man: 4%*
➤ *Amount you reduce your risk of heart attack by reducing your consumption of meat, dairy products and eggs 10%: 9%*
➤ *Amount you reduce your risk of heart attack by reducing your consumption of meat, dairy products and eggs 50%: 45%*
➤ *Amount you reduce your risk of heart attack by reducing your consumption of meat, dairy products and eggs 100%: 90%*
➤ *Rise in blood cholesterol from consuming 1 egg per day: 12%*
➤ *Rise in heart attack risk from 12% rise in blood cholesterol: 24%*
➤ *Meat, dairy and egg industries claim there is no reason to be concerned about your blood cholesterol as long as it is: "normal"*
➤ *Your risk of dying a disease caused by clogged arteries if your blood cholesterol is "normal:" over 50%*
➤ *Your risk of dying of a disease caused by clogged arteries if you do not consume saturated fat and cholesterol: 5%*
➤ *Leading sources of saturated fat and cholesterol in American diets: Meat, dairy products and eggs*
➤ *World populations with high meat intakes who do not have correspondingly high rates of colon cancer: None*

➤ *World populations with low meat intakes who do not have correspondingly low rates of colon cancer: None*

➤ *Increased risk of breast cancer for women who eat meat daily compared to women who eat meat less than once a week: 4 times higher*

➤ *Increased risk of breast cancer for women who eat eggs daily compared to women who eat eggs less than once a week: 3 times higher*

➤ *Increased risk of fatal prostate cancer for men who consume meats, cheese, eggs and milk daily compared to men who eat these foods sparingly or not at all: 3.6 times higher*

➤ *The diseases which are commonly prevented, consistently improved, and sometimes cured by a low-fat vegetarian diet include: Strokes Heart disease Osteoporosis Kidney Stones Breast cancer Colon cancer Prostate cancer Pancreatic cancer Ovarian cancer Cervical cancer Stomach cancer Endometrial cancer Diabetes Hypoglycaemia Kidney disease Peptic ulcers Constipation Haemorrhoids Hiatal hernias Diverticulosis Obesity Gallstones Hypertension Asthma Irritable colon syndrome Salmonellosis Trichinosis*

➤ *Chlorinated hydrocarbon pesticide residues in the U.S. diet supplied by meat: 55%*

➤ *Supplied by Dairy products: 23%*

➤ *Supplied by vegetables: 6%*

➤ *Supplied by fruits: 4%*

➤ *Supplied by grains: 1%*

➤ *Percentage of U.S. mother's milk containing significant levels of DDT: 99%*

➤ *Percentage of U.S. vegetarian mother's milk containing significant levels of DDT: 8%*

➤ *Relative pesticide contamination in breast milk of meat-eating mothers compared to pesticide contamination in breast milk of vegetarian mothers: 35 times as high*

➤ *Percentage of male college students sterile in 1950: .5*

➤ *Percentage of male college students sterile in 1978: 25*

➤ *Sperm count of average American male compared to 30 years ago: Down 30%*

➤ *Principle reason for sterility and sperm count reduction of U.S. males: Chlorinated hydrocarbon pesticides (including dioxin, DDT, etc.)*

➤ *Percentage of hydrocarbon pesticide residues in American diet attributable to meats, dairy products, fish and eggs: 94%*

375

➢ The Meat Board tells us Not to be concerned about the dioxins and other pesticides in today's beef because: the quantities are so small

➢ Less than 1 out of every quarter million slaughtered animals is tested for toxic chemical residues

➢ Wingspan of average Leghorn chicken: 26 inches

➢ Space average leghorn chicken given in egg factories: 6 inches

➢ Number of 700 plus pound pigs confined to space the size of a twin bed in typical factory farm: 3

➢ Reason today's veal is so tender: Calves never allowed to take a single step

➢ Reason today's veal is whitish-pink: Calves force fed on anaemia producing diet

➢ Hamburgers are ground up cows who've had their throats slit by machetes or their brains bashed in by sledgehammers.

➢ Number of animals killed for meat per hour in U.S.: 500,000

➢ Occupation with highest turnover rate in U.S.: Slaughterhouse worker

➢ Occupation with highest employee rate of injury in U.S.: Slaughter-house worker

➢ Cost to render an animal unconscious prior to slaughter with captive bolt pistol so that process is done humanely: 1 penny

➢ Reason given by meat industry for not utilising captive bolt pistol: Too expensive

➢ Percentage of total antibiotics used in U.S. fed routinely to livestock: 55

➢ Percentage of staphylococci infections resistant to penicillin in 1960: 13

➢ Percentage of staphylococci infections resistant to penicillin in 1988: 91

➢ Reason: Breeding of antibiotic resistant bacteria in factory farms due to routine feeding of antibiotics to livestock

➢ Effectiveness of all "wonder-drug" antibiotics: Declining rapidly

➢ Reason: Breeding of antibiotic resistant bacteria in factory farms due to routine feeding of antibiotics to livestock

➢ Response by entire European Economic Community to routine feeding of antibiotics to livestock: Ban

➢ Response by American meat and pharmaceutical industries to routine feeding of antibiotics to livestock: Full and complete support

> ➤ *Only man to win Ironman Triathlon more than twice: Dave Scott (6 time winner)*
> ➤ *Food choices of Dave Scott: Vegetarian*
> ➤ *World record holder for 24 triathlon (Swim 4.8 miles, Cycle 185 miles, Run 52.5): Sixto Linares*
> ➤ *Food choices of Sixto Linares: Strict vegetarian*
> ➤ *Athlete who most totally dominated Olympic sport in track and field history: Edwin Moses (undefeated in 8 years, 400 meter hurdles)*
> ➤ *Food choices of Edwin Moses: Vegetarian*
> ➤ *Other notable vegetarian athletes:*
> ➤ *Stan Price (World record-bench press)*
> ➤ *Robert Sweetgall (World's premier ultra-distance walker)*
> ➤ *Paavo Nurmi (20 World's records in distance running, 9 Olympic medals)*
> ➤ *Bill Pickering (World record – swimming English Channel)*
> ➤ *Murray Rose (World records – 400 and 1500 meter freestyles)*
> ➤ *Andreas Cahling (Winner – Mr. International body-building championships)*
> ➤ *Roy Hilligan (Winner – Mr. America body-building championships)*
> ➤ *Pierro Verot (World's record for downhill endurance skiing)*
> ➤ *Estelle Gray and Cheryl Marek (World's record for cross-country tandem cycling)*
> ➤ *James and Johnathon deDonato (World's record for distance butterfly stroke swimming)*
> ➤ *Ridgely Abele (Winner of 8 national championships in Karate, including U.S. Karate Association World Championships)*
> ➤ *EarthSave, P.O. Box 949, Felton, CA, 95018-0949*
> ➤ *For a larger list of well-known and historical vegetarians, see http://healthyvegetarian.org/vegpeople.html*

## Harmonizing Our Diet

This conscious element leads us right into harmony. Eating with harmony doesn't just mean our harmony. It means we harmonize with those around us. It means that we are harmonizing with those living organisms around us, who are alive as we are.

Each of our bodies is unique. Just as each of us has a distinct combination of fingerprints, retinas, body shape, DNA, mentality, history, and personality, each of us has a particular combination of food that works best for our body.

Every living being has passed through the physical journey with a different history, slightly different tastes, different goals, different aspirations and different desires. Therefore, it would not be logical to gauge someone's eating based upon their blood type, *dosha* type or any other narrow range. While many healers may find this position highly inflammatory, the fact is; there simply are not enough categories to cover all the variances between different body types.

We would practically need at least millions of body types to cover the variances between genetics, personality, and lifestyle. While a person's *dosha* and blood type may well provide some possible explanation in some cases as to why one person might not tolerate certain foods, the fact remains that we simply cannot generalize and categorize billions of people into just three or four types.

In reality, nature gives us all a tremendous amount of leeway in choosing our various food types and diets. This leeway indeed translates itself into very individual selections of diets as our bodies age and accumulate the variances of our choices. As our previous choices provide appropriate reactions in our body types, we each end up with distinctive body shapes and diets. This means we each must make a determination of what foods our bodies are best adjusted to and work from that point. We have to make educated choices.

As our bodies age they become increasingly adapted to whatever diet we have been eating. As a result, a drastic course of change in dietary habits, especially among older people, is not too wise. The drastic change in cuisine can stimulate a variety of reactions. These can include allergic and detoxification responses, as the body tries to clear itself of the unnatural constituents of the previous toxic diet.

A better tactic might be to select our own ultimate diet, and build a gradual bridge between our diet today and that diet goal. This bridge should enable us to make slow, gradual dietary changes. As we make gradual changes, the body will slowly adapt, and gradually detoxify the older diet. For those with medical conditions, these changes may be better overseen by a health professional – particularly one versed in nutrition and detoxification.

Still, we can make gradual adjustments to our diet. The earlier we align our diets to the foods nature has designed for us the better. Following this would be to avoid to the extent possible overly processed foods. These include white flours, white sugars, white salts (white=denatured and bleached); as well as any food packed with chemical preservatives, chemical food dyes, and other synthetic additives. They also include overly-fried foods, especially those cooked in saturated or hydrogenated vegetable oils.

Simplicity is best. The best guideline is to add as many probiotic, fresh, steamed or minimally cooked vegetables, beans, nuts, grains dairy and fruits as possible. This will guarantee good fiber content, probiotic colonies and a wide variety of nutrients. The more of these we can comfortably eat the better.

Should we eat generous amounts of whole nuts, legumes and seeds, we will be gaining important fatty acids and amino acids in their natural states. Seeds are especially important. Let's not spit out the seeds: Sesame seeds, poppy seeds, sunflower seeds (packed with every essential amino acid); and even watermelon seeds, the tiny seeds on strawberries, blackberry seeds and lemon seeds provide important lignans and phytoestrogens. And let's not squeeze out the juice and leave the fiber and peel behind in our fruits. The more peel we can eat the better.

A good strategy is to weekly add a new living, fresh or whole food to our diet. This makes for a fun exploration process. With each addition, we can learn how to prepare that particular food to maximize its taste and nutrition with other foods. This strategy will also allow the body to adapt slowly develop a taste for these foods. With each addition of a whole or fresh food, we can eliminate one denatured, refined or otherwise overly processed food.

For a younger person, changes can be made even faster. Perhaps adding three new whole foods a week might be the way to go. It is best to eliminate systematically, first the more destructive or toxic groups, and then one by one to replace the other food groups with phytonutrient food groups. It might be a good idea to replace a toxic food with a food with a similar mouth feel. For example, there are now a number of great red meat replacement foods which have similar mouth-feel and even taste like some meat dishes.

In other words, going from a plate of sirloin with a few overcooked peas and potatoes on the side, to exclusively salad and soup simply may not work for long. The senses become accustomed to certain diets. Many foods are also considered "comfort foods." Actually, many wonderful-tasting natural foods can also become comfort foods. We simply have to begin to eat them while we are among friends, in a relaxed environment for awhile. Over time, we will associate them with those comfortable surroundings and they too will become "comfort foods."

The bottom line is that our foods should bring us joy. While it might seem odd to consider eating as joyful, it is actually the process of growing, selecting, preparing and offering our food that make them joyful. The eating is simply the icing. The process of preparing and planting our own garden can be joyful as we work with nature's elements and rhythms to determine the right time to plant. Once we dig into the soil to prepare it for planting, we enter the rhythm of nature by becoming part of the process.

As the seeds gently slide from our hands into the soil we experience the joy of being part of the creative process of the Almighty. As we weed, water and defend our garden we bond with the needs of our plants as they beautifully leaf, flower and/or seed into the tomatoes, lettuce, cucumbers, broccoli, beans and other foods. We can ponder their deep resonating colors, reflecting on their start as tiny seeds slipping off our hands. As we harvest them, we share their giving with thankfulness and appreciation. We can then share our bountiful harvests with our neighbors, friends and family. This sharing process brings us joy – the real meaning behind Thanksgiving.

We can also select a local farmer's market or community health food cooperative to shop at. As we shop in these markets, we can connect with the process of growing and producing natural foods by shaking hands with the farmers, or working together with other people in the co-op to share in bulk purchases.

Many community cooperatives work through volunteering at the market. We can volunteer by doing the register, cutting cheese or otherwise working with people in the community. All of these activities can create joy because they involve a sharing of consciousness. Sharing consciousness brings joy – especially when it includes giving of ourselves in some respect.

After harvest or purchase we can then prepare our foods with a humble appreciation for their color, taste and aromas. For most foods we can include the peels to retain color, fiber and nutrition. As we prepare our meals we can create a beautiful painting with each meal. If our meals are whole, they will be colorful. We can place our multi-colored foods upon our plates and our family's plates; each a masterpiece of fragrant color and texture.

There is no coincidence that we receive joy by offering and sharing our food with family and friends before we partake. Most of us consider this simply as being polite – to offer a drink or a sampling of something we eat to our companion before we consume it. However, this can certainly be a joyful act.

The act of sharing our food with not only friends and family, but with those who may be hungry ushers an exchange that our inner selves thrive on: love.

To share food with others creates an inner harmony. Nutrition for the soul. A table of giving is a joyful table, and a table of greed is a sorrowful one.

To extend this harmony on a spiritual level, we can also offer our food to our Creator before partaking. "Saying Grace" before we eat, or creating a devotional offering prior to eating is an ancient practice that has spanned the course of time among our ancestors for thousands of years.

Reaching out spiritually from within harmonizes our food with our inner spiritual consciousness, producing a meal that is nourishing to the soul as well as the body.

# References and Bibliography

Abdureyim S, Amat N, Umar A, Upur H, Berke B, Moore N. Anti-inflammatory, immunomodulatory, and heme oxygenase-1 inhibitory activities of ravan napas, a formulation of uighur traditional medicine, in a rat model of allergic asthma. *Evid Based Complement Alternat Med.* 2011;2011. pii: 725926.

Aberg N, Hesselmar B, Aberg B, Eriksson B. Increase of asthma, allergic rhinitis and eczema in Swedish schoolchildren between 1979 and 1991. *Clin Exp Allergy.* 1995;25:815-819.

Adel-Patient K, Ah-Leung S, Creminon C, Nouaille S, Chatel JM, Langella P, Wal JM. Oral administration of recombinant Lactococcus lactis expressing bovine beta-lactoglobulin partially prevents mice from sensitization. *Clin Exp Allergy.* 2005 Apr;35(4):539-46.

Adoga AS, Otene AA, Yiltok SJ, Adekwu A, Nwaorgu OG. Cervical necrotizing fasciitis: case series and review of literature. *Niger J Med.* 2009 Apr-Jun;18(2):203-7.

Agache I, Ciobanu C. Risk factors and asthma phenotypes in children and adults with seasonal allergic rhinitis. *Phys Sportsmed.* 2010 Dec;38(4):81-6.

Agarwal KN, Bhasin SK, Faridi MM, Mathur M, Gupta S. *Lactobacillus casei* in the control of acute diarrhea – a pilot study. *Indian Pediatr.* 2001 Aug;38(8):905-10.

Agarwal SK, Singh SS, Verma S. Antifungal principle of sesquiterpene lactones from Anamirta cocculus. *Indian Drugs.* 1999;36:754-5.

Agerholm-Larsen L, Raben A, Haulrik N, Hansen AS, Manders M, Astrup A. Effect of 8 week intake of probiotic milk products on risk factors for cardiovascular diseases. *Eur J Clin Nutr.* 2000 Apr;54(4):288-97.

Aggarwal BB, Harikumar KB. Potential therapeutic effects of curcumin, the anti-inflammatory agent, against neurodegenerative, cardiovascular, pulmonary, metabolic, autoimmune and neoplastic diseases. *Int J Biochem Cell Biol.* 2009 Jan;41(1):40-59.

Aggarwal BB, Sung B. Pharmacological basis for the role of curcumin in chronic diseases: an age-old spice with modern targets. *Trends Pharmacol Sci.* 2009 Feb;30(2):85-94.

Agostoni C, Fiocchi A, Riva E, Terracciano L, Sarratud T, Martelli A, Lodi F, D'Auria E, Zuccotti G, Giovannini M. Growth of infants with IgE-mediated cow's milk allergy fed different formulas in the complementary feeding period. *Pediatr Allergy Immunol.* 2007 Nov;18(7):599-606.

Agustina R, Lukito W, Firmansyah A, Suhardjo HN, Murniati D, Bindels J. The effect of early nutritional supplementation with a mixture of probiotic, prebiotic, fiber and micronutrients in infants with acute diarrhea in Indonesia. *Asia Pac J Clin Nutr.* 2007;16(3):435-42.

Ahmed M, Prasad J, Gill H, Stevenson L, Gopal P. Impact of consumption of different levels of *Bifidobacterium lactis* HN019 on the intestinal microflora of elderly human subjects. *J Nutr Health Aging.* 2007 Jan-Feb;11(1):26-31.

Ahmed, AA, McCarthy RD, Porter GA. Effect of of milk constituents on hepatic cholesterogenesis. *Atherosclerosis.* 1979;32:347-57.

Aho K, Koskenvuo M, Tuominen J, Kaprio J. Occurrence of rheumatoid arthritis in a nationwide series of twins. *J Rheumatol.* 1986 Oct;13(5):899-902.

Ahola AJ, Yli-Knuuttila H, Suomalainen T, Poussa T, Ahlström A, Meurman JH, Korpela R. Short-term consumption of probiotic-containing cheese and its effect on dental caries risk factors. *Arch Oral Biol.* 2002 Nov;47(11):799-804.

Aihara K, Kajimoto O, Hirata H, Takahashi R, Nakamura Y. Effect of powdered fermented milk with *Lactobacillus helveticus* on subjects with high-normal blood pressure or mild hypertension. *J Am Coll Nutr.* 2005 Aug;24(4):257-65.

Airola P. How to Get Well. Health Plus Publishers, 1974.

Akil I, Yilmaz O, Kurutepe S, Degerli K, Kavukcu S. Influence of oral intake of *Saccharomyces boulardii* on *Escherichia coli* in enteric flora. *Pediatr Nephrol.* 2006 Jun;21(6):807-10.

Akinbami LJ, Moorman JE, Garbe PL, Sondik EJ. Status of childhood asthma in the United States, 1980-2007. *Pediatrics.* 2009;123:S131-45.

Albarracin SL, Stab B, Casas Z, Sutachan JJ, Samudio I, Gonzalez J, Gonzalo L, Capani F, Morales L, Barreto GE. Effects of natural antioxidants in neurodegenerative disease. Nutr Neurosci. 2012 Jan;15(1):1-9.

Alcalay RN, Gu Y, Mejia-Santana H, Cote L, Marder KS, Scarmeas N. The association between Mediterranean diet adherence and Parkinson's disease. Mov Disord. 2012 May;27(6):771-4.

Alcántar-Aguirre FC, Chagolla A, Tiessen A, Délano JP, González de la Vara LE. ATP produced by oxidative phosphorylation is channeled toward hexokinase bound to mitochondrial porin (VDAC) in beetroots (Beta vulgaris). Planta. 2013 Mar 17.

Alderman MH, Cohen HW. Dietary sodium intake and cardiovascular mortality: controversy resolved? Am J Hypertens. 2012 Jul;25(7):727-34. doi:10.1038/ajh.2012.52.

Aldinucci C, Bellussi L, Monciatti G, Passàli GC, Salerni L, Passàli D, Bocci V. Effects of dietary yoghurt on immunological and clinical parameters of rhinopathic patients. *Eur J Clin Nutr.* 2002 Dec;56(12):1155-61.

Alemán A, Sastre J, Quirce S, de las Heras M, Carnés J, Fernández-Caldas E, Pastor C, Blázquez AB, Vivanco F, Cuesta-Herranz J. Allergy to kiwi: a double-blind, placebo-controlled food challenge study in patients from a birch-free area. *J Allergy Clin Immunol.* 2004 Mar;113(3):543-50.

Alexander DD, Cabana MD. Partially hydrolyzed 100% whey protein infant formula and reduced risk of atopic dermatitis: a meta-analysis. *J Pediatr Gastroenterol Nutr.* 2010 Apr;50(4):422-30.

Alexandrakis M, Letourneau R, Kempuraj D, Kandere-Grzybowska K, Huang M, Christodoulou S, Boucher W, Seretakis D, Theoharides TC. Flavones inhibit proliferation and increase mediator content in human leukemic mast cells (HMC-1). *Eur J Haematol.* 2003 Dec;71(6):448-54.

383

Alfvén T, Braun-Fahrländer C, Brunekreef B, von Mutius E, Riedler J, Scheynius A, van Hage M, Wickman M, Benz MR, Budde J, Michels KB, Schram D, Ublagger E, Waser M, Pershagen G; PARSIFAL study group. Allergic diseases and atopic sensitization in children related to farming and anthroposophic lifestyle – the PARSIFAL study. *Allergy.* 2006 Apr;61(4):414-21. PubMed PMID: 16512802.

Al-Harrasi A, Al-Saidi S. Phytochemical analysis of the essential oil from botanically certified oleogum resin of Boswellia sacra (Omani Luban). *Molecules.* 2008 Sep 16;13(9):2181-9.

Allen SJ, Okoko B, Martinez E, Gregorio G, Dans LF. Probiotics for treating infectious diarrhea. *The Cochrane Library.* 2004;3. Chichester, UK: John Wiley & Sons, Ltd.

Alleva R, Tomasetti M, Bompadre S, Littarru GP. Oxidation of LDL and their subfractions: kinetic aspects and CoQ10 content. *Mol Aspects Med.* 1997;18 Suppl:S105-12.

Almqvist C, Garden F, Xuan W, Mihrshahi S, Leeder SR, Oddy W, Webb K, Marks GB; CAPS team. Omega-3 and omega-6 fatty acid exposure from early life does not affect atopy and asthma at age 5 years. *J Allergy Clin Immunol.* 2007 Jun;119(6):1438-44.

Amato R, Pinelli M, Monticelli A, Miele G, Cocozza S. Schizophrenia and Vitamin D Related Genes Could Have Been Subject to Latitude-driven Adaptation. *BMC Evol Biol.* 2010 Nov 11;10(1):351.

Amenta M, Cascio MT, Di Fiore P, Venturini I. Diet and chronic constipation. Benefits of oral supplementation with symbiotic zir fos (*Bifidobacterium longum* W11 + FOS Actilight). *Acta Biomed.* 2006 Dec;77(3):157-62.

American Conference of Governmental Industrial Hygienists. *Threshold limit values for chemical substances and physical agents in the work environment.* Cincinnati, OH: ACGIH, 1986.

American Dietetic Association; Dietitians of Canada. Position of the American Dietetic Association and Dietitians of Canada: vegetarian diets. *Can J Diet Pract Res.* 2003 Summer;64(2):62-81.

Ammon HP. Boswellic acids (components of frankincense) as the active principle in treatment of chronic inflammatory diseases. *Wien Med Wochenschr.* 2002;152(15-16):373-8.

Ammon HP. Boswellic acids in chronic inflammatory diseases. *Planta Med.* 2006 Oct;72(12):1100-16.

Anand P, Thomas SG, Kunnumakkara AB, Sundaram C, Harikumar KB, Sung B, Tharakan ST, Misra K, Priyadarsini IK, Rajasekharan KN, Aggarwal BB. Biological activities of curcumin and its analogues (Congeners) made by man and Mother Nature. *Biochem Pharmacol.* 2008 Dec 1;76(11):1590-611.

Anderson JL, May HT, Horne BD, Bair TL, Hall NL, Carlquist JF, Lappé DL, Muhlestein JB; Intermountain Heart Collaborative (IHC) Study Group. Relation of vitamin D deficiency to cardiovascular risk factors, disease status, and incident events in a general healthcare population. *Am J Cardiol.* 2010 Oct 1;106(7):963-8.

Anderson JW, Baird P, Davis RH Jr, Ferreri S, Knudtson M, Koraym A, Waters V, Williams CL. Health benefits of dietary fiber. *Nutr Rev.* 2009 Apr;67(4):188-205.

Anderson JW, Gilliland SE. Effect of fermented milk (yogurt) containing *Lactobacillus acidophilus* L1 on serum cholesterol in hypercholesterolemic humans. *J Am Coll Nutr.* 1999 Feb;18(1):43-50.

Anderson M., Grissom C. Increasing the Heavy Atom Effect of Xenon by Adsorption to Zeolites: Photolysis of 2,3-Diazabicyclo[2.2.2]oct-2-ene. *J. Am. Chem. Soc.* 1996;118:9552-9556.

Anderson SD, Charlton B, Weiler JM, Nichols S, Spector SL, Pearlman DS; A305 Study Group. Comparison of mannitol and methacholine to predict exercise-induced bronchoconstriction and a clinical diagnosis of asthma. *Respir Res.* 2009 Jan 23;10:4.

Andoh T, Zhang Q, Yamamoto T, Tayama M, Hattori M, Tanaka K, Kuraishi Y. Inhibitory Effects of the Methanol Extract of Ganoderma lucidum on Mosquito Allergy-Induced Itch-Associated Responses in Mice. *J Pharmacol Sci.* 2010 Oct 8.

André C, André F, Colin L. Effect of allergen ingestion challenge with and without cromoglycate cover on intestinal permeability in atopic dermatitis, urticaria and other symptoms of food allergy. *Allergy.* 1989;44 Suppl 9:47-51.

André C. Food allergy. Objective diagnosis and test of therapeutic efficacy by measuring intestinal permeability. *Presse Med.* 1986 Jan 25;15(3):105-8.

Andre F, Andre C, Feknous M, Colin L, Cavagna S. Digestive permeability to different-sized molecules and to sodium cromoglycate in food allergy. *Allergy Proc.* 1991 Sep-Oct;12(5):293-8.

Andrews RC, Cooper AR, Montgomery AA, Norcross AJ, Peters TJ, Sharp DJ, Jackson N, Fitzsimons K, Bright J, Coulman K, England CY, Gorton J, McLenaghan A, Paxton E, Polet A, Thompson C, Dayan CM. Diet or diet plus physical activity versus usual care in patients with newly diagnosed type 2 diabetes: the Early ACTID randomised controlled trial. *Lancet.* 2011 Jul 9;378(9786):129-39.

Angeli JP, Ribeiro LR, Bellini MF, Mantovani. Anti-clastogenic effect of beta-glucan extracted from barley towards chemically induced DNA damage in rodent cells. *Hum Exp Toxicol.* 2006 Jun;25(6):319-24.

Anim-Nyame N, Sooranna SR, Johnson MR, Gamble J, Steer PJ. Garlic supplementation increases peripheral blood flow: a role for interleukin-6? *J Nutr Biochem.* 2004 Jan;15(1):30-6.

Annweiler C, Schott AM, Berrut G, Chauviré V, Le Gall D, Inzitari M, Beauchet O. Vitamin D and ageing: neurological issues. *Neuropsychobiology.* 2010 Aug;62(3):139-50.

Antczak A, Nowak D, Shariati B, Król M, Piasecka G, Kurmanowska Z. Increased hydrogen peroxide and thiobarbituric acid-reactive products in expired breath condensate of asthmatic patients. *Eur Respir J.* 1997 Jun;10(6):1235-41.

Anukam K, Osazuwa E, Ahonkhai I, Ngwu M, Osemene G, Bruce AW, Reid G. Augmentation of antimicrobial metronidazole therapy of bacterial vaginosis with oral probiotic *Lactobacillus rhamnosus* GR-1 and *Lactobacillus reuteri* RC-14: randomized, double-blind, placebo controlled trial. *Microbes Infect.* 2006 May;8(6):1450-4.

Anukam KC, Osazuwa E, Osemene GI, Ehigiagbe F, Bruce AW, Reid G. Clinical study comparing probiotic Lactobacillus GR-1 and RC-14 with metronidazole vaginal gel to treat symptomatic bacterial vaginosis. *Microbes Infect.* 2006 Oct;8(12-13):2772-6.

# REFERENCES AND BIBLIOGRAPHY

Anukam KC, Osazuwa EO, Osadolor HB, Bruce AW, Reid G. Yogurt containing probiotic *Lactobacillus rhamnosus* GR-1 and *L. reuteri* RC-14 helps resolve moderate diarrhea and increases CD4 count in HIV/AIDS patients. *J Clin Gastroenterol.* 2008 Mar;42(3):239-43.

Aoki T, Usuda Y, Miyakoshi H, Tamura K, Herberman RB. Low natural killer syndrome: clinical and immunologic features. *Nat Immun Cell Growth Regul.* 1987;6(3):116-28.

Apáti P, Houghton PJ, Kite G, Steventon GB, Kéry A. In-vitro effect of flavonoids from Solidago canadensis extract on glutathione S-transferase. *J Pharm Pharmacol.* 2006 Feb;58(2):251-6.

APHA (American Public Health Association). Opposition to the Use of Hormone Growth Promoters in Beef and Dairy Cattle Production. Policy Date: 11/10/2009. Policy Number: 20098. http://www.apha.org/advocacy/policy/id=1379. Accessed Nov. 24, 2010.

Appleby PN, Thorogood M, Mann JI, Key TJ. The Oxford Vegetarian Study: an overview. Am J Clin Nutr. 1999 Sep;70(3 Suppl):525S-531S.

Araki K, Shinozaki T, Irie Y, Miyazawa Y. Trial of oral administration of *Bifidobacterium breve* for the prevention of rotavirus infections. *Kansenshogaku Zasshi.* 1999 Apr;73(4):305-10.

Araujo AC, Aprile LR, Dantas RO, Terra-Filho J, Vianna EO. Bronchial responsiveness during esophageal acid infusion. Lung. 2008 Mar-Apr;186(2):123-8. 2008 Feb 23.

Arbes SJ Jr, Gergen PJ, Vaughn B, Zeldin DC. Asthma cases attributable to atopy: results from the Third National Health and Nutrition Examination Survey. *J Allergy Clin Immunol.* 2007 Nov;120(5):1139-45. 2007 Sep 24.

Argento A, Tiraferri E, Marzaloni M. Oral anticoagulants and medicinal plants. An emerging interaction. *Ann Ital Med Int.* 2000 Apr-Jun;15(2):139-43.

Arif AA, Delclos GL, Colmer-Hamood J. Association between asthma, asthma symptoms and C-reactive protein in US adults: data from the National Health and Nutrition Examination Survey, 1999-2002. *Respirology.* 2007 Sep;12(5):675-82. .

Arif AA, Shah SM. Association between personal exposure to volatile organic compounds and asthma among US adult population. *Int Arch Occup Environ Health.* 2007 Aug;80(8):711-9.

Arjmandi BH, Johnson CD, Campbell SC, Hooshmand S, Chai SC, Akhter MP. Combining fructooligosaccharide and dried plum has the greatest effect on restoring bone mineral density among select functional foods and bioactive compounds. J Med Food. 2010 Apr;13(2):312-9.

Arjmandi, B. H., R. Birnbaum, *et al.* 1998. Bone-sparing effect of soy protein in ovarian hormone-deficient rats is related to its isoflavone content. Am J Clin Nutr 68(6 Suppl): 1364S-1368S.

Armstrong BK. Absorption of vitamin B12 from the human colon. *Am J Clin Nutr.* 1968;21:298-9.

Armuzzi A, Cremonini F, Bartolozzi F, Canducci F, Candelli M, Ojetti V, Cammarota G, Anti M, De Lorenzo A, Pola P, Gasbarrini G, Gasbarrini A. The effect of oral administration of Lactobacillus GG on antibiotic-associated gastrointestinal side-effects during Helicobacter pylori eradication therapy. *Aliment Pharmacol Ther.* 2001 Feb;15(2):163-9.

Arrigo G, D'Angelo A. Achromycin and anaphylactic shock. *Riv Patol Clin.* 1959 Oct;14:719-22.

Arshad SH, Bateman B, Sadeghnejad A, Gant C, Matthews SM. Prevention of allergic disease during childhood by allergen avoidance: the Isle of Wight prevention study. *J Allergy Clin Immunol.* 2007 Feb;119(2):307-13.

Arslanoglu S, Moro GE, Schmitt J, Tandoi L, Rizzardi S, Boehm G. Early dietary intervention with a mixture of prebiotic oligosaccharides reduces the incidence of allergic manifestations and infections during the first two years of life. *J Nutr.* 2008 Jun;138(6):1091-5.

Arterburn LM, Oken HA, Bailey Hall E, Hamersley J, Kuratko CN, Hoffman JP. Algal-oil capsules and cooked salmon: nutritionally equivalent sources of docosahexaenoic acid. *J Am Diet Assoc.* 2008 Jul;108(7):1204-9.

Arterburn LM, Oken HA, Hoffman JP, Bailey-Hall E, Chung G, Rom D, Hamersley J, McCarthy D. Bioequivalence of Docosahexaenoic acid from different algal oils in capsules and in a DHA-fortified food. *Lipids.* 2007 Nov;42(11):1011-24.

Arunachalam K, Gill HS, Chandra RK. Enhancement of natural immune function by dietary consumption of *Bifidobacterium lactis* (HN019). *Eur J Clin Nutr.* 2000 Mar;54(3):263-7.

Arvaniti F, Priftis KN, Panagiotakos DB. Dietary habits and asthma: a review. *Allergy Asthma Proc.* 2010 Mar;31(2):e1-10.

Arvola T, Laiho K, Torkkeli S, Mykkänen H, Salminen S, Maunula L, Isolauri E. Prophylactic Lactobacillus GG reduces antibiotic-associated diarrhea in children with respiratory infections: a randomized study. *Pediatrics.* 1999 Nov;104(5):e64.

Asero R, Antonicelli L, Arena A, Bommarito L, Caruso B, Colombo G, Crivellaro M, De Carli M, Della Torre E, Della Torre F, Heffler E, Lodi Rizzini F, Longo R, Manzotti G, Marcotulli A, Melchiorre A, Minale P, Morandi P, Moreni B, Moschella A, Murzilli F, Nebiolo F, Poppa M, Randazzo S, Rossi G, Senna GE. Causes of food-induced anaphylaxis in Italian adults: a multi-centre study. *Int Arch Allergy Immunol.* 2009;150(3):271-7.

Asero R, Mistrello G, Roncarolo D, Amato S, Caldironi G, Barocci F, van Ree R. Immunological cross-reactivity between lipid transfer proteins from botanically unrelated plant-derived foods: a clinical study. *Allergy.* 2002 Oct;57(10):900-6.

Ashaye A, Gaziano J, Djoussé L. Red meat consumption and risk of heart failure in male physicians. Nutr Metab Cardiovasc Dis. 2010 Jul 30.

Ashrafi K, Chang FY, Watts JL, Fraser AG, Kamath RS, Ahringer J, Ruvkun G. Genome-wide RNAi analysis of Caenorhabditis elegans fat regulatory genes. *Nature.* 2003 Jan 16;421(6920):268-72.

Aso Y, Akaza H, Kotake T, Tsukamoto T, Imai K, Naito S. Preventive effect of a *Lactobacillus casei* preparation on the recurrence of superficial bladder cancer in a double-blind trial. The BLP Study Group. *Eur Urol.* 1995;27(2):104-9.

Aso Y, Akazan H. Prophylactic effect of a *Lactobacillus casei* preparation on the recurrence of superficial bladder cancer. *BLP Study Group. Urol Int.* 1992;49(3):125-9.

Ataie-Jafari A, Larijani B, Alavi Majd H, Tahbaz F. Cholesterol-lowering effect of probiotic yogurt in comparison with ordinary yogurt in mildly to moderately hypercholesterolemic subjects. *Ann Nutr Metab.* 2009;54(1):22-7.

Atkinson W, Harris J, Mills P, Moffat S, White C, Lynch O, Jones M, Cullinan P, Newman Taylor AJ. Domestic aeroallergen exposures among infants in an English town. *Eur Respir J.* 1999 Mar;13(3):583-9.

Atsumi T, Tonosaki K. Smelling lavender and rosemary increases free radical scavenging activity and decreases cortisol level in saliva. *Psychiatry Res.* 2007 Feb 28;150(1):89-96.

Backster C. *Primary Perception: Biocommunication with Plants, Living Foods, and Human Cells.* Anza, CA: White Rose Millennium Press, 2003.

Bacopoulou F, Veltsista A, Vassi I, Gika A, Lekea V, Priftis K, Bakoula C. Can we be optimistic about asthma in childhood? A Greek cohort study. *J Asthma.* 2009 Mar;46(2):171-4.

Badar VA, Thawani VR, Wakode PT, Shrivastava MP, Gharpure KJ, Hingorani LL, Khiyani RM. Efficacy of Tinospora cordifolia in allergic rhinitis. *J Ethnopharmacol.* 2005 Jan 15;96(3):445-9.

Bae GS, Kim MS, Jung WS, Seo SW, Yun SW, Kim SG, Park RK, Kim EC, Song HJ, Park SJ. Inhibition of lipopolysaccharide-induced inflammatory responses by piperine. *Eur J Pharmacol.* 2010 Sep 10;642(1-3):154-62.

Bafadhel M, Singapuri A, Terry S, Hargadon B, Monteiro W, Green RH, Bradding PH, Wardlaw AJ, Pavord ID, Brightling CE. Body mass and fat mass in refractory asthma: an observational 1 year follow-up study. *J Allergy.* 2010;2010:251758. 2010 Dec 1.

Bai AP, Ouyang Q, Xiao XR, Li SF. Probiotics modulate inflammatory cytokine secretion from inflamed mucosa in active ulcerative colitis. *Int J Clin Pract.* 2006 Mar;60(3):284-8.

Baik HW. Nutritional therapy in gastrointestinal disease. *Korean J Gastroenterol.* 2004 Jun;43(6):331-40.

Baker SM. *Detoxification and Healing.* Chicago: Contemporary Books, 2004.

Bakkeheim E, Mowinckel P, Carlsen KH, Håland G, Carlsen KC. Paracetamol in early infancy: the risk of childhood allergy and asthma. *Acta Paediatr.* 2011 Jan;100(1):90-6.

Bakshi A, Stephen S, Borum ML, Doman DB. Emerging therapeutic options for celiac disease: potential alternatives to a gluten-free diet. *Gastroenterol Hepatol (N Y).* 2012 Sep;8(9):582-8.

Balch P, Balch J. *Prescription for Nutritional Healing.* New York: Avery, 2000.

Balimane P, Yong-Haen H, Chong S. Current Industrial Practices of Assessing Permeability and P-Glycoprotein Interaction. *J AAPS* 2006; 8(1).

Ballentine R. *Diet & Nutrition: A holistic approach.* Honesdale, PA: Himalayan Int., 1978.

Ballentine RM. *Radical Healing.* New York: Harmony Books, 1999.

Balli F, Bertolani P, Giberti G, Amarri S. High-dose oral bacteria-therapy for chronic non-specific diarrhea of infancy. *Pediatr Med Chir.* 1992 Jan-Feb;14(1):13-5.

Balliett M, Burke JR. Changes in anthropometric measurements, body composition, blood pressure, lipid profile, and testosterone in patients participating in a low-energy dietary intervention. *J Chiropr Med.* 2013 Mar;12(1):3-14. doi: 10.1016/j.jcm.2012.11.003.

Ballmer-Weber BK, Holzhauser T, Scibilia J, Mittag D, Zisa G, Ortolani C, Oesterballe M, Poulsen LK, Vieths S, Bindslev-Jensen C. Clinical characteristics of soybean allergy in Europe: a double-blind, placebo-controlled food challenge study. *J Allergy Clin Immunol.* 2007 Jun;119(6):1489-96.

Ballmer-Weber BK, Vieths S, Lüttkopf D, Heuschmann P, Wüthrich B. Celery allergy confirmed by double-blind, placebo-controlled food challenge: a clinical study in 32 subjects with a history of adverse reactions to celery root. *J Allergy Clin Immunol.* 2000 Aug;106(2):373-8.

Banno N, Akihisa T, Yasukawa K, Tokuda H, Tabata K, Nakamura Y, Nishimura R, Kimura Y, Suzuki T. Anti-inflammatory activities of the triterpene acids from the resin of Boswellia carteri. *J Ethnopharmacol.* 2006 Sep 19;107(2):249-53.

Bant A, Kruszewski J. Increased sensitization prevalence to common inhalant and food allergens in young adult Polish males. *Ann Agric Environ Med.* 2008 Jun;15(1):21-7.

Barnes M, Cullinan P, Athanasaki P, MacNeill S, Hole AM, Harris J, Kalogeraki S, Chatzinikolaou M, Drakonakis N, Bibaki-Liakou V, Newman Taylor AJ, Bibakis I. Crete: does farming explain urban and rural differences in atopy? *Clin Exp Allergy.* 2001 Dec;31(12):1822-8.

Barnetson RS, Drummond H, Ferguson A. Precipitins to dietary proteins in atopic eczema. *Br J Dermatol.* 1983 Dec;109(6):653-5.

Barnett AG, Williams GM, Schwartz J, Neller AH, Best TL, Petroeschevsky AL, Simpson RW. Air pollution and child respiratory health: a case-crossover study in Australia and New Zealand. *Am J Respir Crit Care Med.* 2005 Jun 1;171(11):1272-8.

Baron M. A patented strain of Bacillus coagulans increased immune response to viral challenge. *Postgrad Med.* 2009 Mar;121(2):114-8.

Barrager E, Veltmann JR Jr, Schauss AG, Schiller RN. A multicentered, open-label trial on the safety and efficacy of methylsulfonylmethane in the treatment of seasonal allergic rhinitis. *J Altern Complement Med.* 2002 Apr;8(2):167-73.

Barros R, Moreira A, Fonseca J, de Oliveira JF, Delgado L, Castel-Branco MG, Haahtela T, Lopes C, Moreira P. Adherence to the Mediterranean diet and fresh fruit intake are associated with improved asthma control. *Allergy.* 2008 Jul;63(7):917-23.

Bartram HP, Scheppach W, Gerlach S, Ruckdeschel G, Kelber E, Kasper H. Does yogurt enriched with *Bifidobacterium longum* affect colonic microbiology and fecal metabolites in health subjects? *Am J Clin Nutr.* 1994 Feb;59(2):428-32.

# REFERENCES AND BIBLIOGRAPHY

Basu A, Devaraj S, Jialal I. Dietary factors that promote or retard inflammation. *Arterioscler Thromb Vasc Biol.* 2006 May;26(5):995-1001.

Basu S, Chatterjee M, Ganguly S, Chandra PK. Effect of *Lactobacillus rhamnosus* GG in persistent diarrhea in Indian children: a randomized controlled trial. *J Clin Gastroenterol.* 2007 Sep;41(8):756-60.

Basu S, Chatterjee M, Ganguly S, Chandra PK. Efficacy of *Lactobacillus rhamnosus* GG in acute watery diarrhoea of Indian children: a randomised controlled trial. *J Paediatr Child Health.* 2007 Dec;43(12):837-42.

Bateman B, Warner JO, Hutchinson E, Dean T, Rowlandson P, Gant C, Grundy J, Fitzgerald C, Stevenson J. The effects of a double blind, placebo controlled, artificial food colourings and benzoate preservative challenge on hyperactivity in a general population sample of preschool children. *Arch Dis Child.* 2004 Jun;89(6):506-11.

Bates DW, Cullen DJ, Laird N, Petersen LA, Small SD, Servi D, Laffel G, Sweitzer BJ, Shea BF, Hallisey R, *et al.* Incidence of adverse drug events and potential adverse drug events. Implications for prevention. ADE Prevention Study Group. *JAMA.* 1995 Jul 5;274(1):29-34.

Batista R, Martins I, Jeno P, Ricardo CP, Oliveira MM. A proteomic study to identify soya allergens – the human response to transgenic versus non-transgenic soya samples. *Int Arch Allergy Immunol.* 2007;144(1):29-38.

Batmanghelidj F. Neurotransmitter histamine: an alternative view point, *Science in Medicine Simplified.* Falls Church, VA: Foundation for the Simple in Medicine, 1990.

Batmanghelidj F. Pain: a need for paradigm change. *Anticancer Res.* 1987 Sep-Oct;7(5B):971-89.

Batmanghelidj F. *Your Body's Many Cries for Water.* 2nd Ed. Vienna, VA: Global Health, 1997.

Bazzan AJ, Newberg AB, Cho WC, Monti DA. Diet and Nutrition in Cancer Survivorship and Palliative Care. Evidence-Based Complementary and Alternative Medicine, vol. 2013, Article ID 917647, 12 pages, 2013.

Beasley R, Clayton T, Crane J, von Mutius E, Lai CK, Montefort S, Stewart A; ISAAC Phase Three Study Group. Association between paracetamol use in infancy and childhood, and risk of asthma, rhinoconjunctivitis, and eczema in children aged 6-7 years: analysis from Phase Three of the ISAAC programme. *Lancet.* 2008 Sep. 20;372(9643):1039-48.

Beaulieu A, Fessele K. Agent Orange: management of patients exposed in Vietnam. *Clin J Oncol Nurs.* 2003 May-Jun;7(3):320-3.

Beausoleil M, Fortier N, Guénette S, L'ecuyer A, Savoie M, Franco M, Lachaine J, Weiss K. Effect of a fermented milk combining *Lactobacillus acidophilus* Cl1285 and *Lactobacillus casei* in the prevention of antibiotic-associated diarrhea: a randomized, double-blind, placebo-controlled trial. *Can J Gastroenterol.* 2007 Nov;21(11):732-6.

Becker DJ, French B, Morris PB, Silvent E, Gordon RY. Phytosterols, red yeast rice, and lifestyle changes instead of statins: a randomized, double-blinded, placebo-controlled trial. Am Heart J. 2013 Jul;166(1):187-96. doi:10.1016/j.ahj.2013.03.019.

Becker DJ, Gordon RY, Halbert SC, French B, Morris PB, Rader DJ. Red yeast rice for dyslipidemia in statin-intolerant patients: a randomized trial. Ann Intern Med. 2009 Jun 16;150(12):830-9, W147-9.

Becker KG, Simon RM, Bailey-Wilson JE, Freidlin B, Biddison WE, McFarland HF, Trent JM. Clustering of non-major histocompatibility complex susceptibility candidate loci in human autoimmune diseases. *Proc Natl Acad Sci U S A.* 1998 Aug 18;95(17):9979-84.

Beddoe AF. *Biologic Ionization as Applied to Human Nutrition.* Warsaw: Wendell Whitman, 2002.

Beecher GR. Phytonutrients' role in metabolism: effects on resistance to degenerative processes. *Nutr Rev.* 1999 Sep;57(9 Pt 2):S3-6.

Behrensmeyer AK. The habitat of Plio-Pleistocene hominids in East Africa: Taphonomic and microstratigraphic evidence. In: Jolly C, editor. Early Hominids of Africa. New York: St. Martin's Press; 1978. pp. 165 – 189.

Bekkali NL, Bongers ME, Van den Berg MM, Liem O, Benninga MA. The role of a probiotics mixture in the treatment of childhood constipation: a pilot study. Nutr J. 2007 Aug 4;6:17.

Belcaro G, Cesarone MR, Errichi S, Zulli C, Errichi BM, Vinciguerra G, Ledda A, Di Renzo A, Stuard S, Dugall M, Pellegrini L, Gizzi G, Ippolito E, Ricci A, Cacchio M, Cipollone G, Ruffini I, Fano F, Hosoi M, Rohdewald P. Variations in C-reactive protein, plasma free radicals and fibrinogen values in patients with osteoarthritis treated with Pycnogenol. *Redox Rep.* 2008;13(6):271-6.

Bell IR, Baldwin CM, Schwartz GE, Illness from low levels of environmental chemicals: relevance to chronic fatigue syndrome and fibromyalgia. *Am J Med.* 1998;105 (suppl 3A).:74-82. S.

Bell SJ, Potter PC. Milk whey-specific immune complexes in allergic and non-allergic subjects. *Allergy.* 1988 Oct;43(7):497-503.

Bellavia A, Larsson SC, Bottai M, Wolk A, Orsini N. Fruit and vegetable consumption and all-cause mortality: a dose-response analysis. Am J Clin Nutr. 2013 Jun 26.

Ben, X.M., Zhou, X.Y., Zhao, W.H., Yu, W.L., Pan, W., Zhang, W.L., Wu, S.M., Van Beusekom, C.M., Schaafsma, A. (2004) Supplementation of milk formula with galactooligosaccharides improves intestinal micro-flora and fermentation in term infants. *Chin Med J.* 117(6):927-931, 2004.

Benard A, Desreumeaux P, Huglo D, Hoorelbeke A, Tonnel AB, Wallaert B. Increased intestinal permeability in bronchial asthma. *J Allergy Clin Immunol.* 1996 Jun;97(6):1173-8.

Bengmark S. Curcumin, an atoxic antioxidant and natural NFkappaB, cyclooxygenase-2, lipooxygenase, and inducible nitric oxide synthase inhibitor: a shield against acute and chronic diseases. *JPEN J Parenter Enteral Nutr.* 2006 Jan-Feb;30(1):45-51.

Bengmark S. Immunonutrition: role of biosurfactants, fiber, and probiotic bacteria. *Nutrition.* 1998 Jul-Aug;14(7-8):585-94.

Benlounes N, Dupont C, Candalh C, Blaton MA, Darmon N, Desjeux JF, Heyman M. The threshold for immune cell reactivity to milk antigens decreases in cow's milk allergy with intestinal symptoms. *J Allergy Clin Immunol.* 1996 Oct;98(4):781-9.

Bennett WD, Zeman KL, Jarabek AM. Nasal contribution to breathing and fine particle deposition in children versus adults. J Toxicol Environ Health A. 2008;71(3):227-37.

Ben-Shoshan M, Harrington DW, Soller L, Fragapane J, Joseph L, St Pierre Y, Godefroy SB, Elliot SJ, Clarke AE. A population-based study on peanut, tree nut, fish, shellfish, and sesame allergy prevalence in Canada. J Allergy Clin Immunol. 2010 Jun;125(6):1327-35.

Ben-Shoshan M, Kagan R, Primeau MN, Alizadehfar R, Turnbull E, Harada L, Dufresne C, Allen M, Joseph L, St Pierre Y, Clarke A. Establishing the diagnosis of peanut allergy in children never exposed to peanut or with an uncertain history: a cross-Canada study. Pediatr Allergy Immunol. 2010 Sep;21(6):920-6.

Bensky D, Gable A, Kaptchuk T (transl.). Chinese Herbal Medicine Materia Medica. Seattle: Eastland Press, 1986.

Benvenuti C, Setnikar I. Effect of Lactobacillus sporogenes on oral isoflavones bioavailability: single dose pharmacokinetic study in menopausal women. Arzneimittelforschung. 2011;61(11):605-9.

Bergner P. The Healing Power of Garlic. Prima Publishing, Rocklin CA 1996.

Berin MC, Yang PC, Ciok L, Waserman S, Perdue MH. Role for IL-4 in macromolecular transport across human intestinal epithelium. Am J Physiol. 1999 May;276(5 Pt 1):C1046-52.

Berkow R., (Ed.) The Merck Manual of Diagnosis and Therapy. 16th Edition. Rahway, N.J.: Merck Research Labs, 1992.

Bernstein AM, Ding EL, Willett WC, Rimm EB. A Meta-Analysis Shows That Docosahexaenoic Acid from Algal Oil Reduces Serum Triglycerides and Increases HDL-Cholesterol and LDL-Cholesterol in Persons without Coronary Heart Disease. J Nutr. 2012 Jan;142(1):99-104.

Bernstein AM, Sun Q, Hu FB, Stampfer MJ, Manson JE, Willett WC. Major dietary protein sources and risk of coronary heart disease in women. Circulation. 2010 Aug 31;122(9):876-83.

Bernstein DI, Epstein T, Murphy-Berendts K, Liss GM. Surveillance of systemic reactions to subcutaneous immunotherapy injections: year 1 outcomes of the ACAAI and AAAAI collaborative study. Ann Allergy Asthma Immunol. 2010 Jun;104(6):530-5. .

Berseth CL, Mitmesser SH, Ziegler EE, Marunycz JD, Vanderhoof J. Tolerance of a standard intact protein formula versus a partially hydrolyzed formula in healthy, term infants. Nutr J. 2009 Jun 19;8:27.

Berteau O and Mulloy B. 2003. Sulfated fucans, fresh perspectives: structures, functions, and biological properties of sulfated fucans and an overview of enzymes active toward this class of polysaccharide. Glycobiology. Jun;13(6):29R-40R.

Bervoets L, Van Hoorenbeeck K, Kortleven I, Van Noten C, Hens N, Vael C, Goossens H, Desager KN, Vankerckhoven V. Differences in gut microbiota composition between obese and lean children: a cross-sectional study. Gut Pathog. 2013 Apr 30;5(1):10. doi: 10.1186/1757-4749-5-10.

Besednova NN, Somova LM, Guliaev SA, Zaporozhets TS. [Neuroprotective effects of sulfated polysaccharides from seaweed]. Vestn Ross Akad Med Nauk. 2013;(5):52-9.

Bevan R, Young C, Holmes P, Fortunato L, Slack R, Rushton L; British Occupational Cancer Burden Study Group. Occupational cancers in Britain. Gastrointestinal cancers: liver, oesophagus, pancreas and stomach. Br J Cancer. 2012 Jun 19;107 Suppl 1:S33-40. doi: 10.1038/bjc.2012.116.

Beyer K, Morrow E, Li XM, Bardina L, Bannon GA, Burks AW, Sampson HA. Effects of cooking methods on peanut allergenicity. J Allergy Clin Immunol. 2001;107:1077-81.

Bezanson G, Delaquis P, Bach S, McKellar R, Topp E, Gill A, Blais B, Gilmour M. Comparative Examination of Escherichia coli O157:H7 Survival on Romaine Lettuce and in Soil at Two Independent Experimental Sites. J Food Prot. 2012 Mar;75(3):480-7.

Bicíková V, Sosvorová L, Bradác O, Pán M, Bicíková M. Phytoestrogens in menopause: working mechanisms and clinical results in 28 patients. Ceska Gynekol. 2012 Feb;77(1):10-4.

Bidulescu A, Chambless LE, Siega-Riz AM, Zeisel SH, Heiss G. Usual choline and betaine dietary intake and incident coronary heart disease: the Atherosclerosis Risk in Communities (ARIC) study. BMC Cardiovasc Disord. 2007;7:20.

Bielory BP, Perez VL, Bielory L. Treatment of seasonal allergic conjunctivitis with ophthalmic corticosteroids: in search of the perfect ocular corticosteroids in the treatment of allergic conjunctivitis. Curr Opin Allergy Clin Immunol. 2010 Oct;10(5):469-77.

Bielory L, Lupoli K. Herbal interventions in asthma and allergy. J Asthma. 1999;36:1-65.

Bielory L, Russin J, Zuckerman GB. Clinical efficacy, mechanisms of action, and adverse effects of complementary and alternative medicine therapies for asthma. Allergy Asthma Proc. 2004;25:283-91.

Bielory L. Complementary and alternative interventions in asthma, allergy, and immunology. Ann Allergy Asthma Immunol. 2004 Aug;93(2 Suppl 1):S45-54.

Billoo AG, Memon MA, Khaskheli SA, Murtaza G, Iqbal K, Saeed Shekhani M, Siddiqi AQ. Role of a probiotic (Saccharomyces boulardii) in management and prevention of diarrhoea. World J Gastroenterol. 2006 Jul 28;12(28):4557-60.

Bindslev-Jensen C, Skov PS, Roggen EL, Hvass P, Brinch DS. Investigation on possible allergenicity of 19 different commercial enzymes used in the food industry. Food Chem Toxicol. 2006 Nov;44(11):1909-15.

Bin-Nun A, Bromiker R, Wilschanski M, Kaplan M, Rudensky B, Caplan M, Hammerman C. Oral probiotics prevent necrotizing enterocolitis in very low birth weight neonates. J Pediatr. 2005 Aug;147(2):192-6.

Birch EE, Khoury JC, Berseth CL, Castañeda YS, Couch JM, Bean J, Tamer R, Harris CL, Mitmesser SH, Scalabrin DM. The impact of early nutrition on incidence of allergic manifestations and common respiratory illnesses in children. J Pediatr. 2010 Jun;156(6):902-6, 906.e1. 2010 Mar 15.

Bisgaard H, Loland L, Holst KK, Pipper CB. Prenatal determinants of neonatal lung function in high-risk newborns. J Allergy Clin Immunol. 2009 Mar;123(3):651-7, 657.e1-4. 2009 Jan 18.

Bisset N.. Herbal Drugs and Phytopharmaceuticals. Stuttgart: CRC, 1994.

# REFERENCES AND BIBLIOGRAPHY

Bjarnason I, MacPherson A, Hollander D. Intestinal permeability: an overview. *Gastroenterology*. 1995 May;108(5):1566-81.

Blackhall K, Appleton S, Cates FJ. Ionisers for chronic asthma. *Cochrane Database Syst Rev* 2003;(3):CD002986.

Blackley, CH. *Experimental Researches on the Causes and Nature of Catarrhus Aestivus (Hay Fever or Hay-Asthma)*. London, 1873.

Bliakher MS, Fedorova IM, Lopatina TK, Arkhipov SN, Kapustin IV, Ramazanova ZK, Karpova NV, Ivanov VA, Sharapov NV. Acilact and improvement of the health status of sickly children. *Vestn Ross Akad Med Nauk.* 2005;(12):32-5.

Blood AJ, Zatorre RJ, Bermudez P, Evans AC. Emotional responses to pleasant and unpleasant music correlate with activity in paralimbic brain regions. *Nat Neurosci.* 1999;2:382-7.

Blumenthal M (ed.) *The Complete German Commission E Monographs.* Boston: Amer Botan Council, 1998.

Blumenthal M, Brinckmann J, Goldberg A (eds). *Herbal Medicine: Expanded Commission E Monographs.* Newton, MA: Integrative Med., 2000.

Bobe G, Sansbury LB, Albert PS, Cross AJ, Kahle L, Ashby J, Slattery ML, Caan B, Paskett E, Iber F, Kikendall JW, Lance P, Daston C, Marshall JR, Schatzkin A, Lanza E. Dietary flavonoids and colorectal adenoma recurrence in the Polyp Prevention Trial. Cancer Epidemiol Biomarkers Prev. 2008 Jun;17(6):1344-53.

Boccafogli A, Vicentini L, Camerani A, Cogliati P, D'Ambrosi A, Scolozzi R. Adverse food reactions in patients with grass pollen allergic respiratory disease. *Ann Allergy.* 1994 Oct;73(4):301-8.

Bode C, Bode JC. Effect of alcohol consumption on the gut. *Best Pract Res Clin Gastroenterol.* 2003 Aug;17(4):575-92.

Bodinier M, Legoux MA, Pineau F, Triballeau S, Segain JP, Brossard C, Denery-Papini S. Intestinal translocation capabilities of wheat allergens using the Caco-2 cell line. *J Agric Food Chem.* 2007 May 30;55(11):4576-83.

Boehm, G., Lidestri, M., Casetta, P., Jelinek, J., Negretti, F., Stahl, B., Martini, A. (2002) Supplementation of a bovine milk formula with an oligosaccharide mixture increases counts of faecal bifidobacteria in preterm infants. *Arch Dis Child Fetal Neonatal Ed.* 86: F178-F181

Boivin DB, Czeisler CA. Resetting of circadian melatonin and cortisol rhythms in humans by ordinary room light. *Neuroreport.* 1998 Mar 30;9(5):779-82.

Boivin DB, Duffy JF, Kronauer RE, Czeisler CA. Dose-response relationships for resetting of human circadian clock by light. *Nature.* 1996 Feb 8;379(6565):540-2.

Bolhaar ST, Tiemessen MM, Zuidmeer L, van Leeuwen A, Hoffmann-Sommergruber K, Bruijnzeel-Koomen CA, Taams LS, Knol EF, van Hoffen E, van Ree R, Knulst AC. Efficacy of birch-pollen immunotherapy on cross-reactive food allergy confirmed by skin tests and double-blind food challenges. *Clin Exp Allergy.* 2004 May;34(5):761-9.

Bolleddula J, Goldfarb J, Wang R, Sampson H, Li XM. Synergistic Modulation Of Eotaxin And Il-4 Secretion By Constituents Of An Anti-asthma Herbal Formula (ASHMI) In Vitro. *J Allergy Clin Immunol.* 2007;119:S172.

Bonfils P, Halimi P, Malinvaud D. Adrenal suppression and osteoporosis after treatment of nasal polyposis. *Acta Otolaryngol.* 2006 Dec;126(11):1195-200.

Bongaerts GP, Severijnen RS. Preventive and curative effects of probiotics in atopic patients. *Med Hypotheses.* 2005;64(6):1089-92.

Bongartz D, Hesse A. Selective extraction of quercetrin in vegetable drugs and urine by off-line coupling of boronic acid affinity chromatography and high-performance liquid chromatography. *J Chromatogr B Biomed Appl.* 1995 Nov 17;673(2):223-30.

Bonsignore MR, La Grutta S, Cibella F, Scichilone N, Cuttitta G, Interrante A, Marchese M, Veca M, Virzi' M, Bonanno A, Profita M, Morici G. Effects of exercise training and montelukast in children with mild asthma. *Med Sci Sports Exerc.* 2008 Mar;40(3):405-12.

Borchers AT, Hackman RM, Keen CL, Stern JS, Gershwin ME. Complementary medicine: a review of immuno-modulatory effects of Chinese herbal medicines. *Am J Clin Nutr.* 1997 Dec;66(6):1303-12.

Borchert VE, Czyborra P, Fetscher C, Goepel M, Michel MC. Extracts from Rhois aromatica and Solidaginis virgaurea inhibit rat and human bladder contraction. *Naunyn Schmiedebergs Arch Pharmacol.* 2004 Mar;369(3):281-6.

Bosetti C, Bravi F, Turati F, Edefonti V, Polesel J, Decarli A, Negri E, Talamini R, Franceschi S, La Vecchia C, Zeegers MP. Nutrient-based dietary patterns and pancreatic cancer risk. Ann Epidemiol. 2013 Mar;23(3):124-8. doi: 10.1016/j.annepidem.2012.12.005.

Böttcher MF, Abrahamsson TR, Fredriksson M, Jakobsson T, Björkstén B. Low breast milk TGF-beta2 is induced by *Lactobacillus reuteri* supplementation and associates with reduced risk of sensitization during infancy. *Pediatr Allergy Immunol.* 2008 Sep;19(6):497-504.

Böttcher MF, Jenmalm MC, Voor T, Julge K, Holt PG, Björkstén B. Cytokine responses to allergens during the first 2 years of life in Estonian and Swedish children. *Clin Exp Allergy.* 2006 May;36(5):619-28.

Bottema RW, Kerkhof M, Reijmerink NE, Thijs C, Smit HA, van Schayck CP, Brunekreef B, van Oosterhout AJ, Postma DS, Koppelman GH. Gene-gene interaction in regulatory T-cell function in atopy and asthma development in childhood. *J Allergy Clin Immunol.* 2010 Aug;126(2):338-46, 346.e1-10.

Bouchez-Mahiout I, Pecquet C, Kerre S, Snégaroff J, Raison-Peyron N, Laurière M. High molecular weight entities in industrial wheat protein hydrolysates are immunoreactive with IgE from allergic patients. *J Agric Food Chem.* 2010 Apr 14;58(7):4207-15.

Bougault V, Turmel J, Boulet LP. Bronchial challenges and respiratory symptoms in elite swimmers and winter sport athletes: Airway hyperresponsiveness in asthma: its measurement and clinical significance. *Chest.* 2010 Aug;138(2 Suppl):31S-37S. 2010 Apr 2.

Boyce JA, Assa'ad A, Burks AW, Jones SM, Sampson HA, Wood RA, Plaut M, Cooper SF, Fenton MJ, Arshad SH, Bahna SL, Beck LA, Byrd-Bredbenner C, Camargo CA Jr, Eichenfield L, Furuta GT, Hanifin JM, Jones C, Kraft M, Levy BD, Lieberman P, Luccioli S, McCall KM, Schneider LC, Simon RA, Simons FE, Teach SJ, Yawn BP, Schwaninger JM. Guidelines for the diagnosis and management of food allergy in the United States: report of the NIAID-sponsored expert panel. *J Allergy Clin Immunol.* 2010 Dec;126(6 Suppl):S1-58.

Boylan R, Li Y, Simeonova L, Sherwin G, Kreismann J, Craig RG, Ship JA, McCutcheon JA. Reduction in bacterial contamination of toothbrushes using the Violight ultraviolet light activated toothbrush sanitizer. *Am J Dent.* 2008 Oct;21(5):313-7.

Bråbäck L, Breborowicz A, Julge K, Knutsson A, Riikjärv MA, Vasar M, Björkstén B. Risk factors for respiratory symptoms and atopic sensitisation in the Baltic area. *Arch Dis Child.* 1995 Jun;72(6):487-93.

Bråbäck L, Kjellman NI, Sandin A, Björkstén B. Atopy among schoolchildren in northern and southern Sweden in relation to pet ownership and early life events. *Pediatr Allergy Immunol.* 2001 Feb;12(1):4-10.

Bradette-Hébert ME, Legault J, Lavoie S, Pichette A. A new labdane diterpene from the flowers of Solidago canadensis. *Chem Pharm Bull.* 2008 Jan;56(1):82-4.

Brandolini R, Vinciguerra G, Dugall M, Griffin M, Ruffini I, Acerbi G, Corsi M,

Brandtzaeg P. The mucosal immune system and its integration with the mammary glands. *J Pediatr.* 2010 Feb;156(2 Suppl):S8-15.

Brasseur JG, Nicosia MA, Pal A, Miller LS. Function of longitudinal vs circular muscle fibers in esophageal peristalsis, deduced with mathematical modeling. *World J Gastroenterol.* 2007 Mar 7;13(9):1335-46.

Bratt K, Sunnerheim K, Bryngelsson S, Fagerlund A, Engman L, Andersson RE, Dimberg LH. Avenanthramides in oats (Avena sativa L.) and structure-antioxidant activity relationships. J Agric Food Chem. 2003 Jan 29;51(3):594-600.

Braun-Fahrländer C, Gassner M, Grize L, Neu U, Sennhauser FH, Varonier HS, Vuille JC, Wüthrich B. Prevalence of hay fever and allergic sensitization in farmer's children and their peers living in the same rural community. SCARPOL team. Swiss Study on Childhood Allergy and Respiratory Symptoms with Respect to Air Pollution. *Clin Exp Allergy.* 1999 Jan;29(1):28-34.

Brehm JM, Schuemann B, Fuhlbrigge AL, Hollis BW, Strunk RC, Zeiger RS, Weiss ST, Litonjua AA; Childhood Asthma Management Program Research Group. Serum vitamin D levels and severe asthma exacerbations in the Childhood Asthma Management Program study. *J Allergy Clin Immunol.* 2010 Jul;126(1):52-8.e5. 2010 Jun 9.

Brighenti F, Valtueña S, Pellegrini N, Ardigò D, Del Rio D, Salvatore S, Piatti P, Serafini M, Zavaroni I. Total antioxidant capacity of the diet is inversely and independently related to plasma concentration of high-sensitivity C-reactive protein in adult Italian subjects. *Br J Nutr.* 2005 May;93(5):619-25.

Brinkhaus B, Witt CM, Jena S, Liecker B, Wegscheider K, Willich SN. Acupuncture in patients with allergic rhinitis: a pragmatic randomized trial. *Ann Allergy Asthma Immunol.* 2008 Nov;101(5):535-43.

Brisman J, Torén K, Lillienberg L, Karlsson G, Ahlstedt S. Nasal symptoms and indices of nasal inflammation in flour-dust-exposed bakers. *Int Arch Occup Environ Health.* 1998 Nov;71(8):525-32.

Brodtkorb TH, Zetterström O, Tinghög G. Cost-effectiveness of clean air administered to the breathing zone in allergic asthma. *Clin Respir J.* 2010 Apr;4(2):104-10.

Brody J. *Jane Brody's Nutrition Book.* New York: WW Norton, 1981.

Broekhuizen BD, Sachs AP, Hoes AW, Moons KG, van den Berg JW, Dalinghaus WH, Lammers E, Verheij TJ. Undetected chronic obstructive pulmonary disease and asthma in people over 50 years with persistent cough. *Br J Gen Pract.* 2010 Jul;60(576):489-94.

Brostoff J, Gamlin L, Brostoff J. *Food Allergies and Food Intolerance: The Complete Guide to Their Identification and Treatment.* Rochester, VT: Healing Arts, 2000.

Brownstein D. *Salt: Your Way to Health.* West Bloomfield, MI: Medical Alternatives, 2006.

Brown-Whitehorn TF, Spergel JM. The link between allergies and eosinophilic esophagitis: implications for management strategies. *Expert Rev Clin Immunol.* 2010 Jan;6(1):101-9.

Bruce S, Nyberg F, Melén E, James A, Pulkkinen V, Orsmark-Pietras C, Bergström A, Dahlén B, Wickman M, von Mutius E, Doekes G, Lauener R, Riedler J, Eder W, van Hage M, Pershagen G, Scheynius A, Kere J. The protective effect of farm animal exposure on childhood allergy is modified by NPSR1 polymorphisms. *J Med Genet.* 2009 Mar;46(3):159-67. 2008 Feb 19.

Bruneton J. *Pharmacognosy, Phytochemistry, Medicinal Plants.* Paris: Lavoisier, 1995.

Bruton A, Lewith GT. The Buteyko breathing technique for asthma: a review. *Complement Ther Med.* 2005 Mar;13(1):41-6. 2005 Apr 18.

Bruton A, Thomas M. The role of breathing training in asthma management. *Curr Opin Allergy Clin Immunol.* 2011 Feb;11(1):53-7.

Bryborn M, Halldén C, Säll T, Cardell LO. CLC- a novel susceptibility gene for allergic rhinitis? *Allergy.* 2010 Feb;65(2):220-8.

Bu LN, Chang MH, Ni YH, Chen HL, Cheng CC. *Lactobacillus casei* rhamnosus Lcr35 in children with chronic constipation. *Pediatr Int.* 2007 Aug;49(4):485-90.

Bublin M, Pfister M, Radauer C, Oberhuber C, Bulley S, Dewitt AM, Lidholm J, Reese G, Vieths S, Breiteneder H, Hoffmann-Sommergruber K, Ballmer-Weber BK. Component-resolved diagnosis of kiwifruit allergy with purified natural and recombinant kiwifruit allergens. *J Allergy Clin Immunol.* 2010 Mar;125(3):687-94, 694.e1.

Buchanan TW, Lutz K, Mirzazade S, Specht K, Shah NJ, Zilles K, *et al.* Recognition of emotional prosody and verbal components of spoken language: an fMRI study. *Cogn Brain Res.* 2000;9:227-38.

Bucher X, Pichler WJ, Dahinden CA, Helbling A. Effect of tree pollen specific, subcutaneous immunotherapy on the oral allergy syndrome to apple and hazelnut. *Allergy*. 2004 Dec;59(12):1272-6.

Budzianowski J. Coumarins, caffeoyltartaric acids and their artifactual methyl esters from Taraxacum officinale leaves. *Planta Med*. 1997 Jun;63(3):288.

Bueso AK, Berntsen S, Mowinckel P, Andersen LF, Lodrup Carlsen KC, Carlsen KH. Dietary intake in adolescents with asthma – potential for improvement. *Pediatr Allergy Immunol*. 2010 Oct 20. doi: 10.1111/j.1399-3038.2010.01013.x.

Bundy R, Walker AF, Middleton RW, Booth J. Turmeric extract may improve irritable bowel syndrome symptomology in otherwise healthy adults: a pilot study. *J Altern Complement Med*. 2004 Dec;10(6):1015-8.

Burdge GC, Jones AE, Wootton SA. Eicosapentaenoic and docosapentaenoic acids are the principal products of alpha-linolenic acid metabolism in young men. *B J Nutr*. 2002 Oct;88(4):355-63.

Buret AG. How stress induces intestinal hypersensitivity. *Am J Pathol*. 2006 Jan;168(1):3-5.

Burgess CD, Bremner P, Thomson CD, Crane J, Siebers RW, Beasley R. Nebulized beta 2-adrenoceptor agonists do not affect plasma selenium or glutathione peroxidase activity in patients with asthma. *Int J Clin Pharmacol Ther*. 1994 Jun;32(6):290-2.

Burke V, Zhao Y, Lee AH, Hunter E, Spargo RM, Gracey M, Smith RM, Beilin LJ, Puddey IB. Health-related behaviours as predictors of mortality and morbidity in Australian Aborigines. *Prev Med*. 2007 Feb;44(2):135-42.

Burke V, Zhao Y, Lee AH, Hunter E, Spargo RM, Gracey M, Smith RM, Beilin LJ, Puddey IB. Health-related behaviours as predictors of mortality and morbidity in Australian Aborigines. *Prev Med*. 2007 Feb;44(2):135-42.

Burks W, Jones SM, Berseth CL, Harris C, Sampson HA, Scalabrin DM. Hypoallergenicity and effects on growth and tolerance of a new amino acid-based formula with docosahexaenoic acid and arachidonic acid. *J Pediatr*. 2008 Aug;153(2):266-71.

Burney PG, Luczynska C, Chinn S, Jarvis D. The European Community Respiratory Health Survey. *Eur Respir J*. 1994;7: 954-960.

Burr ML, Butland BK, King S, Vaughan-Williams E. Changes in asthma prevalence: two surveys 15 years apart. *Arch Dis Child*. 1989;64:1452-1456.

Busse PJ, Wen MC, Huang CK, Srivastava K, Zhang TF, Schofield B, Sampson HA, Li XM. Therapeutic effects of the Chinese herbal formula, MSSM-03d, on persistent airway hyperreactivity and airway remodeling. *J Allergy Clin Immunol*. 2004;113:S220.

Byrne AM, Malka-Rais J, Burks AW, Fleischer DM. How do we know when peanut and tree nut allergy have resolved, and how do we keep it resolved? *Clin Exp Allergy*. 2010 Sep;40(9):1303-11.

Cabanillas B, Pedrosa MM, Rodríguez J, González A, Muzquiz M, Cuadrado C, Crespo JF, Burbano C. Effects of enzymatic hydrolysis on lentil allergenicity. *Mol Nutr Food Res*. 2010 Mar 19.

Caglar E, Cildir SK, Ergeneli S, Sandalli N, Twetman S. Salivary mutans streptococci and lactobacilli levels after ingestion of the probiotic bacterium *Lactobacillus reuteri* ATCC 55730 by straws or tablets. *Acta Odontol Scand*. 2006 Oct;64(5):314-8.

Caglar E, Kavaloglu SC, Kuscu OO, Sandalli N, Holgerson PL, Twetman S. Effect of chewing gums containing xylitol or probiotic bacteria on salivary mutans streptococci and lactobacilli. *Clin Oral Investig*. 2007 Dec;11(4):425-9.

Caglar E, Kuscu OO, Cildir SK, Kuvvetli SS, Sandalli N. A probiotic lozenge administered medical device and its effect on salivary mutans streptococci and lactobacilli. *Int J Paediatr Dent*. 2008 Jan;18(1):35-9.

Caglar E, Kuscu OO, Selvi Kuvvetli S, Kavaloglu Cildir S, Sandalli N, Twetman S. Short-term effect of ice-cream containing *Bifidobacterium lactis* Bb-12 on the number of salivary mutans streptococci and lactobacilli. *Acta Odontol Scand*. 2008 Jun;66(3):154-8.

Cahn J, Borzeix MG. Administration of procyanidolic oligomers in rats. Observed effects on changes in the permeability of the blood-brain barrier. *Sem Hop*. 1983 Jul 7;59(27-28):2031-4.

Calder PC. Dietary modification of inflammation with lipids. *Proc Nutr Soc*. 2002 Aug;61(3):345-58.

Camargo CA Jr, Ingham T, Wickens K, Thadhani R, Silvers KM, Epton MJ, Town GI, Pattemore PK, Espinola JA, Crane J; New Zealand Asthma and Allergy Cohort Study Group. Cord-blood 25-hydroxyvitamin D levels and risk of respiratory infection, wheezing, and asthma. *Pediatrics*. 2011 Jan;127(1):e180-7.

Caminiti L, Passalacqua G, Barberi S, Vita D, Barberio G, De Luca R, Pajno GB. A new protocol for specific oral tolerance induction in children with IgE-mediated cow's milk allergy. *Allergy Asthma Proc*. 2009 Jul-Aug;30(4):443-8.

Campbell TC, Campbell TM. *The China Study*. Dallas, TX: Benbella Books, 2006.

Campbell WW, Tang M. Protein intake, weight loss, and bone mineral density in postmenopausal women. *J Gerontol A Biol Sci Med Sci*. 2010 Oct;65(10):1115-22.

Campieri C, Campieri M, Bertuzzi V, Swennen E, Matteuzzi D, Stefoni S, Pirovano F, Centi C, Ulisse S, Famularo G, De Simone C. Reduction of oxaluria after an oral course of lactic acid bacteria at high concentration. *Kidney Int*. 2001 Sep;60(3):1097-105.

Canakcioglu S, Tahamiler R, Saritzali G, Alimoglu Y, Isildak H, Guvenc MG, Acar GO, Inci E. Evaluation of nasal cytology in subjects with chronic rhinitis: a 7-year study. *Am J Otolaryngol*. 2009 Sep-Oct;30(5):312-7.

Canali R, Comitato R, Schonlau F, Virgili F. The anti-inflammatory pharmacology of Pycnogenol in humans involves COX-2 and 5-LOX mRNA expression in leukocytes. *Int Immunopharmacol*. 2009 Sep;9(10):1145-9.

Canani RB, Cirillo P, Terrin G, Cesarano L, Spagnuolo MI, De Vincenzo A, Albano F, Passariello A, De Marco G, Manguso F, Guarino A. Probiotics for treatment of acute diarrhoea in children: randomised clinical trial of five different preparations. *BMJ.* 2007 Aug 18;335(7615):340.

Canducci F, Armuzzi A, Cremonini F, Cammarota G, Bartolozzi F, Pola P, Gasbarrini G, Gasbarrini A. A lyophilized and inactivated culture of *Lactobacillus acidophilus* increases *Helicobacter pylori* eradication rates. *Aliment Pharmacol Ther.* 2000 Dec;14(12):1625-9.

Canducci F, Cremonini F, Armuzzi A, Di Caro S, Gabrielli M, Santarelli L, Nista E, Lupascu A, De Martini D, Gasbarrini A. Probiotics and Helicobacter pylori eradication. *Dig Liver Dis.* 2002 Sep;34 Suppl 2:S81-3.

Canonica GW, Passalacqua G. Noninjection routes for immunotherapy. *J Allergy Clin Immunol.* 2003 Mar;111(3):437-48; quiz 449.

Cantani A, Micera M. Natural history of cow's milk allergy. An eight-year follow-up study in 115 atopic children. *Eur Rev Med Pharmacol Sci.* 2004 Jul-Aug;8(4):153-64.

Cantani A, Micera M. The prick by prick test is safe and reliable in 58 children with atopic dermatitis and food allergy. *Eur Rev Med Pharmacol Sci.* 2006 May-Jun;10(3):115-20.

Cao G, Alessio HM, Cutler RG. Oxygen-radical absorbance capacity assay for antioxidants. *Free Radic Biol Med.* 1993 Mar;14(3):303-11.

Cao G, Shukitt-Hale B, Bickford PC, Joseph JA, McEwen J, Prior RL. Hyperoxia-induced changes in antioxidant capacity and the effect of dietary antioxidants. *J Appl Physiol.* 1999 Jun;86(6):1817-22.

Cara L, Dubois C, Borel P, Armand M, Senft M, Portugal H, Pauli AM, Bernard PM, Lairon D. Effects of oat bran, rice bran, wheat fiber, and wheat germ on postprandial lipemia in healthy adults. Am J Clin Nutr. 1992 Jan;55(1):81-8.

Caramia G. The essential fatty acids omega-6 and omega-3: from their discovery to their use in therapy. *Minerva Pediatr.* 2008 Apr;60(2):219-33.

Carey DG, Aase KA, Pliego GJ. The acute effect of cold air exercise in determination of exercise-induced bronchospasm in apparently healthy athletes. J Strength Cond Res. 2010 Aug;24(8):2172-8.

Carpita N. C., Kanabus J., Housley T. L. Linkage structure of fructans and fructan oligomers from Triticum aestivum and Festuca arundinacea leaves. *J. Plant Physiol.* 1989;134:162-168

Carroccio A, Cavataio F, Montalto G, D'Amico D, Alabrese L, Iacono G. Intolerance to hydrolysed cow's milk proteins in infants: clinical characteristics and dietary treatment. *Clin Exp Allergy.* 2000 Nov;30(11):1597-603.

Carroll D. *The Complete Book of Natural Medicines.* New York: Summit; 1980.

Caruso M, Frasca G, Di Giuseppe PL, Pennisi A, Tringali G, Bonina FP. Effects of a new nutraceutical ingredient on allergen-induced sulphidoleukotrienes production and CD63 expression in allergic subjects. *Int Immunopharmacol.* 2008 Dec 20;8(13-14):1781-6.

Casale TB, Amin BV. Allergic rhinitis/asthma interrelationship. *Clin Rev Allergy Immunol.* 2001;21:27-49.

Cassidy A, Rimm EB, O'Reilly EJ, Logroscino G, Kay C, Chiuve SE, Rexrode KM. Dietary flavonoids and risk of stroke in women. Stroke. 2012 Apr;43(4):946-51.

Cats A, Kuipers EJ, Bosschaert MA, Pot RG, Vandenbroucke-Grauls CM, Kusters JG. Effect of frequent consumption of a *Lactobacillus casei*-containing milk drink in *Helicobacter pylori*-colonized subjects. *Aliment Pharmacol Ther.* 2003 Feb;17(3):429-35.

Caughey AB, Nicholson JM, Cheng YW, Lyell DJ, Washington AE. Induction of labor and Cesarean delivery by gestational age. *Am J Obstet Gynecol.* 2006 Sep;195(3):700-5.

Celakovská J, Vaněčková J, Ettlerová K, Ettler K, Bukac J. The role of atopy patch test in diagnosis of food allergy in atopic eczema/dermatitis syndrom in patients over 14 years of age. *Acta Medica (Hradec Kralove).* 2010;53(2):101-8.

Celikel S, Karakaya G, Yurtsever N, Sorkun K, Kalyoncu AF. Bee and bee products allergy in Turkish beekeepers: determination of risk factors for systemic reactions. *Allergol Immunopathol (Madr).* 2006 Sep-Oct;34(5):180-4.

Centers for Disease Control and Prevention (CDC). Obesity prevalence among low-income, preschool-aged children – United States, 1998-2008. *MMWR Morb Mortal Wkly Rep.* 2009 Jul 24;58(28):769-73.

Centers for Disease Control and Prevention (CDC). Vital signs: nonsmokers' exposure to secondhand smoke – United States, 1999-2008. *MMWR Morb Mortal Wkly Rep.* 2010 Sep 10;59(35):1141-6.

Centre for Molecular, Environmental, Genetic and Analytic Epidemiology, School of Population Health, The UniverGumowski P, Lech B, Chaves I, Girard JP. Chronic asthma and rhinitis due to Candida albicans, epidermophyton, and trichophyton. *Ann Allergy.* 1987 Jul;59(1):48-51.

Cereijido M, Contreras RG, Flores-Benítez D, Flores-Maldonado C, Larre I, Ruiz A, Shoshani L. New diseases derived or associated with the tight junction. *Arch Med Res.* 2007 Jul;38(5):465-78.

Cerling TE, *et al.* Comment on the paleoenvironment of Ardipithecus ramidus. Science. 2010;328:1105-d. 10.1126/science.1185274.

Cerling TE, Harris JM, Leakey MG. Browsing and grazing in modern and fossil proboscideans. Oecologia. 1999;120:364 – 374.

Cerling TE, Harris JM, Passey BH. Diets of East African Bovidae based on stable isotope analysis. J Mammal. 2003;84:456 – 471.

Cerling TE, Harris JM. Carbon isotope fractionation between diet and bioapatite in ungulate mammals and implications for ecological and paleoecological studies. Oecologia. 1999;120:347 – 363.

Cerling TE, Levin NE, Passey BH. Stable isotope ecology in the Omo-Turkana Basin. Evol Anthropol. 2011 Nov-Dec;20(6):228-37. doi: 10.1002/evan.20326.

Cerling TE, Manthi FK, Mbua EN, Leakey LN, Leakey MG, Leakey RE, Brown FH, Grine FE, Hart JA, Kaleme P, Roche H, Uno KT, Wood BA. Stable isotope-based diet reconstructions of Turkana Basin hominins. Proc Natl Acad Sci U S A. 2013 Jun 25;110(26):10501-6. doi: 10.1073/pnas.1222568110.

Cerling TE, Mbua E, Kirera FM, Manthi FK, Grine FE, Leakey MG, Sponheimer M, Uno KT. Diet of Paranthropus boisei in the early Pleistocene of East Africa. Proc Natl Acad Sci U S A. 2011 Jun 7;108(23):9337-41. doi: 10.1073/pnas.1104627108.

Cerling TE, Mbua E, Kirera FM, Manthi FK, Grine FE, Leakey MG, Sponheimer M, Uno KT. Diet of Paranthropus boisei in the early Pleistocene of East Africa. Proc Natl Acad Sci U S A. 2011 Jun 7;108(23):9337-41. doi: 10.1073/pnas.1104627108.

Cerling TE, Wynn JG, Andanje SA, Bird MI, Korir DK, Levin NE, Mace W, Macharia AN, Quade J, Remien CH. Woody cover and hominin environments in the past 6 million years. Nature. 2011 Aug 3;476(7358):51-6. doi: 10.1038/nature10306.

Cermak NM, Gibala MJ, van Loon LJ. Nitrate supplementation's improvement of 10-km time-trial performance in trained cyclists. Int J Sport Nutr Exerc Metab. 2012 Feb;22(1):64-71.

Cesarone MR, Belcaro G, Nicolaides AN, Ricci A, Geroulakos G, Ippolito E,

Chafen JJ, Newberry SJ, Riedl MA, Bravata DM, Maglione M, Suttorp MJ, Sundaram V, Paige NM, Towfigh A, Hulley BJ, Shekelle PG. Diagnosing and managing common food allergies: a systematic review. *JAMA*. 2010 May 12;303(18):1848-56.

Chahine BG, Bahna SL. The role of the gut mucosal immunity in the development of tolerance versus development of allergy to food. *Curr Opin Allergy Clin Immunol*. 2010 Aug;10(4):394-9.

Chaitow L, Trenev N. *Probiotics: The revolutionary, 'friendly' bacteria way to vital health and well-being*. New York: Thorsons, 1990.

Chaitow L. *Conquer Pain the Natural Way*. San Francisco: Chronicle Books, 2002.

Chakŭrski I, Matev M, Koĭchev A, Angelova I, Stefanov G. Treatment of chronic colitis with an herbal combination of Taraxacum officinale, Hipericum perforatum, Melissa officinaliss, Calendula officinalis and Foeniculum vulgare. *Vutr Boles*. 1981;20(6):51-4.

Chan CK, Kuo ML, Shen JJ, See LC, Chang HH, Huang JL. Ding Chuan Tang, a Chinese herb decoction, could improve airway hyper-responsiveness in stabilized asthmatic children: a randomized, double-blind clinical trial. *Pediatr Allergy Immunol*. 2006;17:316-22.

Chandra RK. Prospective studies of the effect of breast feeding on incidence of infection and allergy. *Acta Paediatr Scand*. 1979 Sep;68(5):691-4.

Chaney M, Ross M. *Nutrition*. New York: Houghton Mifflin, 1971.

Chang HT, Tseng LJ, Hung TJ, Kao BT, Lin WY, Fan TC, Chang MD, Pai TW. Inhibition of the interactions between eosinophil cationic protein and airway epithelial cells by traditional Chinese herbs. *BMC Syst Biol*. 2010 Sep 13;4 Suppl 2:S8.

Chang TT, Huang CC, Hsu CH. Clinical evaluation of the Chinese herbal medicine formula STA-1 in the treatment of allergic asthma. *Phytother Res*. 2006;20:342-7.

Chang TT, Huang CC, Hsu CH. Inhibition of mite-induced immunoglobulin E synthesis, airway inflammation, and hyperreactivity by herbal medicine STA-1. *Immunopharmacol Immunotoxicol*. 2006;28:683-95.

Chao A, Thun MJ, Connell CJ, McCullough ML, Jacobs EJ, Flanders WD, Rodriguez C, Sinha R, Calle EE. Meat consumption and risk of colorectal cancer. *JAMA*. 2005 Jan 12;293(2):172-82.

Chapat L, Chemin K, Dubois B, Bourdet-Sicard R, Kaiserlian D. Lactobacillus casei reduces CD8+ T cell-mediated skin inflammation. *Eur J Immunol*. 2004 Sep;34(9):2520-8.

Chapidze G, Kapanadze S, Dolidze N, Bachutashvili Z, Latsabidze N. Prevention of coronary atherosclerosis by the use of combination therapy with antioxidant coenzyme q10 and statins. *Georgian Med News*. 2005 Jan;(1):20-5.

Characterization and quantitation of Antioxidant Constituents of Sweet Pepper (Capsicum annuum – Cayenne). *J Agric Food Chem*. 2004 Jun 16;52(12):3861-9.

Chatzi L, Apostolaki G, Bibakis I, Skypala I, Bibaki-Liakou V, Tzanakis N, Kogevinas M, Cullinan P. Protective effect of fruits, vegetables and the Mediterranean diet on asthma and allergies among children in Crete. *Thorax*. 2007 Aug;62(8):677-83.

Chatzi L, Torrent M, Romieu I, Garcia-Esteban R, Ferrer C, Vioque J, Kogevinas M, Sunyer J. Mediterranean diet in pregnancy is protective for wheeze and atopy in childhood. *Thorax*. 2008 Jun;63(6):507-13.

Chaves TC, de Andrade e Silva TS, Monteiro SA, Watanabe PC, Oliveira AS, Grossi DB. Craniocervical posture and hyoid bone position in children with mild and moderate asthma and mouth breathing. *Int J Pediatr Otorhinolaryngol*. 2010 Sep;74(9):1021-7.

Chawes BL, Bønnelykke K, Kreiner-Møller E, Bisgaard H. Children with allergic and nonallergic rhinitis have a similar risk of asthma. *J Allergy Clin Immunol*. 2010 Sep;126(3):567-73.e1-8.

Chawes BL, Kreiner-Møller E, Bisgaard H. Objective assessments of allergic and nonallergic rhinitis in young children. *Allergy*. 2009 Oct;64(10):1547-53.

Chehade M, Aceves SS. Food allergy and eosinophilic esophagitis. *Curr Opin Allergy Clin Immunol*. 2010 Jun;10(3):231-7.

Chellini E, Talassi F, Corbo G, Berti G, De Sario M, Rusconi F, Piffer S, Caranci N, Petronio MG, Sestini P, Dell'Orco V, Bonci E, Armenio L, La Grutta S; Gruppo Collaborativo SIDRIA-2. Environmental, social and demographic characteristics of children and adolescents, resident in different Italian areas. *Epidemiol Prev*. 2005 Mar-Apr;29(2 Suppl):14-23.

Chelpanova TI, Vitiazev FV, Mikhaleva NIa, Efimtseva ÉA. Effect of pectin substances on activity of human pancreatic alpha-amylase in vitro. Ross Fiziol Zh Im I M Sechenova. 2012 Jun;98(6):734-43.

393

Chen CY, Milbury PE, Collins FW, Blumberg JB. Avenanthramides are bioavailable and have antioxidant activity in humans after acute consumption of an enriched mixture from oats. J Nutr. 2007 Jun;137(6):1375-82.

Chen CY, Wang FY, Wan HJ, Jin XX, Wei J, Wang ZK, Liu C, Lu H, Shi H, Li DH, Liu J. Amino acid polymorphisms flanking the EPIYA-A motif of Helicobacter pylori CagA C-terminal region is associated with gastric cancer in East China. J Dig Dis. 2013 Mar 21.

Chen HJ, Shih CK, Hsu HY, Chiang W. Mast cell-dependent allergic responses are inhibited by ethanolic extract of adlay (Coix lachryma-jobi L. var. ma-yuen Stapf) testa. J Agric Food Chem. 2010 Feb 24;58(4):2596-601.

Chen JX, Ji B, Lu ZL, Hu LS. Effects of chai hu (radix burpleuri) containing formulation on plasma beta-endorphin, epinephrine and dopamine on patients. Am J Chin Med. 2005;33(5):737-45.

Chen Y, Blaser MJ. Association Between Gastric Helicobacter pylori Colonization and Glycated Hemoglobin Levels. J Infect Dis. 2012 Mar 13.

Chen Y, Blaser MJ. Helicobacter pylori colonization is inversely associated with childhood asthma. J Infect Dis. 2008 Aug 15;198(4):553-60.

Chen Y, Blaser MJ. Inverse associations of Helicobacter pylori with asthma and allergy. Arch Intern Med. 2007 Apr 23;167(8):821-7.

Cheney G, Waxler SH, Miller IJ. Vitamin U therapy of peptic ulcer; experience at San Quentin Prison. Calif Med. 1956 Jan;84(1):39-42.

Chevallier A. Encyclopedia of Medicinal Plants. New York, NY: DK Publishing; 1996.

Chevrier MR, Ryan AE, Lee DY, Zhongze M, Wu-Yan Z, Via CS. Boswellia carterii extract inhibits TH1 cytokines and promotes TH2 cytokines in vitro. Clin Diagn Lab Immunol. 2005 May;12(5):575-80.

Chiang BL, Sheih YH, Wang LH, Liao CK, Gill HS. Enhancing immunity by dietary consumption of a probiotic lactic acid bacterium (Bifidobacterium lactis HN019): optimization and definition of cellular immune responses. Eur J Clin Nutr. 2000 Nov;54(11):849-55.

Chihara G. Recent progress in immunopharmacology and therapeutic effects of polysaccharides. Dev Biol Stand. 1992;77:191-7.

Chilton F, Tucker L. Win the War Within. New York: Rodale, 2006.

Chilton FH, Rudel LL, Parks JS, Arm JP, Seeds MC. Mechanisms by which botanical lipids affect inflammatory disorders. Am J Clin Nutr. 2008 Feb;87(2):498S-503S.

Chilton FH, Tucker L. Win the War Within. New York: Rodale, 2006.

Chin A Paw MJ, de Jong N, Pallast EG, Kloek GC, Schouten EG, Kok FJ. Immunity in frail elderly: a randomized controlled trial of exercise and enriched foods. Med Sci Sports Exerc. 2000 Dec;32(12):2005-11.

Chiquette J, Allison MJ, Rasmussen M. Use of Prevotella bryantii 25A and a commercial probiotic during subacute acidosis challenge in midlactation dairy cows. J Dairy Sci. 2012 Oct;95(10):5985-95. doi: 10.3168/jds.2012-5511.

Chiurillo MA, Moran Y, Cañas M, Valderrama E, Granda N, Sayegh M, Ramírez JL. Genotyping of Helicobacter pylori virulence-associated genes shows high diversity of strains infecting patients in western Venezuela. Int J Infect Dis. 2013 Apr 20.

Chong Neto HJ, Rosário NA; Grupo EISL Curitiba (Estudio Internacional de Sibilancias en Lactantes). Risk factors for wheezing in the first year of life. J Pediatr. 2008 Nov-Dec;84(6):495-502.

Chopra RN, Nayar SL, Chopra IC, eds. Glossary of Indian Medicinal plants. New Delhi: CSIR, 1956.

Choudhry S, Seibold MA, Borrell LN, Tang H, Serebrisky D, Chapela R, Rodriguez-Santana JR, Avila PC, Ziv E, Rodriguez-Cintron W, Risch NJ, Burchard EG. Dissecting complex diseases in complex populations: asthma in latino americans. Proc Am Thorac Soc. 2007 Jul;4(3):226-33.

Chouraqui JP, Grathwohl D, Labaune JM, Hascoet JM, de Montgolfier I, Leclaire M, Giarre M, Steenhout P. Assessment of the safety, tolerance, and protective effect against diarrhea of infant formulas containing mixtures of probiotics or probiotics and prebiotics in a randomized controlled trial. Am J Clin Nutr. 2008 May;87(5):1365-73.

Christensen AS, Viggers L, Hasselström K, Gregersen S. Effect of fruit restriction on glycemic control in patients with type 2 dia-betes – a randomized trial. Nutr J. 2013 Mar 5;12:29.

Christopher JR. School of Natural Healing. Springville UT: Christopher Publ, 1976.

Chu YF, Liu RH. Cranberries inhibit LDL oxidation and induce LDL receptor expression in hepatocytes. Life Sci. 2005;77(15):1892-1901. 27.

Chu YF, Liu RH. Cranberries inhibit LDL oxidation and induce LDL receptor expression in hepatocytes. Life Sci. 2005;77(15):1892-1901.

Chung SY, Butts CL, Maleki SJ, Champagne ET. Linking peanut allergenicity to the processes of maturation, curing, and roasting. J Agric Food Chem. 2003;51: 4273-4277.

Chwirot WB, Popp F. White-light-induced luminescence and mitotic activity of yeast cells. Folia Histochemica et Cytobiologica. 1991;29(4):155.

Cianci A, Giordano R, Delia A, Grasso E, Amodeo A, De Leo V, Caccamo F. Efficacy of Lactobacillus rhamnosus GR-1 and of Lactobacillus reuteri RC-14 in the treatment and prevention of vaginoses and bacterial vaginitis relapses. Minerva Ginecol. 2008 Oct;60(5):369-76.

Cibella F, Cuttitta G. Nocturnal asthma and gastroesophageal reflux. Am J Med. 2001 Dec 3;111 Suppl 8A:31S-36S.

Cingi C, Demirbas D, Songu M. Allergic rhinitis caused by food allergies. Eur Arch Otorhinolaryngol. 2010 Sep;267(9):1327-35.

Ciprandi G, De Amici M, Negrini S, Marseglia G, Tosca MA. TGF-beta and IL-17 serum levels and specific immunotherapy. Int Immunopharmacol. 2009 Sep;9(10):1247-9.

# REFERENCES AND BIBLIOGRAPHY

Cisneros C, García-Río F, Romera D, Villasante C, Girón R, Ancochea J. Bronchial reactivity indices are determinants of health-related quality of life in patients with stable asthma. *Thorax*. 2010 Sep;65(9):795-800.

Clark S, Bock SA, Gaeta TJ, Brenner BE, Cydulka RK, Camargo CA; Multicenter Airway Research Collaboration-8 Investigators. Multicenter study of emergency department visits for food allergies. *J Allergy Clin Immunol*. 2004 Feb;113(2):347-52.

Clement YN, Williams AF, Aranda D, Chase R, Watson N, Mohammed R, Stubbs O, Williamson D. Medicinal herb use among asthmatic patients attending a specialty care facility in Trinidad. *BMC Complement Altern Med*. 2005 Feb 15;5:3.

Clerici M, Balotta C, Meroni L, Ferrario E, Riva C, Trabattoni D, Ridolfo A,Villa M, Shearer GM, Moroni M, Galli M. Type 1 cytokine production and low prevalence of viral isolation correlate with long-term nonprogression in HIV infection. *AIDS Res Hum Retroviruses*. 1996 Jul 20;12(11):1053-61.

Cobo Sanz JM, Mateos JA, Muñoz Conejo A. Effect of *Lactobacillus casei* on the incidence of infectious conditions in children. *Nutr Hosp*. 2006 Jul-Aug;21(4):547-51.

Codispoti CD, Levin L, LeMasters GK, Ryan P, Reponen T, Villareal M, Burkle J, Stanforth S, Lockey JE, Khurana Hershey GK, Bernstein DI. Breast-feeding, aeroallergen sensitization, and environmental exposures during infancy are determinants of childhood allergic rhinitis. *J Allergy Clin Immunol*. 2010 May;125(5):1054-1060.e1.

Cohen RT, Raby BA, Van Steen K, Fuhlbrigge AL, Celedón JC, Rosner BA, Strunk RC, Zeiger RS, Weiss ST; Childhood Asthma Management Program Research Group. In utero smoke exposure and impaired response to inhaled corticosteroids in children with asthma. *J Allergy Clin Immunol*. 2010 Sep;126(3):491-7. 2010 Jul 31. ;

Cohen S, Popp F. Biophoton emission of the human body. *J Photochem & Photobio*. 1997;B 40:187-189.

Colecchia A, Vestito A, La Rocca A, Pasqui F, Nikiforaki A, Festi D; Symbiotic Study Group. Effect of a symbiotic preparation on the clinical manifestations of irritable bowel syndrome, constipation-variant. Results of an open, uncontrolled multicenter study. *Minerva Gastroenterol Dietol*. 2006 Dec;52(4):349-58.

Collipp PJ, Goldzier S 3rd, Weiss N, Soleymani Y, Snyder R. Pyridoxine treatment of childhood bronchial asthma. *Ann Allergy*. 1975 Aug;35(2):93-7.

Colodner R, Edelstein H, Chazan B, Raz R. Vaginal colonization by orally administered *Lactobacillus rhamnosus* GG. *Isr Med Assoc J*. 2003 Nov;5(11):767-9.

Colquhoun DM, Moores D, Somerset SM, Humphries JA. Comparison of the effects on lipoproteins and apolipoproteins of a diet high in monounsaturated fatty acids, enriched with avocado, and a high-carbohydrate diet. *Am J Clin Nutr*. 1992 Oct;56(4):671-7.

Conklin-Brittain NL, Wrangham RW, Smith CC. Ungar PS, Teaford MF. Human Diet: Its Origin and Evolution. Westport: Bergin & Garvey; 2002.

Conquer JA, Holub BJ. Dietary docosahexaenoic acid as a source of eicosapentaenoic acid in vegetarians and omnivores. *Lipids*. 1997 Mar;32(3):341-5.

Constantino PJ, *et al.* Tooth chipping can reveal the diet and bite forces of fossil hominins. Biol Lett. 2010;6:826 – 829.

Consumer Reports. Probiotics: Are enough in your diet? *Cons Rpts Mag*. 2005:34-35.

Conway PL, Gorbach SL, Goldin BR. Survival of lactic acid bacteria in the human stomach and adhesion to intestinal cells. *J Dairy Sci*. 1987 Jan;70(1):1-12.

Cooper GS, Miller FW, Germolec DR. Occupational exposures and autoimmune diseases. *Int Immunopharm* 2002, 2:303-313.

Cooper K. *The Aerobics Program for Total Well-Being*. New York: Evans, 1980.

Corbe C, Boissin JP, Siou A. Light vision and chorioretinal circulation. Study of the effect of procyanidolic oligomers (Endotelon). *J Fr Ophtalmol*. 1988;11(5):453-60.

Corbe C, Boissin JP, Siou A. Light vision and chorioretinal circulation. Study of the effect of procyanidolic oligomers (Endotelon). *J Fr Ophtalmol*. 1988;11(5):453-60.

Corbo GM, Forastiere F, De Sario M, Brunetti L, Bonci E, Bugiani M, Chellini E, La Grutta S, Migliore E, Pistelli R, Rusconi F, Russo A, Simoni M, Talassi F, Galassi C; Sidria-2 Collaborative Group. Wheeze and asthma in children: associations with body mass index, sports, television viewing, and diet. *Epidemiology*. 2008 Sep;19(5):747-55.

Corrêa NB, Péret Filho LA, Penna FJ, Lima FM, Nicoli JR. A randomized formula controlled trial of *Bifidobacterium lactis* and *Streptococcus thermophilus* for prevention of antibiotic-associated diarrhea in infants. *J Clin Gastroenterol*. 2005 May-Jun;39(5):385-9.

Cory S, Ussery-Hall A, Griffin-Blake S, Easton A, Vigeant J, Balluz L, Garvin W, Greenlund K; Centers for Disease Control and Prevention (CDC). Prevalence of selected risk behaviors and chronic diseases and conditions-steps communities, United States, 2006-2007. *MMWR Surveill Summ*. 2010 Sep 24;59(8):1-37.

Cotillard A, Kennedy SP, Kong LC, Prifti E, Pons N, Le Chatelier E, Almeida M, Quinquis B, Levenez F, Galleron N, Gougis S, Rizkalla S, Batto JM, Renault P; ANR MicroObes consortium, Doré J, Zucker JD, Clément K, Ehrlich SD, Blottière H, Leclerc M, Juste C, de Wouters T, Lepage P, Fouqueray C, Basdevant A, Henegar C, Godard C, Fondacci M, Rohia A, Hajduch F, Weissenbach J, Pelletier E, Le Paslier D, Gauchi JP, Gibrat JF, Loux V, Carré W, Maguin E, van de Guchte M, Jamet A, Boumezbeur F, Layec S. Dietary intervention impact on gut microbial gene richness. Nature. 2013 Aug 29;500(7464):585-8. doi: 10.1038/nature12480.

Cottet V, Touvier M, Fournier A, Touillaud MS, Lafay L, Clavel-Chapelon F, Boutron-Ruault MC. Postmenopausal breast cancer risk and dietary patterns in the E3N-EPIC prospective cohort study. Am J Epidemiol. 2009 Nov 15;170(10):1257-67. doi: 10.1093/aje/kwp257.

Courtney R, Cohen M. Investigating the claims of Konstantin Buteyko, M.D., Ph.D.: the relationship of breath holding time to end tidal $CO_2$ and other proposed measures of dysfunctional breathing. *J Altern Complement Med.* 2008 Mar;14(2):115-23.

Couto E, Boffetta P, Lagiou P, Ferrari P, Buckland G, Overvad K, Dahm CC, Tjonneland A, Olsen A, Clavel-Chapelon F, outron-Ruault MC, Cottet V, Trichopoulos D, Naska A, Benetou V, Kaaks R, Rohrmann S, Boeing H, von Ruesten A, Panico S, Pala V, Vineis P, Palli D, Tumino R, May A, Peeters PH, Bueno-de-Mesquita HB, Büchner FL, Lund E, Skeie G, Engeset D, Gonzalez CA, Navarro C, Rodríguez L, Sánchez MJ, Amiano P, Barricarte A, Hallmans G, Johansson I, Manjer J, Wirfärt E, Allen NE, Crowe F, Khaw KT, Wareham N, Moskal A, Slimani N, Jenab M, Romaguera D, Mouw T, Norat T, Riboli E, Trichopoulou A. Mediterranean dietary pattern and cancer risk in the EPIC cohort. Br J Cancer. 2011 Apr 26;104(9):1493-9.

Couto E, Boffetta P, Lagiou P, Ferrari P, Buckland G, Overvad K, Dahm CC, Tjonneland A, Olsen A, Clavel-Chapelon F, Boutron-Ruault MC, Cottet V, Trichopoulos D, Naska A, Benetou V, Kaaks R, Rohrmann S, Boeing H, von Ruesten A, Panico S, Pala V, Vineis P, Palli D, Tumino R, May A, Peeters PH, Bueno-de-Mesquita HB, Büchner FL, Lund E, Skeie G, Engeset D, Gonzalez CA, Navarro C, Rodríguez L, Sánchez MJ, Amiano P, Barricarte A, Hallmans G, Johansson I, Manjer J, Wirfärt E, Allen NE, Crowe F, Khaw KT, Wareham N, Moskal A, Slimani N, Jenab M, Romaguera D, Mouw T, Norat T, Riboli E, Trichopoulou A. Mediterranean dietary pattern and cancer risk in the EPIC cohort. Br J Cancer. 2011 Apr 26;104(9):1493-9.

Couzy F, Kastenmayer P, Vigo M, Clough J, Munoz-Box R, Barclay DV. Calcium bioavailability from a calcium- and sulfate-rich mineral water, compared with milk, in young adult women. *Am J Clin Nutr.* 1995 Dec;62(6):1239-44.

Covar R, Gleason M, Macomber B, Stewart L, Szefler P, Engelhardt K, Murphy J, Liu A, Wood S, DeMichele S, Gelfand EW, Szefler SJ. Impact of a novel nutritional formula on asthma control and biomarkers of allergic airway inflammation in children. *Clin Exp Allergy.* 2010 Aug;40(8):1163-74. 2010 Jun 7.

Crane J, Ellis I, Siebers R, Grimmet D, Lewis S, Fitzharris P. A pilot study of the effect of mechanical ventilation and heat exchange on house-dust mites and Der p 1 in New Zealand homes. *Allergy.* 1998 Aug;53(8):755-62.

Crescente M, Jessen G, Momi S, Höltje HD, Gresele P, Cerletti C, de Gaetano G. Interactions of gallic acid, resveratrol, quercetin and aspirin at the platelet cyclooxygenase-1 level. Functional and modelling studies. *Thromb Haemost.* 2009 Aug;102(2):336-46.

Crinnion WJ. Toxic effects of the easily avoidable phthalates and parabens. *Altern Med Rev.* 2010 Sep;15(3):190-6.

Cross AJ, Ferrucci LM, Risch A, Graubard BI, Ward MH, Park Y, Hollenbeck AR, Schatzkin A, Sinha R. A large prospective study of meat consumption and colorectal cancer risk: an investigation of potential mechanisms underlying this association. Cancer Res. 2010 Mar 15;70(6):2406-14.

Crowley ET, Williams LT, Roberts TK, Dunstan RH, Jones PD. Does milk cause constipation? A crossover dietary trial. Nutrients. 2013 Jan 22;5(1):253-66.

Cserhati E. Current view on the etiology of childhood bronchial asthma. *Orr Hetil.* 2000;141:759-760.

Cuesta-Herranz J, Barber D, Blanco C, Cistero-Bahíma A, Crespo JF, Fernández-Rivas M, Fernández-Sánchez J, Florido JF, Ibáñez MD, Rodríguez R, Salcedo G, Garcia BE, Lombardero M, Quiralte J, Rodriguez J, Sánchez-Monge R, Vereda A, Villalba M, Alonso Díaz de Durana MD, Basagaña M, Carrillo T, Fernández-Nieto M, Tabar AI. Differences among Pollen-Allergic Patients with and without Plant Food Allergy. *Int Arch Allergy Immunol.* 2010 Apr 23;153(2):182-192.

Cummings M. *Human Heredity: Principles and Issues.* St. Paul, MN: West, 1988.

Cusack L, De Buck E, Compernolle V, Vandekerckhove P. Blood type diets lack supporting evidence: a systematic review. Am J Clin Nutr. 2013 Jul;98(1):99-104. doi: 10.3945/ajcn.113.058693.

Custovic A, Simpson BM, Simpson A, Kissen P, Woodcock A; NAC Manchester Asthma and Allergy Study Group. Effect of environmental manipulation in pregnancy and early life on respiratory symptoms and atopy during first year of life: a randomised trial. *Lancet.* 2001 Jul 21;358(9277):188-93.

D'Anneo RW, Bruno ME, Falagiani P. Sublingual allergoid immunotherapy: a new 4-day induction phase in patients allergic to house dust mites. *Int J Immunopathol Pharmacol.* 2010 Apr-Jun;23(2):553-60.

D'Auria E, Sala M, Lodi F, Radaelli G, Riva E, Giovannini M. Nutritional value of a rice-hydrolysate formula in infants with cows' milk protein allergy: a randomized pilot study. *J Int Med Res.* 2003 May-Jun;31(3):215-22.

D'Orazio N, Ficoneri C, Riccioni G, Conti P, Theoharides TC, Bollea MR. Conjugated linoleic acid: a functional food? *Int J Immunopathol Pharmacol.* 2003 Sep-Dec;16(3):215-20.

D'Urbano LE, Pellegrino K, Artesani MC, Donnanno S, Luciano R, Riccardi C, Tozzi AE, Ravà L, De Benedetti F, Cavagni G. Performance of a component-based allergen-microarray in the diagnosis of cow's milk and hen's egg allergy. *Clin Exp Allergy.* 2010 Jul 13.

Dalaly BK, Eitenmiller RR, Friend BA, Shahani KM. Human milk ribonuclease. *Biochim Biophys Acta.* 1980 Oct;615(2):381-91.

Dalaly BK, Eitenmiller RR, Vakil JR, Shahani KM. Simultaneous isolation of human milk ribonuclease and lysozyme. Anal Biochem. 1970 Sep;37(1):208-11.

Dallinga JW, Robroeks CM, van Berkel JJ, Moonen EJ, Godschalk RW, Jöbsis Q, Dompeling E, Wouters EF, van Schooten FJ. Volatile organic compounds in exhaled breath as a diagnostic tool for asthma in children. Clin Exp Allergy. 2010 Jan;40(1):68-76.

Davidson T. *Rhinology: The Collected Writings of Maurice H. Cottle, M.D.* San Diego, CA: American Rhinologic Society, 1987.

Davies G. *Timetables of Medicine.* New York: Black Dog & Leventhal, 2000.

Davin JC, Forget P, Mahieu PR. Increased intestinal permeability to (51 Cr) EDTA is correlated with IgA immune complex-plasma levels in children with IgA-associated nephropathies. *Acta Paediatr Scand.* 1988 Jan;77(1):118-24.

Davis JM, Murphy EA, Brown AS, Carmichael MD, Ghaffar A, Mayer EP. Effects of oat beta-glucan on innate immunity and infection after exercise stress. Med Sci Sports Exerc. 2004 Aug;36(8):1321-7.

de Boissieu D, Dupont C, Badoual J. Allergy to nondairy proteins in mother's milk as assessed by intestinal permeability tests. *Allergy.* 1994 Dec;49(10):882-4.

De Lucca AJ, Bland JM, Vigo CB, Cushion M, Selitrennikoff CP, Peter J, Walsh TJ. CAY-1, a fungicidal saponin from Capsicum sp. fruit. *Med Mycol.* 2002 Apr;40(2):131-7.

De Preter V, Raemen H, Cloetens L, Houben E, Rutgeerts P, Verbeke K. Effect of dietary intervention with different pre- and probiotics on intestinal bacterial enzyme activities. *Eur J Clin Nutr.* 2008 Feb;62(2):225-31.

De Simone C, Ciardi A, Grassi A, Lambert Gardini S, Tzantzoglou S, Trinchieri V, Moretti S, Jirillo E. Effect of *Bifidobacterium bifidum* and *Lactobacillus acidophilus* on gut mucosa and peripheral blood B lymphocytes. *Immunopharmacol Immunotoxicol.* 1992;14(1-2):331-40.

De Smet PA. Herbal remedies. N Engl J Med. 2002;347:2046-2056.

De Stefani E, Boffetta P, Ronco AL, Deneo-Pellegrini H, Correa P, Acosta G, Mendilaharsu M, Luaces ME, Silva C. Processed meat consumption and risk of cancer: a multisite case-control study in Uruguay. Br J Cancer. 2012 Oct 23;107(9):1584-8. doi: 10.1038/bjc.2012.433.

de Vrese M, Rautenberg P, Laue C, Koopmans M, Herremans T, Schrezenmeir J. Probiotic bacteria stimulate virus-specific neutralizing antibodies following a booster polio vaccination. *Eur J Nutr.* 2005 Oct;44(7):406-13.

de Vrese M, Winkler P, Rautenberg P, Harder T, Noah C, Laue C, Ott S, Hampe J, Schreiber S, Heller K, Schrezenmeir J. Effect of *Lactobacillus gasseri* PA 16/8, *Bifidobacterium longum* SP 07/3, B. bifidum MF 20/5 on common cold episodes: a double blind, randomized, controlled trial. *Clin Nutr.* 2005 Aug;24(4):481-91.

Dean C. *Death by Modern Medicine.* Belleville, ON: Matrix Verite-Media, 2005.

Debley JS, Carter ER, Redding GJ. Prevalence and impact of gastroesophageal reflux in adolescents with asthma: a population-based study. *Pediatr Pulmonol.* 2006 May;41(5):475-81.

Dehlink E, Yen E, Leichtner AM, Hait EJ, Fiebiger E. First evidence of a possible association between gastric acid suppression during pregnancy and childhood asthma: a population-based register study. *Clin Exp Allergy.* 2009 Feb;39(2):246-53. 2008 Dec 9.

del Giudice MM, Leonardi S, Maiello N, Brunese FP. Food allergy and probiotics in childhood. *J Clin Gastroenterol.* 2010 Sep;44 Suppl 1:S22-5.

Delacourt C. Bronchial changes in untreated asthma. *Arch Pediatr.* 2004 Jun;11 Suppl 2:71s-73s.

Delia A, Morgante G, Rago G, Musacchio MC, Petraglia F, De Leo V. Effectiveness of oral administration of Lactobacillus paracasei subsp. paracasei F19 in association with vaginal suppositories of Lactobacillus acidofilus in the treatment of vaginosis and in the prevention of recurrent vaginitis. *Minerva Ginecol.* 2006 Jun;58(3):227-31.

Del-Rio-Navarro B, Berber A, Blandón-Vijil V, Ramírez-Aguilar M, Romieu I, Ramírez-Chanona N, Heras-Acevedo S, Serrano-Sierra A, Barraza-Villareal A, Baeza-Bacab M, Sienra-Monge JJ. Identification of asthma risk factors in Mexico City in an International Study of Asthma and Allergy in Childhood survey. *Allergy Asthma Proc.* 2006 Jul-Aug;27(4):325-33.

DeMan, JC, Rogosa M, Sharpe ME. A medium for the cultivation of lactobacilli. *J Bacteriol.* 1960:23;130.

Demidov LV, Manziuk LV, Kharkevitch GY, Pirogova NA, Artamonova EV. Adjuvant fermented wheat germ extract (Avemar) nutraceutical improves survival of high-risk skin melanoma patients: a randomized, pilot, phase II clinical study with a 7-year follow-up. Cancer Biother Radiopharm. 2008 Aug;23(4):477-82. doi:10.1089/cbr.2008.0486. Erratum in: Cancer Biother Radiopharm. 2008 Oct;23(5):669.

Dengate S, Ruben A. Controlled trial of cumulative behavioural effects of a common bread preservative. *J Paediatr Child Health.* 2002 Aug;38(4):373-6.

Dente FL, Bacci E, Bartoli ML, Cianchetti S, Costa F, Di Franco A, Malagrinò L, Vagaggini B, Paggiaro P. Effects of oral prednisone on sputum eosinophils and cytokines in patients with severe refractory asthma. *Ann Allergy Asthma Immunol.* 2010 Jun;104(6):464-70.

Denys GA, Koch KM, Dowzicky MJ. Distribution of resistant gram-positive organisms across the census regions of the United States and in vitro activity of tigecycline, a new glycylcycline antimicrobial. *Am J Infect Control.* 2007 Oct;35(8):521-6.

Depeint F, Tzortzis G, Vulevic J, I'anson K, Gibson GR. Prebiotic evaluation of a novel galactooligosaccharide mixture produced by the enzymatic activity of *Bifidobacterium bifidum* NCIMB 41171, in healthy humans: a randomized, double-blind, crossover, placebo-controlled intervention study. *Am J Clin Nutr.* 2008 Mar;87(3):785-91.

Derebery MJ, Berliner KI. Allergy and its relation to Meniere's disease. *Otolaryngol Clin North Am.* 2010 Oct;43(5):1047-58.

Deriemaeker P, Aerenhouts D, De Ridder D, Hebbelinck M, Clarys P. Health aspects, nutrition and physical characteristics in matched samples of institutionalized vegetarian and non-vegetarian elderly (>65yrs). Nutr Metab (Lond). 2011 Jun 14;8(1):37.

Desbonnet L, Garrett L, Clarke G, Bienenstock J, Dinan TG. The probiotic Bifidobacteria infantis: An assessment of potential antidepressant properties in the rat. *J Psychiatr Res.* 2008 Dec;43(2):164-74.

Desjeux JF, Heyman M. Milk proteins, cytokines and intestinal epithelial functions in children. *Acta Paediatr Jpn.* 1994 Oct;36(5):592-6.

DesRoches A, Infante-Rivard C, Paradis L, Paradis J, Haddad E. Peanut allergy: is maternal transmission of antigens during pregnancy and breastfeeding a risk factor? *J Investig Allergol Clin Immunol.* 2010;20(4):289-94.

Deutsche Gesellschaft für Ernährung. Drink distilled water? *Med. Mo. Pharm.* 1993;16:146.

Devanand D, Lee J, Luchsinger J, Manly J, Marder K, Mayeux R, Scarmeas N, Schupf N, Stern Y. Lessons from Epidemiologic Research about Risk Factors, Modifiers, and Progression of Late Onset Alzheimer's Disease in New York City at Columbia University Medical Center. J Alzheimers Dis. 2012 Jul 24.

Devaraj TL. *Speaking of Ayurvedic Remedies for Common Diseases.* New Delhi: Sterling, 1985.

Devirgiliis C, Zalewski PD, Perozzi G, Murgia C. Zinc fluxes and zinc transporter genes in chronic diseases. *Mutat Res.* 2007 Sep 1;622(1-2):84-93. 2007 Feb 17.

DeWitt RC, Kudsk KA. The gut's role in metabolism, mucosal barrier function, and gut immunology. *Infect Dis Clin North Am.* 1999 Jun;13(2):465-81.

Dharmage SC, Erbas B, Jarvis D, Wjst M, Raherison C, Norbäck D, Heinrich J, Sunyer J, Svanes C. Do childhood respiratory infections continue to influence adult respiratory morbidity? *Eur Respir J.* 2009 Feb;33(2):237-44.

Di Gioacchino M, Cavallucci E, Di Stefano F, Paolini F, Ramondo S, Di Sciascio MB, Ciuffreda S, Riccioni G, Della Vecchia R, Romano A, Boscolo P. Effect of natural allergen exposure on non-specific bronchial reactivity in asthmatic farmers. *Sci Total Environ.* 2001 Apr 10;270(1-3):43-8.

Di Gioacchino M, Cavallucci E, Di Stefano F, Verna N, Ramondo S, Ciuffreda S, Riccioni G, Boscolo P. Influence of total IgE and seasonal increase of eosinophil cationic protein on bronchial hyperreactivity in asthmatic grass-sensitized farmers. *Allergy.* 2000 Nov;55(11):1030-4.

Di Marzio L, Centi C, Cinque B, Masci S, Giuliani M, Arcieri A, Zicari L, De Simone C, Cifone MG. Effect of the lactic acid bacterium *Streptococcus thermophilus* on stratum corneum ceramide levels and signs and symptoms of atopic dermatitis patients. *Exp Dermatol.* 2003 Oct;12(5):615-20.

Dierksen KP, Moore CJ, Inglis M, Wescombe PA, Tagg JR. The effect of ingestion of milk supplemented with salivaricin A-producing Streptococcus salivarius on the bacteriocin-like inhibitory activity of streptococcal populations on the tongue. *FEMS Microbiol Ecol.* 2007 Mar;59(3):584-91.

Diğrak M, Ilçim A, Hakki Alma M. Antimicrobial activities of several parts of Pinus brutia, Juniperus oxycedrus, Abies cilicia, Cedrus libani and Pinus nigra. *Phytother Res.* 1999 Nov;13(7):584-7.

DiMango E, Holbrook JT, Simpson E, Reibman J, Richter J, Narula S, Prusakowski N, Mastronarde JG, Wise RA; American Lung Association Asthma Clinical Research Centers. Effects of asymptomatic proximal and distal gastroesophageal reflux on asthma severity. *Am J Respir Crit Care Med.* 2009 Nov 1;180(9):809-16. 2009 Aug 6.

Dimitonova SP, Danova ST, Serkedjieva JP, Bakalov BV. Antimicrobial activity and protective properties of vaginal lactobacilli from healthy Bulgarian women. *Anaerobe.* 2007 Oct-Dec;13(5-6):178-84.

Din FV, Theodoratou E, Farrington SM, Tenesa A, Barnetson RA, Cetnarskyj R, Stark L, Porteous ME, Campbell H, Dunlop MG. Effect of aspirin and NSAIDs on risk and survival from colorectal cancer. *Gut.* 2010 Dec;59(12):1670-9.

Dinleyici EC, Eren M, Yargic ZA, Dogan N, Vandenplas Y. Clinical efficacy of *Saccharomyces boulardii* and metronidazole compared to metronidazole alone in children with acute bloody diarrhea caused by amebiasis: a prospective, randomized, open label study. *Am J Trop Med Hyg.* 2009 Jun;80(6):953-5.

Diop L, Guillou S, Durand H. Probiotic food supplement reduces stress-induced gastrointestinal symptoms in volunteers: a double-blind, placebo-controlled, randomized trial. *Nutr Res.* 2008 Jan;28(1):1-5.

Dixon AE, Kaminsky DA, Holbrook JT, Wise RA, Shade DM, Irvin CG. Allergic rhinitis and sinusitis in asthma: differential effects on symptoms and pulmonary function. *Chest.* 2006 Aug;130(2):429-35.

Dona A, Arvanitoyannis IS. Health risks of genetically modified foods. *Crit Rev Food Sci Nutr.* 2009 Feb;49(2):164-75.

Donato F, Monarca S, Premi S., and Gelatti, U. Drinking water hardness and chronic degenerative diseases. Part III. Tumors, urolithiasis, fetal malformations, deterioration of the cognitive function in the aged and atopic eczema. *Ann. Ig.* 2003;15:57-70.

Dooley, M.A. and Hogan S.L. Environmental epidemiology and risk factors for autoimmune disease. *Curr Opin Rheum.* 2003;15(2):99-103.

dos Santos LH, Ribeiro IO, Sánchez PG, Hetzel JL, Felicetti JC, Cardoso PF. Evaluation of pantoprazol treatment response of patients with asthma and gastroesophageal reflux: a randomized prospective double-blind placebo-controlled study. *J Bras Pneumol.* 2007 Apr;33(2):119-27.

Dotolo Institute. *The Study of Colon Hydrotherapy.* Pinellas Park, FL: Dotolo, 2003.

Dove MS, Dockery DW, Connolly GN. Smoke-free air laws and asthma prevalence, symptoms, and severity among nonsmoking youth. *Pediatrics.* 2011 Jan;127(1):102-9. 2010 Dec 13.

Dowd JB, Zajacova A, Aiello A. Early origins of health disparities: burden of infection, health, and socioeconomic status in U.S. children. *Soc Sci Med.* 2009 Feb;68(4):699-707. 2009 Jan 17.

Drago L, De Vecchi E, Nicola L, Zucchetti E, Gismondo MR, Vicariotto F. Activity of a *Lactobacillus acidophilus*-based douche for the treatment of bacterial vaginosis. *J Altern Complement Med.* 2007 May;13(4):435-8.

Drouault-Holowacz S, Bieuvelet S, Burckel A, Cazaubiel M, Dray X, Marteau P. A double blind randomized controlled trial of a probiotic combination in 100 patients with irritable bowel syndrome. *Gastroenterol Clin Biol.* 2008 Feb;32(2):147-52.

Drubaix I, Maraval M, Robert L, Robert AM. Hyaluronic acid (hyaluronan) levels in pathological human saphenous veins. Effects of procyanidol oligomers, *Pathol Biol* 1997 Jan;45(1):86-91.

Drubaix I, Robert L, Maraval M, Robert AM. Synthesis of glycoconjugates by human diseased veins: modulation by procyanidolic oligomers. *Int J Exp Pathol.* 1997 Apr;78(2):117-21.

Ducrotté P. Irritable bowel syndrome: from the gut to the brain-gut. *Gastroenterol Clin Biol.* 2009 Aug-Sep;33(8-9):703-12.

Duffey KJ, Gordon-Larsen P, Shikany JM, Guilkey D, Jacobs DR Jr, Popkin BM. Food price and diet and health outcomes: 20 years of the CARDIA Study. Arch Intern Med. 2010 Mar 8;170(5):420-6. Erratum in: Arch Intern Med. 2010 Jun 28;170(12):1089.

Duke J. CRC Handbook of Medicinal Herbs. Boca Raton: CRC; 1989.

Duke J. The Green Pharmacy. New York: St. Martins, 1997.

Dunn R. Human Ancestors were nearly all vegetarians. Sci Am. 2012. Jul 12. http://blogs.scientificamerican.com/guest-blog/2012/07/23/human-ancestors-were-nearly-all-vegetarians. Acc. Oct 21, 2013.

Dunstan JA, Roper J, Mitoulas L, Hartmann PE, Simmer K, Prescott SL. The effect of supplementation with fish oil during pregnancy on breast milk immunoglobulin A, soluble CD14, cytokine levels and fatty acid composition. Clin Exp Allergy. 2004 Aug;34(8):1237-42.

Duong M, Subbarao P, Adelroth E, Obminski G, Strinich T, Inman M, Pedersen S, O'Byrne PM. Sputum eosinophils and the response of exercise-induced bronchoconstriction to corticosteroid in asthma. Chest. 2008 Feb;133(2):404-11. 2007 Dec 10.

Dupont C, Barau E, Molkhou P, Raynaud F, Barbet JP, Dehennin L. Food-induced alterations of intestinal permeability in children with cow's milk-sensitive enteropathy and atopic dermatitis. J Pediatr Gastroenterol Nutr. 1989 May;8(4):459-65.

Dupont C, Barau E, Molkhou P. Intestinal permeability disorders in children. Allerg Immunol. 1991 Mar;23(3):95-103.

Dupont C, Soulaines P, Lapillonne A, Donne N, Kalach N, Benhamou P. Atopy patch test for early diagnosis of cow's milk allergy in preterm infants. J Pediatr Gastroenterol Nutr. 2010 Apr;50(4):463-4.

Dupuy P, Cassé M, André F, Dhivert-Donnadieu H, Pinton J, Hernandez-Pion C. Low-salt water reduces intestinal permeability in atopic patients. Dermatology. 1999;198(2):153-5.

Duran-Tauleria E, Vignati G, Guedan MJ, Petersson CJ. The utility of specific immunoglobulin E measurements in primary care. Allergy. 2004 Aug;59 Suppl 78:35-41.

Duwiejua M, Zeitlin IJ, Waterman PG, Chapman J, Mhango GJ, Provan GJ. Anti-inflammatory activity of resins from some species of the plant family Burseraceae. Planta Med. 1993 Feb;59(1):12-6.

Dykewicz MS, Lemmon JK, Keaney DL. Comparison of the Multi-Test II and Skintestor Omni allergy skin test devices. Ann Allergy Asthma Immunol. 2007 Jun;98(6):559-62.

E.R. Farnworth, I. Mainville, M.-P. Desjardins, N. Gardner, I. Fliss and C. Champagne. 2006. Growth of probiotic bacteria and bifidobacteria in a soy yogurt formulation. Internl Jnl Food Microbiology. 10.1016.

Eastham EJ, Walker WA. Effect of cow's milk on the gastrointestinal tract: a persistent dilemma for the pediatrician. Pediatrics. 1977 Oct;60(4):477-81.

Eaton KK, Howard M, Howard JM. Gut permeability measured by polyethylene glycol absorption in abnormal gut fermentation as compared with food intolerance. J R Soc Med. 1995 Feb;88(2):63-6.

Ebers GC, Kukay K, Bulman DE, Sadovnick AD, Rice G, Anderson C, Armstrong H, Cousin K, Bell RB, Hader W, Paty DW, Hashimoto S, Oger J, Duquette P, Warren S, Gray T, O'Connor P, Nath A, Auty A, Metz L, Francis G, Paulseth JE, Murray TJ, Pryse-Phillips W, Nelson R, Freedman M, Brunet D, Bouchard JP, Hinds D, Risch N. A full genome search in multiple sclerosis. Nat Genet. 1996 Aug;13(4):472-6.

Eccles R. Menthol and related cooling compounds. J Pharm Pharmacol. 1994 Aug;46(8):618-30.

ECRHS (2002) The European Community Respiratory Health Survey II. Eur Respir J. 20: 1071-1079.

Edgecombe K, Latter S, Peters S, Roberts G. Health experiences of adolescents with uncontrolled severe asthma. Arch Dis Child. 2010 Dec;95(12):985-91. 2010 Jul 30.

Edgell PG. The psychology of asthma. Can Med Assoc J. 1952 Aug;67(2):121-5.

Egashira Y, Nagano H. A multicenter clinical trial of TJ-96 in patients with steroid-dependent bronchial asthma. A comparison of groups allocated by the envelope method. Ann N Y Acad Sci. 1993 Jun 23;685:580-3.

Ege MJ, Frei R, Bieli C, Schram-Bijkerk D, Waser M, Benz MR, Weiss G, Nyberg F, van Hage M, Pershagen G, Brunekreef B, Riedler J, Lauener R, Braun-Fahrländer C, von Mutius E; PARSIFAL Study team. Not all farming environments protect against the development of asthma and wheeze in children. J Allergy Clin Immunol. 2007 May;119(5):1140-7.

Ege MJ, Herzum I, Büchele G, Krauss-Etschmann S, Lauener RP, Roponen M, Hyvärinen A, Vuitton DA, Riedler J, Brunekreef B, Dalphin JC, Braun-Fahrländer C, Pekkanen J, Renz H, von Mutius E; Protection Against Allergy Study in Rural Environments (PASTURE) Study group. Prenatal exposure to a farm environment modifies atopic sensitization at birth. J Allergy Clin Immunol. 2008 Aug;122(2):407-12, 412.e1-4.

Eggermont E. Cow's milk protein allergy. Tijdschr Kindergeneeskd. 1981 Feb;49(1):16-20.

Ehling S, Hengel M, and Shibamoto T. Formation of acrylamide from lipids. Adv Exp Med Biol 2005, 561:223-233.

Ehling S, Hengel M, and Shibamoto T. Formation of acrylamide from lipids. Adv Exp Med Biol 2005, 561:223-233.

Ehnert B, Lau-Schadendorf S, Weber A, Buettner P, Schou C, Wahn U. Reducing domestic exposure to dust mite allergen reduces bronchial hyperreactivity in sensitive children with asthma. J Allergy Clin Immunol. 1992 Jul;90(1):135-8.

Ehren J, Morón B, Martin E, Bethune MT, Gray GM, Khosla C. A food-grade enzyme preparation with modest gluten detoxification properties. PLoS One. 2009 Jul 21;4(7):e6313.

Eijkemans M, Mommers M, de Vries SI, van Buuren S, Stafleu A, Bakker I, Thijs C. Asthmatic symptoms, physical activity, and overweight in young children: a cohort study. Pediatrics. 2008 Mar;121(3):e666-72.

Eldridge MW, Peden DB. Allergen provocation augments endotoxin-induced nasal inflammation in subjects with atopic asthma. J Allergy Clin Immunol. 2000 Mar;105(3):475-81.

el-Ghazaly M, Khayyal MT, Okpanyi SN, Arens-Corell M. Study of the anti-inflammatory activity of Populus tremula, Solidago virgaurea and Fraxinus excelsior. Arzneimittelforschung. 1992 Mar;42(3):333-6.

Ellingwood F. *American Materia Medica, Therapeutics and Pharmacognosy.* Portland: Eclectic Medical Publ., 1983.

Elliott RB, Harris DP, Hill JP, Bibby NJ, Wasmuth HE. Type I (insulin-dependent) diabetes mellitus and cow milk: casein variant consumption. *Diabetologia.* 1999 Mar;42(3):292-6.

Elmer GW, McFarland LV, Surawicz CM, Danko L, Greenberg RN. Behaviour of *Saccharomyces boulardii* in recurrent *Clostridium difficile* disease patients. *Aliment Pharmacol Ther.* 1999 Dec;13(12):1663-8.

Elwood PC. Epidemiology and trace elements. *Clin Endocrinol Metab.* 1985 Aug;14(3):617-28.

Emberlin JC, Lewis RA. Pollen challenge study of a phototherapy device for reducing the symptoms of hay fever. *Curr Med Res Opin.* 2009 Jul;25(7):1635-44.

Emmanouil E, Manios Y, Grammatikaki E, Kondaki K, Oikonomou E, Papadopoulos N, Vassilopoulou E. Association of nutrient intake and wheeze or asthma in a Greek pre-school population. *Pediatr Allergy Immunol.* 2010 Feb;21(1 Pt 1):90-5. 2009 Sep 9.

Engan HK, Jones AM, Ehrenberg F, Schagatay E. Acute dietary nitrate supplementation improves dry static apnea performance. *Respir Physiol Neurobiol.* 2012 Jul 1;182(2-3):53-9.

Engler RJ. Alternative and complementary medicine: a source of improved therapies for asthma? A challenge for redefining the specialty? *J Allergy Clin Immunol.* 2000;106:627-9.

Environmental Working Group. *Human Toxome Project.* 2007. http://www.ewg.org/sites/humantoxome/. Accessed: 2007 Sep.

EPA. *A Brief Guide to Mold, Moisture and Your Home.* Environmental Protection Agency, Office of Air and Radiation/Indoor Environments Division. EPA 2002;402-K-02-003.

Epstein GN, Halper JP, Barrett EA, Birdsall C, McGee M, Baron KP, Lowenstein S. A pilot study of mind-body changes in adults with asthma who practice mental imagery. *Altern Ther Health Med.* 2004 Jul-Aug;10(4):66-71.

Epstein SS. Potential public health hazards of biosynthetic milk hormones. *Int J Health Serv.* 1990;20(1):73-84.

Ercan N, Nuttall FQ, Gannon MC, Lane JT, Burmeister LA, Westphal SA. Plasma glucose and insulin responses to bananas of varying ripeness in persons with noninsulin-dependent diabetes mellitus. *J Am Coll Nutr.* 1993 Dec;12(6):703-9.

Erkkola M, Kaila M, Nwaru BI, Kronberg-Kippilä C, Ahonen S, Nevalainen J, Veijola R, Pekkanen J, Ilonen J, Simell O, Knip M, Virtanen SM. Maternal vitamin D intake during pregnancy is inversely associated with asthma and allergic rhinitis in 5-year-old children. *Clin Exp Allergy.* 2009 Jun;39(6):875-82.

Ernst E. Frankincense: systematic review. *BMJ.* 2008 Dec 17;337:a2813.

Erwin EA, James HR, Gutekunst HM, Russo JM, Kelleher KJ, Platts-Mills TA. Serum IgE measurement and detection of food allergy in pediatric patients with eosinophilic esophagitis. *Ann Allergy Asthma Immunol.* 2010 Jun;104(6):496-502.

Esposito K., Kastorini C.M., Panagiotakos D.B., Giugliano D. Mediterranean diet and weight loss: meta-analysis of randomized controlled trials. Metab Syndr Relat Disord. 2011;9:1 – 12.

Estruch R, *et al.* Primary Prevention of Cardiovascular Disease with a Mediterranean Diet. NE Jour. Med. 2013. Jan 25. DOI: 10.1056/NEJMoa1200303

EuroPrevall. *WP 1.1 Birth Cohort Update.* 1st Quarter 2006. Berlin, Germany: Charité University Medical Centre.

Evans P, Forte D, Jacobs C, Fredhoi C, Aitchison E, Hucklebridge F, Clow A. Cortisol secretory activity in older people in relation to positive and negative well-being. *Psychoneuroendocrinology.* 2007 Aug 7

Everhart JE. *Digestive Diseases in the United States.* Darby, PA: Diane Pub, 1994.

FAAN. *Public Comment on 2005 Food Safety Survey: Docket No. 2004N-0516 (2005 FSS).* Fairfax, VA: Food Allergy & Anaphylaxis Network.

Fabian E, Elmadfa I. Influence of daily consumption of probiotic and conventional yoghurt on the plasma lipid profile in young healthy women. *Ann Nutr Metab.* 2006;50(4):387-93.

Fabian E, Majchrzak D, Dieminger B, Meyer E, Elmadfa I. Influence of probiotic and conventional yoghurt on the status of vitamins B1, B2 and B6 in young healthy women. *Ann Nutr Metab.* 2008;52(1):29-36.

Fairchild SS, Shannon K, Kwan E, Mishell RI. T cell-derived glucosteroid response-modifying factor (GRMFT): a unique lymphokine made by normal T lymphocytes and a T cell hybridoma. *J Immunol.* 1984 Feb;132(2):821-7.

Fälth-Magnusson K, Kjellman NI, Magnusson KE, Sundqvist T. Intestinal permeability in healthy and allergic children before and after sodium-cromoglycate treatment assessed with different-sized polyethyleneglycols (PEG 400 and PEG 1000). *Clin Allergy.* 1984 May;14(3):277-86.

Fälth-Magnusson K, Kjellman NI, Odelram H, Sundqvist T, Magnusson KE. Gastrointestinal permeability in children with cow's milk allergy: effect of milk challenge and sodium cromoglycate as assessed with polyethyleneglycols (PEG 400 and PEG 1000). *Clin Allergy.* 1986 Nov;16(6):543-51.

Famularo G, De Simone C, Pandey V, Sahu AR, Minisola G. Probiotic lactobacilli: an innovative tool to correct the malabsorption syndrome of vegetarians? Med Hypotheses. 2005;65(6):1132-5.

Fan AY, Lao L, Zhang RX, Zhou AN, Wang LB, Moudgil KD, Lee DY, Ma ZZ, Zhang WY, Berman BM. Effects of an acetone extract of Boswellia carterii Birdw. (Burseraceae) gum resin on adjuvant-induced arthritis in lewis rats. *J Ethnopharmacol.* 2005 Oct 3;101(1-3):104-9.

Fanaro S, Marten B, Bagna R, Vigi V, Fabris C, Peña-Quintana L, Argüelles F, Scholz-Ahrens KE, Sawatzki G, Zelenka R, Schrezenmeir J, de Vrese M and Bertino E. Galacto-oligosaccharides are bifidogenic and safe at weaning: A double-blind Randomized Multicenter study. *J Pediatr Gastroent Nutr.* 2009 48; 82-88

Fang H, Elina T, Heikki A, Seppo S. Modulation of humoral immune response through probiotic intake. *FEMS Immunol Med Microbiol.* 2000 Sep;29(1):47-52.

Fang SP, Tanaka T, Tago F, Okamoto T, Kojima S. Immunomodulatory effects of gyokuheifusan on INF-gamma/IL-4 (Th1/Th2) balance in ovalbumin (OVA)-induced asthma model mice. *Biol Pharm Bull.* 2005;28:829-33.

# REFERENCES AND BIBLIOGRAPHY

Fanigliulo L, Comparato G, Aragona G, Cavallaro L, Iori V, Maino M, Cavestro GM, Soliani P, Sianesi M, Franzè A, Di Mario F. Role of gut microflora and probiotic effects in the irritable bowel syndrome. *Acta Biomed.* 2006 Aug;77(2):85-9.

FAO/WHO Expert Committee. *Fats and Oils in Human Nutrition.* Food and Nutrition Paper. 1994;(57).

Farber JE, Ross J, Stephens G. Antibiotic anaphylaxis. *Calif Med.* 1954 Jul;81(1):9-11.

Farber JE, Ross J. Antibiotic anaphylaxis; a note on the treatment and prevention of severe reactions to penicillin, streptomycin and dihydrostreptomycin. *Med Times.* 1952 Jan;80(1):28-30.

Farkas E. [Fermented wheat germ extract in the supportive therapy of colorectal cancer]. *Orv Hetil.* 2005 Sep 11;146(37):1925-31.

Fasano A, Shea-Donohue T. Mechanisms of disease: the role of intestinal barrier function in the pathogenesis of gastrointestinal autoimmune diseases. *Nat Clin Pract Gastroenterol Hepatol.* 2005 Sep;2(9):416-22.

Fawell J, Nieuwenhuijsen MJ. Contaminants in drinking water. *Br Med Bull.* 2003;68:199-208.

Féart C, Pérès K, Samieri C, Letenneur L, Dartigues JF, Barberger-Gateau P. Adherence to a Mediterranean diet and onset of disability in older persons. *Eur J Epidemiol.* 2011 Sep;26(9):747-56. doi: 10.1007/s10654-011-9611-4.

Fecka I. Qualitative and quantitative determination of hydrolysable tannins and other polyphenols in herbal products from meadowsweet and dog rose. *Phytochem Anal.* 2009 May;20(3):177-90.

Feibel CS, Harris JM, Brown FH. Palaeoenvironmental context for the Late Neogene of the Turkana Basin. In: Harris JM, editor. Koobi Fora Research Project. Vol. 3. Oxford: Clarendon Press; 1991. pp. 321 – 346.

Felley CP, Corthésy-Theulaz I, Rivero JL, Sipponen P, Kaufmann M, Bauerfeind P, Wiesel PH, Brassart D, Pfeifer A, Blum AL, Michetti P. Favourable effect of an acidified milk (LC-1) on *Helicobacter pylori* gastritis in man. *Eur J Gastroenterol Hepatol.* 2001 Jan;13(1):25-9.

Ferencík M, Ebringer L, Mikes Z, Jahnová E, Ciznár I. Successful modification of human intestinal microflora with oral administration of lactic acid bacteria. *Bratisl Lek Listy.* 1999 May;100(5):238-45.

Ferguson BJ. Categorization of eosinophilic chronic rhinosinusitis. *Curr Opin Otolaryngol Head Neck Surg.* 2004 Jun;12(3):237-42.

Ferrari M, Benini L, Brotto E, Locatelli F, De Iorio F, Bonella F, Tacchella N, Corradini G, Lo Cascio V, Vantini I. Omeprazole reduces the response to capsaicin but not to methacholine in asthmatic patients with proximal reflux. *Scand J Gastroenterol.* 2007 Mar;42(3):299-307.

Ferreira LF, Behnke BJ. A toast to health and performance! Beetroot juice lowers blood pressure and the O2 cost of exercise. J Appl Physiol. 2011 Mar;110(3):585-6.

Ferrier L, Berard F, Debrauwer L, Chabo C, Langella P, Bueno L, Fioramonti J. Impairment of the intestinal barrier by ethanol involves enteric microflora and mast cell activation in rodents. *Am J Pathol.* 2006 Apr;168(4):1148-54.

Ferrier L, Berard F, Debrauwer L, Chabo C, Langella P, Bueno L, Fioramonti J. Impairment of the intestinal barrier by ethanol involves enteric microflora and mast cell activation in rodents. *Am J Pathol.* 2006 Apr;168(4):1148-54.

Field RW, Krewski D, Lubin JH, Zielinski JM, Alavanja M, Catalan VS, Klotz JB, Létourneau EG, Lynch CF, Lyon JL, Sandler DP, Schoenberg JB, Steck DJ, Stolwijk JA, Weinberg C, Wilcox HB. An overview of the North American residential radon and lung cancer case-control studies. *J Toxicol Environ Health A.* 2006 Apr;69(7):599-631.

Field T, Henteleff T, Hernandez-Reif M, Martinez E, Mavunda K, Kuhn C, Schanberg S. Children with asthma have improved pulmonary functions after massage therapy. *J Pediatr.* 1998 May;132(5):854-8.

File SE, Hartley DE, Elsabagh S, Duffy R, Wiseman H. 2005. Cognitive improvement after 6 weeks of soy supplements in postmenopausal women is limited to frontal lobe function. Menopause. Mar;12(2):193-201.

Finkelman FD, Boyce JA, Vercelli D, Rothenberg ME. Key advances in mechanisms of asthma, allergy, and immunology in 2009. *J Allergy Clin Immunol.* 2010 Feb;125(2):312-8.

Fiocchi, A; Restani, P; Riva, E; Qualizza, R; Bruni, P; Restelli, AR; Galli, CL. Meat allergy: I. Specific IgE to BSA and OSA in atopic, beef sensitive children. *J Am Coll Nutr.* 1995 14: 239-244.

Firmesse O, Alvaro E, Mogenet A, Bresson JL, Lemée R, Le Ruyet P, Bonhomme C, Lambert D, Andrieux C, Doré J, Corthier G, Furet JP, Rigottier-Gois L. Fate and effects of Camembert cheese micro-organisms in the human colonic microbiota of healthy volunteers after regular Camembert consumption. *Int J Food Microbiol.* 2008 Jul 15;125(2):176-81.

Fjeld T, Veiersted B, Sandvik L, Riise G, Levy F. The Effect of Indoor Foliage Plants on Health and Discomfort Symptoms among Office Workers. *Ind Built Environ.* 1998 July;7(4): 204-209.

Flandrin, J, Montanari M. (eds.). *Food: A Culinary History from Antiquity to the Present.* New York: Penguin Books, 1999.

Fleischer DM, Conover-Walker MK, Christie L, Burks AW, Wood RA. Peanut allergy: recurrence and its management. *J Allergy Clin Immunol.* 2004 Nov;114(5):1195-201.

Flinterman AE, van Hoffen E, den Hartog Jager CF, Koppelman S, Pasmans SG, Hoekstra MO, Bruijnzeel-Koomen CA, Knulst AC, Knol EF. Children with peanut allergy recognize predominantly Ara h2 and Ara h6, which remains stable over time. *Clin Exp Allergy.* 2007 Aug;37(8):1221-8.

Fogarty MC, Hughes CM, Burke G, Brown JC, Davison GW. Acute and chronic watercress supplementation attenuates exercise-induced peripheral mononuclear cell DNA damage and lipid peroxidation. Br J Nutr. 2012 Apr 5:1-9.

Foliaki S, Annesi-Maesano I, Tuuau-Potoi N, Waqatakirewa L, Cheng S, Douwes J, Pearce N. Risk factors for symptoms of childhood asthma, allergic rhinoconjunctivitis and eczema in the Pacific: an ISAAC Phase III study. *Int J Tuberc Lung Dis.* 2008 Jul;12(7):799-806.

Food and Drug Administration, HHS. Food labeling: health claims; soluble dietary fiber from certain foods and coronary heart disease. Interim final rule. Fed Regist. 2002 Oct 2;67(191):61773-83.

Forbes EE, Groschwitz K, Abonia JP, Brandt EB, Cohen E, Blanchard C, Ahrens R, Seidu L, McKenzie A, Strait R, Finkelman FD, Foster PS, Matthaei KI, Rothenberg ME, Hogan SP. IL-9- and mast cell-mediated intestinal permeability predisposes to oral antigen hypersensitivity. *J Exp Med.* 2008 Apr 14;205(4):897-913.

Forestier C, Guelon D, Cluytens V, Gillart T, Sirot J, De Champs C. Oral probiotic and prevention of Pseudomonas aeruginosa infections: a randomized, double-blind, placebo-controlled pilot study in intensive care unit patients. *Crit Care.* 2008;12(3):R69.

Forestier C, Guelon D, Cluytens V, Gillart T, Sirot J, De Champs C. Oral probiotic and prevention of Pseudomonas aeruginosa infections: a randomized, double-blind, placebo-controlled pilot study in intensive care unit patients. *Crit Care.* 2008;12(3):R69.

Forget-Dubois N, Boivin M, Dionne G, Pierce T, Tremblay RE, Pérusse D. A longitudinal twin study of the genetic and environmental etiology of maternal hostile-reactive behavior during infancy and toddlerhood. *Infant Behav Dev.* 2007

Foster S, Hobbs C. *Medicinal Plants and Herbs.* Boston: Houghton Mifflin, 2002.

Fox RD, *Algoculture.* Doctorate Disseration, 1983 Jul.

Francavilla R, Lionetti E, Castellaneta SP, Magistà AM, Maurogiovanni G, Bucci N, De Canio A, Indrio F, Cavallo L, Ierardi E, Miniello VL. Inhibition of Helicobacter pylori infection in humans by Lactobacillus reuteri ATCC 55730 and effect on eradication therapy: a pilot study. *Helicobacter.* 2008 Apr;13(2):127-34.

Francavilla R, Lionetti E, Castellaneta SP, Magistà AM, Maurogiovanni G, Bucci N, De Canio A, Indrio F, Cavallo L, Ierardi E, Miniello VL. Inhibition of *Helicobacter pylori* infection in humans by *Lactobacillus reuteri* ATCC 55730 and effect on eradication therapy: a pilot study. *Helicobacter.* 2008 Apr;13(2):127-34.

Francey RJ, *et al.* A 1000-year high precision record of δ13C in atmospheric CO2. Tellus. 1999;51:170 – 193.

Francis H, Fletcher G, Anthony C, Pickering C, Oldham L, Hadley E, Custovic A, Niven R. Clinical effects of air filters in homes of asthmatic adults sensitized and exposed to pet allergens. *Clin Exp Allergy.* 2003 Jan;33(1):101-5.

Frank PI, Morris JA, Hazell ML, Linehan MF, Frank TL. Long term prognosis in preschool children with wheeze: longitudinal postal questionnaire study 1993-2004. *BMJ.* 2008 Jun 21;336(7658):1423-6. 2008 Jun 16.

Frawley D, Lad V. *The Yoga of Herbs.* Sante Fe: Lotus Press, 1986.

Freedman BJ. A dietary free from additives in the management of allergic disease. *Clin Allergy.* 1977 Sep;7(5):417-21.

Fremont S, Moneret-Vautrin DA, Franck P, Morisset M, Croizier A, Codreanu F, Kanny G. Prospective study of sensitization and food allergy to flaxseed in 1317 subjects. *Eur Ann Allergy Clin Immunol.* 2010 Jun;42(3):103-11.

Frias J, Song YS, Martínez-Villaluenga C, González de Mejia E, Vidal-Valverde C. Immunoreactivity and amino acid content of fermented soybean products. *J Agric Food Chem.* 2008 Jan 9;56(1):99-105.

Friedman LS, Harvard Health Publ. Ed. *Controlling GERD and Chronic Heartburn.* Boston: Harvard Health, 2008.

Friend BA, Shahani KM, Long CA, Vaughn LA. The effect of processing and storage on key enzymes, B vitamins, and lipids of mature human milk. Evaluation of fresh samples and effects of freezing and frozen storage. *Pediatr Res.* 1983 Jan;17(1):61-4.

Friend BA, Shahani KM. Characterization and evaluation of Aspergillus oryzae lactase coupled to a regenerable support. *Biotechnol Bioeng.* 1982 Feb;24(2):329-45.

Frumkin H. Beyond toxicity: human health and the natural environment. *Am J Prev Med.* 2001;20(3):234-40.

Fu G, Zhong Y, Li C, Li Y, Lin X, Liao B, Tsang EW, Wu K, Huang S. Epigenetic regulation of peanut allergen gene Ara h 3 in developing embryos. *Planta.* 2010 Apr;231(5):1049-60.

Fu JX. Measurement of MEFV in 66 cases of asthma in the convalescent stage and after treatment with Chinese herbs. *Zhong Xi Yi Jie He Za Zhi.* 1989 Nov;9(11):658-9, 644.

Fuiano N, Fusilli S, Passalacqua G, Incorvaia C. Allergen-specific immunoglobulin E in the skin and nasal mucosa of symptomatic and asymptomatic children sensitized to aeroallergens. *J Investig Allergol Clin Immunol.* 2010;20(5):425-30.

Fujii T, Ohtsuka Y, Lee T, Kudo T, Shoji H, Sato H, Nagata S, Shimizu T, Yamashiro Y. Bifidobacterium breve enhances transforming growth factor beta1 signaling by regulating Smad7 expression in preterm in-fants. *J Pediatr Gastroenterol Nutr.* 2006 Jul;43(1):83-8.

Fujii T, Ohtsuka Y, Lee T, Kudo T, Shoji H, Sato H, Nagata S, Shimizu T, Yamashiro Y. *Bifidobacterium breve* enhances transforming growth factor beta1 signaling by regulating Smad7 expression in preterm infants. *J Pediatr Gastroenterol Nutr.* 2006 Jul;43(1):83-8.

Fujimori S, Gudis K, Mitsui K, Seo T, Yonezawa M, Tanaka S, Tatsuguchi A, Sakamoto C. A randomized controlled trial on the efficacy of synbiotic versus probiotic or prebiotic treatment to improve the quality of life in patients with ulcerative colitis. *Nutrition.* 2009 May;25(5):520-5.

Fulgoni VL 3rd. Current protein intake in America: analysis of the National Health and Nutrition Examination Survey, 2003-2004. *Am J Clin Nutr.* 2008 May;87(5):1554S-1557S.

Fung TT, Schulze M, Manson JE, Willett WC, Hu FB. Dietary patterns, meat intake, and the risk of type 2 diabetes in women. Arch Intern Med. 2004 Nov 8;164(20):2235-40.

Fung TT, Stampfer MJ, Manson JE, Rexrode KM, Willett WC, Hu FB. Prospective study of major dietary patterns and stroke risk in women. Stroke. 2004 Sep;35(9):2014-9.

Furrie E, Macfarlane S, Kennedy A, Cummings JH, Walsh SV, O'neil DA, Macfarlane GT. Synbiotic therapy (*Bifidobacterium longum*/Synergy 1) initiates resolution of inflammation in patients with active ulcerative colitis: a randomised controlled pilot trial. *Gut.* 2005 Feb;54(2):242-9.

# REFERENCES AND BIBLIOGRAPHY

Furrie E. Probiotics and allergy. *Proc Nutr Soc.* 2005 Nov;64(4):465-9.

Furuhjelm C, Warstedt K, Larsson J, Fredriksson M, Böttcher MF, Fälth-Magnusson K, Duchén K. Fish oil supplementation in pregnancy and lactation may decrease the risk of infant allergy. *Acta Paediatr.* 2009 Sep;98(9):1461-7.

Gabory A, Attig L, Junien C. Sexual dimorphism in environmental epigenetic programming. *Mol Cell Endocrinol.* 2009 May 25;304(1-2):8-18. 2009 Mar 9.

Gaddy JA, Radin JN, Loh JT, Zhang F, Washington MK, Peek RM Jr, Algood HM, Cover TL. High dietary salt intake exacerbates Helicobacter pylori-induced gastric carcinogenesis. Infect Immun. 2013 Apr 8.

Gamboa PM, Cáceres O, Antepara I, Sánchez-Monge R, Ahrazem O, Salcedo G, Barber D, Lombardero M, Sanz ML. Two different profiles of peach allergy in the north of Spain. *Allergy.* 2007 Apr;62(4):408-14.

Gao X, Wang W, Wei S, Li W. Review of pharmacological effects of Glycyrrhiza radix and its bioactive compounds. *Zhongguo Zhong Yao Za Zhi.* 2009 Nov;34(21):2695-700.

Gaón D, Doweck Y, Gómez Zavaglia A, Ruiz Holgado A, Oliver G. Lactose digestion by milk fermented with *Lactobacillus acidophilus* and *Lactobacillus casei* of human origin. *Medicina (B Aires).* 1995;55(3):237-42.

Gaón D, Winter L, Rodríguez N, Quintás R, González SN, Oliver G. Effect of Lactobacillus strains and *Saccharomyces boulardii* on persistent diarrhea in children. *Medicina (B Aires).* 2003;63(4):293-8.

Gaón D, Garmendia C, Murrielo NO, de Cucco Games A, Cerchio A, Quintas R, González SN, Oliver G. Effect of Lactobacillus strains (L. casei and L. Acidophilus Strains cerela) on bacterial overgrowth-related chronic diarrhea. *Medicina.* 2002;62(2):159-63.

Garaczi E, Boros-Gyevi M, Bella Z, Csoma Z, Kemény L, Koreck A. Intranasal phototherapy is more effective than fexofenadine hydrochloride in the treatment of seasonal allergic rhinitis: results of a pilot study. *Photochem Photobiol.* 2011 Mar-Apr;87(2):474-7.

Garavello W, Somigliana E, Acaia B, Gaini L, Pignataro L, Gaini RM. Nasal lavage in pregnant women with seasonal allergic rhinitis: a randomized study. *Int Arch Allergy Immunol.* 2010;151(2):137-41. 2009 Sep 15. 19752567.

Garcia Gomez LJ, Sanchez-Muniz FJ. Review: cardiovascular effect of garlic (Allium sativum). *Arch Latinoam Nutr.* 2000 Sep;50(3):219-29.

Garcia Vilela E, De Lourdes De Abreu Ferrari M, Oswaldo Da Gama Torres H, Guerra Pinto A, Carolina Carneiro Aguirre A, Paiva Martins F, Marcos Andrade Goulart E, Sales Da Cunha A. Influence of *Saccharomyces boulardii* on the intestinal permeability of patients with Crohn's disease in remission. *Scand J Gastroenterol.* 2008;43(7):842-8.

García-Compeán D, González MV, Galindo G, Mar DA, Treviño JL, Martínez R, Bosques F, Maldonado H. Prevalence of gastroesophageal reflux disease in patients with extraesophageal symptoms referred from otolaryngology, allergy, and cardiology practices: a prospective study. *Dig Dis.* 2000;18(3):178-82.

Garcia-Marcos L, Canflanca IM, Garrido JB, Varela AL, Garcia-Hernandez G, Guillen Grima F, Gonzalez-Diaz C, Carvajal-Urueña I, Arnedo-Pena A, Busquets-Monge RM, Morales Suarez-Varela M, Blanco-Quiros A. Relationship of asthma and rhinoconjunctivitis with obesity, exercise and Mediterranean diet in Spanish school-children. *Thorax.* 2007 Jun;62(6):503-8.

Gardener S, Gu Y, Rainey-Smith SR, Keogh JB, Clifton PM, Mathieson SL, Taddei K, Mondal A, Ward VK, Scarmeas S, Barnes M, Ellis KA, Head R, Masters CL, Ames D, Macaulay SL, Rowe CC, Szoeke C, Martins RN; AIBL Research Group. Adherence to a Mediterranean diet and Alzheimer's disease risk in an Australian population. Transl Psychiatry. 2012 Oct 2;2:e164. doi: 10.1038/tp.2012.91.

Gardener S, Gu Y, Rainey-Smith SR, Keogh JB, Clifton PM, Mathieson SL, Taddei K, Mondal A, Ward VK, Scarmeas S, Barnes M, Ellis KA, Head R, Masters CL, Ames D, Macaulay SL, Rowe CC, Szoeke C, Martins RN; AIBL Research Group. Adherence to a Mediterranean diet and Alzheimer's disease risk in an Australian population. Transl Psychiatry. 2012 Oct 2;2:e164.

Gardner CD, Fortmann SP, Krauss RM. Association of small low-density lipoprotein particles with the incidence of coronary artery disease in men and women. *JAMA.* 1996 Sep 18;276(11):875-81.

Gardner ML. Gastrointestinal absorption of intact proteins. *Annu Rev Nutr.* 1988;8:329-50.

Gary WK, Fanny WS, David SC. Factors associated with difference in prevalence of asthma in children from three cities in China: multicentre epidemiological survey. *BMJ.* 2004;329:1-4.

Garzi A, Messina M, Frati F, Carfagna L, Zagordo L, Belcastro M, Parmiani S, Sensi L, Marcucci F. An extensively hydrolysed cow's milk formula improves clinical symptoms of gastroesophageal reflux and reduces the gastric emptying time in infants. *Allergol Immunopathol (Madr).* 2002 Jan-Feb;30(1):36-41.

Gawrońska A, Dziechciarz P, Horvath A, Szajewska H. A randomized double-blind placebo-controlled trial of Lactobacillus GG for abdominal pain disorders in children. *Aliment Pharmacol Ther.* 2007 Jan 15;25(2):177-84.

Gazdik F, Horvathova M, Gazdikova K, Jahnova E. The influence of selenium supplementation on the immunity of corticoid-dependent asthmatics. *Bratisl Lek Listy.* 2002;103(1):17-21.

Gazdik F, Kadrabova J, Gazdikova K. Decreased consumption of corticosteroids after selenium supplementation in corticoid-dependent asthmatics. *Bratisl Lek Listy.* 2002;103(1):22-5.

Geha RS, Beiser A, Ren C, Patterson R, Greenberger PA, Grammer LC, Ditto AM, Harris KE, Shaughnessy MA, Yarnold PR, Corren J, Saxon A. Multicenter, double-blind, placebo-controlled, multiple-challenge evaluation of reported reactions to monosodium glutamate. *J Allergy Clin Immunol.* 2000 Nov;106(5):973-80.

Geidl W, Pfeifer K. Physical activity and exercise for rehabilitation of type 2 diabetes. Rehabilitation. 2011 Aug;50(4):255-65.

Gerez IF, Shek LP, Chng HH, Lee BW. Diagnostic tests for food allergy. *Singapore* Med J. 2010 Jan;51(1):4-9.

403

Gergen PJ, Arbes SJ Jr, Calatroni A, Mitchell HE, Zeldin DC. Total IgE levels and asthma prevalence in the US population: results from the National Health and Nutrition Examination Survey 2005-2006. *J Allergy Clin Immunol.* 2009 Sep;124(3):447-53. 2009 Aug 3.

Ghadioungui P. (transl.) The Ebers Papyrus. Academy of Scientific Research. Cairo, 1987.

Giampietro PG, Kjellman NI, Oldaeus G, Wouters-Wesseling W, Businco L. Hypoallergenicity of an extensively hydrolyzed whey formula. *Pediatr Allergy Immunol.* 2001 Apr;12(2):83-6.

Gibbons E. *Stalking the Healthful Herbs.* New York: David McKay, 1966.

Gibson RA. Docosa-hexaenoic acid (DHA) accumulation is regulated by the polyunsaturated fat content of the diet: Is it synthesis or is it incorporation? *Asia Pac J Clin Nutr.* 2004;13(Suppl):S78.

Gilbert CR, Arum SM, Smith CM. Vitamin D deficiency and chronic lung disease. *Can Respir J.* 2009 May-Jun;16(3):75-80.

Gill HS, Rutherfurd KJ, Cross ML, Gopal PK. Enhancement of immunity in the elderly by dietary supplementation with the probiotic Bifidobacterium lactis HN019. *Am J Clin Nutr.* 2001 Dec;74(6):833-9.

Gill HS, Rutherfurd KJ, Cross ML. Dietary probiotic supplementation enhances natural killer cell activity in the elderly: an investigation of age-related immunological changes. *J Clin Immunol.* 2001 Jul;21(4):264-71.

Gillman A, Douglass JA. What do asthmatics have to fear from food and additive allergy? *Clin Exp Allergy.* 2010 Sep;40(9):1295-302.

Ginde AA, Mansbach JM, Camargo CA Jr. Association between serum 25-hydroxyvitamin D level and upper respiratory tract infection in the Third National Health and Nutrition Examination Survey. *Arch Intern Med.* 2009 Feb 23;169(4):384-90.

Gionchetti P, Rizzello F, Venturi A, Brigidi P, Matteuzzi D, Bazzocchi G, Poggioli G, Miglioli M, Campieri M. Oral bacteriotherapy as maintenance treatment in patients with chronic pouchitis: a double-blind, placebo-controlled trial. *Gastroenterology.* 2000 Aug;119(2):305-9.

Gironés-Vilaplana A, Valentão P, Moreno DA, Ferreres F, García-Viguera C, Andrade PB. New beverages of lemon juice enriched with the exotic berries Maqui, Açaí, and Blackthorn: bioactive components and in vitro biological properties. J Agric Food Chem. 2012 May 29.

Gittleman AL. *Guess What Came to Dinner.* New York: Avery, 2001.

Glück U, Gebbers J. Ingested probiotics reduce nasal colonization with pathogenic bacteria (Staphylococcus aureus, Streptococcus pneumoniae, and b-hemolytic streptococci. *Am J. Clin. Nutr.* 2003;77:517-520.

Glück U, Gebbers J. Ingested probiotics reduce nasal colonization with pathogenic bacteria (*Staphylococcus aureus, Streptococcus pneumoniae,* and b-hemolytic streptococci. *Am J. Clin. Nutr.* 2003;77:517-520.

Goedsche K, Förster M, Kroegel C, Uhlemann C. Repeated cold water stimulations (hydrotherapy according to Kneipp) in patients with COPD. *Forsch Komplementmed.* 2007 Jun;14(3):158-66.

Goel V, Dolan RJ. The functional anatomy of humor: segregating cognitive and affective components. *Nat Neurosci.* 2001;4:237-8.

Gohil K, Packer L. Bioflavonoid-Rich Botanical Extracts Show Antioxidant and Gene Regulatory Activity. *Ann N Y Acad Sci.* 2002:957:70-7.

Goldin BR, Adlercreutz H, Dwyer JT, Swenson L, Warram JH, Gorbach SL. Effect of diet on excretion of estrogens in pre- and postmenopausal women. *Cancer Res.* 1981 Sep;41(9 Pt 2):3771-3.

Goldin BR, Adlercreutz H, Gorbach SL, Warram JH, Dwyer JT, Swenson L, Woods MN. Estrogen excretion patterns and plasma levels in vegetarian and omnivorous women. *N Engl J Med.* 1982 Dec 16;307(25):1542-7.

Goldin BR, Adlercreutz H, Gorbach SL, Warram JH, Dwyer JT, Swenson L, Woods MN. Estrogen excretion patterns and plasma levels in vegetarian and omnivorous women. *N Engl J Med.* 1982 Dec 16;307(25):1542-7.

Goldin BR, Swenson L, Dwyer J, Sexton M, Gorbach SL. Effect of diet and Lactobacillus acidophilus supplements on human fecal bacterial enzymes. *J Natl Cancer Inst.* 1980 Feb;64(2):255-61.

Goldin BR, Swenson L, Dwyer J, Sexton M, Gorbach SL. Effect of diet and *Lactobacillus acidophilus* supplements on human fecal bacterial enzymes. *J Natl Cancer Inst.* 1980 Feb;64(2):255-61.

Goldstein JL, Aisenberg J, Zakko SF, Berger MF, Dodge WE. Endoscopic ulcer rates in healthy subjects associated with use of aspirin (81 mg q.d.) alone or coadministered with celecoxib or naproxen: a randomized, 1-week trial. *Dig Dis Sci.* 2008 Mar;53(3):647-56.

Golub E. *The Limits of Medicine.* New York: Times Books, 1994.

Gonzales M, Malcoe LH, Myers OB, Espinoza J. Risk factors for asthma and cough among Hispanic children in the southwestern United States of America, 2003-2004. *Rev Panam Salud Publica.* 2007 May;21(5):274-81.

González Alvarez R, Arruzazabala ML. Current views of the mechanism of action of prophylactic antiallergic drugs. *Allergol Immunopathol (Madr).* 1981 Nov-Dec;9(6):501-8.

Gonzalez CA, Riboli E. Diet and cancer prevention: Contributions from the European Prospective Investigation into Cancer and Nutrition (EPIC) study. *Eur J Cancer.* 2010 Sep;46(14):2555-62.

Gonzalez CA, Riboli E. Diet and cancer prevention: Contributions from the European Prospective Investigation into Cancer and Nutrition (EPIC) study. *Eur J Cancer.* 2010 Sep;46(14):2555-62.

González J, Fernández M, García Fragoso L. Exclusive breastfeeding reduces asthma in a group of children from the Caguas municipality of Puerto Rico. *Bol Asoc Med P R.* 2010 Jan-Mar;102(1):10-2.

González Morales JE, Leal de Hernández L, González Spencer D. Asthma associated with gastroesophageal reflux. *Rev Alerg Mex.* 1998 Jan-Feb;45(1):16-21.

Gonzalez V, Huen K, Venkat S, Pratt K, Xiang P, Harley KG, Kogut K, Trujillo CM, Bradman A, Eskenazi B, Holland NT. Cholinesterase and paraoxonase (PON1) enzyme activities in Mexi-can-American mothers and children from an agricultural commu-nity. J Expo Sci Environ Epidemiol. 2012 Jul 4.

# REFERENCES AND BIBLIOGRAPHY

González-Pérez A, Aponte Z, Vidaurre CF, Rodríguez LA. Anaphylaxis epidemiology in patients with and patients without asthma: a United Kingdom database review. *J Allergy Clin Immunol*. 2010 May;125(5):1098-1104.e1.

González-Sánchez R, Trujillo X, Trujillo-Hernández B, Vásquez C, Huerta M, Elizalde A. Forskolin versus sodium cromoglycate for prevention of asthma attacks: a single-blinded clinical trial. *J Int Med Res*. 2006 Mar-Apr;34(2):200-7.

Goossens D, Jonkers D, Russel M, Stobberingh E, Van Den Bogaard A, StockbrUgger R. The effect of *Lactobacillus plantarum* 299v on the bacterial composition and metabolic activity in faeces of healthy volunteers: a placebo-controlled study on the onset and duration of effects. *Aliment Pharmacol Ther*. 2003 Sep 1;18(5):495-505.

Goossens DA, Jonkers DM, Russel MG, Stobberingh EE, Stockbrügger RW. The effect of a probiotic drink with *Lactobacillus plantarum* 299v on the bacterial composition in faeces and mucosal biopsies of rectum and ascending colon. *Aliment Pharmacol Ther*. 2006 Jan 15;23(2):255-63.

Gopinath K, Prakash D, Sudhandiran G. Neuroprotective effect of naringin, a dietary flavonoid against 3-nitropropionic acid-induced neuronal apoptosis. Neurochem Int. 2011 Dec;59(7):1066-73.

Gordon BR. Patch testing for allergies. *Curr Opin Otolaryngol Head Neck Surg*. 2010 Jun;18(3):191-4.

Gore KV, Rao AK, Guruswamy MN. Physiological studies with Tylophora asthmatica in bronchial asthma. *Indian J Med Res*. 1980 Jan;71:144-8.

Goren AI, Hellmann S. Changes prevalence of asthma among schoolchildren in Israel. *Eur Respir J*. 1997;10:2279-2284.

Gotteland M, Poliak L, Cruchet S, Brunser O. Effect of regular ingestion of Saccharomyces boulardii plus inulin or Lactobacillus acidophilus LB in children colonized by Helicobacter pylori. *Acta Paediatr*. 2005 Dec;94(12):1747-51.

Gotteland M, Poliak L, Cruchet S, Brunser O. Effect of regular ingestion of *Saccharomyces boulardii* plus inulin or *Lactobacillus acidophilus* LB in children colonized by *Helicobacter pylori*. Acta Paediatr. 2005 Dec;94(12):1747-51.

Govindan S, Viswanathan S, Vijayasekaran V, Alagappan R. A pilot study on the clinical efficacy of Solanum xanthocarpum and Solanum trilobatum in bronchial asthma. *J Ethnopharmacol*. 1999 Aug;66(2):205-10.

Govindan S, Viswanathan S, Vijayasekaran V, Alagappan R. Further studies on the clinical efficacy of Solanum xanthocarpum and Solanum trilobatum in bronchial asthma. *Phytother Res*. 2004 Oct;18(10):805-9.

Gowlett JAJ, Harris JWK, Walton D, Wood BA. Early archaeological sites, hominid remains and traces of fire from Chesowanja, Kenya. Nature. 1981;294:125 – 129.

Grant J, Mahanty S, Khadir A, MacLean JD, Kokoskin E, Yeager B, Joseph L, Diaz J, Gotuzzo E, Mainville N, Ward BJ. Wheat germ supplement reduces cyst and trophozoite passage in people with giardiasis. Am J Trop Med Hyg. 2001 Dec;65(6):705-10.

Grant WB, Holick MF. Benefits and requirements of vitamin D for optimal health: a review. *Altern Med Rev*. 2005 Jun;10(2):94-111.

Grant WB. Hypothesis – ultraviolet-B irradiance and vitamin D reduce the risk of viral infections and thus their sequelae, including autoimmune diseases and some cancers. *Photochem Photobiol*. 2008 Mar-Apr;84(2):356-65. 2008 Jan 7.

Grasso F, Grillo C, Musumeci F, Triglia A, Rodolico G, Cammisuli F, Rinzivillo C, Fragati G, Santuccio A, Rodolico M. Photon emission from normal and tumour human tissues. *Experientia*. 1992;48:10-13.

Gray H. *Anatomy, Descriptive and Surgical*. 15th Edition. New York: Random House, 1977.

Gray-Davison F. *Ayurvedic Healing*. New York: Keats, 2002.

Greskevitch M, Kullman G, Bang KM, Mazurek JM. Respiratory disease in agricultural workers: mortality and morbidity statistics. J Agromedicine. 2007;12(3):5-10.

Griffith HW. *Healing Herbs: The Essential Guide*. Tucson: Fisher Books, 2000.

Grimm T, Chovanová Z, Muchová J, Sumegová K, Liptáková A, Duracková Z, Högger P. Inhibition of NF-kappaB activation and MMP-9 secretion by plasma of human volunteers after ingestion of maritime pine bark extract (Pycnogenol). J Inflamm (Lond). 2006 Jan 27;3:1.

Grimm T, Schäfer A, Högger P. Antioxidant activity and inhibition of matrix metalloproteinases by metabolites of maritime pine bark extract (pycnogenol). *Free Radic Biol Med*. 2004 Mar 15;36(6):811-22.

Grimm T, Skrabala R, Chovanová Z, Muchová J, Sumegová K, Liptáková A, Duracková Z, Högger P. Single and multiple dose pharmacokinetics of maritime pine bark extract (pycnogenol) after oral administration to healthy volunteers. *BMC Clin Pharmacol*. 2006 Aug 3;6:4.

Grimshaw KE, Maskell J, Oliver EM, Morris RC, Foote KD, Mills EN, Margetts BM, Roberts G. Diet and food allergy development during infancy: Birth cohort study findings using prospective food diary data. J Allergy Clin Immunol. 2013 Jul 23.

Grine FE, Kay RF. Early hominid diets from quantitative image analysis of dental microwear. Nature. 1988;333:765 – 768.

Grine FE, Kay RF. Early hominid diets from quantitative image analysis of dental microwear. Nature. 1988;333:765 – 768.

Grine FE, Ungar PS, Teaford MF, El Zaatari S. Molar microwear in Praeanthropus afarensis: Evidence for dietary stasis through time and under diverse paleoecological conditions. J Hum Evol. 2006;51:297 – 319.

Grine FE, Ungar PS, Teaford MF. Was the Early Pliocene hominin 'Australopithecus' anamensis a hard object feeder? S Afr J Sci. 2006;102:301 – 310.

Grönlund MM, Gueimonde M, Laitinen K, Kociubinski G, Grönroos T, Salminen S, Isolauri E. Maternal breast-milk and intestinal bifidobacteria guide the compositional development of the *Bifidobacterium* microbiota in infants at risk of allergic disease. *Clin Exp Allergy*. 2007 Dec;37(12):1764-72.

Gropper SS, Smith JL, Groff JL. *Advanced nutrition and human metabolism*. Belmonth, CA: Wadsworth Publ, 2008.

Groppo FC, Ramacciato JC, Simões RP, Flório FM, Sartoratto A. Antimicrobial activity of garlic, tea tree oil, and chlorhexidine against oral microorganisms. *Int Dent J*. 2002 Dec;52(6):433-7.

Groschwitz KR, Ahrens R, Osterfeld H, Gurish MF, Han X, Abrink M, Finkelman FD, Pejler G, Hogan SP. Mast cells regulate homeostatic intestinal epithelial migration and barrier function by a chymase/Mcpt4-dependent mechanism. *Proc Natl Acad Sci U S A*. 2009 Dec 29;106(52):22381-6.

Grosser BI, Monti-Bloch L, Jennings-White C, Berliner DL. Behavioral and electrophysiological effects of androstadienone, a human pheromone. *Psychoneuroendocrinology*. 2000 Apr;25(3):289-99.

Grzanna R, Lindmark L, Frondoza CG. Ginger – an herbal medicinal product with broad anti-inflammatory actions. *J Med Food*. 2005 Summer;8(2):125-32.

Gu Y, Nieves JW, Stern Y, Luchsinger JA, Scarmeas N. Food combination and Alzheimer disease risk: a protective diet. *Arch Neurol*. 2010 Jun;67(6):699-706.

Gu Y, Scarmeas N. Dietary patterns in Alzheimer's disease and cognitive aging. *Curr Alzheimer Res*. 2011 Aug;8(5):510-9.

Guajardo-Flores D, Serna-Saldívar SO, Gutiérrez-Uribe JA. Evaluation of the antioxidant and antiproliferative activities of extracted saponins and flavonols from germinated black beans (Phaseolus vulgaris L.). *Food Chem*. 2013 Nov 15;141(2):1497-503.

Guajardo-Flores D, Serna-Saldívar SO, Gutiérrez-Uribe JA. Evaluation of the antioxidant and antiproliferative activities of extracted saponins and flavonols from germinated black beans (Phaseolus vulgaris L.). *Food Chem*. 2013 Nov 15;141(2):1497-503.

Guallar-Castillón P, Rodríguez-Artalejo F, Tormo MJ, Sánchez MJ, Rodríguez L, Quirós JR, Navarro C, Molina E, Martínez C, Marín P, Lopez-Garcia E, Larrañaga N, Huerta JM, Dorronsoro M, Chirlaque MD, Buckland G, Barricarte A, Banegas JR, Arriola L, Ardanaz E, González CA, Moreno-Iribas C. Major dietary patterns and risk of coronary heart disease in middle-aged persons from a Mediterranean country: The EPIC-Spain cohort study. *Nutr Metab Cardiovasc Dis*. 2010 Aug 11.

Guandalini S. The influence of gluten: weaning recommendations for healthy children and children at risk for celiac disease. *Nestle Nutr Workshop Ser Pediatr Program*. 2007;60:139-51; discussion 151-5.

Guarino A, Canani RB, Spagnuolo MI, Albano F, Di Benedetto L. Oral bacterial therapy reduces the duration of symptoms and of viral excretion in children with mild diarrhea. *J Pediatr Gastroenterol Nutr*. 1997 Nov;25(5):516-9.

Guerin M, Huntley ME, Olaizola M. Haematococcus astaxanthin: applications for human health and nutrition. *Trends Biotechnol*. 2003 May;21(5):210-6.

Guerin-Danan C, Chabanet C, Pedone C, Popot F, Vaissade P, Bouley C, Szylit O, Andrieux C. Milk fermented with yogurt cultures and *Lactobacillus casei* compared with yogurt and gelled milk: influence on intestinal microflora in healthy infants. *Am J Clin Nutr*. 1998 Jan;67(1):111-7.

Guinot P, Brambilla C, Duchier J, Braquet P, Bonvoisin B, Cournot A. Effect of BN 52063, a specific PAF-acether antagonist, on bronchial provocation test to allergens in asthmatic patients. A preliminary study. *Prostaglandins*. 1987 Nov;34(5):723-31.

Gundermann KJ, Müller J. Phytodolor – effects and efficacy of a herbal medicine. *Wien Med Wochenschr*. 2007;157(13-14):343-7.

Gupta I, Gupta V, Parihar A, Gupta S, Lüdtke R, Safayhi H, Ammon HP. Effects of Boswellia serrata gum resin in patients with bronchial asthma: results of a double-blind, placebo-controlled, 6-week clinical study. *Eur J Med Res*. 1998 Nov 17;3(11):511-4.

Guslandi M, Giollo P, Testoni PA. A pilot trial of *Saccharomyces boulardii* in ulcerative colitis. *Eur J Gastroenterol Hepatol*. 2003 Jun;15(6):697-8.

Guslandi M, Mezzi G, Sorghi M, Testoni PA. *Saccharomyces boulardii* in maintenance treatment of Crohn's disease. *Dig Dis Sci*. 2000 Jul;45(7):1462-4.

Gutmanis J. *Hawaiian Herbal Medicine*. Waipahu, HI: Island Heritage, 2001.

Guyonnet D, Woodcock A, Stefani B, Trevisan C, Hall C. Fermented milk containing Bifidobacterium lactis DN-173 010 improved self-reported digestive comfort amongst a general population of adults. A randomized, open-label, controlled, pilot study. *J Dig Dis*. 2009 Feb;10(1):61-70.

Haarman M, Knol J. Quantitative real-time PCR to identify and quantify fecal *Bifidobacterium* species in infants receiving a prebiotic infant formula. *Appl Environ Microbiol*. 2005 May;71(5):2318-24.

Haggag EG, Abou-Moustafa MA, Boucher W, Theoharides TC. The effect of a herbal water-extract on histamine release from mast cells and on allergic asthma. *J Herb Pharmacother*. 2003;3(4):41-54.

Haines JL, Ter-Minassian M, Bazyk A, Gusella JF, Kim DJ, Terwedow H, Pericak-Vance MA, Rimmler JB, Haynes CS, Roses AD, Lee A, Shaner B, Menold M, Seboun E, Fitoussi RP, Gartioux C, Reyes C, Ribierre F, Gyapay G, Weissenbach J, Hauser SL, Goodkin DE, Lincoln R, Usuku K, Oksenberg JR, et al. A complete genomic screen for multiple sclerosis underscores a role for the major histocompatability complex. The Multiple Sclerosis Genetics Group. *Nat Genet*. 1996 Aug;13(4):469-71..

Halász A, Cserháti E. The prognosis of bronchial asthma in childhood in Hungary: a long-term follow-up. *J Asthma*. 2002 Dec;39(8):693-9.

Halbert SC, French B, Gordon RY, Farrar JT, Schmitz K, Morris PB, Thompson PD, Rader DJ, Becker DJ. Tolerability of red yeast rice (2,400 mg twice daily) versus pravastatin (20 mg twice daily) in patients with previous statin intolerance. Am J Cardiol. 2010 Jan 15;105(2):198-204. doi: 10.1016/j.amjcard.2009.08.672.

Halken S, Hansen KS, Jacobsen HP, Estmann A, Faelling AE, Hansen LG, Kier SR, Lassen K, Lintrup M, Mortensen S, Ibsen KK, Osterballe O, Host A. Comparison of a partially hydrolyzed infant formula with two extensively hydrolyzed formulas for allergy prevention: a prospective, randomized study. *Pediatr Allergy Immunol.* 2000 Aug;11(3):149-61.

Hallén A, Jarstrand C, Påhlson C. Treatment of bacterial vaginosis with lactobacilli. Sex Transm Dis. 1992 May-Jun;19(3):146-8.

Hallmann E, Rembialkowska E. Characterisation of antioxidant compounds in sweet bell pepper (Capsicum annuum L.) under organic and conventional growing systems. J Sci Food Agric. 2012 Feb 24.

Hallmann E. The influence of organic and conventional cultivation systems on the nutritional value and content of bioactive compounds in selected tomato types. J Sci Food Agric. 2012 Feb 20.

Halloran BP, Wronski TJ, VonHerzen DC, Chu V, Xia X, Pingel JE, Williams AA, Smith BJ. Dietary dried plum increases bone mass in adult and aged male mice. J Nutr. 2010 Oct;140(10):1781-7.

Halpern GM, Miller AH. *Medicinal Mushrooms: Ancient Remedies for Modern Ailments.* New York: M. Evans, 2002.

Hamasaki Y, Kobayashi I, Hayasaki R, Zaitu M, Muro E, Yamamoto S, Ichimaru T, Miyazaki S. The Chinese herbal medicine, shinpi-to, inhibits IgE-mediated leukotriene synthesis in rat basophilic leukemia-2H3 cells. *J Ethnopharmacol.* 1997 Apr;56(2):123-31.

Hamelmann E, Beyer K, Gruber C, Lau S, Matricardi PM, Nickel R, Niggemann B, Wahn U. Primary prevention of allergy: avoiding risk or providing protection? *Clin Exp Allergy.* 2008 Feb;38(2):233-45.

Hamilton RG. Clinical laboratory assessment of immediate-type hypersensitivity. *J Allergy Clin Immunol.* 2010 Feb;125(2 Suppl 2):S284-96.

Hammond BG, Mayhew DA, Kier LD, Mast RW, Sander WJ. Safety assessment of DHA-rich microalgae from Schizochytrium sp. *Regul Toxicol Pharmacol.* 2002 Apr;35(2 Pt 1):255-65.

Han ER, Choi IS, Kim HK, Kang YW, Park JG, Lim JR, Seo JH, Choi JH. Inhaled corticosteroid-related tooth problems in asthmatics. *J Asthma.* 2009 Mar;46(2):160-4.

Han SN, Leka LS, Lichtenstein AH, Ausman LM, Meydani SN. Effect of a therapeutic lifestyle change diet on immune functions of moderately hypercholesterolemic humans. *J Lipid Res.* 2003 Dec;44(12):2304-10.

Hansen KS, Ballmer-Weber BK, Lüttkopf D, Skov PS, Wüthrich B, Bindslev-Jensen C, Vieths S, Poulsen LK. Roasted hazelnuts – allergenic activity evaluated by double-blind, placebo-controlled food challenge. *Allergy.* 2003 Feb;58(2):132-8.

Hansen KS, Ballmer-Weber BK, Sastre J, Lidholm J, Andersson K, Oberhofer H, Lluch-Bernal M, Ostling J, Mattsson L, Schocker F, Vieths S, Poulsen LK. Component-resolved in vitro diagnosis of hazelnut allergy in Europe. *J Allergy Clin Immunol.* 2009 May;123(5):1134-41, 1141.e1-3.

Hansen KS, Khinchi MS, Skov PS, Bindslev-Jensen C, Poulsen LK, Malling HJ. Food allergy to apple and specific immunotherapy with birch pollen. *Mol Nutr Food Res.* 2004 Nov;48(6):441-8.

Haranath PS, Shyamalakumari S. Experimental study on mode of action of Tylophora asthmatica in bronchial asthma. *Indian J Med Res.* 1975 May;63(5):661-70.

Hardy K, Buckley S, Collins MJ, Estalrrich A, Brothwell D, Copeland L, García-Tabernero A, García-Vargas S, de la Rasilla M, Lalueza-Fox C, Huguet R, Bastir M, Santamaría D, Madella M, Wilson J, Cortés AF, Rosas A. Neanderthal medics? Evidence for food, cooking, and medicinal plants entrapped in dental calculus. Naturwissenschaften. 2012 Aug;99(8):617-26. doi: 10.1007/s00114-012-0942-0.

Harrington JJ, Lee-Chiong T Jr. Sleep and older patients. *Clin Chest Med.* 2007 Dec;28(4):673-84, v.

Harris LA, Chang L. Irritable bowel syndrome: new and emerging therapies. *Curr Opin Gastroenterol.* 2006 Mar;22(2):128-35.

Hartz C, Lauer I, Del Mar San Miguel Moncin M, Cistero-Bahima A, Foetisch K, Lidholm J, Vieths S, Scheurer S. Comparison of IgE-Binding Capacity, Cross-Reactivity and Biological Potency of Allergenic Non-Specific Lipid Transfer Proteins from Peach, Cherry and Hazelnut. *Int Arch Allergy Immunol.* 2010 Jun 17;153(4):335-346.

Harvald B, Hauge M: Hereditary factors elucidated by twin studies. *In Genetics and the Epidemiology of Chronic Disease.* Edited by Neel JV, Shaw MV, Schull WJ. Washington, DC: Dept Health, Education and Welfare, 1965:64-76.

Harvey HP, Solomon HJ. Acute anaphylactic shock due to para-aminosalicyic acid. *Am Rev Tuberc.* 1958 Mar;77(3):492-5.

Hassan AM. Selenium status in patients with aspirin-induced asthma. *Ann Clin Biochem.* 2008 Sep;45(Pt 5):508-12.

Hasselmark L, Malmgren R, Zetterström O, Unge G. Selenium supplementation in intrinsic asthma. *Allergy.* 1993 Jan;48(1):30-6.

Hata K, Ishikawa K, Hori K, Konishi T. Differentiation-inducing activity of lupeol, a lupane-type triterpene from Chinese dandelion root (Hokouei-kon), on a mouse melanoma cell line. *Biol Pharm Bull.* 2000 Aug;23(8):962-7.

Hata Y, Yamamoto M, Ohni M, Nakajima K, Nakamura Y, Takano T. A placebo-controlled study of the effect of sour milk on blood pressure in hypertensive subjects. *Am J Clin Nutr.* 1996 Nov;64(5):767-71.

Hatakka K, Holma R, El-Nezami H, Suomalainen T, Kuisma M, Saxelin M, Poussa T, Mykkänen H, Korpela R. The influence of *Lactobacillus rhamnosus* LC705 together with Propionibacterium freudenreichii ssp. shermanii JS on potentially carcinogenic bacterial activity in human colon. *Int J Food Microbiol.* 2008 Dec 10;128(2):406-10.

Hattori K, Sasai M, Yamamoto A, Taniuchi S, Kojima T, Kobayashi Y, Iwamoto H, Yaeshima T, Hayasawa H. Intestinal flora of infants with cow milk hypersensitivity fed on casein-hydrolyzed formula supplemented raffinose. *Arerugi.* 2000 Dec;49(12):1146-55.

Hattori K, Yamamoto A, Sasai M, Taniuchi S, Kojima T, Kobayashi Y, Iwamoto H, Namba K, Yaeshima T. Effects of administration of bifidobacteria on fecal microflora and clinical symptoms in infants with atopic dermatitis. *Arerugi.* 2003 Jan;52(1):20-30.

Hawser SP, Bouchillon SK, Hoban DJ, Badal RE, Hsueh PR, Paterson DL. Emergence of high levels of extended-spectrum-beta-lactamase-producing gram-negative bacilli in the Asia-Pacific region: data from the Study for

Monitoring Antimicrobial Resistance Trends (SMART) program, 2007. Antimicrob Agents Chemother. 2009 Aug;53(8):3280-4. doi: 10.1128/AAC.00426-09.

He M, Antoine JM, Yang Y, Yang J, Men J, Han H. Influence of live flora on lactose digestion in male adult lactose-malabsorbers after dairy products intake. Wei Sheng Yan Jiu. 2004 Sep;33(5):603-5.

He T, Priebe MG, Zhong Y, Huang C, Harmsen HJ, Raangs GC, Antoine JM, Welling GW, Vonk RJ. Effects of yogurt and bifidobacteria supplementation on the colonic microbiota in lactose-intolerant subjects. J Appl Microbiol. 2008 Feb;104(2):595-604.

Heaney LG, Brightling CE, Menzies-Gow A, Stevenson M, Niven RM; British Thoracic Society Difficult Asthma Network. Refractory asthma in the UK: cross-sectional findings from a UK multicentre registry. Thorax. 2010 Sep;65(9):787-94.

Heaney RP, Dowell MS. Absorbability of the calcium in a high-calcium mineral water. Osteoporos Int. 1994 Nov;4(6):323-4.

Heap GA, van Heel DA. Genetics and pathogenesis of coeliac disease. Semin Immunol. May 13 2009.

Heine RG, Nethercote M, Rosenbaum J, Allen KJ. Emerging management concepts for eosinophilic esophagitis in children. J Gastroenterol Hepatol. 2011 May 4.

Hemmer W, Focke M, Marzban G, Swoboda I, Jarisch R, Laimer M. Identification of Bet v 1-related allergens in fig and other Moraceae fruits. Clin Exp Allergy. 2010 Apr;40(4):679-87.

Hendel B, Ferreira P. Water & Salt: The Essence of Life. Gaithersburg: Natural Resources, 2003.

Henderson ST, Vogel JL, Barr LJ, Garvin F, Jones JJ, Costantini LC. Study of the ketogenic agent AC-1202 in mild to moderate Alzheimer's disease: a randomized, double-blind, placebo-controlled, multicenter trial. Nutr Metab (Lond). 2009 Aug 10;6:31.

Herbert V. Vitamin B12: Plant sources, requirements, and assay. Am J Clin Nutr. 1988;48:852-858.

Herman PM, Drost LM. Evaluating the clinical relevance of food sensitivity tests: a single subject experiment. Altern Med Rev. 2004 Jun;9(2):198-207.

Herzog AM, Black KA, Fountaine DJ, Knotts TR. Reflection and attentional recovery as two distinctive benefits of restorative environments. J Environ Psychol. 1997;17:165-70.

Hess-Kosa K. Indoor Air Quality: Sampling Methodologies. Boca Rataon: CRC Press, 2002.

Heyman M, Grasset E, Ducroc R, Desjeux JF. Antigen absorption by the jejunal epithelium of children with cow's milk allergy. Pediatr Res. 1988 Aug;24(2):197-202.

Hickson M, D'Souza AL, Muthu N, Rogers TR, Want S, Rajkumar C, Bulpitt CJ. Use of probiotic Lactobacillus preparation to prevent diarrhoea associated with antibiotics: randomised double blind placebo controlled trial. BMJ. 2007 Jul 14;335(7610):80.

Hide DW, Matthews S, Tariq S, Arshad SH. Allergen avoidance in infancy and allergy at 4 years of age. Allergy. 1996 Feb;51(2):89-93.

Hijazi Z, Molla AM, Al-Habashi H, Muawad WM, Molla AM, Sharma PN. Intestinal permeability is increased in bronchial asthma. Arch Dis Child. 2004 Mar;89(3):227-9.

Hildebrand F, Nguyen TL, Brinkman B, Yunta RG, Cauwe B, Vandenabeele P, Liston A, Raes J. Inflammation-associated enterotypes, host genotype, cage and inter-individual effects drive gut microbiota variation in common laboratory mice. Genome Biol. 2013 Jan 24;14(1):R4.

Hill J, Micklewright A, Lewis S, Britton J. Investigation of the effect of short-term change in dietary magnesium intake in asthma. Eur Respir J. 1997 Oct;10(10):2225-9.

Hilton E, Isenberg HD, Alperstein P, France K, Borenstein MT. Ingestion of yogurt containing Lactobacillus acidophilus as prophylaxis for Candida vaginitis. Ann Intern Med. 1992 Mar 1;116(5):353-7.

Hirose Y, Murosaki S, Yamamoto Y, Yoshikai Y, Tsuru T. Daily intake of heat-killed Lactobacillus plantarum L-137 augments acquired immunity in healthy adults. J Nutr. 2006 Dec;136(12):3069-73.

Hlivak P, Jahnova E, Odraska J, Ferencik M, Ebringer L, Mikes Z. Long-term (56-week) oral administration of probiotic Enterococcus faecium M-74 decreases the expression of sICAM-1 and monocyte CD54, and increases that of lymphocyte CD49d in humans. Bratisl Lek Listy. 2005;106(4-5):175-81.

Hlivak P, Odraska J, Ferencik M, Ebringer L, Jahnova E, Mikes Z. One-year application of probiotic strain Enterococcus faecium M-74 decreases serum cholesterol levels. Bratisl Lek Listy. 2005;106(2):67-72.

Hobbs C. Kombucha Manchurian Tea Mushroom: The Essential Guide. Santa Cruz, CA: Botanica Press, 1995.

Hobbs C. Medicinal Mushrooms. Summertown, TN: Botanica Press, 2003.

Hobbs C. Stress & Natural Healing. Loveland, CO: Interweave Press, 1997.

Hobbs C, Kaffa N, George TW, Methven L, Lovegrove JA. Blood pressure-lowering effects of beetroot juice and novel beetroot-enriched bread products in normotensive male subjects. Br J Nutr. 2012 Dec 14;108(11):2066-74.

Hoff S, Seiler H, Heinrich J, Kompauer I, Nieters A, Becker N, Nagel G, Gedrich K, Karg G, Wolfram G, Linseisen J. Allergic sensitisation and allergic rhinitis are associated with n-3 polyunsaturated fatty acids in the diet and in red blood cell membranes. Eur J Clin Nutr. 2005 Sep;59(9):1071-80.

Hoffmann D. Holistic Herbal. London: Thorsons, 2002.

Hofmann D, Hecker M, Völp A. Efficacy of dry extract of ivy leaves in children with bronchial asthma-a review of randomized controlled trials. Phytomedicine. 2003 Mar;10(2-3):213-20.

Höiby AS, Strand V, Robinson DS, Sager A, Rak S. Efficacy, safety, and immunological effects of a 2-year immunotherapy with Depigoid birch pollen extract: a randomized, double-blind, placebo-controlled study. Clin Exp Allergy. 2010 Jul;40(7):1062-70.

Holick MF. Sunlight and vitamin D for bone health and prevention of autoimmune diseases, cancers, and cardiovascular disease. Am J Clin Nutr. 2004 Dec;80(6 Suppl):1678S-88S.

# REFERENCES AND BIBLIOGRAPHY

Holick MF. The vitamin D deficiency pandemic and consequences for nonskeletal health: mechanisms of action. *Mol Aspects Med.* 2008 Dec;29(6):361-8

Holick MF. Vitamin D status: measurement, interpretation, and clinical application. *Ann Epidemiol.* 2009 Feb;19(2):73-8.

Holladay, S.D. Prenatal Immunotoxicant Exposure and Postnatal Autoimmune Disease. *Environ Health Perspect.* 1999; 107(suppl 5):687-691.

Holmes HC, Burns SP, Michelakakis H, Kordoni V, Bain MD, Chalmers RA, Rafter JE, Iles RA. Choline and L-carnitine as precursors of trimethylamine. Biochem Soc Trans. 1997 Feb;25(1):96S.

Holt GA. Food & Drug Interactions. Chicago: Precept Press, 1998, 83.

Holtrop G, Johnstone AM, Fyfe C, Gratz SW. Diet composition is associated with endogenous formation of N-nitroso compounds in obese men. J Nutr. 2012 Sep;142(9):1652-8.

Homma M, Oka K, Niitsuma T, Itoh H. A novel 11 beta-hydroxysteroid dehydrogenase inhibitor contained in saiboku-to, a herbal remedy for steroid-dependent bronchial asthma. *J Pharm Pharmacol.* 1994 Apr;46(4):305-9.

Hönscheid A, Rink L, Haase H. T-lymphocytes: a target for stimulatory and inhibitory effects of zinc ions. *Endocr Metab Immune Disord Drug Targets.* 2009 Jun;9(2):132-44.

Hooper R, Calvert J, Thompson RL, Deetlefs ME, Burney P. Urban/rural differences in diet and atopy in South Africa. *Allergy.* 2008 Apr;63(4):425-31.

Hooshmand S, Arjmandi BH. Viewpoint: dried plum, an emerging functional food that may effectively improve bone health. Ageing Res Rev. 2009 Apr;8(2):122-7.

Hooshmand S, Chai SC, Saadat RL, Payton ME, Brummel-Smith K, Arjmandi BH. Comparative effects of dried plum and dried apple on bone in postmenopausal women. Br J Nutr. 2011 Sep;106(6):923-30.

Hope BE, Massey DG, Fournier-Massey G. Hawaiian materia medica for asthma. *Hawaii Med J.* 1993 Jun;52(6):160-6.

Horak E, Morass B, Ulmer H. Association between environmental tobacco smoke exposure and wheezing disorders in Austrian preschool children. *Swiss Med Wkly.* 2007 Nov 3;137(43-44):608-13.

Horrobin DF. Effects of evening primrose oil in rheumatoid arthritis. *Ann Rheum Dis.* 1989 Nov;48(11):965-6.

Hospers IC, de Vries-Vrolijk K, Brand PL. Double-blind, placebo-controlled cow's milk challenge in children with alleged cow's milk allergies, performed in a general hospital: diagnosis rejected in two-thirds of the children. *Ned Tijdschr Geneeskd.* 2006 Jun 10;150(23):1292-7.

Hosseini S, Pishnamazi S, Sadrzadeh SM, Farid F, Farid R, Watson RR. Pycnogenol((R)) in the Management of Asthma. *J Med Food.* 2001 Winter;4(4):201-209.

Hota B, Ellenbogen C, Hayden MK, Aroutcheva A, Rice TW, Weinstein RA. Community-associated methicillin-resistant *Staphylococcus aureus* skin and soft tissue infections at a public hospital: do public housing and incarceration amplify transmission? *Arch Intern Med.* 2007 May 28;167(10):1026-33.

Hougee S, Vriesema AJ, Wijering SC, Knippels LM, Folkerts G, Nijkamp FP, Knol J, Garssen J. Oral treatment with probiotics reduces allergic symptoms in ovalbumin-sensitized mice: a bacterial strain comparative study. *Int Arch Allergy Immunol.* 2010;151(2):107-17. 2009 Sep 15.

Houle CR, Leo HL, Clark NM. A developmental, community, and psychosocial approach to food allergies in children. *Curr Allergy Asthma Rep.* 2010 Sep;10(5):381-6.

Houssen ME, Ragab A, Mesbah A, El-Samanoudy AZ, Othman G, Moustafa AF, Badria FA. Natural anti-inflammatory products and leukotriene inhibitors as complementary therapy for bronchial asthma. *Clin Biochem.* 2010 Jul;43(10-11):887-90.

Howard AL, Robinson M, Smith GJ, Ambrosini GL, Piek JP, Oddy WH. ADHD is associated with a "Western" dietary pattern in adolescents. J Atten Disord. 2011 Jul;15(5):403-11.

Hoyme UB, Saling E. Efficient prematurity prevention is possible by pH-self measurement and immediate therapy of threatening ascending infection. *Eur J Obstet Gynecol Reprod Biol.* 2004 Aug 10;115(2):148-53.

Hoyos AB. Reduced incidence of necrotizing enterocolitis associated with enteral administration of *Lactobacillus acidophilus* and *Bifidobacterium infantis* to neonates in an intensive care unit. *Int J Infect Dis.* 1999 Summer;3(4):197-202.

Hsieh KH. Evaluation of efficacy of traditional Chinese medicines in the treatment of childhood bronchial asthma: clinical trial, immunological tests and animal study. Taiwan Asthma Study Group. *Pediatr Allergy Immunol.* 1996 Aug;7(3):130-40.

Hsu CH, Lu CM, Chang TT. Efficacy and safety of modified Mai-Men-Dong-Tang for treatment of allergic asthma. *Pediatr Allergy Immunol.* 2005;16:76-81.

Hu C, Kitts DD. Antioxidant, prooxidant, and cytotoxic activities of solvent-fractionated dandelion (Taraxacum officinale) flower extracts in vitro. *J Agric Food Chem.* 2003 Jan 1;51(1):301-10.

Hu C, Kitts DD. Dandelion (Taraxacum officinale) flower extract suppresses both reactive oxygen species and nitric oxide and prevents lipid oxidation in vitro. *Phytomedicine.* 2005 Aug;12(8):588-97.

Hu C, Kitts DD. Luteolin and luteolin-7-O-glucoside from dandelion flower suppress iNOS and COX-2 in RAW264.7 cells. *Mol Cell Biochem.* 2004 Oct;265(1-2):107-13.

Hu FB, Willett WC. Optimal diets for prevention of coronary heart disease. *JAMA.* 2002 Nov 27;288(20):2569-78.

Huang D, Ou B, Prior RL. The chemistry behind antioxidant capacity assays. *J Agric Food Chem.* 2005 Mar 23;53(6):1841-56.

Huang M, Wang W, Wei S. Investigation on medicinal plant resources of Glycyrrhiza uralensis in China and chemical assessment of its underground part. *Zhongguo Zhong Yao Za Zhi.* 2010 Apr;35(8):947-52.

Human Microbiome Project Consortium. A framework for human microbiome research. Nature. 2012 Jun 13;486(7402):215-21. doi: 10.1038/nature11209.

Hun L. Bacillus coagulans significantly improved abdominal pain and bloating in patients with IBS. *Postgrad Med.* 2009 Mar;121(2):119-24.

Huntley A, Ernst E: Herbal medicines for asthma: a systematic review. *Thorax.* 2000, 55:925-929.

Hur YM, Rushton JP. Genetic and environmental contributions to prosocial behaviour in 2- to 9-year-old South Korean twins. *Biol Lett.* 2007 Dec 22;3(6):664-6.

Husby S. Dietary antigens: uptake and humoral immunity in man. *APMIS Suppl.* 1988;1:1-40.

Hye-Seung J, Sung-Eun K, Mi-Kyung S. 2002. Protective Effect of Soybean Saponins and Major Antioxidants Against Aflatoxin B1-Induced Mutagenicity and DNA-Adduct Formation. Journal of Medicinal Food. Dec, Vol. 5, No. 4 : 235 -240.

Hylander WL. Incisor size and diet in anthropoids with special reference to Cercopithecidae. Science. 1975;189:1095 – 1098.

Hyndman SJ, Vickers LM, Htut T, Maunder JW, Peock A, Higenbottam TW. A randomized trial of dehumidification in the control of house dust mite. Clin Exp Allergy. 2000 Aug;30(8):1172-80.

Ibero M, Boné J, Martín B, Martínez J. Evaluation of an extensively hydrolysed casein formula (Damira 2000) in children with allergy to cow's milk proteins. *Allergol Immunopathol (Madr).* 2010 Mar-Apr;38(2):60-8.

Ibrahim AR, Kawamoto S, Nishimura M, Pak S, Aki T, Diaz-Perales A, Salcedo G, Asturias JA, Hayashi T, Ono K. A new lipid transfer protein homolog identified as an IgE-binding antigen from Japanese cedar pollen. *Biosci Biotechnol Biochem.* 2010;74(3):504-9.

Ikeda Y, Tsuji S, Satoh A, Ishikura M, Shirasawa T, Shimizu T. Protec-tive effects of astaxanthin on 6-hydroxydopamine-induced apoptosis in human neuroblastoma SH-SY5Y cells. J Neurochem. 2008 Dec;107(6):1730-40.

Imase K, Tanaka A, Tokunaga K, Sugano H, Ishida H, Takahashi S. *Lactobacillus reuteri* tablets suppress *Helicobacter pylori* infection – a double-blind randomised placebo-controlled cross-over clinical study. *Kansenshogaku Zasshi.* 2007 Jul;81(4):387-93.

Inbar O, Dotan R, Dlin RA, Neuman I, Bar-Or O. Breathing dry or humid air and exercise-induced asthma during swimming. *Eur J Appl Physiol Occup Physiol.* 1980;44(1):43-50.

Indrio F, Ladisa G, Mautone A, Montagna O. Effect of a fermented formula on thymus size and stool pH in healthy term infants. *Pediatr Res.* 2007 Jul;62(1):98-100.

Indrio F, Riezzo G, Raimondi F, Bisceglia M, Cavallo L, Francavilla R. The effects of probiotics on feeding tolerance, bowel habits, and gastrointestinal motility in preterm newborns. *J Pediatr.* 2008 Jun;152(6):801-6.

Innis SM, Hansen JW. Plasma fatty acid responses, metabolic effects, and safety of microalgal and fungal oils rich in arachidonic and docosahexaenoic acids in adults. *Am J Clin Nutr.* 1996 Aug;64(2):159-67.

Innis SM, Hansen JW. Plasma fatty acid responses, metabolic effects, and safety of microalgal and fungal oils rich in arachidonic and docosahexaenoic acids in healthy adults. *Am J Clin Nutr.* 1996 Aug;64(2):159-67.

Ionescu JG. New insights in the pathogenesis of atopic disease. *J Med Life.* 2009 Apr-Jun;2(2):146-54.

Iovieno A, Lambiase A, Sacchetti M, Stampachiacchiere B, Micera A, Bonini S. Preliminary evidence of the efficacy of probiotic eye-drop treatment in patients with vernal keratoconjunctivitis. *Graefes Arch Clin Exp Ophthalmol.* 2008 Mar;246(3):435-41.

Iribarren C, Tolstykh IV, Miller MK, Eisner MD. Asthma and the prospective risk of anaphylactic shock and other allergy diagnoses in a large integrated health care delivery system. *Ann Allergy Asthma Immunol.* 2010 May;104(5):371-7.

ISAAC. The International Study of Asthma and Allergies in Childhood (ISAAC) Steering Committee. Worldwide variation in prevalence of symptoms of asthma, allergic rhinoconjunctivitis, and atopic eczema: ISAAC. *Lancet.* 1998;351:1225-1232.

Ishida Y, Nakamura F, Kanzato H, Sawada D, Hirata H, Nishimura A, Kajimoto O, Fujiwara S. Clinical effects of *Lactobacillus acidophilus* strain L-92 on perennial allergic rhinitis: a double-blind, placebo-controlled study. *J Dairy Sci.* 2005 Feb;88(2):527-33.

Ishida Y, Nakamura F, Kanzato H, Sawada D, Hirata H, Nishimura A, Kajimoto O, Fujiwara S. Clinical effects of *Lactobacillus acidophilus* strain L-92 on perennial allergic rhinitis: a double-blind, placebo-controlled study. *J Dairy Sci.* 2005 Feb;88(2):527-33.

Ishida Y, Nakamura F, Kanzato H, Sawada D, Yamamoto N, Kagata H, Oh-Ida M, Takeuchi H, Fujiwara S. Effect of milk fermented with *Lactobacillus acidophilus* strain L-92 on symptoms of Japanese cedar pollen allergy: a randomized placebo-controlled trial. *Biosci Biotechnol Biochem.* 2005 Sep;69(9):1652-60.

Ishikawa H, Akedo I, Otani T, Suzuki T, Nakamura T, Takeyama I, Ishiguro S, Miyaoka E, Sobue T, Kakizoe T. Randomized trial of dietary fiber and *Lactobacillus casei* administration for prevention of colorectal tumors. *Int J Cancer.* 2005 Sep 20;116(5):762-7.

Ishtiaq M, Hanif W, Khan MA, Ashraf M, Butt AM. An ethnomedicinal survey and documentation of important medicinal folklore food phytonims of flora of Samahni valley, (Azad Kashmir) Pakistan. *Pak J Biol Sci.* 2007 Jul 1;10(13):2241-56.

Isoflavone supplements containing predominantly genistein reduce hot flash. Menopause. Sep-Oct;13(5):831-9.

Isolauri E, Joensuu J, Suomalainen H, Luomala M, Vesikari T. Improved immunogenicity of oral D x RRV reassortant rotavirus vaccine by *Lactobacillus casei* GG. *Vaccine.* 1995 Feb;13(3):310-2.

Isolauri E, Juntunen M, Rautanen T, Sillanaukee P, Koivula T. A human Lactobacillus strain (*Lactobacillus casei* sp strain GG) promotes recovery from acute diarrhea in children. *Pediatrics.* 1991 Jul;88(1):90-7.

Isolauri E, Kaila M, Mykkänen H, Ling WH, Salminen S. Oral bacteriotherapy for viral gastroenteritis. *Dig Dis Sci.* 1994 Dec;39(12):2595-600.

Itokawa Y. Magnesium intake and cardiovascular disease. *Clin Calcium.* 2005 Feb;15(2):154-9.

# REFERENCES AND BIBLIOGRAPHY

Ivory K, Chambers SJ, Pin C, Prieto E, Arqués JL, Nicoletti C. Oral delivery of *Lactobacillus casei* Shirota modifies allergen-induced immune responses in allergic rhinitis. *Clin Exp Allergy.* 2008 Aug;38(8):1282-9.

Izbicki G, Chavko R, Banauch GI, Weiden MD, Berger KI, Aldrich TK, Hall C, Kelly KJ, Prezant DJ. World trade center "sarcoid-like" granulomatous pulmonary disease in New York City fire department rescue workers. *Chest.* 2007 May;131(5):1414-23.

Izquierdo JL, Martín A, de Lucas P, Rodríguez-González-Moro JM, Almonacid C, Paravisini A. Misdiagnosis of patients receiving inhaled therapies in primary care. *Int J Chron Obstruct Pulmon Dis.* 2010 Aug 9;5:241-9.

Izumi K, Aihara M, Ikezawa Z. Effects of non steroidal antiinflammatory drugs (NSAIDs) on immediate-type food allergy analysis of Japanese cases from 1998 to 2009. *Arerugi.* 2009 Dec;58(12):1629-39.

Jaber R. Respiratory and allergic diseases: from upper respiratory tract infections to asthma. *Prim Care.* 2002 Jun;29(2):231-61.

Jackson DJ, Lemanske RF Jr. The role of respiratory virus infections in childhood asthma inception. *Immunol Allergy Clin North Am.* 2010 Nov;30(4):513-22, vi.

Jacobs DE, Wilson J, Dixon SL, Smith J, Evens A. The relationship of housing and population health: a 30-year retrospective analysis. *Environ Health Perspect.* 2009 Apr;117(4):597-604. 2008 Dec 16.

Jacobsen CN, Rosenfeldt Nielsen V, Hayford AE, Moller PL, Michaelsen KF, Paerregaard A, Sandström B, Tvede M, Jakobsen M. Screening of probiotic activities of forty-seven strains of Lactobacillus spp. by in vitro techniques and evaluation of the colonization ability of five selected strains in humans. *Appl Environ Microbiol.* 1999 Nov;65(11):4949-56.

Jagetia GC, Aggarwal BB. "Spicing up" of the immune system by curcumin. *J Clin Immunol.* 2007 Jan;27(1):19-35.

Jagetia GC, Nayak V, Vidyasagar MS. Evaluation of the antineoplastic activity of guduchi (Tinospora cordifolia) in cultured HeLa cells. *Cancer Lett.* 1998 May 15;127(1-2):71-82.

Jagetia GC, Rao SK. Evaluation of Cytotoxic Effects of Dichloromethane Extract of Guduchi (Tinospora cordifolia Miers ex Hook F & THOMS) on Cultured HeLa Cells. *Evid Based Complement Alternat Med.* 2006 Jun;3(2):267-72.

Jahnova E, Horvathova M, Gazdik F, Weissova S. Effects of selenium supplementation on expression of adhesion molecules in corticoid-dependent asthmatics. *Bratisl Lek Listy.* 2002;103(1):12-6.

Jain PK, McNaught CE, Anderson AD, MacFie J, Mitchell CJ. Influence of synbiotic containing *Lactobacillus acidophilus* La5, *Bifidobacterium lactis* Bb 12, *Streptococcus thermophilus*, *Lactobacillus bulgaricus* and oligofructose on gut barrier function and sepsis in critically ill patients: a randomised controlled trial. *Clin Nutr.* 2004 Aug;23(4):467-75.

Jaiswal M, Prajapati PK, Patgiri BJ Ravishankar B. A Comparative Pharmaco – Clinical Study on Anti-Asthmatic Effect of Shirisharishta Prepared by Bark, Sapwood and Heartwood of Albizia Lebbeck. *J Res Ayurv.* 2006;27(3):67-74.

Jaiswal M, Prajapati PK, Patgiri BJ, Ravishankar B. Clinical Study on Anti-Asthmatic Effect of Shirisharishta Prepared by Bark, Sapwood and Heartwood of Albizia Lebbeck. *Pharmaco.* 2006 27(3): 67-74

Janelle KC, Barr SI. Nutrient intakes and eating behavior scores of vegetarian and nonvegetarian women. *J Am Diet Assoc.* 1995 Feb;95(2):180-6, 189, quiz 187-8.

Janson C, Anto J, Burney P, Chinn S, de Marco R, Heinrich J, Jarvis D, Kuenzli N, Leynaert B, Luczynska C, Neukirch F, Svanes C, Sunyer J, Wjst M; European Community Respiratory Health Survey II. The European Community Respiratory Health Survey: what are the main results so far? European Community Respiratory Health Survey II. *Eur Respir J.* 2001 Sep;18(3):598-611.

Jarocka-Cyrta E, Baniukiewicz A, Wasilewska J, Pawlak J, Kaczmarski M. Focal villous atrophy of the duodenum in children who have outgrown cow's milk allergy. Chromoendoscopy and magnification endoscopy evaluation. *Med Wieku Rozwoj.* 2007 Apr-Jun;11(2 Pt 1):123-7.

Jauhiainen T, Vapaatalo H, Poussa T, Kyrönpalo S, Rasmussen M, Korpela R. *Lactobacillus helveticus* fermented milk lowers blood pressure in hypertensive subjects in 24-h ambulatory blood pressure measurement. *Am J Hypertens.* 2005 Dec;18(12 Pt 1):1600-5.

Jayaprakasam B, Doddaga S, Wang R, Holmes D, Goldfarb J, Li XM. Licorice flavonoids inhibit eotaxin-1 secretion by human fetal lung fibroblasts in vitro. *J Agric Food Chem.* 2009 Feb 11;57(3):820-5.

Jenkins DJ, Jones PJ, Lamarche B, Kendall CW, Faulkner D, Cermakova L, Gigleux I, Ramprasath V, de Souza R, Ireland C, Patel D, Srichaikul K, Abdulnour S, Bashyam B, Collier C, Hoshizaki S, Josse RG, Leiter LA, Connelly PW, Frohlich J. Effect of a dietary portfolio of cholesterol-lowering foods given at 2 levels of intensity of dietary advice on serum lipids in hyperlipidemia: a randomized controlled trial. JAMA. 2011 Aug 24;306(8):831-9.

Jennings S, Prescott SL. Early dietary exposures and feeding practices: role in pathogenesis and prevention of allergic disease? *Postgrad Med J.* 2010 Feb;86(1012):94-9.

Jensen B. *Foods that Heal.* Garden City Park, NY: Avery Publ, 1988, 1993.

Jensen B. *Nature Has a Remedy.* Los Angeles: Keats, 2001.

Jensen HK. The molecular genetic basis and diagnosis of familial hypercholesterolemia in Denmark. *Dan Med Bull.* 2002 Nov;49(4):318-45.

Jeon HJ, Kang HJ, Jung HJ, Kang YS, Lim CJ, Kim YM, Park EH. Anti-inflammatory activity of Taraxacum officinale. J Ethnopharmacol. 2008 Jan 4;115(1):82-8.

Jernelöv S, Höglund CO, Axelsson J, Axén J, Grönneberg R, Grunewald J, Stierna P, Lekander M. Effects of examination stress on psychological responses, sleep and allergic symptoms in atopic and non-atopic students. *Int J Behav Med.* 2009;16(4):305-10.

Jiang T, Mustapha A, Savaiano DA. Improvement of lactose digestion in humans by ingestion of unfermented milk containing *Bifidobacterium longum*. *J Dairy Sci*. 1996 May;79(5):750-7.

Jiménez E, Fernández L, Maldonado A, Martín R, Olivares M, Xaus J, Rodríguez JM. Oral administration of Lactobacillus strains isolated from breast milk as an alternative for the treatment of infectious mastitis during lactation. *Appl Environ Microbiol*. 2008 Aug;74(15):4650-5.

Jiménez F, Barbaglia Y, Bucci P, Tedeschi FA, Zalazar FE. Molecular detection and genotypification of Helicobacter pylori in gastric biopsies from symptomatic adult patients in Santa Fe, Argentina. Rev Argent Microbiol. 2013 Jan-Mar;45(1):39-43.

Jin H, Leng Q, Li C. Dietary flavonoid for preventing colorectal neoplasms. Cochrane Database Syst Rev. 2012 Aug 15;8:CD009350.

Johansson G, Holmén A, Persson L, Högstedt B, Wassén C, Ottova L, Gustafsson JA. Dietary influence on some proposed risk factors for colon cancer: fecal and urinary mutagenic activity and the activity of some intestinal bacterial enzymes. Cancer Detect Prev. 1997;21(3):258-66.

Johansson G, Holmén A, Persson L, Högstedt B, Wassén C, Ottova L, Gustafsson JA. Long-term effects of a change from a mixed diet to a lacto-vegetarian diet on human urinary and faecal mutagenic activity. *Mutagenesis*. 1998 Mar;13(2):167-71.

Johansson G, Holmén A, Persson L, Högstedt B, Wassén C, Ottova L, Gustafsson JA. Dietary influence on some proposed risk factors for colon cancer: fecal and urinary mutagenic activity and the activity of some intestinal bacterial enzymes. *Cancer Detect Prev*. 1997;21(3):258-66.

Johansson G, Holmén A, Persson L, Högstedt R, Wassén C, Ottova L, Gustafsson JA. The effect of a shift from a mixed diet to a lacto-vegetarian diet on human urinary and fecal mutagenic activity. Carcinogenesis. 1992 Feb;13(2):153-7.

Johansson G, Holmén A, Persson L, Högstedt R, Wassén C, Ottova L, Gustafsson JA. The effect of a shift from a mixed diet to a lacto-vegetarian diet on human urinary and fecal mutagenic activity. *Carcinogenesis*. 1992 Feb;13(2):153-7.

Johansson G, Ravald N. Comparison of some salivary variables between vegetarians and omnivores. *Eur J Oral Sci*. 1995 Apr;103(2 ( Pt 1)):95-8.

Johansson GK, Ottova L, Gustafsson JA. Shift from a mixed diet to a lactovegetarian diet: influence on some cancer-associated intestinal bacterial enzyme activities. Nutr Cancer. 1990;14(3-4):239-46.

Johansson GK, Ottova L, Gustafsson JA. Shift from a mixed diet to a lactovegetarian diet: influence on some cancer-associated intestinal bacterial enzyme activities. *Nutr Cancer*. 1990;14(3-4):239-46. PubMed PMID: 2128119.

Johansson ML, Nobaek S, Berggren A, Nyman M, Björck I, Ahrné S, Jeppsson B, Molin G. Survival of *Lactobacillus plantarum* DSM 9843 (299v), and effect on the short-chain fatty acid content of faeces after ingestion of a rose-hip drink with fermented oats. *Int J Food Microbiol*. 1998 Jun 30;42(1-2):29-38.

Johari H. *Ayurvedic Massage: Traditional Indian Techniques for Balancing Body and Mind*. Rochester, VT: Healing Arts, 1996.

Johnson CD, Lucas EA, Hooshmand S, Campbell S, Akhter MP, Arjmandi BH. Addition of fructooligosaccharides and dried plum to soy-based diets reverses bone loss in the ovariectomized rat. Evid Based Complement Alternat Med. 2011;2011:836267.

Johnson LM. Gitksan medicinal plants – cultural choice and efficacy. *J Ethnobiol Ethnomed*. 2006 Jun 21;2:29.

Jolliffe N., Archer M. Statistical associations between international coronary heart disease death rates and certain environmental factors. J. Chronic Dis. 1959; 9;636-652,

Jolly CJ. The seed eaters: A new model of hominid differentiation based on a baboon analogy. Man. 1970;5:5 – 26.

Jones MA, Silman AJ, Whiting S, *et al.* Occurrence of rheumatoid arthritis is not increased in the first degree relatives of a population based inception cohort of inflammatory polyarthritis. *Ann Rheum Dis*. 1996;55(2): 89-93.

Jones SE, Versalovic J. Probiotic Lactobacillus reuteri biofilms produce antimicrobial and anti-inflammatory factors. *BMC Microbiol*. 2009 Feb 11;9:35.

José RJ, Roberts J, Bakerly ND. The effectiveness of a social marketing model on case-finding for COPD in a deprived inner city population. *Prim Care Respir J*. 2010 Jun;19(2):104-8.

Joseph SP, Borrell LN, Shapiro A. Self-reported lifetime asthma and nativity status in U.S. children and adolescents: results from the National Health and Nutrition Examination Survey 1999-2004. *J Health Care Poor Underserved*. 2010 May;21(2 Suppl):125-39.

Jou HJ, Wu SC, Chang FW, Ling PY, Chu KS, Wu WH. Effect of intestinal production of equol on menopausal symptoms in women treated with soy isoflavones. Int J Gynaecol Obstet. 2008 Jul;102(1):44-9.

Journoud M, Jones PJ. Red yeast rice: a new hypolipidemic drug. Life Sci. 2004 Apr 16;74(22):2675-83.

Juergens UR, Dethlefsen U, Steinkamp G, Gillissen A, Repges R, Vetter H. Anti-inflammatory activity of 1.8-cineol (eucalyptol) in bronchial asthma: a double-blind placebo-controlled trial. *Respir Med*. 2003 Mar;97(3):250-6.

Julkunen-Tiitto R. A chemotaxonomic survey of phenolics in leaves of northern Salicaceae species. Phytochemistry. 1986;25(3):663-667.

Jung HA, Yokozawa T, Kim BW, Jung JH, Choi JS. Selective inhibition of prenylated flavonoids from Sophora flavescens against BACE1 and cholinesterases. *Am J Chin Med*. 2010;38(2):415-29.

Jung UJ, Lee MK, Jeong KS, Choi MS. The hypoglycemic effects of hesperidin and naringin are partly mediated by hepatic glucose-regulating enzymes in C57BL/KsJ-db/db mice. J Nutr. 2004 Oct;134(10):2499-503.

Jurenka JS. Anti-inflammatory properties of curcumin, a major constituent of Curcuma longa: a review of preclinical and clinical research. *Altern Med Rev*. 2009 Feb;14(2):141-153.

Juvonen R, Bloigu A, Peitso A, Silvennoinen-Kassinen S, Saikku P, Leinonen M, Hassi J, Harju T. Training improves physical fitness and decreases CRP also in asthmatic conscripts. *J Asthma*. 2008 Apr;45(3):237-42.

# REFERENCES AND BIBLIOGRAPHY

Kähkönen MP, Hopia AI, Vuorela HJ, Rauha JP, Pihlaja K, Kujala TS, Heinonen M. Antioxidant activity of plant extracts containing phenolic compounds. *J Agric Food Chem.* 1999 Oct;47(10):3954-62.

Kaila M, Isolauri E, Saxelin M, Arvilommi H, Vesikari T. Viable versus inactivated lactobacillus strain GG in acute rotavirus diarrhoea. *Arch Dis Child.* 1995 Jan;72(1):51-3.

Kaila M, Vanto T, Valovirta E, Koivikko A, Juntunen-Backman K. Diagnosis of food allergy in Finland: survey of pediatric practices. *Pediatr Allergy Immunol.* 2000 Nov;11(4):246-9.

Kajander K, Hatakka K, Poussa T, Färkkilä M, Korpela R. A probiotic mixture alleviates symptoms in irritable bowel syndrome patients: a controlled 6-month intervention. *Aliment Pharmacol Ther.* 2005 Sep 1;22(5):387-94.

Kajander K, Korpela R. Clinical studies on alleviating the symptoms of irritable bowel syndrome. *Asia Pac J Clin Nutr.* 2006;15(4):576-80.

Kajander K, Krogius-Kurikka L, Rinttilä T, Karjalainen H, Palva A, Korpela R. Effects of multispecies probiotic supplementation on intestinal microbiota in irritable bowel syndrome. *Aliment Pharmacol Ther.* 2007 Aug 1;26(3):463-73.

Kajander K, Myllyluoma E, Rajilić-Stojanović M, Kyrönpalo S, Rasmussen M, Järvenpää S, Zoetendal EG, de Vos WM, Vapaatalo H, Korpela R. Clinical trial: multispecies probiotic supplementation alleviates the symptoms of irritable bowel syndrome and stabilizes intestinal microbiota. *Aliment Pharmacol Ther.* 2008 Jan 1;27(1):48-57.

Kalach N, Benhamou PH, Campeotto F, Dupont Ch. Anemia impairs small intestinal absorption measured by intestinal permeability in children. *Eur Ann Allergy Clin Immunol.* 2007 Jan;39(1):20-2.

Kaliner M, Shelhamer JH, Borson B, Nadel J, Patow C, Marom Z. Human respiratory mucus. *Am Rev Respir Dis.* 1986 Sep;134(3):612-21.

Kalliomäki M, Salminen S, Arvilommi H, Kero P, Koskinen P, Isolauri E. Probiotics in primary prevention of atopic disease: a randomised placebo-controlled trial. *Lancet.* 2001 Apr 7;357(9262):1076-9.

Kalliomäki M, Salminen S, Poussa T, Arvilommi H, Isolauri E. Probiotics and prevention of atopic disease: 4-year follow-up of a randomised placebo-controlled trial. *Lancet.* 2003 May 31;361(9372):1869-71.

Kalliomäki M, Salminen S, Poussa T, Isolauri E. Probiotics during the first 7 years of life: a cumulative risk reduction of eczema in a randomized, placebo-controlled trial. *J Allergy Clin Immunol.* 2007 Apr;119(4):1019-21.

Kanazawa H, Nagino M, Kamiya S, Komatsu S, Mayumi T, Takagi K, Asahara T, Nomoto K, Tanaka R, Nimura Y. Synbiotics reduce postoperative infectious complications: a randomized controlled trial in biliary cancer patients undergoing hepatectomy. *Langenbecks Arch Surg.* 2005 Apr;390(2):104-13.

Kang SK, Kim JK, Ahn SH, Oh JE, Kim JH, Lim DH, Son BK. Relationship between silent gastroesophageal reflux and food sensitization in infants and young children with recurrent wheezing. *J Korean Med Sci.* 2010 Mar;25(3):425-8.

Kankaanpää PE, Yang B, Kallio HP, Isolauri E, Salminen SJ. Influence of probiotic supplemented infant formula on composition of plasma lipids in atopic infants. *J Nutr Biochem.* 2002 Jun;13(6):364-369.

Kanny G, Grignon G, Dauca M, Guedenet JC, Moneret-Vautrin DA. Ultrastructural changes in the duodenal mucosa induced by ingested histamine in patients with chronic urticaria. *Allergy.* 1996 Dec;51(12):935-9.

Kano H, Mogami O, Uchida M. Oral administration of milk fermented with Lactobacillus delbrueckii ssp. bulgaricus OLL1073R-1 to DBA/1 mice inhibits secretion of proinflammatory cytokines. *Cytotechnology.* 2002 Nov;40(1-3):67-73.

Kapil A, Sharma S. Immunopotentiating compounds from Tinospora cordifolia. *J Ethnopharmacol.* 1997 Oct;58(2):89-95.

Kaplan C. Indoor air pollution from unprocessed solid fuels in developing countries. *Rev Environ Health.* 2010 Jul-Sep;25(3):221-42.

Kaplan M, Mutlu EA, Benson M, Fields JZ, Banan A, Keshavarzian A. Use of herbal preparations in the treatment of oxidant-mediated inflammatory disorders. *Complement Ther Med.* 2007 Sep;15(3):207-16. 2006 Aug 21.

Kaplan R. The nature of the view from home: psychological benefits. *Environ Behav.* 2001;33(4):507-42.

Kaplan R. Wilderness perception and psychological benefits: an analysis of a continuing program. *Leisure Sci.* 1984;6(3):271-90.

Kaptan K, Beyan C, Ural AU, Cetin T, Avcu F, Gülşen M, Finci R, Yalçin A. Helicobacter pylori--is it a novel causative agent in Vitamin B12 deficiency? Arch Intern Med. 2000 May 8;160(9):1349-53.

Karkoulias K, Patouchas D, Alahiotis S, Tsiamita M, Vrodakis K, Spiropoulos K. Specific sensitization in wheat flour and contributing factors in traditional bakers. *Eur Rev Med Pharmacol Sci.* 2007 May-Jun;11(3):141-8.

Karlsson CL, Onnerfält J, Xu J, Molin G, Ahrné S, Thorngren-Jerneck K. The microbiota of the gut in preschool children with normal and excessive body weight. Obesity (Silver Spring). 2012 Nov;20(11):2257-61. doi: 10.1038/oby.2012.110.

Karpińska J, Mikołuć B, Motkowski R, Piotrowska-Jastrzębska J. HPLC method for simultaneous determination of retinol, alpha-tocopherol and coenzyme Q10 in human plasma. *J Pharm Biomed Anal.* 2006 Sep 18;42(2):232-6.

Kashiwada Y, Takanaka K, Tsukada H, Miwa Y, Taga T, Tanaka S, Ikeshiro Y. Sesquiterpene glucosides from anti-leukotriene B4 release fraction of Taraxacum officinale. *J Asian Nat Prod Res.* 2001;3(3):191-7.

Katagiri M, Satoh A, Tsuji S, Shirasawa T. Effects of astaxanthin-rich Haematococcus pluvialis extract on cognitive function: a randomised, double-blind, placebo-controlled study. J Clin Biochem Nutr. 2012 Sep;51(2):102-7.

Katial RK, Strand M, Prasertsuntarasai T, Leung R, Zheng W, Alam R. The effect of aspirin desensitization on novel biomarkers in aspirin-exacerbated respiratory diseases. *J Allergy Clin Immunol.* 2010 Oct;126(4):738-44. 2010 Aug 21.

Kattan JD, Srivastava KD, Sampson HA, Li XM. Pharmacologic and Immunologic Effects of Individual Herbs of Food Allergy Herbal Formula 2 in a Murine Model of Peanut Allergy. *J Allergy Clin Immunol.* 2006;117(2):S34.

413

Kattan JD, Srivastava KD, Zou ZM, Goldfarb J, Sampson HA, Li XM. Pharmacological and immunological effects of individual herbs in the Food Allergy Herbal Formula-2 (FAHF-2) on peanut allergy. *Phytother Res.* 2008 May;22(5):651-9.

Katz DL, Cushman D, Reynolds J, Njike V, Treu JA, Walker J, Smith E, Katz C. Putting physical activity where it fits in the school day: preliminary results of the ABC (Activity Bursts in the Classroom) for fitness program. *Prev Chronic Dis.* 2010 Jul;7(4):A82. 2010 Jun 15.

Katz Y, Rajuan N, Goldberg MR, Eisenberg E, Heyman E, Cohen A, Leshno M. Early exposure to cow's milk protein is protective against IgE-mediated cow's milk protein allergy. *J Allergy Clin Immunol.* 2010 Jul;126(1):77-82.e1.

Kawase M, Hashimoto H, Hosoda M, Morita H, Hosono A. Effect of administration of fermented milk containing whey protein concentrate to rats and healthy men on serum lipids and blood pressure. *J Dairy Sci.* 2000 Feb;83(2):255-63.

Kazaks AG, Uriu-Adams JY, Albertson TE, Shenoy SF, Stern JS. Effect of oral magnesium supplementation on measures of airway resistance and subjective assessment of asthma control and quality of life in men and women with mild to moderate asthma: a randomized placebo controlled trial. *J Asthma.* 2010 Feb;47(1):83-92.

Kazansky DB. MHC restriction and allogeneic immune responses. *J Immunotoxicol.* 2008 Oct;5(4):369-84.

Kazlowska K, Hsu T, Hou CC, Yang WC, Tsai GJ. Anti-inflammatory properties of phenolic compounds and crude extract from Porphyra dentata. *J Ethnopharmacol.* 2010 Mar 2;128(1):123-30.

Ke X, Qian D, Zhu L, Hong S. [Analysis on quality of life and personality characteristics of allergic rhinitis]. *Lin Chung Er Bi Yan Hou Tou Jing Wai Ke Za Zhi.* 2010 Mar;24(5):200-2.

Keast DR, O'Neil CE, Jones JM. Dried fruit consumption is associated with improved diet quality and reduced obesity in US adults: National Health and Nutrition Examination Survey, 1999-2004. *Nutr Res.* 2011 Jun;31(6):460-7.

Kecskés G, Belágyi T, Oláh A. Early jejunal nutrition with combined pre- and probiotics in acute pancreatitis – prospective, randomized, double-blind investigations. *Magy Seb.* 2003 Feb;56(1):3-8.

Keeling RF, Piper SC, Bollenbacher AF, Walker SJ. Trends: A Compendium of Data on Global Change. Oak Ridge, TN: Carbon Dioxide Information Analysis Center, Oak Ridge National Laboratory, US Department of Energy; 2010. Monthly atmospheric 13C/12C isotopic ratios for 11 SIO stations.

Keenan JM, Goulson M, Shamliyan T, Knutson N, Kolberg L, Curry L. The effects of concentrated barley beta-glucan on blood lipids in a population of hypercholesterolaemic men and women. *Br J Nutr.* 2007 Jun;97(6):1162-8.

Keita AV, Söderholm JD. The intestinal barrier and its regulation by neuroimmune factors. *Neurogastroenterol Motil.* 2010 Jul;22(7):718-33.

Kekkonen RA, Lummela N, Karjalainen H, Latvala S, Tynkkynen S, Jarvenpaa S, Kautiainen H, Julkunen I, Vapaatalo H, Korpela R. Probiotic intervention has strain-specific anti-inflammatory effects in healthy adults. *World J Gastroenterol.* 2008 Apr 7;14(13):2029-36.

Kekkonen RA, Sysi-Aho M, Seppanen-Laakso T, Julkunen I, Vapaatalo H, Oresic M, Korpela R. Effect of probiotic *Lactobacillus rhamnosus* GG intervention on global serum lipidomic profiles in healthy adults. *World J Gastroenterol.* 2008 May 28;14(20):3188-94.

Kekkonen RA, Vasankari TJ, Vuorimaa T, Haahtela T, Julkunen I, Korpela R. The effect of probiotics on respiratory infections and gastrointestinal symptoms during training in marathon runners. *Int J Sport Nutr Exerc Metab.* 2007 Aug;17(4):352-63.

Kekkonen RA, Vasankari TJ, Vuorimaa T, Haahtela T, Julkunen I, Korpela R. The effect of probiotics on respiratory infections and gastrointestinal symptoms during training in marathon runners. *Int J Sport Nutr Exerc Metab.* 2007 Aug;17(4):352-63.

Kelder P. *Ancient Secret of the Fountain of Youth.* New York: Doubleday, 1998.

Kelly HW, Van Natta ML, Covar RA, Tonascia J, Green RP, Strunk RC; CAMP Research Group. Effect of long-term corticosteroid use on bone mineral density in children: a prospective longitudinal assessment in the childhood Asthma Management Program (CAMP) study. *Pediatrics.* 2008 Jul;122(1):e53-61.

Kelly J, Fulford J, Vanhatalo A, Blackwell JR, French O, Bailey SJ, Gilchrist M, Winyard PG, Jones AM. Effects of short-term dietary nitrate supplementation on blood pressure, O2 uptake kinetics, and muscle and cognitive function in older adults. *Am J Physiol Regul Integr Comp Physiol.* 2013 Jan 15;304(2):R73-83.

Kelly J, Vanhatalo A, Wilkerson DP, Wylie LJ, Jones AM. Effects of Nitrate on the Power-Duration Relationship for Severe-Intensity Exercise. *Med Sci Sports Exerc.* 2013 Mar 7

Kelly SA, Summerbell CD, Brynes A, Whittaker V, Frost G. Wholegrain cereals for coronary heart disease. *Cochrane Database Syst Rev.* 2007 Apr 18;(2):CD005051.

Kelly-Pieper K, Patil SP, Busse P, Yang N, Sampson H, Li XM, Wisnivesky JP, Kattan M. Safety and tolerability of an antiasthma herbal Formula (ASHMI) in adult subjects with asthma: a randomized, double-blinded, placebo-controlled, dose-escalation phase I study. *J Altern Complement Med.* 2009 Jul;15(7):735-43.

Kelsey NA, Wilkins HM, Linseman DA. Nutraceutical antioxidants as novel neuroprotective agents. Molecules. 2010 Nov 3;15(11):7792-814. doi: 10.3390/molecules15117792.

Kenia P, Houghton T, Beardsmore C. Does inhaling menthol affect nasal patency or cough? *Pediatr Pulmonol.* 2008 Jun;43(6):532-7.

Keogh JB, Grieger JA, Noakes M, Clifton PM. Flow-Mediated Dilatation Is Impaired by a High-Saturated Fat Diet but Not by a High-Carbohydrate Diet. *Arterioscler Thromb Vasc Biol.* 2005 Mar 17

Keogh JB, Grieger JA, Noakes M, Clifton PM. Flow-Mediated Dilatation Is Impaired by a High-Saturated Fat Diet but Not by a High-Carbohydrate Diet. *Arterioscler Thromb Vasc Biol.* 2005 Mar 17

414

Kerckhoffs DA, Brouns F, Hornstra G, Mensink RP. Effects on the human serum lipoprotein profile of beta-glucan, soy protein and isoflavones, plant sterols and stanols, garlic and tocotrienols. *J Nutr.* 2002 Sep;132(9):2494-505.

Kerckhoffs DA, Brouns F, Hornstra G, Mensink RP. Effects on the human serum lipoprotein profile of beta-glucan, soy protein and isoflavones, plant sterols and stanols, garlic and tocotrienols. *J Nutr.* 2002 Sep;132(9):2494-505.

Kerkhof M, Postma DS, Brunekreef B, Reijmerink NE, Wijga AH, de Jongste JC, Gehring U, Koppelman GH. Toll-like receptor 2 and 4 genes influence susceptibility to adverse effects of traffic-related air pollution on child-hood asthma. *Thorax.* 2010 Aug;65(8):690-7.

Key T, Appleby P, Davey G, Allen N, Spencer E, Travis R. Mortality in British vegetarians: review and preliminary results from EPIC-Oxford. *Amer. Jour. Clin. Nutr. Suppl.* 2003;78(3): 533S-538S.

Kiecolt-Glaser JK, Heffner KL, Glaser R, Malarkey WB, Porter K, Atkinson C, Laskowski B, Lemeshow S, Marshall GD. How stress and anxiety can alter immediate and late phase skin test responses in allergic rhinitis. *Psycho-neuroendocrinology.* 2009 Jun;34(5):670-80.

Kiefte-de Jong JC, Escher JC, Arends LR, Jaddoe VW, Hofman A, Raat H, Moll HA. Infant nutritional factors and functional constipation in childhood: the Generation R study. *Am J Gastroenterol.* 2010 Apr;105(4):940-5.

Kiessling G, Schneider J, Jahreis G. Long-term consumption of fermented dairy products over 6 months increases HDL cholesterol. *Eur J Clin Nutr.* 2002 Sep;56(9):843-9.

Kilara A, Shahani KM. The use of immobilized enzymes in the food industry: a review. *CRC Crit Rev Food Sci Nutr.* 1979 Dec;12(2):161-98.

Kim HM, Shin HY, Lim KH, Ryu ST, Shin TY, Chae HJ, Kim HR, Lyu YS, An NH, Lim KS. Taraxacum officinale inhibits tumor necrosis factor-alpha production from rat astrocytes. *Immunopharmacol Immunotoxicol.* 2000 Aug;22(3):519-30.

Kim JH, An S, Kim JE, Choi GS, Ye YM, Park HS. Beef-induced anaphylaxis confirmed by the basophil activation test. *Allergy Asthma Immunol Res.* 2010 Jul;2(3):206-8.

Kim JH, Ellwood PE, Asher MI. Diet and asthma: looking back, moving forward. *Respir Res.* 2009 Jun 12;10:49.

Kim JH, Kim JE, Choi GS, Hwang EK, An S, Ye YM, Park HS. A case of occupational rhinitis caused by rice powder in the grain industry. *Allergy Asthma Immunol Res.* 2010 Apr;2(2):141-3.

Kim JH, Lee SY, Kim HB, Jin HS, Yu JH, Kim BJ, Kim BS, Kang MJ, Jang SO, Hong SJ. TBXA2R gene polymor-phism and responsiveness to leukotriene receptor antagonist in children with asthma. *Clin Exp Allergy.* 2008 Jan;38(1):51-9.

Kim JI, Lee MS, Jung SY, Choi JY, Lee S, Ko JM, Zhao H, Zhao J, Kim AR, Shin MS, Kang KW, Jung HJ, Kim TH, Liu B, Choi SM. Acupuncture for persistent allergic rhinitis: a multi-centre, randomised, controlled trial protocol. *Trials.* 2009 Jul 14;10:54.

Kim JY, Kim DY, Lee YS, Lee BK, Lee KH, Ro JY. DA-9601, Artemisia asiatica herbal extract, ameliorates airway inflammation of allergic asthma in mice. *Mol Cells.* 2006;22:104-12.

Kim LS, Waters RF, Burkholder PM. Immunological activity of larch arabinogalactan and Echinacea: a preliminary, randomized, double-blind, placebo-controlled trial. *Altern Med Rev.* 2002 Apr;7(2):138-49.

Kim MN, Kim N, Lee SH, Hwang JH, Kim JW, Jeong SH, Lee DH, Kim JS, Jung HC, Song IS. The effects of probiotics on PPI-triple therapy for *Helicobacter pylori* eradication. *Helicobacter.* 2008 Aug;13(4):261-8.

Kim MS, Hwang SS, Park EJ, Bae JW. Strict vegetarian diet improves the risk factors associated with metabolic diseases by modulating gut microbiota and reducing intestinal inflammation. Environ Microbiol Rep. 2013 Oct;5(5):765-75. doi: 10.1111/1758-2229.12079.

Kim MS, Hwang SS, Park EJ, Bae JW. Strict vegetarian diet improves the risk factors associated with metabolic diseases by modulating gut microbiota and reducing intestinal inflammation. Environ Microbiol Rep. 2013 Oct;5(5):765-75. doi: 10.1111/1758-2229.12079.

Kim NI, Jo Y, Ahn SB, Son BK, Kim SH, Park YS, Kim SH, Ju JE. A case of eosinophilic esophagitis with food hypersensitivity. *J Neurogastroenterol Motil.* 2010 Jul;16(3):315-8.

Kim SJ, Jung JY, Kim HW, Park T. Anti-obesity effects of Juniperus chinensis extract are associated with increased AMP-activated protein kinase expression and phosphorylation in the visceral adipose tissue of rats. *Biol Pharm Bull.* 2008 Jul;31(7):1415-21.

Kim TE, Park SW, Noh G, Lee S. Comparison of skin prick test results between crude allergen extracts from foods and commercial allergen extracts in atopic dermatitis by double-blind placebo-controlled food challenge for milk, egg, and soybean. *Yonsei Med J.* 2002 Oct;43(5):613-20.

Kim YG, Moon JT, Lee KM, Chon NR, Park H. The effects of probiotics on symptoms of irritable bowel syn-drome. *Korean J Gastroenterol.* 2006 Jun;47(6):413-9.

Kim YH, Kim KS, Han CS, Yang HC, Park SH, Ko KI, Lee SH, Kim KH, Lee NH, Kim JM, Son K. Inhibitory effects of natural plants of Jeju Island on elastase and MMP-1 expression. *Int J Cosmet Sci.* 2007 Dec;29(6):487-8.

Kimata H. Differential effects of laughter on allergen-specific immunoglobulin and neurotrophin levels in tears. *Percept Mot Skills.* 2004 Jun;98(3 Pt 1):901-8.

Kimata H. Effect of viewing a humorous vs. nonhumorous film on bronchial responsiveness in patients with bronchial asthma. *Physiol Behav.* 2004 Jun;81(4):681-4.

Kimata H. Emotion with tears decreases allergic responses to latex in atopic eczema patients with latex allergy. *J Psychosom Res.* 2006 Jul;61(1):67-9.

Kimata H. Increase in dermcidin-derived peptides in sweat of patients with atopic eczema caused by a humorous video. *J Psychosom Res.* 2007 Jan;62(1):57-9.

Kimata H. Laughter counteracts enhancement of plasma neurotrophin levels and allergic skin wheal responses by mobile phone-mediated stress. *Behav Med.* 2004 Winter;29(4):149-52.

Kimata H. Modulation of fecal polyamines by viewing humorous films in patients with atopic dermatitis. *Eur J Gastroenterol Hepatol.* 2010 Jun;22(6):724-8.

Kimata H. Reduction of allergic responses in atopic infants by mother's laughter. *Eur J Clin Invest.* 2004 Sep;34(9):645-6.

Kimata H. Viewing a humorous film decreases IgE production by seminal B cells from patients with atopic eczema. *J Psychosom Res.* 2009 Feb;66(2):173-5.

Kimata H. Viewing humorous film improves nighttime wakening in children with atopic dermatitis. *Indian Pediatr.* 2007 Apr;44(4):281-5.

Kimata M, Inagaki N, Nagai H. Effects of luteolin and other flavonoids on IgE-mediated allergic reactions. *Planta Med.* 2000 Feb;66(1):25-9.

Kimata M, Shichijo M, Miura T, Serizawa I, Inagaki N, Nagai H. Effects of luteolin, quercetin and baicalein on immunoglobulin E-mediated mediator release from human cultured mast cells. *Clin Exp Allergy.* 2000 Apr;30(4):501-8.

Kimbel WH, Delezene LK. "Lucy" redux: A review of research on Australopithecus afarensis. Am J Phys Anthropol. 2009;140(Suppl 49):2 – 48.

Kimmatkar N, Thawani V, Hingorani L, Khiyani R. Efficacy and tolerability of Boswellia serrata extract in treatment of osteoarthritis of knee – a randomized double blind placebo controlled trial. *Phytomedicine.* 2003 Jan;10(1):3-7.

Kimura-Kuroda J, Komuta Y, Kuroda Y, Hayashi M, Kawano H. Nicotine-like effects of the neonicotinoid insecticides acetami-prid and imidacloprid on cerebellar neurons from neonatal rats. PLoS One. 2012;7(2):e32432.

Kinaciyan T, Jahn-Schmid B, Radakovics A, Zwölfer B, Schreiber C, Francis JN, Ebner C, Bohle B. Successful sublingual immunotherapy with birch pollen has limited effects on concomitant food allergy to apple and the immune response to the Bet v 1 homolog Mal d 1. *J Allergy Clin Immunol.* 2007 Apr;119(4):937-43.

Kinross JM, von Roon AC, Holmes E, Darzi A, Nicholson JK. The human gut microbiome: implications for future health care. *Curr Gastroenterol Rep.* 2008 Aug;10(4):396-403.

Kippelen P, Larsson J, Anderson SD, Brannan JD, Dahlén B, Dahlén SE. Effect of sodium cromoglycate on mast cell mediators during hyperpnea in athletes. *Med Sci Sports Exerc.* 2010 Oct;42(10):1853-60.

Kirjavainen PV, Arvola T, Salminen SJ, Isolauri E. Aberrant composition of gut microbiota of allergic infants: a target of bifidobacterial therapy at weaning? *Gut.* 2002 Jul;51(1):51-5.

Kirjavainen PV, Salminen SJ, Isolauri E. Probiotic bacteria in the management of atopic disease: underscoring the importance of viability. *J Pediatr Gastroenterol Nutr.* 2003 Feb;36(2):223-7.

Kirpich IA, Solovieva NV, Leikhter SN, Shidakova NA, Lebedeva OV, Sidorov PI, Bazhukova TA, Soloviev AG, Barve SS, McClain CJ, Cave M. Probiotics restore bowel flora and improve liver enzymes in human alcohol-induced liver injury: a pilot study. *Alcohol.* 2008 Dec;42(8):675-82.

Kisiel W, Barszcz B. Further sesquiterpenoids and phenolics from Taraxacum officinale. *Fitoterapia.* 2000 Jun;71(3):269-73.

Kisiel W, Michalska K. Sesquiterpenoids and phenolics from Taraxacum hondoense. *Fitoterapia.* 2005 Sep;76(6):520-4.

Kitajima H, Sumida Y, Tanaka R, Yuki N, Takayama H, Fujimura M. Early administration of Bifidobacterium breve to preterm infants: randomised controlled trial. *Arch Dis Child Fetal Neonatal Ed.* 1997 Mar;76(2):F101-7.

Klarin B, Johansson ML, Molin G, Larsson A, Jeppsson B. Adhesion of the probiotic bacterium Lactobacillus plantarum 299v onto the gut mucosa in critically ill patients: a randomised open trial. *Crit Care.* 2005 Jun;9(3):R285-93.

Klarin B, Molin G, Jeppsson B, Larsson A. Use of the probiotic Lactobacillus plantarum 299 to reduce pathogenic bacteria in the oropharynx of intubated patients: a randomised controlled open pilot study. *Crit Care.* 2008;12(6):R136.

Klein A, Friedrich U, Vogelsang H, Jahreis G. Lactobacillus acidophilus 74-2 and Bifidobacterium animalis subsp lactis DGCC 420 modulate unspecific cellular immune response in healthy adults. *Eur J Clin Nutr.* 2008 May;62(5):584-93.

Klein E, Smith D, Laxminarayan R. Trends in Hospitalizations and Deaths in the United States Associated with Infections Caused by Staphylococcus aureus and MRSA, 1999-2004. *Emerging Infectious Diseases. University of Florida Rel.* 2007 Dec 3.

Klein R, Landau MG. *Healing: The Body Betrayed.* Minneapolis: DCI:Chronimed, 1992.

Klein U, Kanellis MJ, Drake D. Effects of four anticaries agents on lesion depth progression in an in vitro caries model. *Pediatr Dent.* 1999 May-Jun;21(3):176-80.

Klein-Galczinsky C. Pharmacological and clinical effectiveness of a fixed phytogenic combination trembling poplar (Populus tremula), true goldenrod (Solidago virgaurea) and ash (Fraxinus excelsior) in mild to moderate rheumatic complaints. *Wien Med Wochenschr.* 1999;149(8-10):248-53.

Klemola T, Vanto T, Juntunen-Backman K, Kalimo K, Korpela R, Varjonen E. Allergy to soy formula and to extensively hydrolyzed whey formula in infants with cow's milk allergy: a prospective, randomized study with a follow-up to the age of 2 years. *J Pediatr.* 2002 Feb;140(2):219-24.

Klima H, Haas O, Roschger P. Photon emission from blood cells and its possible role in immune system regulation. In: Jezowska-Trzebiatowska B. (ed.): *Photon Emission from Biological Systems. Singapore: World Sci.* 1987:153-169.

# REFERENCES AND BIBLIOGRAPHY

Klingberg TD, Budde BB. The survival and persistence in the human gastrointestinal tract of five potential probiotic lactobacilli consumed as freeze-dried cultures or as probiotic sausage. *Int J Food Microbiol.* 2006 May 25;109(1-2):157-9.

Kloss J. *Back to Eden.* Twin Oaks, WI: Lotus Press, 1939-1999.

Knutson TW, Bengtsson U, Dannaeus A, Ahlstedt S, Knutson L. Effects of luminal antigen on intestinal albumin and hyaluronan permeability and ion transport in atopic patients. *J Allergy Clin Immunol.* 1996 Jun;97(6):1225-32.

Ko J, Busse PJ, Shek L, Noone SA, Sampson HA, Li XM. Effect of Chinese Herbal Formulas on T Cell Responses in Patients with Peanut Allergy or Asthma. *J Allergy Clin Immunol.*2005;115:S34.

Ko J, Lee JI, Munoz-Furlong A, Li XM, Sicherer SH. Use of complementary and alternative medicine by food-allergic patients. *Ann Allergy Asthma Immunol.* 2006;97:365-9.

Kobayashi I, Hamasaki Y, Sato R, Zaitu M, Muro E, Yamamoto S, Ichimaru T, Miyazaki S. Saiboku-To, a herbal extract mixture, selectively inhibits 5-lipoxygenase activity in leukotriene synthesis in rat basophilic leukemia-1 cells. *J Ethnopharmacol.* 1995 Aug 11;48(1):33-41.

Koeth RA, Wang Z, Levison BS, Buffa JA, Org E, Sheehy BT, Britt EB, Fu X, Wu Y, Li L, Smith JD, Didonato JA, Chen J, Li H, Wu GD, Lewis JD, Warrier M, Brown JM, Krauss RM, Tang WH, Bushman FD, Lusis AJ, Hazen SL. Intestinal microbiota metabolism of l-carnitine, a nutrient in red meat, promotes atherosclerosis. Nat Med. 2013 Apr 7.

Kohlhammer Y, Döring A, Schäfer T, Wichmann HE, Heinrich J; KORA Study Group. Swimming pool attendance and hay fever rates later in life. *Allergy.* 2006 Nov;61(11):1305-9. PubMed PMID: 17002706.

Kohlhammer Y, Zutavern A, Rzehak P, Woelke G, Heinrich J. Influence of physical inactivity on the prevalence of hay fever. *Allergy.* 2006 Nov;61(11):1310-5.

Kohn MJ, Schoeninger MJ, Valley JW. Herbivore tooth oxygen isotope compositions: Effects of diet and physiology. Geochim Cosmochim Acta. 1996;60:3889 – 3896.

Kokwaro JO. *Medicinal Plants of East Africa.* Nairobi: Univ of Neirobi Press, 2009.

Koletzko B, Sauerwald U, Keicher U, Saule H, Wawatschek S, Böhles H, Bervoets K, Fleith M, Crozier-Willi G. Fatty acid profiles, antioxidant status, and growth of preterm infants fed diets without or with long-chain polyunsaturated fatty acids. A randomized clinical trial. Eur J Nutr. 2003 Oct;42(5):243-53.

Kollaritsch H, Holst H, Grobara P, Wiedermann G. Prevention of traveler's diarrhea with *Saccharomyces boulardii.* Results of a placebo controlled double-blind study. *Fortschr Med.* 1993 Mar 30;111(9):152-6.

Kong LF, Guo LH, Zheng XY. Effect of yiqi bushen huoxue herbs in treating children asthma and on levels of nitric oxide, endothelin-1 and serum endothelial cells. *Zhongguo Zhong Xi Yi Jie He Za Zhi.* 2001 Sep;21(9):667-9.

Koo HN, Hong SH, Song BK, Kim CH, Yoo YH, Kim HM. Taraxacum officinale induces cytotoxicity through TNF-alpha and IL-1alpha secretion in Hep G2 cells. *Life Sci.* 2004 Jan 16;74(9):1149-57.

Koop H, Bachem MG. Serum iron, ferritin, and vitamin B12 during prolonged omeprazole therapy. *J Clin Gastroenterol.* 1992;14:288-92.

Kootstra HS, Vlieg-Boerstra BJ, Dubois AE. Assessment of the reduced allergenic properties of the Santana apple. *Ann Allergy Asthma Immunol.* 2007 Dec;99(6):522-5.

Koren O, Knights D, Gonzalez A, Waldron L, Segata N, Knight R, Huttenhower C, Ley RE. A guide to enterotypes across the human body: meta-analysis of microbial community structures in human microbiome datasets. PLoS Comput Biol. 2013;9(1):e1002863. doi: 10.1371/journal.pcbi.1002863.

Korschunov VM, Smeianov VV, Efimov BA, Tarabrina NP, Ivanov AA, Baranov AE. Therapeutic use of an antibiotic-resistant *Bifidobacterium* preparation in men exposed to high-dose gamma-irradiation. *J Med Microbiol.* 1996 Jan;44(1):70-4.

Kositz C, Schroecksnadel K, Grander G, Schennach H, Kofler H, Fuchs D. High serum tryptophan concentration in pollinosis patients is associated with unresponsiveness to pollen extract therapy. *Int Arch Allergy Immunol.* 2008;147(1):35-40.

Kotowska M, Albrecht P, Szajewska H. *Saccharomyces boulardii* in the prevention of antibiotic-associated diarrhoea in children: a randomized double-blind placebo-controlled trial. *Aliment Pharmacol Ther.* 2005 Mar 1;21(5):583-90.

Kotzampassi K, Giamarellos-Bourboulis EJ, Voudouris A, Kazamias P, Eleftheriadis E. Benefits of a synbiotic formula (Synbiotic 2000Forte) in critically Ill trauma patients: early results of a randomized controlled trial. *World J Surg.* 2006 Oct;30(10):1848-55.

Kotzampassi K, Giamarellos-Bourboulis EJ, Voudouris A, Kazamias P, Eleftheriadis E. Benefits of a synbiotic formula (Synbiotic 2000Forte) in critically Ill trauma patients: early results of a randomized controlled trial. *World J Surg.* 2006 Oct;30(10):1848-55.

Kovács T, Mette H, Per B, Kun L, Schmelczer M, Barta J, Jean-Claude D, Nagy J. Relationship between intestinal permeability and antibodies against food antigens in IgA nephropathy. *Orv Hetil.* 1996 Jan 14;137(2):65-9.

Kowalchik C, Hylton W (eds). *Rodale's Illustrated Encyclopedia of Herbs.* Emmaus, PA: 1987.

Kowalczyk E, Krzesiński P, Kura M, Niedworok J, Kowalski J, Błaszczyk J. Pharmacological effects of flavonoids from Scutellaria baicalensis. *Przegl Lek.* 2006;63(2):95-6.

Kozlowski LT, Mehta NY, Sweeney CT, Schwartz SS, Vogler GP, Jarvis MJ, West RJ. Filter ventilation and nicotine content of tobacco in cigarettes from Canada, the United Kingdom, and the United States. *Tob Control.* 1998 Winter;7(4):369-75.

Krasse P, Carlsson B, Dahl C, Paulsson A, Nilsson A, Sinkiewicz G. Decreased gum bleeding and reduced gingivitis by the probiotic *Lactobacillus reuteri. Swed Dent J.* 2006;30(2):55-60.

Kreig M. *Black Market Medicine.* New York: Bantam, 1968.

417

Kremmyda LS, Vlachava M, Noakes PS, Diaper ND, Miles EA, Calder PC. Atopy Risk in Infants and Children in Relation to Early Exposure to Fish, Oily Fish, or Long-Chain Omega-3 Fatty Acids: A Systematic Review. *Clin Rev Allergy Immunol.* 2009 Dec 9.

Krogulska A, Dynowski J, Wasowska-Królikowska K. Bronchial reactivity in schoolchildren allergic to food. *Ann Allergy Asthma Immunol.* 2010 Jul;105(1):31-8.

Krogulska A, Wasowska-Królikowska K, Dynowski J. Evaluation of bronchial hyperreactivity in children with asthma undergoing food challenges. *Pol Merkur Lekarski.* 2007 Jul;23(133):30-5.

Krogulska A, Wasowska-Królikowska K, Polakowska E, Chrul S. Cytokine profile in children with asthma undergoing food challenges. *J Investig Allergol Clin Immunol.* 2009;19(1):43-8.

Krogulska A, Wasowska-Królikowska K, Polakowska E, Chrul S. Evaluation of receptor expression on immune system cells in the peripheral blood of asthmatic children undergoing food challenges. Int Arch Allergy Immunol. 2009;150(4):377-88. 2009 Jul 1.

Krogulska A, Wasowska-Królikowska K, Trzeźwińska B. Food challenges in children with asthma. *Pol Merkur Lekarski.* 2007 Jul;23(133):22-9.

Kroidl RF, Schwichtenberg U, Frank E. Bronchial asthma due to storage mite allergy. Pneumologie. 2007 Aug;61(8):525-30.

Krueger AP, Reed EJ. Biological impact of small air ions. Science. 1976 Sep 24;193(4259):1209-13.

Kruger K, Kamilli I, Schattenkirchner M. Blastocystis hominis as a rare arthritogenic pathogen. *Z Rheumatol.* 1994 Mar-Apr;53(2):83-5.

Krüger P, Kanzer J, Hummel J, Fricker G, Schubert-Zsilavecz M, Abdel-Tawab M. Permeation of Boswellia extract in the Caco-2 model and possible interactions of its constituents KBA and AKBA with OATP1B3 and MRP2. *Eur J Pharm Sci.* 2009 Feb 15;36(2-3):275-84.

Krzysiek-Maczka G, Targosz A, Ptak-Belowska A, Korbut E, Szczyrk U, Strzalka M, Brzozowski T. Molecular alterations in fibroblasts exposed to Helicobacter pylori: a missing link in bacterial inflammation progressing into gastric carcinogenesis? J Physiol Pharmacol. 2013 Feb;64(1):77-87.

Kubota A, He F, Kawase M, Harata G, Hiramatsu M, Iino H. Diversity of intestinal bifidobacteria in patients with Japanese cedar pollinosis and possible influence of probiotic intervention. *Curr Microbiol.* 2011 Jan;62(1):71-7.

Kubota A, He F, Kawase M, Harata G, Hiramatsu M, Salminen S, Iino H. Lactobacillus strains stabilize intestinal microbiota in Japanese cedar pollinosis patients. *Microbiol Immunol.* 2009 Apr;53(4):198-205.

Kuitunen M, Kukkonen K, Juntunen-Backman K, Korpela R, Poussa T, Tuure T, Haahtela T, Savilahti E. Probiotics prevent IgE-associated allergy until age 5 years in Cesarean-delivered children but not in the total cohort. *J Allergy Clin Immunol.* 2009 Feb;123(2):335-41.

Kuitunen M, Savilahti E, Sarnesto A. Human alpha-lactalbumin and bovine beta-lactoglobulin absorption in infants. *Allergy.* 1994 May;49(5):354-60.

Kuitunen M, Savilahti E. Mucosal IgA, mucosal cow's milk antibodies, serum cow's milk antibodies and gastrointestinal permeability in infants. *Pediatr Allergy Immunol.* 1995 Feb;6(1):30-5.

Kukkonen K, Kuitunen M, Haahtela T, Korpela R, Poussa T, Savilahti E. High intestinal IgA associates with reduced risk of IgE-associated allergic diseases. *Pediatr Allergy Immunol.* 2010 Feb;21(1 Pt 1):67-73.

Kukkonen K, Nieminen T, Poussa T, Savilahti E, Kuitunen M. Effect of probiotics on vaccine antibody responses in infancy – a randomized placebo-controlled double-blind trial. *Pediatr Allergy Immunol.* 2006 Sep;17(6):416-21.

Kukkonen K, Savilahti E, Haahtela T, Juntunen-Backman K, Korpela R, Poussa T, Tuure T, Kuitunen M. Probiotics and prebiotic galacto-oligosaccharides in the prevention of allergic diseases: a randomized, double-blind, placebo-controlled trial. *J Allergy Clin Immunol.* 2007 Jan;119(1):192-8.

Kukkonen K, Savilahti E, Haahtela T, Juntunen-Backman K, Korpela R, Poussa T, Tuure T, Kuitunen M. Long-term safety and impact on infection rates of postnatal probiotic and prebiotic (synbiotic) treatment: randomized, double-blind, placebo-controlled trial. *Pediatrics.* 2008 Jul;122(1):8-12.

Kukkonen K, Savilahti E, Haahtela T, Juntunen-Backman K, Korpela R, Poussa T, Tuure T, Kuitunen M. Probiotics and prebiotic galacto-oligosaccharides in the prevention of allergic diseases: a randomized, double-blind, placebo-controlled trial. *J Allergy Clin Immunol.* 2007 Jan;119(1):192-8.

Kulka M. The potential of natural products as effective treatments for allergic inflammation: implications for allergic rhinitis. *Curr Top Med Chem.* 2009;9(17):1611-24.

Kull I, Bergström A, Lilja G, Pershagen G, Wickman M. Fish consumption during the first year of life and development of allergic diseases during childhood. *Allergy.* 2006 Aug;61(8):1009-15.

Kull I, Melen E, Alm J, Hallberg J, Svartengren M, van Hage M, Pershagen G, Wickman M, Bergström A. Breastfeeding in relation to asthma, lung function, and sensitization in young schoolchildren. *J Allergy Clin Immunol.* 2010 May;125(5):1013-9.

Kullo IJ, Ballantyne CM. Conditional risk factors for atherosclerosis. *Mayo Clin Proc.* 2005 Feb;80(2):219-30.

Kulvinskas V. 1978. Nutritional Evaluation of Sprouts and Grasses. Omango D' Press, Wethersfield, CT.

Kumar A, Panghal S, Mallapur SS, Kumar M, Ram V, Singh BK. Antiinflammatory Activity of Piper longum Fruit Oil. *Indian J Pharm Sci.* 2009 Jul;71(4):454-6.

Kumar A, Saluja AK, Shah UD, Mayavanshi AV. Pharmacological potential of Albizzia lebbeck: A Review. *Pharmacog.* 2007 Jan-May; 1(1) 171-174.

Kumar J, Garg G, Sundaramoorthy E, Prasad PV, Karthikeyan G, Ramakrishnan L, Ghosh S, Sengupta S. Vitamin B12 deficiency is associated with coronary artery disease in an Indian population. Clin Chem Lab Med. 2009;47(3):334-8.

Kumar P, Kumar A. Protective effect of hesperidin and naringin against 3-nitropropionic acid induced Huntington's like symptoms in rats: possible role of nitric oxide. Behav Brain Res. 2010 Jan 5;206(1):38-46.

# REFERENCES AND BIBLIOGRAPHY

Kumar R, Singh BP, Srivastava P, Sridhara S, Arora N, Gaur SN. Relevance of serum IgE estimation in allergic bronchial asthma with special reference to food allergy. *Asian Pac J Allergy Immunol.* 2006 Dec;24(4):191-9.

Kummeling I, Mills EN, Clausen M, Dubakiene R, Pérez CF, Fernández-Rivas M, Knulst AC, Kowalski ML, Lidholm J, Le TM, Metzler C, Mustakov T, Popov T, Potts J, van Ree R, Sakellariou A, Töndury B, Tzannis K, Burney P. The EuroPrevall surveys on the prevalence of food allergies in children and adults: background and study methodology. *Allergy.* 2009 Oct;64(10):1493-7.

Kung HC, Hoyert DL, Xu J, Murphy SL. Deaths: Final Data for 2005. *National Vital Statistics Reports.* 2008;56(10). http://www.cdc.gov/nchs/data/ nvsr/nvsr56/nvsr56_10.pdf. Accessed: 2008 Jun.

Kunisawa J, Kiyono H. Aberrant interaction of the gut immune system with environmental factors in the development of food allergies. *Curr Allergy Asthma Rep.* 2010 May;10(3):215-21.

Kurth T, Barr RG, Gaziano JM, Buring JE. Randomised aspirin assignment and risk of adult-onset asthma in the Women's Health Study. *Thorax.* 2008 Jun;63(6):514-8. 2008 Mar 13.

Kurugöl Z, Koturoğlu G. Effects of *Saccharomyces boulardii* in children with acute diarrhoea. *Acta Paediatr.* 2005 Jan;94(1):44-7.

Kusunoki T, Morimoto T, Nishikomori R, Yasumi T, Heike T, Mukaida K, Fujii T, Nakahata T. Breastfeeding and the prevalence of allergic diseases in schoolchildren: Does reverse causation matter? *Pediatr Allergy Immunol.* 2010 Feb;21(1 Pt 1):60-6.

Kuvaeva IB. Permeability of the gastronintestinal tract for macromolecules in health and disease. *Hum Physiol.* 1979 Mar-Apr;4(2):272-83.

Kuz'mina IaS, Vavilova NN. Kinesitherapy of patients with bronchial asthma and excessive body weight at the early stage of rehabilitation treatment. *Vopr Kurortol Fizioter Lech Fiz Kult.* 2009 Sep-Oct;(5):17-20.

Kuznetsov VF, Iushchuk ND, Iurko LP, Nabokova NIu. Intestinal dysbacteriosis in yersiniosis patients and the possibility of its correction with biopreparations. *Ter Arkh.* 1994;66(11):17-8.

Kuznetsova TA, Shevchenko NM, Zviagintseva TN, Besednova NN. Biological activity of fucoidans from brown algae and the prospects of their use in medicine]. *Antibiot Khimioter.* 2004;49(5):24-30.

Kwan ML, Weltzien E, Kushi LH, Castillo A, Slattery ML, Caan BJ. Dietary patterns and breast cancer recurrence and survival among women with early-stage breast cancer. J Clin Oncol. 2009 Feb 20;27(6):919-26.

Kvamme JM, Wilsgaard T, Florholmen J, Jacobsen BK. Body mass index and disease burden in elderly men and women: the Tromso Study. *Eur J Epidemiol.* 2010 Mar;25(3):183-93. 2010 Jan 20.

L.G. Howes, J.B. Howes and D.C. Knight . Isoflavone therapy for menopausal flushes: A systematic review and meta-analysis. Maturitas. Vol 55, P 203-211.

Lacruz RS, Dean MC, Ramirez-Rozzi F, Bromage TG. Megadontia, striae periodicity and patterns of enamel secretion in Plio-Pleistocene fossil hominins. J Anat. 2008 Aug;213(2):148-58.

Lad V. *Ayurveda: The Science of Self-Healing.* Twin Lakes, WI: Lotus Press.

Laitinen K, Isolauri E. Management of food allergy: vitamins, fatty acids or probiotics? *Eur J Gastroenterol Hepatol.* 2005 Dec;17(12):1305-11.

Laitinen K, Poussa T, Isolauri E; Nutrition, Allergy, Mucosal Immunology and Intestinal Microbiota Group. Probiotics and dietary counselling contribute to glucose regulation during and after pregnancy: a randomised controlled trial. *Br J Nutr.* 2009 Jun;101(11):1679-87.

Lamaison JL, Carnat A, Petitjean-Freytet C. Tannin content and inhibiting activity of elastase in Rosaceae. *Ann Pharm Fr.* 1990;48(6):335-40.

Landmark K, Reikvam A. Do vitamins C and E protect against the development of carotid stenosis and cardiovascular disease? *Tidsskr Nor Laegeforen.* 2005 Jan 20;125(2):159-62.

Laney AS, Cragin LA, Blevins LZ, Sumner AD, Cox-Ganser JM, Kreiss K, Moffatt SG, Lohff CJ. Sarcoidosis, asthma, and asthma-like symptoms among occupants of a historically water-damaged office building. *Indoor Air.* 2009 Feb;19(1):83-90.

Lang CJ, Hansen M, Roscioli E, Jones J, Murgia C, Leigh Ackland M, Zalewski P, Anderson G, Ruffin R. Dietary zinc mediates inflammation and protects against wasting and metabolic derangement caused by sustained cigarette smoke exposure in mice. *Biometals.* 2011 Feb;24(1):23-39. 2010 Aug 29.

Lange NE, Rifas-Shiman SL, Camargo CA Jr, Gold DR, Gillman MW, Litonjua AA. Maternal dietary pattern during pregnancy is not associated with recurrent wheeze in children. *J Allergy Clin Immunol.* 2010 Aug;126(2):250-5, 255.e1-4.

Langhendries JP, Detry J, Van Hees J, Lamboray JM, Darimont J, Mozin MJ, Secretin MC, Senterre J. Effect of a fermented infant formula containing viable bifidobacteria on the fecal flora composition and pH of healthy full-term infants. *J Pediatr Gastroenterol Nutr.* 1995 Aug;21(2):177-81.

Lansley KE, Winyard PG, Bailey SJ, Vanhatalo A, Wilkerson DP, Blackwell JR, Gilchrist M, Benjamin N, Jones AM. Acute dietary nitrate supplementation improves cycling time trial performance. Med Sci Sports Exerc. 2011 Jun;43(6):1125-31.

Lappe FM. *Diet for a Small Planet.* New York: Ballantine, 1971.

Lara-Villoslada F, Sierra S, Boza J, Xaus J, Olivares M. Beneficial effects of consumption of a dairy product containing two probiotic strains, Lactobacillus coryniformis CECT5711 and *Lactobacillus gasseri* CECT5714 in healthy children. *Nutr Hosp.* 2007 Jul-Aug;22(4):496-502.

Larenas-Linnemann D, Matta JJ, Shah-Hosseini K, Michels A, Mösges R. Skin prick test evaluation of Dermatophagoides pteronyssinus diagnostic extracts from Europe, Mexico, and the United States. *Ann Allergy Asthma Immunol.* 2010 May;104(5):420-5.

Larsson SC, Wolk A. Red and processed meat consumption and risk of pancreatic cancer: meta-analysis of prospective studies. Br J Cancer. 2012 Jan 12.

419

Lau BH, Riesen SK, Truong KP, Lau EW, Rohdewald P, Barreta RA. Pycnogenol as an adjunct in the management of childhood asthma. *J Asthma*. 2004;41(8):825-32.

Laubereau B, Filipiak-Pittroff B, von Berg A, Grübl A, Reinhardt D, Wichmann HE, Koletzko S; GINI Study Group. Caesarean section and gastrointestinal symptoms, atopic dermatitis, and sensitisation during the first year of life. *Arch Dis Child*. 2004 Nov;89(11):993-7.

Laurière M, Pecquet C, Bouchez-Mahiout I, Snégaroff J, Bayrou O, Raison-Peyron N, Vigan M. Hydrolysed wheat proteins present in cosmetics can induce immediate hypersensitivities. *Contact Dermatitis*. 2006 May;54(5):283-9.

LaValle JB. *The Cox-2 Connection*. Rochester, VT: Healing Arts, 2001.

Lavilla-Lerma L, Pérez-Pulido R, Martínez-Bueno M, Maqueda M, Valdivia E. Characterization of functional, safety, and gut survival related characteristics of Lactobacillus strains isolated from farmhouse goat's milk cheeses. *Int J Food Microbiol*. 2013 May 15;163(2-3):136-45. doi: 10.1016/j.ijfoodmicro.2013.02.015.

Lazarou J, Pomeranz BH, Corey PN. Incidence of adverse drug reactions in hospitalized patients: a meta-analysis of prospective studies. *JAMA*. 1998 Apr.

Le Chatelier E, Nielsen T, Qin J, Prifti E, Hildebrand F, Falony G, Almeida M, Arumugam M, Batto JM, Kennedy S, Leonard P, Li J, Burgdorf K, Grarup N, Jørgensen T, Brandslund I, Nielsen HB, Juncker AS, Bertalan M, Levenez F, Pons N, Rasmussen S, Sunagawa S, Tap J, Tims S, Zoetendal EG, Brunak S, Clément K, Doré J, Kleerebezem M, Kristiansen K, Renault P, Sicheritz-Ponten T, de Vos WM, Zucker JD, Raes J, Hansen T; MetaHIT consortium, Bork P, Wang J, Ehrlich SD, Pedersen O, Guedon E, Delorme C, Layec S, Khaci G, van de Guchte M, Vandemeulebrouck G, Jamet A, Dervyn R, Sanchez N, Maguin E, Haimet F, Winogradski Y, Cultrone A, Leclerc M, Juste C, Blottière H, Pelletier E, LePaslier D, Artiguenave F, Bruls T, Weissenbach J, Turner K, Parkhill J, Antolin M, Manichanh C, Casellas F, Boruel N, Varela E, Torrejon A, Guarner F, Denariaz G, Derrien M, van Hylckama Vlieg JE, Veiga P, Oozeer R, Knol J, Rescigno M, Brechot C, M'Rini C, Mérieux A, Yamada T. Richness of human gut microbiome correlates with metabolic markers. *Nature*. 2013 Aug 29;500(7464):541-6.

Leal AL, Eslava-Schmalbach J, Alvarez C, Buitrago G, Méndez M; Grupo para el Control de la Resistencia Bacteriana en Bogotá. Endemic tendencies and bacterial resistance markers in third-level hospitals in Bogotá, Colombia. *Rev Salud Publica* (Bogota). 2006 May;8 Suppl 1:59-70.

Lean G. US study links more than 200 diseases to pollution. *London Independent*. 2004 Nov 14.

Leander M, Cronqvist A, Janson C, Uddenfeldt M, Rask-Andersen A. Health-related quality of life predicts onset of asthma in a longitudinal population study. *Respir Med*. 2009 Feb;103(2):194-200.

Lecheler J, Pfannebecker B, Nguyen DT, Petzold U, Munzel U, Kremer HJ, Maus J. Prevention of exercise-induced asthma by a fixed combination of disodium cromoglycate plus reproterol compared with montelukast in young patients. *Arzneimittelforschung*. 2008;58(6):303-9.

Lee E, Haa K, Yook JM, Jin MH, Seo CS, Son KH, Kim HP, Bae KH, Kang SS, Son JK, Chang HW. Anti-asthmatic activity of an ethanol extract from Saururus chinensis. *Biol Pharm Bull*. 2006 Feb;29(2):211-5.

Lee JH, Noh J, Noh G, Kim HS, Mun SH, Choi WS, Cho S, Lee S. Allergen-specific B cell subset responses in cow's milk allergy of late eczematous reactions in atopic dermatitis. *Cell Immunol*. 2010;262(1):44-51.

Lee JY, Kim CJ. Determination of allergenic egg proteins in food by protein-, mass spectrometry-, and DNA-based methods. *J AOAC Int*. 2010 Mar-Apr;93(2):462-77.

Lee KH, Yeh MH, Kao ST, Hung CM, Chen BC, Liu CJ, Yeh CC. Xia-bai-san inhibits lipopolysaccharide-induced activation of intercellular adhesion molecule-1 and nuclear factor-kappa B in human lung cells. *J Ethnopharmacol*. 2009 Jul 30;124(3):530-8.

Lee MC, Lin LH, Hung KL, Wu HY. Oral bacterial therapy promotes recovery from acute diarrhea in children. *Acta Paediatr Taiwan*. 2001 Sep-Oct;42(5):301-5.

Lee SJ, Cho SJ, Park EA. Effects of probiotics on enteric flora and feeding tolerance in preterm infants. *Neonatology*. 2007;91(3):174-9.

Lee SJ, Shim YH, Cho SJ, Lee JW. Probiotics prophylaxis in children with persistent primary vesicoureteral reflux. *Pediatr Nephrol*. 2007 Sep;22(9):1315-20.

Lee TH, Hsueh PR, Yeh WC, Wang HP, Wang TH, Lin JT. Low frequency of bacteremia after endoscopic mucosal resection. *Gastrointest Endosc*. 2000 Aug;52(2):223-5.

Lee YS, Kim SH, Jung SH, Kim JK, Pan CH, Lim SS. Aldose reductase inhibitory compounds from Glycyrrhiza uralensis. *Biol Pharm Bull*. 2010;33(5):917-21.

Lee-Thorp JA, Sponheimer M, Passey BH, de Ruiter DJ, Cerling TE. Stable isotopes in fossil hominin tooth enamel suggest a fundamental dietary shift in the Pliocene. *Philos Trans R Soc Lond B Biol Sci*. 2010 Oct 27;365(1556):3389-96. doi: 10.1098/rstb.2010.0059.

Léger D, Annesi-Maesano I, Carat F, Rugina M, Chanal I, Pribil C, El Hasnaoui A, Bousquet J. Allergic rhinitis and its consequences on quality of sleep: An unexplored area. *Arch Intern Med*. 2006 Sep 18;166(16):1744-8.

Lehmann B. The vitamin D3 pathway in human skin and its role for regulation of biological processes. *Photochem Photobiol*. 2005 Nov-Dec;81(6):1246-51.

Lehto M, Airaksinen L, Puustinen A, Tillander S, Hannula S, Nyman T, Toskala E, Alenius H, Lauerma A. Thaumatin-like protein and baker's respiratory allergy. *Ann Allergy Asthma Immunol*. 2010 Feb;104(2):139-46.

Leistner R, Meyer E, Gastmeier P, Pfeifer Y, Eller C, Dem P, Schwab F. Risk Factors Associated with the Community-Acquired Colonization of Extended-Spectrum Beta-Lactamase (ESBL) Positive Escherichia Coli. An Exploratory Case-Control Study. *PLoS One*. 2013 Sep 11;8(9):e74323. doi: 10.1371/journal.pone.0074323.

Leistner R, Meyer E, Gastmeier P, Pfeifer Y, Eller C, Dem P, Schwab F. Risk Factors Associated with the Community-Acquired Colonization of Extended-Spectrum Beta-Lactamase (ESBL) Positive Escherichia Coli. An Exploratory Case-Control Study. PLoS One. 2013 Sep 11;8(9):e74323. doi: 10.1371/journal.pone.0074323.

Leitzmann C. Vegetarian diets: what are the advantages? *Forum Nutr.* 2005;(57):147-56.

Léonard R, Wopfner N, Pabst M, Stadlmann J, Petersen BO, Duus JO, Himly M, Radauer C, Gadermaier G, Razzazi-Fazeli E, Ferreira F, Altmann F. A new allergen from ragweed (Ambrosia artemisiifolia) with homology to art v 1 from mugwort. *J Biol Chem.* 2010 Aug 27;285(35):27192-200.

Lerman RH, Minich DM, Darland G, Lamb JJ, Chang JL, Hsi A, Bland JS, Tripp ML. Subjects with elevated LDL cholesterol and metabolic syndrome benefit from supplementation with soy protein, phytosterols, hops rho iso-alpha acids, and Acacia nilotica proanthocyanidins. J Clin Lipidol. 2010 Jan-Feb;4(1):59-68.

Lerman-Garber I, Ichazo-Cerro S, Zamora-González J, Cardoso-Saldaña J, Posadas-Romero C. Effect of a high-monounsaturated fat diet enriched with avocado in NIDDM patients. Diabetes Care. 1994 Apr;17(4):311-5.

Leu YL, Shi LS, Damu AG. Chemical constituents of Taraxacum formosanum. Chem *Pharm Bull.* 2003 May;51(5):599-601.

Leu YL, Wang YL, Huang SC, Shi LS. Chemical constituents from roots of Taraxacum formosanum. *Chem Pharm Bull.* 2005 Jul;53(7):853-5.

Leung DY, Sampson HA, Yunginger JW, Burks AW Jr, Schneider LC, Wortel CH, Davis FM, Hyun JD, Shanahan WR Jr, Avon Longitudinal Study of Parents and Children Study Team. Effect of anti-IgE therapy in patients with peanut allergy. N Engl J Med. 2003 Mar 13;348(11):986-93.

Leung DY, Shanahan WR Jr, Li XM, Sampson HA. New approaches for the treatment of anaphylaxis. *Novartis Found Symp.* 2004;257:248-60; discussion 260-4, 276-85.

Levin NE, Cerling TE, Passey BH, Harris JM, Ehleringer JR. Stable isotopes as a proxy for paleoaridity. Proc Natl Acad Sci USA. 2006;103:11201 – 11205.

Levin NE, *et al.* Quade J, Wynn JG, editors. Herbivore enamel carbon isotopic composition and the environmental context of Ardipithecus at Gona, Ethiopia. Geol Soc Am Special Paper. 2008;446:215 – 234.

Levin NE, *et al.* Quade J, Wynn JG, editors. Herbivore enamel carbon isotopic composition and the environmental context of Ardipithecus at Gona, Ethiopia. Geol Soc Am Special Paper. 2008;446:215 – 234.

Lewerin C, Jacobsson S, Lindstedt G, Nilsson-Ehle H. Serum biomarkers for atrophic gastritis and antibodies against Helicobacter pylori in the elderly: Implications for vitamin B12, folic acid and iron status and response to oral vitamin therapy. Scand J Gastroenterol. 2008;43(9):1050-6.

Lewerin C, Jacobsson S, Lindstedt G, Nilsson-Ehle H. Serum biomarkers for atrophic gastritis and antibodies against Helicobacter pylori in the elderly: Implications for vitamin B12, folic acid and iron status and response to oral vitamin therapy. *Scand J Gastroenterol.* 2008;43(9):1050-6.

Lewis SA, Grimshaw KE, Warner JO, Hourihane JO. The promiscuity of immunoglobulin E binding to peanut allergens, as determined by Western blotting, correlates with the severity of clinical symptoms. *Clin Exp Allergy.* 2005 Jun;35(6):767-73.

Lewis WH, Elvin-Lewis MPF. *Medical Botany: Plants Affecting Man's Health.* New York: Wiley, 1977.

Lewontin R. *The Genetic Basis of Evolutionary Change.* New York: Columbia Univ Press, 1974.

Ley RE, Turnbaugh PJ, Klein S, Gordon JI. Microbial ecology: human gut microbes associated with obesity. Nature. 2006;444:1022 – 1023.

Leyel CF. *Culpeper's English Physician & Complete Herbal.* Hollywood, CA: Wilshire, 1971.

Leynadier F. Mast cells and basophils in asthma. Ann Biol Clin (Paris). 1989;47(6):351-6.

Leyva DR, Zahradka P, Ramjiawan B, Guzman R, Aliani M, Pierce GN. The effect of dietary flaxseed on improving symptoms of cardiovascular disease in patients with peripheral artery disease: rationale and design of the FLAX-PAD randomized controlled trial. Contemp Clin Trials. 2011 Sep;32(5):724-30.

Li J, Sun B, Huang Y, Lin X, Zhao D, Tan G, Wu J, Zhao H, Cao L, Zhong N. A multicentre study assessing the prevalence of sensitizations in patients with asthma and/or rhinitis in China. *Allergy.* 2009;64:1083-1092.

Li MH, Zhang HL, Yang BY. Effects of ginkgo leaf concentrated oral liquor in treating asthma. *Zhongguo Zhong Xi Yi Jie He Za Zhi.* 1997 Apr;17(4):216-8. 5.

Li Q, Li XL, Yang X, Bao JM, Shen XH. Effects of antiallergic herbal agents on cystic fibrosis transmembrane conductance regulator in nasal mucosal epithelia of allergic rhinitis rabbits. *Chin Med J (Engl).* 2009 Dec 20;122(24):3020-4.

Li S, Li W, Wang Y, Asada Y, Koike K. Prenylflavonoids from Glycyrrhiza uralensis and their protein tyrosine phosphatase-1B inhibitory activities. *Bioorg Med Chem Lett.* 2010 Sep 15;20(18):5398-401.

Li XM, Huang CK, Zhang TF, Teper AA, Srivastava K, Schofield BH, Sampson HA. The chinese herbal medicine formula MSSM-002 suppresses allergic airway hyperreactivity and modulates TH1/TH2 responses in a murine model of allergic asthma. *J Allergy Clin Immunol.* 2000;106:660-8.

Li XM, Srivastava K. Traditional Chinese medicine for the therapy of allergic disorders. *Curr Opin Otolaryngol Head Neck Surg.* 2006 Jun;14(3):191-6.

Li XM, Zhang TF, Huang CK, Srivastava K, Teper AA, Zhang L, Schofield BH, Sampson HA. Food Allergy Herbal Formula-1 (FAHF-1) blocks peanut-induced anaphylaxis in a murine model. *J Allergy Clin Immunol.* 2001;108:639-46.

Li XM, Zhang TF, Sampson H, Zou ZM, Beyer K, Wen MC, Schofield B. The potential use of Chinese herbal medicines in treating allergic asthma. *Ann Allergy Asthma Immunol.* 2004;93:S35-S44.

Li XM. Beyond allergen avoidance: update on developing therapies for peanut allergy. *Curr Opin Allergy Clin Immunol.* 2005;5:287-92.

421

Li YQ, Yuan W, Zhang SL. Clinical and experimental study of xiao er ke cuan ling oral liquid in the treatment of infantile bronchopneumonia. *Zhongguo Zhong Xi Yi Jie He Za Zhi.* 1992 Dec;12(12):719-21, 737, 708.

Lied GA, Lillestol K, Valeur J, Berstad A. Intestinal B cell-activating factor: an indicator of non-IgE-mediated hypersensitivity reactions to food? *Aliment Pharmacol Ther.* 2010 Jul;32(1):66-73.

Lieske JC, Goldfarb DS, De Simone C, Regnier C. Use of a probiotic to decrease enteric hyperoxaluria. *Kidney Int.* 2005 Sep;68(3):1244-9.

Lillestol K, Berstad A, Lind R, Florvaag E, Arslan Lied G, Tangen T. Anxiety and depression in patients with self-reported food hypersensitivity. *Gen Hosp Psychiatry.* 2010 Jan-Feb;32(1):42-8.

Lima JA, Fischer GB, Sarria EE, Mattiello R, Solé D. Prevalence of and risk factors for wheezing in the first year of life. *J Bras Pneumol.* 2010 Oct;36(5):525-31. English, Portuguese.

Limb SL, Brown KC, Wood RA, Wise RA, Eggleston PA, Tonascia J, Hamilton RG, Adkinson NF Jr. Adult asthma severity in individuals with a history of childhood asthma. *J Allergy Clin Immunol.* 2005 Jan;115(1):61-6.

Lin HC, Hsu CH, Chen HL, Chung MY, Hsu JF, Lien RI, Tsao LY, Chen CH, Su BH. Oral probiotics prevent necrotizing enterocolitis in very low birth weight preterm infants: a multicenter, randomized, controlled trial. *Pediatrics.* 2008 Oct;122(4):693-700.

Lin HC, Su BH, Chen AC, Lin TW, Tsai CH, Yeh TF, Oh W. Oral probiotics reduce the incidence and severity of necrotizing enterocolitis in very low birth weight infants. *Pediatrics.* 2005 Jan;115(1):1-4.

Lin JS, Chiu YH, Lin NT, Chu CH, Huang KC, Liao KW, Peng KC. Different effects of probiotic species/strains on infections in preschool children: A double-blind, randomized, controlled study. *Vaccine.* 2009 Feb 11;27(7):1073-9.

Lin PY, Lai HM. 2006. Bioactive compounds in legumes and their germinated products. J Agric Food Chem. 2006 May 31;54(11):3807-14.

Lin SY, Ayres JW, Winkler W Jr, Sandine WE. Lactobacillus effects on cholesterol: in vitro and in vivo results. *J Dairy Sci.* 1989 Nov;72(11):2885-99.

Lindahl O, Lindwall L, Spångberg A, Stenram A, Ockerman PA. Vegan regimen with reduced medication in the treatment of bronchial asthma. *J Asthma.* 1985;22(1):45-55.

Lindfors K, Blomqvist T, Juuti-Uusitalo K, Stenman S, Venäläinen J, Mäki M, Kaukinen K. Live probiotic Bifido-bacterium lactis bacteria inhibit the toxic effects induced by wheat gliadin in epithelial cell culture. Clin Exp Immunol. 2008 Jun;152(3):552-8. doi: 10.1111/j.1365-2249.2008.03635.x.

Ling WH, Hänninen O. Shifting from a conventional diet to an uncooked vegan diet reversibly alters fecal hydrolytic activities in humans. *J Nutr.* 1992 Apr;122(4):924-30.

Lininger S, Gaby A, Austin S, Brown D, Wright J, Duncan A. *The Natural Pharmacy.* New York: Three Rivers, 1999.

Link LB, Canchola AJ, Bernstein L, Clarke CA, Stram DO, Ursin G, Horn-Ross PL. Dietary patterns and breast cancer risk in the California Teachers Study cohort. Am J Clin Nutr. 2013 Oct 9.

Linsalata M, Russo F, Berloco P, Caruso ML, Matteo GD, Cifone MG, Simone CD, Ierardi E, Di Leo A. The influence of *Lactobacillus brevis* on ornithine decarboxylase activity and polyamine profiles in *Helicobacter pylori*-infected gastric mucosa. *Helicobacter.* 2004 Apr;9(2):165-72.

Lipkind M. Registration of spontaneous photon emission from virus-infected cell cultures: development of experimental system. *Indian J Exp Biol.* 2003 May;41(5):457-72.

Lipski E. *Digestive Wellness.* Los Angeles, CA: Keats, 2000.

Liu AH, Jaramillo R, Sicherer SH, Wood RA, Bock SA, Burks AW, Massing M, Cohn RD, Zeldin DC. National prevalence and risk factors for food allergy and relationship to asthma: results from the National Health and Nutrition Examination Survey 2005-2006. *J Allergy Clin Immunol.* 2010 Oct;126(4):798-806.e13.

Liu F, Zhang J, Liu Y, Zhang N, Holtappels G, Lin P, Liu S, Bachert C. Inflammatory profiles in nasal mucosa of patients with persistent vs intermittent allergic rhinitis. *Allergy.* 2010 Sep;65(9):1149-57.

Liu GM, Cao MJ, Huang YY, Cai QF, Weng WY, Su WJ. Comparative study of in vitro digestibility of major allergen tropomyosin and other food proteins of Chinese mitten crab (Eriocheir sinensis). *J Sci Food Agric.* 2010 Aug 15;90(10):1614-20.

Liu HY, Giday Z, Moore BF. Possible pathogenetic mechanisms producing bovine milk protein inducible malab-sorption: a hypothesis. *Ann Allergy.* 1977 Jul;39(1):1-7.

Liu J, Zhang J, Shi Y, Grimsgaard S, Alraek T, Fønnebø V. Chinese red yeast rice (Monascus purpureus) for primary hyperlipidemia: a meta-analysis of randomized controlled trials. *Chin Med.* 2006 Nov 23;1:4.

Liu JY, Hu JH, Zhu QG, Li FQ, Wang J, Sun HJ. Effect of matrine on the expression of substance P receptor and inflammatory cytokines production in human skin keratinocytes and fibroblasts. *Int Immunopharmacol.* 2007 Jun;7(6):816-23.

Liu L, Zubik L, Collins FW, Marko M, Meydani M. The antiatherogenic potential of oat phenolic compounds. *Atherosclerosis.* 2004 Jul;175(1):39-49.

Liu Q, Chen X, Yang G, Min X, Deng M. Apigenin inhibits cell migration through MAPK pathways in human bladder smooth muscle cells. *Biocell.* 2011 Dec;35(3):71-9.

Liu T, Valdez R, Yoon PW, Crocker D, Moonesinghe R, Khoury MJ. The association between family history of asthma and the prevalence of asthma among US adults: National Health and Nutrition Examination Survey, 1999-2004. *Genet Med.* 2009 May;11(5):323-8.

Liu X, Beaty TH, Deindl P, Huang SK, Lau S, Sommerfeld C, Fallin MD, Kao WH, Wahn U, Nickel R. Associations between specific serum IgE response and 6 variants within the genes IL4, IL13, and IL4RA in German chil-dren: the German Multicenter Atopy Study. *J Allergy Clin Immunol.* 2004 Mar;113(3):489-95.

Liu XJ, Cao MA, Li WH, Shen CS, Yan SQ, Yuan CS. Alkaloids from Sophora flavescens Aition. *Fitoterapia.* 2010 Sep;81(6):524-7.

Liu Z, Bhattacharyya S, Ning B, Midoro-Horiuti T, Czerwinski EW, Goldblum RM, Mort A, Kearney CM. Plant-expressed recombinant mountain cedar allergen Jun a 1 is allergenic and has limited pectate lyase activity. *Int Arch Allergy Immunol.* 2010;153(4):347-58.

Lloyd JU. *American Materia Medica, Therapeutics and Pharmacognosy.* Portland, OR: Eclectic Medical Publications, 1989-1983.

Lloyd Spencer J. Immunization via the anal mucosa and adjacent skin to protect against respiratory virus infections and allergic rhinitis: a hypothesis. *Med Hypotheses.* 2010 Mar;74(3):542-6.

Lloyd-Still JD, Powers CA, Hoffman DR, Boyd-Trull K, Lester LA, Benisek DC, Arterburn LM. Bioavailability and safety of a high dose of docosahexaenoic acid triacylglycerol of algal origin in cystic fibrosis patients: a randomized, controlled study. *Nutrition.* 2006 Jan;22(1):36-46.

Locke GR 3rd, Talley NJ, Fett SL, Zinsmeister AR, Melton LJ 3rd. Prevalence and clinical spectrum of gastroesophageal reflux: a population-based study in Olmsted County, Minnesota. *Gastroenterology.* 1997 May;112(5):1448-56.

Loguercio C, Abbiati R, Rinaldi M, Romano A, Del Vecchio Blanco C, Coltorti M. Long-term effects of *Enterococcus faecium* SF68 versus lactulose in the treatment of patients with cirrhosis and grade 1-2 hepatic encephalopathy. *J Hepatol.* 1995 Jul;23(1):39-46.

Loguercio C, Del Vecchio Blanco C, Coltorti M. Enterococcus lactic acid bacteria strain SF68 and lactulose in hepatic encephalopathy: a controlled study. *J Int Med Res.* 1987 Nov-Dec;15(6):335-43.

Loizzo MR, Saab AM, Tundis R, Statti GA, Menichini F, Lampronti I, Gambari R, Cinatl J, Doerr HW. Phytochemical analysis and in vitro antiviral activities of the essential oils of seven Lebanon species. *Chem Biodivers.* 2008 Mar;5(3):461-70.

Lomax AR, Calder PC. Probiotics, immune function, infection and inflammation: a review of the evidence from studies conducted in humans. *Curr Pharm Des.* 2009;15(13):1428-518.

Longo G, Barbi E, Berti I, Meneghetti R, Pittalis A, Ronfani L, Ventura A. Specific oral tolerance induction in children with very severe cow's milk-induced reactions. *J Allergy Clin Immunol.* 2008 Feb;121(2):343-7.

Lopes EA, Fanelli-Galvani A, Prisco CC, Gonçalves RC, Jacob CM, Cabral AL, Martins MA, Carvalho CR. Assessment of muscle shortening and static posture in children with persistent asthma. *Eur J Pediatr.* 2007 Jul;166(7):715-21.

López A, El-Naggar T, Dueñas M, Ortega T, Estrella I, Hernández T, Gómez-Serranillos MP, Palomino OM, Carretero ME. Effect of cooking and germination on phenolic composition and biological properties of dark beans (Phaseolus vulgaris L.). Food Chem. 2013 May 1;138(1):547-55.

López A, El-Naggar T, Dueñas M, Ortega T, Estrella I, Hernández T, Gómez-Serranillos MP, Palomino OM, Carretero ME. Effect of cooking and germination on phenolic composition and biological properties of dark beans (Phaseolus vulgaris L.). Food Chem. 2013 May 1;138(1):547-55.

López N, de Barros-Mazón S, Vilela MM, Silva CM, Ribeiro JD. Genetic and environmental influences on atopic immune response in early life. *J Investig Allergol Clin Immunol.* 1999 Nov-Dec;9(6):392-8.

Lopez-Garcia E, Schulze MB, Meigs JB, Manson JE, Rifai N, Stampfer MJ, Willett WC, Hu FB. Consumption of trans fatty acids is related to plasma biomarkers of inflammation and endothelial dysfunction. *J Nutr.* 2005 Mar;135(3):562-6.

Lopez-Garcia E, Schulze MB, Meigs JB, Manson JE, Rifai N, Stampfer MJ, Willett WC, Hu FB. Consumption of trans fatty acids is related to plasma biomarkers of inflammation and endothelial dysfunction. *J Nutr.* 2005 Mar;135(3):562-6.

Lorea Baroja M, Kirjavainen PV, Hekmat S, Reid G. Anti-inflammatory effects of probiotic yogurt in inflammatory bowel disease patients. *Clin Exp Immunol.* 2007 Sep;149(3):470-9.

Lu J, Wang CM, Xu ST, Song LL, Zhao XM, Wang QY, Sheng GY. Role of helicobacter pylori infection in the pathogenesis and clinical outcome of childhood acute idiopathic thrombocytopenic purpura. Zhonghua Xue Ye Xue Za Zhi. 2013 Jan;34(1):41-4.

Lu MK, Shih YW, Chang Chien TT, Fang LH, Huang HC, Chen PS. α-Solanine inhibits human melanoma cell migration and invasion by reducing matrix metalloproteinase-2/9 activities. *Biol Pharm Bull.* 2010;33(10):1685-91.

Lu Y, Zhang C, Bucheli P, Wei D. Citrus flavonoids in fruit and traditional Chinese medicinal food ingredients in China. Plant Foods Hum Nutr. 2006 Jun;61(2):57-65.

Lucas A, Brooke OG, Cole TJ, Morley R, Bamford MF. Food and drug reactions, wheezing, and eczema in preterm infants. *Arch Dis Child.* 1990 Apr;65(4):411-5. 8; .

Lucendo AJ, Lucendo B. An update on the immunopathogenesis of eosinophilic esophagitis. *Expert Rev Gastroenterol Hepatol.* 2010 Apr;4(2):141-8.

Lunardi AC, Marques da Silva CC, Rodrigues Mendes FA, Marques AP, Stelmach R, Fernandes Carvalho CR. Musculoskeletal dysfunction and pain in adults with asthma. *J Asthma.* 2011 Feb;48(1):105-10.

Lustig RH, Schmidt LA, Brindis CD. Public health: The toxic truth about sugar. Nature. 2012 Feb 1;482(7383):27-9.

Lv X, Xi L, Han D, Zhang L. Evaluation of the psychological status in seasonal allergic rhinitis patients. *ORL J Otorhinolaryngol Relat Spec.* 2010;72(2):84-90.

Lykken DT, Tellegen A, DeRubeis R: Volunteer bias in twin research: the rule of two-thirds. *Soc Biol* 1978, 25(1): 1-9. Phillips DI: Twin studies in medical research: can they tell us whether diseases are genetically determined? *Lancet* 1993;341(8851): 1008-1009.

Lythcott GI. Anaphylaxis to viomycin. *Am Rev Tuberc.* 1957 Jan;75(1):135-8.

Ma J, Xiao L, Knowles SB. Obesity, insulin resistance and the prevalence of atopy and asthma in US adults. Allergy. 2010 Nov;65(11):1455-63.

Ma XP, Muzhapaer D. Efficacy of sublingual immunotherapy in children with dust mite allergic asthma. *Zhongguo Dang Dai Er Ke Za Zhi.* 2010 May;12(5):344-7.

Mabey R, ed. *The New Age Herbalist.* New York: Simon & Schuster, 1941.

MacDonald R, Guo J, Copeland J, Browning J, Sleper D, Rottinghaus G, Berhow M. 2005. Environmental Influences on Isoflavones and Saponins in Soybeans and Their Role in Colon Cancer. J. Nutr. 135:1239-1242, May.

Macdonald TT, Monteleone G. Immunity, inflammation, and allergy in the gut. *Science.* 2005 Mar 25;307(5717):1920-5.

Macho GA, Shimizu D, Jiang Y, Spears IR. Australopithecus anamensis: A finite-element approach to studying the functional adaptations of extinct hominins. Anat Rec. 2005;283A:310 – 318.

Macho GA, Shimizu D. Kinematic parameters inferred from enamel microstructure: new insights into the diet of Australopithecus anamensis. J Hum Evol. 2010 Jan;58(1):23-32.

Maciorkowska E, Kaczmarski M, Andrzej K. Endoscopic evaluation of upper gastrointestinal tract mucosa in children with food hypersensitivity. *Med Wieku Rozwoj.* 2000 Jan-Mar;4(1):37-48.

Mackerras D, Cunningham J, Hunt A, Brent P. Re: "effect of supplemental folic acid in pregnancy on childhood asthma: a prospective birth cohort study". *Am J Epidemiol.* 2010 Mar 15;171(6):746-7; author reply 747. 2010 Feb 9.

MacRedmond R, Singhera G, Attridge S, Bahzad M, Fava C, Lai Y, Hallstrand TS, Dorscheid DR. Conjugated linoleic acid improves airway hyper-reactivity in overweight mild asthmatics. *Clin Exp Allergy.* 2010 Jul;40(7):1071-8.

Macsali F, Real FG, Omenaas ER, Bjorge L, Janson C, Franklin K, Svanes C. Oral contraception, body mass index, and asthma: a cross-sectional Nordic-Baltic population survey. *J Allergy Clin Immunol.* 2009 Feb;123(2):391-7.

Madden JA, Plummer SF, Tang J, Garaiova I, Plummer NT, Herbison M, Hunter JO, Shimada T, Cheng L, Shirakawa T. Effect of probiotics on preventing disruption of the intestinal microflora following antibiotic therapy: a double-blind, placebo-controlled pilot study. *Int Immunopharmacol.* 2005 Jun;5(6):1091-7.

Madupu R, Szpakowski S, Nelson KE. Microbiome in human health and disease. Sci Prog. 2013;96(Pt 2):153-70.

Maeda N, Inomata N, Morita A, Kirino M, Ikezawa Z. Correlation of oral allergy syndrome due to plant-derived foods with pollen sensitization in Japan. *Ann Allergy Asthma Immunol.* 2010 Mar;104(3):205-10.

Maes HH, Silberg JL, Neale MC, Eaves LJ. Genetic and cultural transmission of antisocial behavior: an extended twin parent model. *Twin Res Hum Genet.* 2007 Feb;10(1):136-50.

Mah KW, Chin VI, Wong WS, Lay C, Tannock GW, Shek LP, Aw MM, Chua KY, Wong HB, Panchalingham A, Lee BW. Effect of a milk formula containing probiotics on the fecal microbiota of asian infants at risk of atopic diseases. Pediatr Res. 2007 Dec;62(6):674-9.

Mai XM, Kull I, Wickman M, Bergström A. Antibiotic use in early life and development of allergic diseases: respiratory infection as the explanation. *Clin Exp Allergy.* 2010 Aug;40(8):1230-7.

Mainardi T, Kapoor S, Bielory L. Complementary and alternative medicine: herbs, phytochemicals and vitamins and their immunologic effects. *J Allergy Clin Immunol.* 2009 Feb;123(2):283-94; quiz 295-6.

Majamaa H, Isolauri E, Saxelin M, Vesikari T. Lactic acid bacteria in the treatment of acute rotavirus gastroenteritis. *J Pediatr Gastroenterol Nutr.* 1995 Apr;20(3):333-8.

Majamaa H, Isolauri E. Probiotics: a novel approach in the management of food allergy. *J Allergy Clin Immunol.* 1997 Feb;99(2):179-85.

Maki KC, Gibson GR, Dickmann RS, Kendall CW, Oliver Chen CY, Costabile A, Comelli EM, McKay DL, Almeida NG, Jenkins D, Zello GA, Blumberg JB. Digestive and physiologic effects of a wheat bran extract, arabino-xylan-oligosaccharide, in breakfast cereal. Nutrition. 2012 Jul 6.

Maki KC, Gibson GR, Dickmann RS, Kendall CW, Oliver Chen CY, Costabile A, Comelli EM, McKay DL, Almeida NG, Jenkins D, Zello GA, Blumberg JB. Digestive and physiologic effects of a wheat bran extract, arabino-xylan-oligosaccharide, in breakfast cereal. Nutrition. 2012 Jul 6.

Mäkivuokko H, Lahtinen SJ, Wacklin P, Tuovinen E, Tenkanen H, Nikkilä J, Björklund M, Aranko K, Ouwehand AC, Mättö J. Association between the ABO blood group and the human intestinal microbiota composition. BMC Microbiol. 2012 Jun 6;12:94. doi: 10.1186/1471-2180-12-94.

Makrides M, Neumann M, Gibson R. Effect of maternal docosahexaenoic acid (DHA) supplementation on breast milk composition. *Europ Jrnl of Clin Nutr.* 1996;50:352-357.

Maliakal PP, Wanwimolruk S. Effect of herbal teas on hepatic drug metabolizing enzymes in rats. *J Pharm Pharmacol.* 2001 Oct;53(10):1323-9.

Mälkönen T, Alanko K, Jolanki R, Luukkonen R, Aalto-Korte K, Lauerma A, Susitaival P. Long-term follow-up study of occupational hand eczema. Br J Dermatol. 2010 Aug 13.

Mallol J, Solé D, Baeza-Bacab M, Aguirre-Camposano V, Soto-Quiros M, Baena-Cagnani C; Latin American ISAAC Group. Regional variation in asthma symptom prevalence in Latin American children. *J Asthma.* 2010 Aug;47(6):644-50.

Maneechotesuwan K, Supawita S, Kasetsinsombat K, Wongkajornsilp A, Barnes PJ. Sputum indoleamine-2, 3-dioxygenase activity is increased in asthmatic airways by using inhaled corticosteroids. *J Allergy Clin Immunol.* 2008 Jan;121(1):43-50.

Manley KJ, Fraenkel MB, Mayall BC, Power DA. Probiotic treatment of vancomycin-resistant enterococci: a randomised controlled trial. *Med J Aust.* 2007 May 7;186(9):454-7.

Mansfield LE, Posey CR. Daytime sleepiness and cognitive performance improve in seasonal allergic rhinitis treated with intranasal fluticasone propionate. *Allergy Asthma Proc.* 2007 Mar-Apr;28(2):226-9.

Månsson HL. Fatty acids in bovine milk fat. *Food Nutr Res.* 2008;52. doi: 10.3402/fnr.v52i0.1821.

424

Manthey JA, Bendele P. Anti-inflammatory activity of an orange peel polymethoxylated flavone, 3',4',3,5,6,7,8-heptamethoxyflavone, in the rat carrageenan/paw edema and mouse lipopolysaccharide-challenge assays. *J Agric Food Chem.* 2008 Oct 22;56(20):9399-403.

Manz F. Hydration and disease. *J Am Coll Nutr.* 2007 Oct;26(5 Suppl):535S-541S.

Manzoni P, Mostert M, Leonessa ML, Priolo C, Farina D, Monetti C, Latino MA, Gomirato G. Oral supplementation with *Lactobacillus casei* subspecies *rhamnosus* prevents enteric colonization by *Candida* species in preterm neonates: a randomized study. *Clin Infect Dis.* 2006 Jun 15;42(12):1735-42.

Marcos A, Wärnberg J, Nova E, Gómez S, Alvarez A, Alvarez R, Mateos JA, Cobo JM. The effect of milk fermented by yogurt cultures plus *Lactobacillus casei* DN-114001 on the immune response of subjects under academic examination stress. *Eur J Nutr.* 2004 Dec;43(6):381-9.

Marcucci F, Duse M, Frati F, Incorvaia C, Marseglia GL, La Rosa M. The future of sublingual immunotherapy. *Int J Immunopathol Pharmacol.* 2009 Oct-Dec;22(4 Suppl):31-3.

Marder K, Gu Y, Eberly S, Tanner CM, Scarmeas N, Oakes D, Shoulson I. Relationship of Mediterranean Diet and Caloric Intake to Phenoconversion in Huntington Disease. *JAMA Neurol.* 2013 Sep 2.

Margioris AN. Fatty acids and postprandial inflammation. *Curr Opin Clin Nutr Metab Care.* 2009 Mar;12(2):129-37.

Maria KW, Behrens T, Brasky TM. Are asthma and allergies in children and adolescents increasing? Results from ISAAC Phase I and Phase II surveys in Munster, Germany. *Allergy.* 2003;58:572-579.

Marin C, Ramirez R, Delgado-Lista J, Yubero-Serrano EM, Perez-Martinez P, Carracedo J, Garcia-Rios A, Rodriguez F, Gutierrez-Mariscal FM, Gomez P, Perez-Jimenez F, Lopez-Miranda J. Mediterranean diet reduces endothelial damage and improves the regenerative capacity of endothelium. *Am J Clin Nutr.* 2011 Feb;93(2):267-74.

Marteau P, Pochart P, Bouhnik Y, Zidi S, Goderel I, Rambaud JC. Survival of *Lactobacillus acidophilus* and *Bifidobacterium* sp. in the small intestine following ingestion in fermented milk. A rational basis for the use of probiotics in man. *Gastroenterol Clin Biol.* 1992;16(1):25-8.

Marth K, Novatchkova M, Focke-Tejkl M, Jenisch S, Jäger S, Kabelitz D, Valenta R. Tracing antigen signatures in the human IgE repertoire. *Mol Immunol.* 2010 Aug;47(14):2323-9.

Martin IR, Wickens K, Patchett K, Kent R, Fitzharris P, Siebers R, Lewis S, Crane J, Holbrook N, Town GI, Smith S. Cat allergen levels in public places in New Zealand. *N Z Med J.* 1998 Sep 25;111(1074):356-8.

Martinez M. Docosahexaenoic acid therapy in docosahexaenoic acid-deficient patients with disorders of peroxisomal biogenesis. *Versicherungsmedizin.* 1996;31 Suppl:145-152

Martínez-Augustin O, Boza JJ, Del Pino JI, Lucena J, Martínez-Valverde A, Gil A. Dietary nucleotides might influence the humoral immune response against cow's milk proteins in preterm neonates. *Biol Neonate.* 1997;71(4):215-23.

Martin-Venegas R, Roig-Perez S, Ferrer R, Moreno JJ. Arachidonic acid cascade and epithelial barrier function during Caco-2 cell differentiation. *J Lipid Res.* 2006 Apr;3.

Martin-Venegas R, Roig-Perez S, Ferrer R, Moreno JJ. Arachidonic acid cascade and epithelial barrier function during Caco-2 cell differentiation. *J Lipid Res.* 2006 Apr;3.

Marushko IuV. The development of a treatment method for streptococcal tonsillitis in children. *Lik Sprava.* 2000 Jan-Feb;(1):79-82.

Maslowski KM, Mackay CR. Diet, gut microbiota and immune responses. *Nat Immunol.* 2011 Jan;12(1):5-9.

Masoli M, Fabian D, Holt S, Beasley R. The global burden of asthma: executive summary of the GINA Dissemination Committee Report. *Allergy.* 2004;59:469-478.

Massey DG, Chien YK, Fournier-Massey G. Mamane: scientific therapy for asthma? *Hawaii Med J.* 1994;53:350-1. 363.

Massicot JG, Cohen SG. Epidemiologic and socioeconomic aspects of allergic diseases. *J Allergy Clin Immunol.* 1986 Nov;78(5 Pt 2):954-8.

Masuno T, Kishimoto S, Ogura T, Honma T, Niitani H, Fukuoka M, Ogawa N. A comparative trial of LC9018 plus doxorubicin and doxorubicin alone for the treatment of malignant pleural effusion secondary to lung cancer. *Cancer.* 1991 Oct 1;68(7):1495-500.

Matasar MJ, Neugut AI. Epidemiology of anaphylaxis in the United States. *Curr Allergy Asthma Rep.* 2003;3:30-35.

Mater DD, Bretigny L, Firmesse O, Flores MJ, Mogenet A, Bresson JL, Corthier G. *Streptococcus thermophilus* and *Lactobacillus delbrueckii* subsp. bulgaricus survive gastrointestinal transit of healthy volunteers consuming yogurt. *FEMS Microbiol Lett.* 2005 Sep 15;250(2):185-7.

Matheson MC, Haydn Walters E, Burgess JA, Jenkins MA, Giles GG, Hopper JL, Abramson MJ, Dharmage SC. Childhood immunization and atopic disease into middle-age – a prospective cohort study. *Pediatr Allergy Immunol.* 2010 Mar;21(2 Pt 1):301-6.

Mathur BN, Shahani KM. Use of total whey constituents for human food. *J Dairy Sci.* 1979 Jan;62(1):99-105.

Matricardi PM, Bockelbrink A, Beyer K, Keil T, Niggemann B, Grüber C, Wahn U, Lau S. Primary versus secondary immunoglobulin E sensitization to soy and wheat in the Multi-Centre Allergy Study cohort. *Clin Exp Allergy.* 2008 Mar;38(3):493-500.

Matsui EC, Matsui W. Higher serum folate levels are associated with a lower risk of atopy and wheeze. *J Allergy Clin Immunol.* 2009 Jun;123(6):1253-9.e2. 2009 May 5.

Matsumoto M, Benno Y. Anti-inflammatory metabolite production in the gut from the consumption of probiotic yogurt containing *Bifidobacterium animalis* subsp. *lactis* LKM512. *Biosci Biotechnol Biochem.* 2006 Jun;70(6):1287-92.

Matsumoto M, Benno Y. Consumption of *Bifidobacterium lactis* LKM512 yogurt reduces gut mutagenicity by increasing gut polyamine contents in healthy adult subjects. *Mutat Res.* 2004 Dec 21;568(2):147-53.

Matsumoto Y, Noguchi E, Imoto Y, Nanatsue K, Takeshita K, Shibasaki M, Arinami T, Fujieda S. Upregulation of IL17RB during natural allergen exposure in patients with seasonal allergic rhinitis. *Allergol Int.* 2011 Mar;60(1):87-92.

Matsuzaki T, Saito M, Usuku K, Nose H, Izumo S, Arimura K, Osame M. A prospective uncontrolled trial of fermented milk drink containing viable *Lactobacillus casei* strain Shirota in the treatment of HTLV-1 associated myelopathy/tropical spastic paraparesis. *J Neurol Sci.* 2005 Oct 15;237(1-2):75-81.

Matthies A, Loh G, Blaut M, Braune A. Daidzein and genistein are converted to equol and 5-hydroxy-equol by human intestinal Slackia isoflavoniconvertens in gnotobiotic rats. *J Nutr.* 2012 Jan;142(1):40-6.

Mattila P, Pihlava JM, Hellström J. Contents of phenolic acids, alkyl- and alkenylresorcinols, and avenanthramides in commercial grain products. *J Agric Food Chem.* 2005 Oct 19;53(21):8290-5.

Mattila P, Renkonen J, Toppila-Salmi S, Parviainen V, Joenväärä S, Alff-Tuomala S, Nicorici D, Renkonen R. Time-series nasal epithelial transcriptomics during natural pollen exposure in healthy subjects and allergic patients. *Allergy.* 2010 Feb;65(2):175-83.

Maurer HR. Bromelain: biochemistry, pharmacology and medical use. *Cell Mol Life Sci.* 2001 Aug;58(9):1234-45.

Mayes MD. Epidemiologic studies of environmental agents and systemic autoimmune diseases. *Environ Health Perspect.* 1999 Oct;107 Suppl 5:743-8.

McAlindon TE. Nutraceuticals: do they work and when should we use them? *Best Pract Res Clin Rheumatol.* 2006 Feb;20(1):99-115.

McCarney RW, Lasserson TJ, Linde K, Brinkhaus B. An overview of two Cochrane systematic reviews of complementary treatments for chronic asthma: acupuncture and homeopathy. *Respir Med.* 2004 Aug;98(8):687-96.

McCarney RW, Linde K, Lasserson TJ. Homeopathy for chronic asthma. *Cochrane Database Syst Rev.* 2004;(1):CD000353.

McConnaughey E. *Sea Vegetables.* Happy Camp, CA: Naturegraph, 1985.

McCullough ML, Gapstur SM, Shah R, Jacobs EJ, Campbell PT. Association between red and processed meat intake and mortality among colorectal cancer survivors. *J Clin Oncol.* 2013 Aug 1;31(22):2773-82. doi: 10.1200/JCO.2013.49.1126.

McDougall J, McDougall M. *The McDougal Plan.* Clinton, NJ: New Win, 1983.

McGuire BW, Sia LL, Haynes JD, Kisicki JC, Gutierrez ML, Stokstad EL. Absorption kinetics of orally administered leucovorin calcium. *NCI Monogr.* 1987;(5):47-56.

McGuire BW, Sia LL, Leese PT, Gutierrez ML, Stokstad EL. Pharmacokinetics of leucovorin calcium after intravenous, intramuscular, and oral administration. *Clin Pharm.* 1988 Jan;7(1):52-8.

McHugh MK, Symanski E, Pompeii LA, Delclos GL. Prevalence of asthma by industry and occupation in the U.S. working population. *Am J Ind Med.* 2010 May;53(5):463-75.

McHugh MK, Symanski E, Pompeii LA, Delclos GL. Prevalence of asthma among adult females and males in the United States: results from the National Health and Nutrition Examination Survey (NHANES), 2001-2004. *J Asthma.* 2009 Oct;46(8):759-66.

McKeever TM, Lewis SA, Cassano PA, Ocké M, Burney P, Britton J, Smit HA. Patterns of dietary intake and relation to respiratory disease, forced expiratory volume in 1 s, and decline in 5-y forced expiratory volume. *Am J Clin Nutr.* 2010 Aug;92(2):408-15. 2010 Jun 16.

McKenzie H, Main J, Pennington CR, Parratt D. Antibody to selected strains of Saccharomyces cerevisiae (baker's and brewer's yeast) and Candida albicans in Crohn's disease. *Gut.* 1990 May;31(5):536-8.

McLachlan CN. beta-casein A1, ischaemic heart disease mortality, and other illnesses. *Med Hypotheses.* 2001 Feb;56(2):262-72.

McNally ME, Atkinson SA, Cole DE. Contribution of sulfate and sulfoesters to total sulfur intake in infants fed human milk. *J Nutr.* 1991 Aug;121(8):1250-4.

McNaught CE, Woodcock NP, Anderson AD, MacFie J. A prospective randomised trial of probiotics in critically ill patients. *Clin Nutr.* 2005 Apr;24(2):211-9.

McNaught CE, Woodcock NP, Anderson AD, MacFie J. A prospective randomised trial of probiotics in critically ill patients. *Clin Nutr.* 2005 Apr;24(2):211-9.

McNaught CE, Woodcock NP, MacFie J, Mitchell CJ. A prospective randomised study of the probiotic *Lactobacillus plantarum* 299V on indices of gut barrier function in elective surgical patients. *Gut.* 2002 Dec;51(6):827-31.

McQuistan TJ, Simonich MT, Pratt MM, Pereira CB, Hendricks JD, Dashwood RH, Williams DE, Bailey GS. Cancer chemoprevention by dietary chlorophylls: A 12,000-animal dose-dose matrix biomarker and tumor study. *Food Chem Toxicol.* 2011 Nov 3.

Meglio P, Bartone E, Plantamura M, Arabito E, Giampietro PG. A protocol for oral desensitization in children with IgE-mediated cow's milk allergy. *Allergy.* 2004 Sep;59(9):980-7.

Mehra PN, Puri HS. Studies on Gaduchi satwa. *Indian J Pharm.* 1969;31:180-2.

Meier B, Shao Y, Julkunen-Tiitto R, Bettschart A, Sticher O. A chemotaxonomic survey of phenolic compounds in Swiss willow species. *Planta Med.* 1992;58:A698.

Meier B, Sticher O, Julkunen-Tiitto R. Pharmaceutical aspects of the use of willows in herbal remedies. *Planta Med.* 1988;54(6):559-560.

Melcion C, Verroust P, Baud L, Ardaillou N, Morel-Maroger L, Ardaillou R. Protective effect of procyanidolic oligomers on the heterologous phase of glomerulonephritis induced by anti-glomerular basement membrane antibodies. *C R Seances Acad Sci III.* 1982 Dec 6;295(12):721-6.

Melcion C, Verroust P, Baud L, Ardaillou N, Morel-Maroger L, Ardaillou R. Protective effect of procyanidolic oligomers on the heterologous phase of glomerulonephritis induced by anti-glomerular basement membrane antibodies. *C R Seances Acad Sci III.* 1982 Dec 6;295(12):721-6.

# REFERENCES AND BIBLIOGRAPHY

Men, Research, And The History Of Hay Fever. *OldAndSold.com*, 1943; Accessed May 16, 2011

Merchant RE and Andre CA. 2001. A review of recent clinical trials of the nutritional supplement Chlorella pyrenoidosa in the treatment of fibromyalgia, hypertension, and ulcerative colitis. *Altern Ther Health Med*. May-Jun;7(3):79-91.

Messina M. Insights gained from 20 years of soy research. *J Nutr*. 2010 Dec;140(12):2289S-2295S. 2010 Oct 27.

Metsälä J, Lundqvist A, Kaila M, Gissler M, Klaukka T, Virtanen SM. Maternal and perinatal characteristics and the risk of cow's milk allergy in infants up to 2 years of age: a case-control study nested in the Finnish population. *Am J Epidemiol*. 2010 Jun 15;171(12):1310-6.

Meyer A, Kirsch H, Domergue F, Abbadi A, Sperling P, Bauer J, Cirpus P, Zank TK, Moreau H, Roscoe TJ, Zahringer U, Heinz E. Novel fatty acid elongases and their use for the reconstitution of docosahexaenoic acid biosynthesis. *J Lipid Res*. 2004 Oct;45(10):1899-909.

Meyer AL, Elmadfa I, Herbacek I, Micksche M. Probiotic, as well as conventional yogurt, can enhance the stimulated production of proinflammatory cytokines. *J Hum Nutr Diet*. 2007 Dec;20(6):590-8.

Meyer AL, Elmadfa I, Herbacek I, Micksche M. Probiotic, as well as conventional yogurt, can enhance the stimulated production of proinflammatory cytokines. *J Hum Nutr Diet*. 2007 Dec;20(6):590-8.

Micha R, Wallace SK, Mozaffarian D. Red and processed meat consump-tion and risk of incident coronary heart disease, stroke, and diabetes mellitus: a systematic review and meta-analysis. *Circulation*. 2010 Jun 1;121(21):2271-83.

Michaelsen KF. Probiotics, breastfeeding and atopic eczema. *Acta Derm Venereol Suppl (Stockh)*. 2005 Nov;(215):21-4.

Michail S. The role of probiotics in allergic diseases. *Allergy Asthma Clin Immunol*. 2009 Oct 22;5(1):5.

Michalska K, Kisiel W. Sesquiterpene lactones from Taraxacum obovatum. *Planta Med*. 2003 Feb;69(2):181-3.

Michelson PH, Williams LW, Benjamin DK, Barnato AE. Obesity, inflammation, and asthma severity in childhood: data from the National Health and Nutrition Examination Survey 2001-2004. *Ann Allergy Asthma Immunol*. 2009 Nov;103(5):381-5.

Michetti P, Dorta G, Wiesel PH, Brassart D, Verdu E, Herranz M, Felley C, Porta N, Rouvet M, Blum AL, Corthésy-Theulaz I. Effect of whey-based culture supernatant of *Lactobacillus acidophilus* (johnsonii) La1 on *Helicobacter pylori* infection in humans. *Digestion*. 1999;60(3):203-9.

Michielutti F, Bertini M, Presciuttini B, Andreotti G. Clinical assessment of a new oral bacterial treatment for children with acute diarrhea. *Minerva Med*. 1996 Nov;87(11):545-50.

Mickleborough TD, Lindley MR, Ray S. Dietary salt, airway inflammation, and diffusion capacity in exercise-induced asthma. *Med Sci Sports Exerc*. 2005 Jun;37(6):904-14.

Mikoluc B, Motkowski R, Karpinska J, Piotrowska-Jastrzebska J. Plasma levels of vitamins A and E, coenzyme Q10, and anti-ox-LDL antibody titer in children treated with an elimination diet due to food hypersensitivity. *Int J Vitam Nutr Res*. 2009 Sep;79(5-6):328-36.

Milgrom P, Ly KA, Roberts MC, Rothen M, Mueller G, Yamaguchi DK. Mutans streptococci dose response to xylitol chewing gum. *J Dent Res*. 2006 Feb;85(2):177-81.

Miller AL. The etiologies, pathophysiology, and alternative/complementary treatment of asthma. *Altern Med Rev*. 2001 Feb;6(1):20-47.

Miller GT. *Living in the Environment*. Belmont, CA: Wadsworth, 1996.

Miller JD, Morin LP, Schwartz WJ, Moore RY. New insights into the mammalian circadian clock. *Sleep*. 1996 Oct;19(8):641-67.

Miller K. Cholesterol and In-Hospital Mortality in Elderly Patients. *Am Family Phys*. 2004 May.

Mindell E, Hopkins V. *Prescription Alternatives*. New Canaan, CT: Keats, 1998.

Miranda H, Outeiro TF. The sour side of neurodegenerative disorders: the effects of protein glycation. *J Pathol*. 2010 May;221(1):13-25.

Mitchell AE, Hong YJ, Koh E, Barrett DM, Bryant DE, Denison RF, Kaffka S. Ten-year comparison of the influence of organic and conventional crop management practices on the content of flavonoids in tomatoes. *J Agric Food Chem*. 2007 Jul 25;55(15):6154-9.

Mittag D, Akkerdaas J, Ballmer-Weber BK, Vogel L, Wensing M, Becker WM, Koppelman SJ, Knulst AC, Helbling A, Hefle SL, Van Ree R, Vieths S. Ara h 8, a Bet v 1-homologous allergen from peanut, is a major allergen in patients with combined birch pollen and peanut allergy. *J Allergy Clin Immunol*. 2004 Dec;114(6):1410-7.

Mittag D, Vieths S, Vogel L, Becker WM, Rihs HP, Helbling A, Wüthrich B, Ballmer-Weber BK. Soybean allergy in patients allergic to birch pollen: clinical investigation and molecular characterization of allergens. *J Allergy Clin Immunol*. 2004 Jan;113(1):148-54.

Miyake Y, Sasaki S, Tanaka K, Hirota Y. Dairy food, calcium and vitamin D intake in pregnancy, and wheeze and eczema in infants. *Eur Respir J*. 2010 Jun;35(6):1228-34. 2009 Oct 19.

Miyazaki T, Kohno S, Mitsutake K, Maesaki S, Tanaka K, Ishikawa N, Hara K. Plasma (1 → >3)-beta-D-glucan and fungal antigenemia in patients with candidemia, aspergillosis, and cryptococcosis. *J Clin Microbiol*. 1995 Dec;33(12):3115-8.

Miyazawa T, Itahashi K, Imai T. Management of neonatal cow's milk allergy in high-risk neonates. *Pediatr Int*. 2009 Aug;51(4):544-7.

Moattari A, Aleyasin S, Arabpour M, Sadeghi S. Prevalence of Human Metapneumovirus (hMPV) in Children with Wheezing in Shiraz-Iran. *Iran J Allergy Asthma Immunol*. 2010 Dec;9(4):250-4.

*Modern Biology*. Austin: Harcourt Brace, 1993.

Moeller AH, Ochman H. Factors that drive variation among gut microbial communities. *Gut Microbes*. 2013 Aug 9;4(5).

427

Mohammad MA, Molloy A, Scott J, Hussein L. Plasma cobalamin and folate and their metabolic markers methylmalonic acid and total homocysteine among Egyptian children before and after nutritional supplementation with the probiotic bacteria *Lactobacillus acidophilus* in yoghurt matrix. *Int J Food Sci Nutr.* 2006 Nov-Dec;57(7-8):470-80.

Mohammed AE, Smit I, Pawelzik E, Keutgen AJ, Horneburg B. Organically grown tomato (Lycopersicon esculentum Mill.): bioactive compounds in the fruit and infection with Phytophthora infestans. J Sci Food Agric. 2011 Dec 7.

Mohan R, Koebnick C, Schildt J, Mueller M, Radke M, Blaut M. Effects of *Bifidobacterium lactis* Bb12 supplementation on body weight, fecal pH, acetate, lactate, calprotectin, and IgA in preterm infants. *Pediatr Res.* 2008 Oct;64(4):418-22.

Mohan R, Koebnick C, Schildt J, Schmidt S, Mueller M, Possner M, Radke M, Blaut M. Effects of *Bifidobacterium lactis* Bb12 supplementation on intestinal microbiota of preterm infants: a double-blind, placebo-controlled, randomized study. *J Clin Microbiol.* 2006 Nov;44(11):4025-31.

Mokhtar N, Chan SC. Use of complementary medicine amongst asthmatic patients in primary care. *Med J Malaysia.* 2006 Mar;61(1):125-7.

Monarca S. Zerbini I, Simonati C, Gelatti U. Drinking water hardness and chronic degenerative diseases. Part II. Cardiovascular diseases. *Ann. Ig.* 2003;15:41-56.

Moneret-Vautrin DA, Kanny G, Thévenin F. Asthma caused by food allergy. *Rev Med Interne.* 1996;17(7):551-7.

Moneret-Vautrin DA, Morisset M. Adult food allergy. *Curr Allergy Asthma Rep.* 2005 Jan;5(1):80-5.

Monks H, Gowland MH, Mackenzie H, Erlewyn-Lajeunesse M, King R, Lucas JS, Roberts G. How do teenagers manage their food allergies? *Clin Exp Allergy.* 2010 Aug 2.

Moorhead KJ, Morgan HC. *Spirulina: Nature's Superfood.* Kailua-Kona, HI: Nutrex, 1995.

Moreira A, Delgado L, Haahtela T, Fonseca J, Moreira P, Lopes C, Mota J, Santos P, Rytilä P, Castel-Branco MG. Physical training does not increase allergic inflammation in asthmatic children. Eur Respir J. 2008 Dec;32(6):1570-5.

Moreira P, Moreira A, Padrão P, Delgado L. The role of economic and educational factors in asthma: evidence from the Portuguese health survey. *Public Health.* 2008 Apr;122(4):434-9. 2007 Oct 17.

Morel AF, Dias GO, Porto C, Simionatto E, Stuker CZ, Dalcol II. Antimicrobial activity of extractives of Solidago microglossa. *Fitoterapia.* 2006 Sep;77(6):453-5.

Morimoto K, Takeshita T, Nanno M, Tokudome S, Nakayama K. Modulation of natural killer cell activity by supplementation of fermented milk containing *Lactobacillus casei* in habitual smokers. *Prev Med.* 2005 May;40(5):589-94.

Morisset M, Moneret-Vautrin DA, Kanny G, Guénard L, Beaudouin E, Flabbée J, Hatahet R. Thresholds of clinical reactivity to milk, egg, peanut and sesame in immunoglobulin E-dependent allergies: evaluation by double-blind or single-blind placebo-controlled oral challenges. *Clin Exp Allergy.* 2003 Aug;33(8):1046-51.

Moss M. *E. coli* Path Shows Flaws in Ground Beef Inspection. NY Times 2009 Oct 3.

Moussaieff A, Shein NA, Tsenter J, Grigoriadis S, Simeonidou C, Alexandrovich AG, Trembovler V, Ben-Neriah Y, Schmitz ML, Fiebich BL, Munoz E, Mechoulam R, Shohami E. Incensole acetate: a novel neuroprotective agent isolated from Boswellia carterii. *J Cereb Blood Flow Metab.* 2008 Jul;28(7):1341-52.

Moyle A. *Nature Cure for Asthma and Hay Fever.* Wellingborough, U.K.: Thorsons, 1978.

Mozafar A. Is there vitamin B12 in plants or not? A plant nutritionist's view. *Veg Nutr.* 1997;1/2:50-52.

Mozaffarian D, Aro A, Willett WC. Health effects of trans-fatty acids: experimental and observational evidence. *Eur J Clin Nutr.* 2009 May;63 Suppl 2:S5-21.

Mugie SM, Di Lorenzo C, Benninga MA. Constipation in childhood. Nat Rev Gastroenterol Hepatol. 2011 Aug 2;8(9):502-11.

Muller H, Lindman AS, Blomfeldt A, Seljeflot I, Pedersen JI. A diet rich in coconut oil reduces diurnal postprandial variations in circulating tissue plasminogen activator antigen and fasting lipoprotein (a) compared with a diet rich in unsaturated fat in women. *J Nutr.* 2003 Nov;133(11):3422-7.

Müller S, Pühl S, Vieth M, Stolte M. Analysis of symptoms and endoscopic findings in 117 patients with histological diagnoses of eosinophilic esophagitis. *Endoscopy.* 2007 Apr;39(4):339-44.

Mullié C, Yazourh A, Thibault H, Odou MF, Singer E, Kalach N, Kremp O, Romond MB. Increased poliovirus-specific intestinal antibody response coincides with promotion of Bifidobacterium longum-infantis and Bifidobacterium breve in infants: a randomized, double-blind, placebo-controlled trial. *Pediatr Res.* 2004 Nov;56(5):791-5.

Mulvihill EE, Assini JM, Lee JK, Allister EM, Sutherland BG, Koppes JB, Sawyez CG, Edwards JY, Telford DE, Charbonneau A, St-Pierre P, Marette A, Huff MW. Nobiletin attenuates VLDL overproduction, dyslipidemia, and atherosclerosis in mice with diet-induced insulin resistance. *Diabetes.* 2011 May;60(5):1446-57.

Munro, I. C., Harwood, M., Hlywka, J. J., Stephen, A. M., Doull, J., Flamm, W. G. & Adlercreutz, H. 2005. Soy isoflavones: a safety review. Nutr. Rev. 61:1-33. J Pediatr Gastroenterol Nutr. Nov;41(5):660-6.

Muralikrishna G, Rao MV. Cereal non-cellulosic polysaccharides: structure and function relationship – an overview. Crit Rev Food Sci Nutr. 2007;47(6):599-610.

Murphy EA, Davis JM, Brown AS, Carmichael MD, Ghaffar A, Mayer EP. Oat beta-glucan effects on neutrophil respiratory burst activity following exercise. Med Sci Sports Exerc. 2007 Apr;39(4):639-44.

Murphy M, Eliot K, Heuertz RM, Weiss E. Whole beetroot consumption acutely improves running performance. J Acad Nutr Diet. 2012 Apr;112(4):548-52.

Murray M and Pizzorno J. *Encyclopedia of Natural Medicine.* 2nd Edition. Roseville, CA: Prima Publishing, 1998.

Murray M, Pizzorno J. 1998. Encyclopedia of Natural Medicine. Prima Publishing, Roseville, CA.

Murray M, Pizzorno J. *Encyclopedia of Natural Medicine.* 2nd Edition. Roseville, CA: Prima Publishing, 1998.

# REFERENCES AND BIBLIOGRAPHY

Murri M, Leiva I, Gomez-Zumaquero JM, Tinahones FJ, Cardona F, Soriguer F, Queipo-Ortuño MI. Gut microbiota in children with type 1 diabetes differs from that in healthy children: a case-control study. BMC Med. 2013 Feb 21;11:46. doi: 10.1186/1741-7015-11-46.

Mustapha A, Jiang T, Savaiano DA. Improvement of lactose digestion by humans following ingestion of unfermented acidophilus milk: influence of bile sensitivity, lactose transport, and acid tolerance of *Lactobacillus acidophilus*. J Dairy Sci. 1997 Aug;80(8):1537-45.

Myllyluoma E, Ahonen AM, Korpela R, Vapaatalo H, Kankuri E. Effects of multispecies probiotic combination on helicobacter pylori infection in vitro. *Clin Vaccine Immunol.* 2008 Sep;15(9):1472-82.

Nadkarni AK, Nadkarni KM. *Indian Materia Medica.* (Vols 1 and 2). Bombay, India: Popular Pradashan, 1908, 1976.

Nagai T, Arai Y, Emori M, Nunome SY, Yabe T, Takeda T, Yamada H. Anti-allergic activity of a Kampo (Japanese herbal) medicine "Sho-seiryu-to (Xiao-Qing-Long-Tang)" on airway inflammation in a mouse model. *Int Immunopharmacol.* 2004 Oct;4(10-11):1353-65.

Nagel G, Linseisen J. Dietary intake of fatty acids, antioxidants and selected food groups and asthma in adults. *Eur J Clin Nutr.* 2005 Jan;59(1):8-15.

Nagel G, Weinmayr G, Kleiner A, Garcia-Marcos L, Strachan DP; ISAAC Phase Two Study Group. Effect of diet on asthma and allergic sensitisation in the International Study on Allergies and Asthma in Childhood (ISAAC) Phase Two. Thorax. 2010 Jun;65(6):516-22.

Naghii MR, Samman S. The role of boron in nutrition and metabolism. *Prog Food Nutr Sci.* 1993 Oct-Dec;17(4):331-49.

Nair PK, Rodriguez S, Ramachandran R, Alamo A, Melnick SJ, Escalon E, Garcia PI Jr, Wnuk SF, Ramachandran C. Immune stimulating properties of a novel polysaccharide from the medicinal plant Tinospora cordifolia. *Int Immunopharmacol.* 2004 Dec 15;4(13):1645-59.

Naito S, Koga H, Yamaguchi A, Fujimoto N, Hasui Y, Kuramoto H, Iguchi A, Kinukawa N; Kyushu University Urological Oncology Group. Prevention of recurrence with epirubicin and *Lactobacillus casei* after transurethral resection of bladder cancer. *J Urol.* 2008 Feb;179(2):485-90.

Nakano T, Shimojo N, Morita Y, Arima T, Tomiita M, Kohno Y. Sensitization to casein and beta-lactoglobulin (BLG) in children with cow's milk allergy (CMA). *Arerugi.* 2010 Feb;59(2):117-22.

Nalepa B, Siemianowska E, Skibniewska KA. Influence of Bifidobacterium bifidum on release of minerals from bread with differing bran content. J Toxicol Environ Health A. 2012;75(1):1-5. doi: 10.1080/15287394.2011.615106.

Napoli, J.E., Brand-Miller, J.C., Conway, P. (2003) Bifidogenic effects of feeding infant formula containing galactooligosaccharides in healthy formula-fed infants. *Asia Pac J Clin Nutr.* 12(Suppl): S60

Nariya M, Shukla V, Jain S, Ravishankar B. Comparison of enteroprotective efficacy of triphala formulations (Indian Herbal Drug) on methotrexate-induced small intestinal damage in rats. *Phytother Res.* 2009 Aug;23(8):1092-8.

Naruszewicz M, Daniewski M, Nowicka G, Kozłowska-Wojciechowska M. Trans-unsaturated fatty acids and acrylamide in food as potential atherosclerosis progression factors. Based on own studies. *Acta Microbiol Pol.* 2003;52 Suppl:75-81.

Naruszewicz M, Johansson ML, Zapolska-Downar D, Bukowska H. Effect of Lactobacillus plantarum 299v on cardiovascular disease risk factors in smokers. *Am J Clin Nutr.* 2002 Dec;76(6):1249-55.

Naruszewicz M, Johansson ML, Zapolska-Downar D, Bukowska H. Effect of *Lactobacillus plantarum* 299v on cardiovascular disease risk factors in smokers. *Am J Clin Nutr.* 2002 Dec;76(6):1249-55.

Narva M, Nevala R, Poussa T, Korpela R. The effect of *Lactobacillus helveticus* fermented milk on acute changes in calcium metabolism in postmenopausal women. *Eur J Nutr.* 2004 Apr;43(2):61-8.

Näse L, Hatakka K, Savilahti E, Saxelin M, Pönkä A, Poussa T, Korpela R, Meurman JH. Effect of long-term consumption of a probiotic bacterium, *Lactobacillus rhamnosus* GG, in milk on dental caries and caries risk in children. *Caries Res.* 2001 Nov-Dec;35(6):412-20.

National Cooperation Group on Childhood Asthma. A nationwide survey in China on prevalence of asthma in urban children. Chin J Pediatr. pp. 123-127.

National Institutes of Health. Third Report of the National Cholesterol Education Program (NCEP) Expert Panel on Detection, Evaluation, and Treatment of High Blood Cholesterol in Adults (PDF), July 2004, The National Institutes of Heath: The National Heart, Lung, and Blood Institute.

National Toxicology Program. Final Report on Carcinogens Background Document for Formaldehyde. *Rep Carcinog Backgr Doc.* 2010 Jan;(10-5981):i-512.

NDL, BHNRC, ARS, USDA. *Oxygen Radical Absorbance Capacity (ORAC) of Selected Foods – 2007.* Beltsville, MD: USDA-ARS. 2007.

Neal EG, Chaffe H, Schwartz RH, Lawson MS, Edwards N, Fitzsimmons G, Whitney A, Cross JH. The ketogenic diet for the treatment of childhood epilepsy: a randomised controlled trial. Lancet Neurol. 2008;7:500–506.

Neff LM, Culiner J, Cunningham-Rundles S, Seidman C, Meehan D, Maturi J, Wittkowski KM, Levine B, Breslow JL. Algal docosahexaenoic acid affects plasma lipoprotein particle size distribution in overweight and obese adults. J Nutr. 2011 Feb;141(2):207-13.

Nentwich I, Michková E, Nevoral J, Urbanek R, Szépfalusi Z. Cow's milk-specific cellular and humoral immune responses and atopy skin symptoms in infants from atopic families fed a partially (pHF) or extensively (eHF) hydrolyzed infant formula. *Allergy.* 2001 Dec;56(12):1144-56.

Nestel PJ. Adulthood – prevention: Cardiovascular disease. Med J Aust. 2002 Jun 3;176(11 Suppl):S118-9.

Nettleton JA, Greany KA, Thomas W, Wangen KE, Adlercreutz H, Kurzer MS. Plasma phytoestrogens are not altered by probiotic consumption in postmenopausal women with and without a history of breast cancer. J Nutr. 2004 Aug;134(8):1998-2003.

Newall CA, Anderson LA, Phillipson JD (eds). *Herbal Medicines: A Guide for Health-Care Professionals.* London: Pharmaceut Press; 1996.

Newmark T, Schulick P. *Beyond Aspirin.* Prescott, AZ: Holm, 2000.

Neyestani TR, Shariatzadeh N, Gharavi A, Kalayi A, Khalaji N. Physiological dose of lycopene suppressed oxidative stress and enhanced serum levels of immunoglobulin M in patients with Type 2 diabetes mellitus: a possible role in the prevention of long-term complications. *J Endocrinol Invest.* 2007 Nov;30(10):833-8.

Ngai SP, Jones AY, Hui-Chan CW, Ko FW, Hui DS. Effect of Acu-TENS on post-exercise expiratory lung volume in subjects with asthma-A randomized controlled trial. *Respir Physiol Neurobiol.* 2009 Jul 31;167(3):348-53. 2009 Jun 18.

Nicholls SJ, Lundman P, Harmer JA, Cutri B, Griffiths KA, Rye KA, Barter PJ, Celermajer DS. Consumption of saturated fat impairs the anti-inflammatory properties of high-density lipoproteins and endothelial function. *J Am Coll Cardiol.* 2006 Aug 15;48(4):715-20.

Nicolaou N, Poorafshar M, Murray C, Simpson A, Winell H, Kerry G, Härlin A, Woodcock A, Ahlstedt S, Custovic A. Allergy or tolerance in children sensitized to peanut: prevalence and differentiation using component-resolved diagnostics. *J Allergy Clin Immunol.* 2010 Jan;125(1):191-7.e1-13.

Nie L, Wise M, Peterson D, Meydani M. Mechanism by which avenanthramide-c, a polyphenol of oats, blocks cell cycle progression in vascular smooth muscle cells. *Free Radic Biol Med.* 2006 Sep 1;41(5):702-8.

Nie L, Wise ML, Peterson DM, Meydani M. Avenanthramide, a polyphenol from oats, inhibits vascular smooth muscle cell proliferation and enhances nitric oxide production. *Atherosclerosis.* 2006 Jun;186(2):260-6.

Niederau C, Göpfert E. The effect of chelidonium- and turmeric root extract on upper abdominal pain due to functional disorders of the biliary system. Results from a placebo-controlled double-blind study. *Med Klin.* 1999 Aug 15;94(8):425-30.

Niedzielin K, Kordecki H, Birkenfeld B. A controlled, double-blind, randomized study on the efficacy of *Lactobacillus plantarum* 299V in patients with irritable bowel syndrome. *Eur J Gastroenterol Hepatol.* 2001 Oct;13(10):1143-7.

Nielsen OH, Jørgensen S, Pedersen N, Justesen T. Microbiological evaluation of jejunal aspirates and faecal samples after oral administration of bifidobacteria and lactic acid bacteria. *J Appl Bacteriol.* 1994 May;76(5):469-74.

Nielsen RG, Bindslev-Jensen C, Kruse-Andersen S, Husby S. Severe gastroesophageal reflux disease and cow milk hypersensitivity in infants and children: disease association and evaluation of a new challenge procedure. *J Pediatr Gastroenterol Nutr.* 2004 Oct;39(4):383-91.

Nies LK, Cymbala AA, Kasten SL, Lamprecht DG, Olson KL. Complementary and alternative therapies for the management of dyslipidemia. *Ann Pharmacother.* 2006 Nov;40(11):1984-92.

Niggemann B, von Berg A, Bollrath C, Berdel D, Schauer U, Rieger C, Haschke-Becher E, Wahn U. Safety and efficacy of a new extensively hydrolyzed formula for infants with cow's milk protein allergy. *Pediatr Allergy Immunol.* 2008 Jun;19(4):348-54.

Nightingale JA, Rogers DF, Hart LA, Kharitonov SA, Chung KF, Barnes PJ. Effect of inhaled endotoxin on induced sputum in normal, atopic, and atopic asthmatic subjects. *Thorax.* 1998 Jul;53(7):563-71.

Niimi A, Nguyen LT, Usmani O, Mann B, Chung KF. Reduced pH and chloride levels in exhaled breath condensate of patients with chronic cough. *Thorax.* 2004 Jul;59(7):608-12.

Nilson HW, Vakil JR, Shahani KM. B-complex vitamin content of cheddar cheese. *J Nutr.* 1965 Aug;86:362-8.

Nimptsch K, Bernstein AM, Giovannucci E, Fuchs CS, Willett WC, Wu K. Dietary intakes of red meat, poultry, and fish during high school and risk of colorectal adenomas in women. *Am J Epidemiol.* 2013 Jul 15;178(2):172-83. doi: 10.1093/aje/kwt099.

Ninan TK, Russell G. Respiratory symptoms and atopy in Aberdeen schoolchildren: evidence from two surveys 25 years apart. *BMJ.* 1992;304:873-875.

Njoroge GN, Bussmann RW. Traditional management of ear, nose and throat (ENT) diseases in Central Kenya. *J Ethnobiol Ethnomed.* 2006 Dec 27;2:54.

Nobaek S, Johansson ML, Molin G, Ahrné S, Jeppsson B. Alteration of intestinal microflora is associated with reduction in abdominal bloating and pain in patients with irritable bowel syndrome. *Am J Gastroenterol.* 2000 May;95(5):1231-8.

Nodake Y, Fukumoto S, Fukasawa M, Sakakibara R, Yamasaki N. Reduction of the immunogenicity of beta-lactoglobulin from cow's milk by conjugation with a dextran derivative. *Biosci Biotechnol Biochem.* 2010;74(4):721-6.

Noh J, Lee JH, Noh G, Bang SY, Kim HS, Choi WS, Cho S, Lee SS. Characterisation of allergen-specific responses of IL-10-producing regulatory B cells (Br1) in Cow Milk Allergy. *Cell Immunol.* 2010;264(2):143-9.

Noone EJ, Roche HM, Nugent AP, Gibney MJ. The effect of dietary supplementation using isomeric blends of conjugated linoleic acid on lipid metabolism in healthy human subjects. *Br J Nutr.* 2002 Sep;88(3):243-51.

Noorbakhsh R, Mortazavi SA, Sankian M, Shahidi F, Assarehzadegan MA, Varasteh A. Cloning, expression, characterization, and computational approach for cross-reactivity prediction of manganese superoxide dismutase allergen from pistachio nut. *Allergol Int.* 2010 Sep;59(3):295-304.

Nopchinda S, Varavithya W, Phuapradit P, Sangchai R, Suthutvoravut U, Chantraruksa V, Haschke F. Effect of bifidobacterium Bb12 with or without *Streptococcus thermophilus* supplemented formula on nutritional status. *J Med Assoc Thai.* 2002 Nov;85 Suppl 4:S1225-31.

Nordmann P, Poirel L. Emerging carbapenemases in Gram-negative aerobes. *Clin Microbiol Infect.* 2002 Jun;8(6):321-31.

Norris R. "Flush-free niacin": Dietary supplement may be "benefit-free." *Prev Cardio.* 2006 Winter: 64.

Nova E, Toro O, Varela P, López-Vidriero I, Morandé G, Marcos A. Effects of a nutritional intervention with yogurt on lymphocyte subsets and cytokine production capacity in anorexia nervosa patients. *Eur J Nutr.* 2006 Jun;45(4):225-33.

Novembre E, Dini L, Bernardini R, Resti M, Vierucci A. Unusual reactions to food additives. *Pediatr Med Chir.* 1992 Jan-Feb;14(1):39-42.

Nowak-Wegrzyn A, Fiocchi A. Is oral immunotherapy the cure for food allergies? *Curr Opin Allergy Clin Immunol.* 2010 Jun;10(3):214-9.

Nsouli TM. Long-term use of nasal saline irrigation: harmful or helpful? *Amer Acad of Allergy, Asthma and Immunol.* 2009; Abstract O32.

Nurmatov U, Devereux G, Sheikh A. Nutrients and foods for the primary prevention of asthma and allergy: Systematic review and meta-analysis. *J Allergy Clin Immunol.* 2010 Dec 23.

Nusem D, Panasoff J. Beer anaphylaxis. *Isr Med Assoc J.* 2009 Jun;11(6):380-1.

Nwaru BI, Erkkola M, Ahonen S, Kaila M, Haapala AM, Kronberg-Kippilä C, Salmelin R, Veijola R, Ilonen J, Simell O, Knip M, Virtanen SM. Age at the introduction of solid foods during the first year and allergic sensitization at age 5 years. *Pediatrics.* 2010 Jan;125(1):50-9. 2009 Dec 7.

O'Connor J., Bensky D. (ed). *Shanghai College of Traditional Chinese Medicine: Acupuncture: A Comprehensive Text.* Seattle: Eastland Press, 1981.

O'Donnell MJ, Yusuf S, Mente A, Gao P, Mann JF, Teo K, McQueen M, Sleight P, Sharma AM, Dans A, Probstfield J, Schmieder RE. Urinary sodium and potassium excretion and risk of cardiovascular events. JAMA. 2011 Nov 23;306(20):2229-38. doi: 10.1001/jama.2011.1729.

O'Neil C, Helbling AA, Lehrer SB. Allergic reactions to fish. *Clin Rev Allergy.* 1993 Summer;11(2):183-200.

O'Neil C, Helbling AA, Lehrer SB. Allergic reactions to fish. *Clin Rev Allergy.* 1993;11(2):183-200.

O'Neil CE, Nicklas TA, Rampersaud GC, Fulgoni VL 3rd. One hundred percent orange juice consumption is associated with better diet quality, improved nutrient adequacy, and no increased risk for overweight/obesity in children. Nutr Res. 2011 Sep;31(9):673-82.

O'Brien SJ, Shannon JE, Gail MH. A molecular approach to the identification and individualization of human and animal cells in culture: isozyme and allozyme genetic signatures. *In Vitro.* 1980 Feb;16(2):119-35.

Odamaki T, Xiao JZ, Iwabuchi N, Sakamoto M, Takahashi N, Kondo S, Miyaji K, Iwatsuki K, Togashi H, Enomoto T, Benno Y. Influence of Bifidobacterium longum BB536 intake on faecal microbiota in individuals with Japanese cedar pollinosis during the pollen season. *J Med Microbiol.* 2007 Oct;56(Pt 10):1301-8.

Odamaki T, Xiao JZ, Iwabuchi N, Sakamoto M, Takahashi N, Kondo S, Iwatsuki K, Kokubo S, Togashi H, Enomoto T, Benno Y. Fluctuation of fecal microbiota in individuals with Japanese cedar pollinosis during the pollen season and influence of probiotic intake. *J Investig Allergol Clin Immunol.* 2007;17(2):92-100.

Oehme FW (ed.). *Toxicity of heavy metals in the environment. Part 1.* New York: M.Dekker, 1979.

Ogawa T, Hashikawa S, Asai Y, Sakamoto H, Yasuda K, Makimura Y. A new synbiotic, Lactobacillus casei subsp. casei together with dextran, reduces murine and human allergic reaction. *FEMS Immunol Med Microbiol.* 2006 Apr;46(3):400-9.

Ogawa T, Hashikawa S, Asai Y, Sakamoto H, Yasuda K, Makimura Y. A new synbiotic, *Lactobacillus casei* subsp. casei together with dextran, reduces murine and human allergic reaction. *FEMS Immunol Med Microbiol.* 2006 Apr;46(3):400-9.

Oh CK, Lücker PW, Wetzelsberger N, Kuhlmann F. The determination of magnesium, calcium, sodium and potassium in assorted foods with special attention to the loss of electrolytes after various forms of food preparations. *Mag.-Bull.* 1986;8:297-302.

Oh SY, Chung J, Kim MK, Kwon SO, Cho BH. Antioxidant nutrient intakes and corresponding biomarkers associated with the risk of atopic dermatitis in young children. *Eur J Clin Nutr.* 2010 Mar;64(3):245-52. 2010 Jan 27.

Ohara T, Doi Y, Ninomiya T, Hirakawa Y, Hata J, Iwaki T, Kanba S, Kiyohara Y. Glucose tolerance status and risk of dementia in the community: The Hisayama Study. Neurology. 2011 Sep 20;77(12):1126-34.

Ohashi Y, Nakai S, Tsukamoto T, Masumori N, Akaza H, Miyanaga N, Kitamura T, Kawabe K, Kotake T, Kuroda M, Naito S, Koga H, Saito Y, Nomata K, Kitagawa M, Aso Y. Habitual intake of lactic acid bacteria and risk reduction of bladder cancer. *Urol Int.* 2002;68(4):273-80.

Ok IS, Kim SH, Kim BK, Lee JC, Lee YC. Pinellia ternata, Citrus reticulata, and their combinational prescription inhibit eosinophil infiltration and airway hyperresponsiveness by suppressing CCR3+ and Th2 cytokines production in the ovalbumin-induced asthma model. *Mediators Inflamm.* 2009;2009:413270.

Okamura T, Maehara Y, Sugimachi K. Phase II clinical study of LC9018 on carcinomatous peritonitis of gastric cancer. Subgroup for Carcinomatous Peritonitis, Cooperative, Study Group of LC9018. *Gan To Kagaku Ryoho.* 1989 Jun;16(6):2257-62.

Okawa T, Niibe H, Arai T, Sekiba K, Noda K, Takeuchi S, Hashimoto S, Ogawa N. Effect of LC9018 combined with radiation therapy on carcinoma of the uterine cervix. A phase III, multicenter, randomized, controlled study. *Cancer.* 1993 Sep 15;72(6):1949-54.

Okazaki Y, Isobe T, Iwata Y, Matsukawa T, Matsuda F, Miyagawa H, Ishihara A, Nishioka T, Iwamura H. Metabolism of avenanthramide phytoalexins in oats. *Plant J.* 2004 Aug;39(4):560-72.

Oláh A, Belágyi T, Issekutz A, Gamal ME, Bengmark S. Randomized clinical trial of specific lactobacillus and fibre supplement to early enteral nutrition in patients with acute pancreatitis. *Br J Surg.* 2002 Sep;89(9):1103-7.

Oldak E, Kurzatkowska B, Stasiak-Barmuta A. Natural course of sensitization in children: follow-up study from birth to 6 years of age, I. Evaluation of total serum IgE and specific IgE antibodies with regard to atopic family history. *Rocz Akad Med Bialymst.* 2000;45:87-95.

Oleĭnichenko EV, Mitrokhin SD, Nonikov VE, Minaev VI. Effectiveness of acipole in prevention of enteric dysbacteriosis due to antibacterial therapy. *Antibiot Khimioter.* 1999;44(1):23-5.

Olivares M, Díaz-Ropero MA, Gómez N, Lara-Villoslada F, Sierra S, Maldonado JA, Martín R, López-Huertas E, Rodríguez JM, Xaus J. Oral administration of two probiotic strains, *Lactobacillus gasseri* CECT5714 and Lactobacillus coryniformis CECT5711, enhances the intestinal function of healthy adults. *Int J Food Microbiol.* 2006 Mar 15;107(2):104-11.

Olivares M, Paz Díaz-Ropero M, Gómez N, Sierra S, Lara-Villoslada F, Martín R, Miguel Rodríguez J, Xaus J. Dietary deprivation of fermented foods causes a fall in innate immune response. Lactic acid bacteria can counteract the immunological effect of this deprivation. *J Dairy Res.* 2006 Nov;73(4):492-8.

Oliveira AB, Moura CF, Gomes-Filho E, Marco CA, Urban L, Miranda MR. The Impact of Organic Farming on Quality of To-matoes Is Associated to Increased Oxidative Stress during Fruit Development. PLoS One. 2013;8(2):e56354.

O'Mahony L, McCarthy J, Kelly P, Hurley G, Luo F, Chen K, O'Sullivan GC, Kiely B, Collins JK, Shanahan F, Quigley EM. Lactobacillus and bifidobacterium in irritable bowel syndrome: symptom responses and relationship to cytokine profiles. *Gastroenterology.* 2005 Mar;128(3):541-51.

Onbasi K, Sin AZ, Doganavsargil B, Onder GF, Bor S, Sebik F. Eosinophil infiltration of the oesophageal mucosa in patients with pollen allergy during the season. *Clin Exp Allergy.* 2005 Nov;35(11):1423-31.

Onder G, *et al.* Serum cholesterol levels and in-hospital mortality in the elderly. *Am J Med.* 2003 Sept;115:265-71.

Onwulata CI, Rao DR, Vankineni P. Relative efficiency of yogurt, sweet acidophilus milk, hydrolyzed-lactose milk, and a commercial lactase tablet in alleviating lactose maldigestion. *Am J Clin Nutr.* 1989 Jun;49(6):1233-7.

Oozeer R, Leplingard A, Mater DD, Mogenet A, Michelin R, Seksek I, Marteau P, Doré J, Bresson JL, Corthier G. Survival of *Lactobacillus casei* in the human digestive tract after consumption of fermented milk. *Appl Environ Microbiol.* 2006 Aug;72(8):5615-7.

Oreskovic NM, Sawicki GS, Kinane TB, Winickoff JP, Perrin JM. Travel patterns to school among children with asthma. *Clin Pediatr.* 2009 Jul;48(6):632-40. 2009 May 6.

Ortiz-Andrellucchi A, Sánchez-Villegas A, Rodríguez-Gallego C, Lemes A, Molero T, Soria A, Peña-Quintana L, Santana M, Ramírez O, García J, Cabrera F, Cobo J, Serra-Majem L. Immunomodulatory effects of the intake of fermented milk with Lactobacillus casei DN114001 in lactating mothers and their children. *Br J Nutr.* 2008 Oct;100(4):834-45.

Osguthorpe JD. Immunotherapy. *Curr Opin Otolaryngol Head Neck Surg.* 2010 Jun;18(3):206-12.

Ostlund RE Jr, Racette SB, Stenson WF. Inhibition of cholesterol absorption by phytosterol-replete wheat germ compared with phytosterol-depleted wheat germ. Am J Clin Nutr. 2003 Jun;77(6):1385-9.

Otto SJ, van Houwelingen AC, Hornstra G. The effect of supplementation with docosahexaenoic and arachidonic acid derived from single cell oils on plasma and erythrocyte fatty acids of pregnant women in the second trimester. *Prostaglandins Leukot Essent Fatty Acids.* 2000 Nov;63(5):323-8.

Ou CC, Tsao SM, Lin MC, Yin MC. Protective action on human LDL against oxidation and glycation by four organosulfur compounds derived from garlic. *Lipids.* 2003 Mar;38(3):219-24.

Ou J, Carbonero F, Zoetendal EG, DeLany JP, Wang M, Newton K, Gaskins HR, O'Keefe SJ. Diet, microbiota, and microbial metabolites in colon cancer risk in rural Africans and African Americans. Am J Clin Nutr. 2013 Jul;98(1):111-20. doi: 10.3945/ajcn.112.056689.

Ou J, DeLany JP, Zhang M, Sharma S, O'Keefe SJ. Association between low colonic short-chain fatty acids and high bile acids in high colon cancer risk populations. Nutr Cancer. 2012;64(1):34-40. doi: 10.1080/01635581.2012.630164.

Ouwehand AC, Bergsma N, Parhiala R, Lahtinen S, Gueimonde M, Finne-Soveri H, Strandberg T, Pitkälä K, Salminen S. *Bifidobacterium* microbiota and parameters of immune function in elderly subjects. *FEMS Immunol Med Microbiol.* 2008 Jun;53(1):18-25.

Ouwehand AC, Nermes M, Collado MC, Rautonen N, Salminen S, Isolauri E. Specific probiotics alleviate allergic rhinitis during the birch pollen season. *World J Gastroenterol.* 2009 Jul 14;15(26):3261-8.

Ouwehand AC, Tiihonen K, Saarinen M, Putaala H, Rautonen N. Influence of a combination of *Lactobacillus acidophilus* NCFM and lactitol on healthy elderly: intestinal and immune parameters. *Br J Nutr.* 2009 Feb;101(3):367-75.

Ouwehand AC. Antiallergic effects of probiotics. *J Nutr.* 2007 Mar;137(3 Suppl 2):794S-7S.

Ozawa M, Ninomiya T, Ohara T, Doi Y, Uchida K, Shirota T, Yonemoto K, Kitazono T, Kiyohara Y. Dietary patterns and risk of dementia in an elderly Japanese population: the Hisayama Study. Am J Clin Nutr. 2013 May;97(5):1076-82. doi: 10.3945/ajcn.112.045575.

Ozdemir O. Any benefits of probiotics in allergic disorders? *Allergy Asthma Proc.* 2010 Mar;31(2):103-11.

Ozkan TB, Sahin E, Erdemir G, Budak F. Effect of *Saccharomyces boulardii* in children with acute gastroenteritis and its relationship to the immune response. *J Int Med Res.* 2007 Mar-Apr;35(2):201-12.

Paganelli R, Pallone F, Montano S, Le Moli S, Matricardi PM, Fais S, Paoluzi P, D'Amelio R, Aiuti F. Isotypic analysis of antibody response to a food antigen in inflammatory bowel disease. *Int Arch Allergy Appl Immunol.* 1985;78(1):81-5.

Pahud JJ, Schwarz K. Research and development of infant formulae with reduced allergenic properties. *Ann Allergy.* 1984 Dec;53(6 Pt 2):609-14.

Paineau D, Carcano D, Leyer G, Darquy S, Alyanakian MA, Simoneau G, Bergmann JF, Brassart D, Bornet F, Ouwehand AC. Effects of seven potential probiotic strains on specific immune responses in healthy adults: a double-blind, randomized, controlled trial. *FEMS Immunol Med Microbiol.* 2008 Jun;53(1):107-13.

Pakhale S, Doucette S, Vandemheen K, Boulet LP, McIvor RA, Fitzgerald JM, Hernandez P, Lemiere C, Sharma S, Field SK, Alvarez GG, Dales RE, Aaron SD. A comparison of obese and nonobese people with asthma: exploring an asthma-obesity interaction. *Chest.* 2010 Jun;137(6):1316-23. 2010 Feb 12.

Palacin A, Bartra J, Muñoz R, Diaz-Perales A, Valero A, Salcedo G. Anaphylaxis to wheat flour-derived foodstuffs and the lipid transfer protein syndrome: a potential role of wheat lipid transfer protein Tri a 14. *Int Arch Allergy Immunol.* 2010;152(2):178-83.

Palacios R, Sugawara I. Hydrocortisone abrogates proliferation of T cells in autologous mixed lymphocyte reaction by rendering the interleukin-2 Producer T cells unresponsive to interleukin-1 and unable to synthesize the T-cell growth factor. *Scand J Immunol.* 1982 Jan;15(1):25-31. 7.

Palacios R. HLA-DR antigens render interleukin-2-producer T lymphocytes sensitive to interleukin-1. *Scand J Immunol.* 1981 Sep;14(3):321-6.

Palmer DJ, Gold MS, Makrides M. Effect of cooked and raw egg consumption on ovalbumin content of human milk: a randomized, double-blind, cross-over trial. *Clin Exp Allergy.* 2005 Feb;35(2):173-8.

Paluszkiewicz P, Smolińska K, Dębińska I, Turski WA. Main dietary compounds and pancreatic cancer risk. The quantitative analysis of case-control and cohort studies. Cancer Epidemiol. 2012 Feb;36(1):60-7.

Pan A, Chen M, Chowdhury R, Wu JH, Sun Q, Campos H, Mozaffarian D, Hu FB. α-Linolenic acid and risk of cardiovascular disease: a systematic review and meta-analysis. Am J Clin Nutr. 2012 Oct 17.

Pan A, Sun Q, Bernstein AM, Manson JE, Willett WC, Hu FB. Changes in red meat consumption and subsequent risk of type 2 diabetes mellitus: three cohorts of US men and women. JAMA Intern Med. 2013 Jul 22;173(14):1328-35. doi: 10.1001/jamainternmed.2013.6633.

Pan A, Sun Q, Bernstein AM, Schulze MB, Manson JE, Stampfer MJ, Willett WC, Hu FB. Red meat consumption and mortality: results from 2 prospective cohort studies. Arch Intern Med. 2012 Apr 9;172(7):555-63. doi: 10.1001/archinternmed.2011.2287.

Pan A, Sun Q, Bernstein AM, Schulze MB, Manson JE, Willett WC, Hu FB. Red meat consumption and risk of type 2 diabetes: 3 cohorts of US adults and an updated meta-analysis. Am J Clin Nutr. 2011 Oct;94(4):1088-96.

Panghal S, Mallapur SS, Kumar M, Ram V, Singh BK. Antiinflammatory Activity of Piper longum Fruit Oil. *Indian J Pharm Sci.* 2009 Jul;71(4):454-6.

Panigrahi P, Parida S, Pradhan L, Mohapatra SS, Misra PR, Johnson JA, Chaudhry R, Taylor S, Hansen NI, Gewolb IH. Long-term colonization of a *Lactobacillus plantarum* synbiotic preparation in the neonatal gut. *J Pediatr Gastroenterol Nutr.* 2008 Jul;47(1):45-53.

Pant H, Ferguson BJ, Macardle PJ. The role of allergy in rhinosinusitis. *Curr Opin Otolaryngol Head Neck Surg.* 2009 Jun;17(3):232-8.

Pant H, Kette FE, Smith WB, Wormald PJ, Macardle PJ. Fungal-specific humoral response in eosinophilic mucus chronic rhinosinusitis. *Laryngoscope.* 2005 Apr;115(4):601-6.

Panunzio MF, Caporizzi R, Antoniciello A, Cela EP, Ferguson LR, D'Ambrosio P. Randomized, controlled nutrition education trial promotes a Mediterranean diet and improves anthropometric, dietary, and metabolic parameters in adults. Ann Ig. 2011 Jan-Feb;23(1):13-25.

Panunzio MF, Caporizzi R, Antoniciello A, Cela EP, Ferguson LR, D'Ambrosio P. Randomized, controlled nutrition education trial promotes a Mediterranean diet and improves anthropometric, dietary, and metabolic parameters in adults. Ann Ig. 2011 Jan-Feb;23(1):13-25.

Panzani R, Ariano R, Mistrello G. Cypress pollen does not cross-react to plant-derived foods. *Eur Ann Allergy Clin Immunol.* 2010 Jun;42(3):125-6.

Pápay ZE, Kósa A, Boldizsár I, Ruszkai A, Balogh E, Klebovich I, Antal I. Pharmaceutical and formulation aspects of Petroselinum crispum extract. Acta Pharm Hung. 2012;82(1):3-14.

Parcell S. Sulfur in human nutrition and applications in medicine. *Altern Med Rev.* 2002 Feb;7(1):22-44.

Park BJ, Tsunetsugu Y, Kasetani T, Kagawa T, Miyazaki Y. The physiological effects of Shinrin-yoku (taking in the forest atmosphere or forest bathing): evidence from field experiments in 24 forests across Japan. *Environ Health Prev Med.* 2010 Jan;15(1):18-26.

Parra D, De Morentin BM, Cobo JM, Mateos A, Martinez JA. Monocyte function in healthy middle-aged people receiving fermented milk containing *Lactobacillus casei. J Nutr Health Aging.* 2004;8(4):208-11.

Parra MD, Martínez de Morentin BE, Cobo JM, Mateos A, Martínez JA. Daily ingestion of fermented milk containing Lactobacillus casei DN114001 improves innate-defense capacity in healthy middle-aged people. *J Physiol Biochem.* 2004 Jun;60(2):85-91.

Parra MD, Martínez de Morentin BE, Cobo JM, Mateos A, Martínez JA. Daily ingestion of fermented milk containing *Lactobacillus casei* DN114001 improves innate-defense capacity in healthy middle-aged people. *J Physiol Biochem.* 2004 Jun;60(2):85-91.

Partridge MR, Dockrell M, Smith NM: The use of complementary medicines by those with asthma. Respir Med 2003, 97:436-438.

Passeron T, Lacour JP, Fontas E, Ortonne JP. Prebiotics and synbiotics: two promising approaches for the treatment of atopic dermatitis in children above 2 years. *Allergy.* 2006 Apr;61(4):431-7.

Passey BH, Cerling TE, Levin NE. Temperature dependence of acid fractionation for modern and fossil tooth enamels. Rapid Commun Mass Spectrom. 2007;21:2853 – 2859.

Passey BH, Levin NE, Cerling TE, Brown FH, Eiler J. High temperature environments of human evolution in East Africa based on bond ordering in paleosol carbonates. Proc Natl Acad Sci USA. 2010;107:11245 – 11249.

Pastorello EA, Farioli L, Conti A, Pravettoni V, Bonomi S, Iametti S, Fortunato D, Scibilia J, Bindslev-Jensen C, Ballmer-Weber B, Robino AM, Ortolani C. Wheat IgE-mediated food allergy in European patients: alpha-

433

amylase inhibitors, lipid transfer proteins and low-molecular-weight glutenins. Allergenic molecules recognized by double-blind, placebo-controlled food challenge. *Int Arch Allergy Immunol.* 2007;144(1):10-22.

Pastorello EA, Pompei C, Pravettoni V, Farioli L, Calamari AM, Scibilia J, Robino AM, Conti A, Iametti S, Fortunato D, Bonomi S, Ortolani C. Lipid-transfer protein is the major maize allergen maintaining IgE-binding activity after cooking at 100 degrees C, as demonstrated in anaphylactic patients and patients with positive double-blind, placebo-controlled food challenge results. *J Allergy Clin Immunol.* 2003 Oct;112(4):775-83.

Patchett K, Lewis S, Crane J, Fitzharris P. Cat allergen (Fel d 1) levels on school children's clothing and in primary school classrooms in Wellington, New Zealand. *J Allergy Clin Immunol.* 1997 Dec;100(6 Pt 1):755-9.

Patel DS, Rafferty GF, Lee S, Hannam S, Greenough A. Work of breathing and volume targeted ventilation in respiratory distress. *Arch Dis Child Fetal Neonatal Ed.* 2010 Nov;95(6):F443-6.

Patriarca G, Nucera E, Pollastrini E, Roncallo C, De Pasquale T, Lombardo C, Pedone C, Gasbarrini G, Buonomo A, Schiavino D. Oral specific desensitization in food-allergic children. *Dig Dis Sci.* 2007 Jul;52(7):1662-72.

Patriarca G, Nucera E, Roncallo C, Pollastrini E, Bartolozzi F, De Pasquale T, Buonomo A, Gasbarrini G, Di Campli C, Schiavino D. Oral desensitizing treatment in food allergy: clinical and immunological results. *Aliment Pharmacol Ther.* 2003 Feb;17(3):459-65.

Patterson DB. Anaphylactic shock from chloromycetin. Northwest Med. 1950 May;49(5):352-3. Agarwal KN, Bhasin SK. Feasibility studies to control acute diarrhoea in children by feeding fermented milk preparations Actimel and Indian Dahi. *Eur J Clin Nutr.* 2002 Dec;56 Suppl 4:S56-9.

Patwardhan B, Gautam M. Botanical immunodrugs: scope and opportunities. *Drug Discov Today.* 2005 Apr 1;10(7):495-502.

Paul M, Somkuti GA. Hydrolytic breakdown of lactoferricin by lactic acid bacteria. J Ind Microbiol Biotechnol. 2010 Feb;37(2):173-8. Epub 2009 Nov 19

Payment P, Franco E, Richardson L, Siemiatyck, J. Gastrointestinal health effects associated with the consumption of drinking water produced by point-of-use domestic reverse-osmosis filtration units. *Appl. Environ. Microbiol.* 1991;57:945-948.

Peat JK, van den Berg RH, Green WF, Mellis CM, Leeder SR, Woolcock AJ. Changing prevalence of asthma in Australian children. *BMJ.* 1994;308:1591-1596.

Peat JK. The rising trend in allergic illness: which environmental factors are important? Clin Exp Allergy. 1994 Sep;24(9):797-800.

Pedersen AN, Kondrup J, Borsheim E. Health effects of protein intake in healthy adults: a systematic literature review. Food Nutr Res. 2013 Jul 30;57.

Pedone CA, Arnaud CC, Postaire ER, Bouley CF, Reinert P. Multicentric study of the effect of milk fermented by *Lactobacillus casei* on the incidence of diarrhoea. *Int J Clin Pract.* 2000 Nov;54(9):568-71.

Pedone CA, Bernabeu AO, Postaire ER, Bouley CF, Reinert P. The effect of supplementation with milk fermented by *Lactobacillus casei* (strain DN-114 001) on acute diarrhoea in children attending day care centres. *Int J Clin Pract.* 1999 Apr-May;53(3):179-84.

Pedrosa MC, Golner BB, Goldin BR, Barakat S, Dallal GE, Russell RM. Survival of yogurt-containing organisms and *Lactobacillus gasseri* (ADH) and their effect on bacterial enzyme activity in the gastrointestinal tract of healthy and hypochlorhydric elderly subjects. *Am J Clin Nutr.* 1995 Feb;61(2):353-9.

Pehowich DJ, Gomes AV, Barnes JA. Fatty acid composition and possible health effects of coconut constituents. *West Indian Med J.* 2000 Jun;49(2):128-33.

Pelsser LM, Frankena K, Toorman J, Savelkoul HF, Dubois AE, Pereira RR, Haagen TA, Rommelse NN, Buitelaar JK. Effects of a restricted elimination diet on the behaviour of children with attention-deficit hyperactivity disorder (INCA study): a randomised controlled trial. Lancet. 2011 Feb 5;377(9764):494-503.

Peng Y, Yang X, Zhang Y. 2005. Microbial fibrinolytic enzymes: an overview of source, production, properties, and thrombolytic activity in vivo. Appl Microbiol Biotechnol. Nov;69(2):126-32.

Peral MC, Martinez MA, Valdez JC. Bacteriotherapy with *Lactobacillus plantarum* in burns. *Int Wound J.* 2009 Feb;6(1):73-81.

Perez-Galvez A, Martin HD, Sies H, Stahl W. Incorporation of carotenoids from paprika oleoresin into human chylomicrons. *Br J Nutr.* 2003 Jun;89(6):787-93.

Perez-Pena R. Secrets of the Mummy's Medicine Chest. *NY Times.* 2005 Sept 10.

Perry G, Phelix CF, Nunomura A, Colom LV, Castellani RJ, Petersen RB, Lee HG, Zhu X. Untangling the vascular web from Alzheimer disease and oxidative stress. Can J Neurol Sci. 2012 Jan;39(1):4.

Persson R, Orbaek P, Kecklund G, Akerstedt T. Impact of an 84-hour workweek on biomarkers for stress, metabolic processes and diurnal rhythm. *Scand J Work Environ Health.* 2006 Oct;32(5):349-58.

Pescuma M, Espeche Turbay MB, Mozzi F, Font de Valdez G, Savoy de Giori G, Hebert EM. Diversity in proteinase specificity of thermophilic lactobacilli as revealed by hydrolysis of dairy and vegetable proteins. Appl Microbiol Biotechnol. 2013 Jul 9.

Pessi T, Sütas Y, Hurme M, Isolauri E. Interleukin-10 generation in atopic children following oral *Lactobacillus rhamnosus* GG. *Clin Exp Allergy.* 2000 Dec;30(12):1804-8.

Peter JJ, Beecher GR, Bhagwat SA, Dwyer JT, Gebhardt SE, Haytowitz DB, Holden JM. Flavanones in grapefruit, lemons, and limes: A compilation and review of the data from the analytical literature. Jrnl Food Comp and Anal. 2006;19:S74-S80.

Peters CR, Vogel JC. Africa's wild C4 plant foods and possible early hominid diets. J Hum Evol. 2005;48:219 – 236.

Peters JI, McKinney JM, Smith B, Wood P, Forkner E, Galbreath AD. Impact of obesity in asthma: evidence from a large prospective disease management study. *Ann Allergy Asthma Immunol.* 2011 Jan;106(1):30-5.

Peterson CG, Hansson T, Skott A, Bengtsson U, Ahlstedt S, Magnussons J. Detection of local mast-cell activity in patients with food hypersensitivity. *J Investig Allergol Clin Immunol.* 2007;17(5):314-20.

Peterson KA, Samuelson WM, Ryujin DT, Young DC, Thomas KL, Hilden K, Fang JC. The role of gastroesophageal reflux in exercise-triggered asthma: a randomized controlled trial. *Dig Dis Sci.* 2009 Mar;54(3):564-71. 2008 Aug 8.

Petlevski R, Hadzija M, Slijepcević M, Juretić D, Petrik J. Glutathione S-transferases and malondialdehyde in the liver of NOD mice on short-term treatment with plant mixture extract P-9801091. *Phytother Res.* 2003 Apr;17(4):311-4.

Petricevic L, Unger FM, Viernstein H, Kiss H. Randomized, double-blind, placebo-controlled study of oral lactobacilli to improve the vaginal flora of postmenopausal women. *Eur J Obstet Gynecol Reprod Biol.* 2008 Nov;141(1):54-7.

Petricevic L, Witt A. The role of *Lactobacillus casei* rhamnosus Lcr35 in restoring the normal vaginal flora after antibiotic treatment of bacterial vaginosis. *BJOG.* 2008 Oct;115(11):1369-74.

Petrunov B, Marinova S, Markova R, Nenkov P, Nikolaeva S, Nikolova M, Taskov H, Cvetanov J. Cellular and humoral systemic and mucosal immune responses stimulated in volunteers by an oral polybacterial immunomodulator "Dentavax". *Int Immunopharmacol.* 2006 Jul;6(7):1181-93.

Petti S, Tarsitani G, D'Arca AS. A randomized clinical trial of the effect of yoghurt on the human salivary microflora. *Arch Oral Biol.* 2001 Aug;46(8):705-12.

Pfefferle PI, Sel S, Ege MJ, Büchele G, Blümer N, Krauss-Etschmann S, Herzum I, Albers CE, Lauener RP, Roponen M, Hirvonen MR, Vuitton DA, Riedler J, Brunekreef B, Dalphin JC, Braun-Fahrländer C, Pekkanen J, von Mutius E, Renz H; PASTURE Study Group. Cord blood allergen-specific IgE is associated with reduced IFN-gamma production by cord blood cells: the Protection against Allergy-Study in Rural Environments (PASTURE) Study. *J Allergy Clin Immunol.* 2008 Oct;122(4):711-6.

Pfundstein B, El Desouky SK, Hull WE, Haubner R, Erben G, Owen RW. Polyphenolic compounds in the fruits of Egyptian medicinal plants (Terminalia bellerica, Terminalia chebula and Terminalia horrida): characterization, quantitation and determination of antioxidant capacities. *Phytochemistry.* 2010 Jul;71(10):1132-48.

Phuapradit P, Varavithya W, Vathanophas K, Sangchai R, Podhipak A, Suthutvoravut U, Nopchinda S, Chantraruksa V, Haschke F. Reduction of rotavirus infection in children receiving bifidobacteria-supplemented formula. *J Med Assoc Thai.* 1999 Nov;82 Suppl 1:S43-8.

*Physicians' Desk Reference.* Montvale, NJ: Thomson, 2003-2008.

Picard C, Fioramonti J, Francois A, Robinson T, Neant F, Matuchansky C. Review article: bifidobacteria as probiotic agents -- physiological effects and clinical benefits. Aliment Pharmacol Ther. 2005 Sep 15;22(6):495-512.

Picherit, C., C. Bennetau-Pelissero, *et al.* 2001. Soybean isoflavones dose-dependently reduce bone turnover but do not reverse established osteopenia in adult ovariectomized rats. J Nutr 131(3): 723-8.

Pierce SK, Klinman NR. Antibody-specific immunoregulation. *J Exp Med.* 1977 Aug 1;146(2):509-19.

Pieterse Z, Jerling JC, Oosthuizen W, Kruger HS, Hanekom SM, Smuts CM, Schutte AE. Substitution of high monounsaturated fatty acid avocado for mixed dietary fats during an energy-restricted diet: effects on weight loss, serum lipids, fibrinogen, and vascular function. Nutrition. 2005 Jan;21(1):67-75

Piirainen L, Haahtela S, Helin T, Korpela R, Haahtela T, Vaarala O. Effect of Lactobacillus rhamnosus GG on rBet v1 and rMal d1 specific IgA in the saliva of patients with birch pollen allergy. *Ann Allergy Asthma Immunol.* 2008 Apr;100(4):338-42.

Piirainen L, Haahtela S, Helin T, Korpela R, Haahtela T, Vaarala O. Effect of *Lactobacillus rhamnosus* GG on rBet v1 and rMal d1 specific IgA in the saliva of patients with birch pollen allergy. *Ann Allergy Asthma Immunol.* 2008 Apr;100(4):338-42.

Pike MG, Heddle RJ, Boulton P, Turner MW, Atherton DJ. Increased intestinal permeability in atopic eczema. *J Invest Dermatol.* 1986 Feb;86(2):101-4.

Pimentel D. Environmental and Economic Costs of the Appli-cation of Pesticides Primarily in the United States. Environment, Development and Sustainability. 2005. 7: 229-252.

Pines JM, Prabhu A, Hilton JA, Hollander JE, Datner EM. The effect of emergency department crowding on length of stay and medication treatment times in discharged patients with acute asthma. *Acad Emerg Med.* 2010 Aug;17(8):834-9.

Pitkala KH, Strandberg TE, Finne Soveri UH, Ouwehand AC, Poussa T, Salminen S. Fermented cereal with specific bifidobacteria normalizes bowel movements in elderly nursing home residents. A randomized, controlled trial. *J Nutr Health Aging.* 2007 Jul-Aug;11(4):305-11.

Pitten FA, Scholler M, Krüger U, Effendy I, Kramer A. Filamentous fungi and yeasts on mattresses covered with different encasings. Eur J Dermatol. 2001 Nov-Dec;11(6):534-7.

Pitt-Rivers R, Trotter WR. *The Thyroid Gland.* London: Butterworth Publ, 1954.

Plaschke P, Janson C, Norrman E, Björnsson E, Ellbjär S, Järvholm B. Association between atopic sensitization and asthma and bronchial hyperresponsiveness in swedish adults: pets, and not mites, are the most important allergens. *J Allergy Clin Immunol.* 1999 Jul;104(1):58-65.

Plaut M, Valentine MD. Clinical practice. Allergic rhinitis. *N Engl J Med.* 2005 Nov 3;353(18):1934-44.

Plaut TE, Jones TB. *Dr. Tom Plaut's Asthma guide for people of all ages.* Amherst, MA: Pedipress, 1999.

Plaza V, Miguel E, Bellido-Casado J, Lozano MP, Ríos L, Bolibar I. [Usefulness of the Guidelines of the Spanish Society of Pulmonology and Thoracic Surgery (SEPAR) in identifying the causes of chronic cough]. Arch Bronconeumol. 2006 Feb;42(2):68-73.

Plein K, Hotz J. Therapeutic effects of *Saccharomyces boulardii* on mild residual symptoms in a stable phase of Crohn's disease with special respect to chronic diarrhea -- a pilot study. *Z Gastroenterol.* 1993 Feb;31(2):129-34.

Plohmann B, Bader G, Hiller K, Franz G. Immunomodulatory and antitumoral effects of triterpenoid saponins. *Pharmazie*. 1997 Dec;52(12):953-7.

Poblocka-Olech I, Krauze-Baranowska M. SPE-HPTLC of procyanidins from the barks of different species and clones of Salix. *J Pharm Biomed Anal*. 2008 Nov 4;48(3):965-8.

Pohjavuori E, Viljanen M, Korpela R, Kuitunen M, Tiittanen M, Vaarala O, Savilahti E. Lactobacillus GG effect in increasing IFN-gamma production in infants with cow's milk allergy. *J Allergy Clin Immunol*. 2004 Jul;114(1):131-6.

Pohjavuori E, Viljanen M, Korpela R, Kuitunen M, Tiittanen M, Vaarala O, Savilahti E. Lactobacillus GG effect in increasing IFN-gamma production in infants with cow's milk allergy. *J Allergy Clin Immunol*. 2004 Jul;114(1):131-6.

Polito A, Aboab J, Annane D. The hypothalamic pituitary adrenal axis in sepsis. *Novartis Found Symp*. 2007;280:182-203.

Polk S, Sunyer J, Muñoz-Ortiz L, Barnes M, Torrent M, Figueroa C, Harris J, Vall O, Antó JM, Cullinan P. A prospective study of Fel d1 and Der p1 exposure in infancy and childhood wheezing. *Am J Respir Crit Care Med*. 2004 Aug 1;170(3):273-8.

Pollini F, Capristo C, Boner AL. Upper respiratory tract infections and atopy. *Int J Immunopathol Pharmacol*. 2010 Jan-Mar;23(1 Suppl):32-7.

Ponsonby AL, McMichael A, van der Mei I. Ultraviolet radiation and autoimmune disease: insights from epidemiological research. *Toxicology*. 2002 Dec 27;181-182:71-8.

Poppitt SD, van Drunen JD, McGill AT, Mulvey TB, Leahy FE. Supplementation of a high-carbohydrate breakfast with barley beta-glucan improves postprandial glycaemic response for meals but not beverages. *Asia Pac J Clin Nutr*. 2007;16(1):16-24.

Postlethwait EM. Scavenger receptors clear the air. *J Clin Invest*. 2007 Mar;117(3):601-4.

Postma DS. Gender Differences in Asthma Development and Progression. *Gender Medicine*. 2007;4:S133-146.

Postolache TT, Lapidus M, Sander ER, Langenberg P, Hamilton RG, Soriano JJ, McDonald JS, Furst N, Bai J, Scrandis DA, Cabassa JA, Stiller JW, Balis T, Guzman A, Togias A, Tonelli LH. Changes in allergy symptoms and depression scores are positively correlated in patients with recurrent mood disorders exposed to seasonal peaks in aeroallergens. *ScientificWorldJournal*. 2007 Dec 17;7:1968-77.

Potterton D. (Ed.) *Culpeper's Color Herbal*. New York: Sterling, 1983.

Poulos LM, Waters AM, Correll PK, Loblay RH, Marks GB. Trends in hospitalizations for anaphylaxis, angioedema, and urticaria in Australia, 1993-1994 to 2004-2005. *J Allergy Clin Immunol*. 2007 Oct;120(4):878-84.

Powe DG, Groot Kormelink T, Sisson M, Blokhuis BJ, Kramer MF, Jones NS, Redegeld FA. Evidence for the involvement of free light chain immunoglobulins in allergic and nonallergic rhinitis. *J Allergy Clin Immunol*. 2010 Jan;125(1):139-45.e1-3.

Pregliasco F, Anselmi G, Fonte L, Giussani F, Schieppati S, Soletti L. A new chance of preventing winter diseases by the administration of synbiotic formulations. *J Clin Gastroenterol*. 2008 Sep;42 Suppl 3 Pt 2:S224-33.

Prescott SL, Wickens K, Westcott L, Jung W, Currie H, Black PN, Stanley TV, Mitchell EA, Fitzharris P, Siebers R, Wu L, Crane J; Probiotic Study Group. Supplementation with Lactobacillus rhamnosus or Bifidobacterium lactis probiotics in pregnancy increases cord blood interferon-gamma and breast milk transforming growth factor-beta and immunoglobin A detection. *Clin Exp Allergy*. 2008 Oct;38(10):1606-14.

Prescott SL, Wickens K, Westcott L, Jung W, Currie H, Black PN, Stanley TV, Mitchell EA, Fitzharris P, Siebers R, Wu L, Crane J; Probiotic Study Group. Supplementation with *Lactobacillus rhamnosus* or *Bifidobacterium lactis* probiotics in pregnancy increases cord blood interferon-gamma and breast milk transforming growth factor-beta and immunoglobin A detection. *Clin Exp Allergy*. 2008 Oct;38(10):1606-14.

Priftis KN, Panagiotakos DB, Anthracopoulos MB, Papadimitriou A, Nicolaidou P. Aims, methods and preliminary findings of the Physical Activity, Nutrition and Allergies in Children Examined in Athens (PANACEA) epidemiological study. *BMC Public Health*. 2007 Jul 4;7:140.

Prioult G, Fliss I, Pecquet S. Effect of probiotic bacteria on induction and maintenance of oral tolerance to beta-lactoglobulin in gnotobiotic mice. *Clin Diagn Lab Immunol*. 2003 Sep;10(5):787-92.

Prucksunand C, Indrasukhsri B, Leethochawalit M, Hungsprugs K. Phase II clinical trial on effect of the long turmeric (Curcuma longa Linn) on healing of peptic ulcer. *Southeast Asian J Trop Med Public Health*. 2001 Mar;32(1):208-15.

Pruthi S, Thapa MM. Infectious and inflammatory disorders. *Magn Reson Imaging Clin N Am*. 2009 Aug;17(3):423-38, v.

Psaltopoulou T, Sergentanis TN, Panagiotakos DB, Sergentanis IN, Kosti R, Scarmeas N. Mediterranean diet, stroke, cognitive impairment, and depression: A meta-analysis. Ann Neurol. 2013 May 30.

Pyle GG, Paaso B, Anderson BE, Allen DD, Marti T, Li Q, Siegel M, Khosla C, Gray GM. Effect of pretreatment of food gluten with prolyl endopeptidase on gluten-induced malabsorption in celiac sprue. Clin Gastroenterol Hepatol. 2005 Jul;3(7):687-94.

Qin HL, Zheng JJ, Tong DN, Chen WX, Fan XB, Hang XM, Jiang YQ. Effect of Lactobacillus plantarum enteral feeding on the gut permeability and septic complications in the patients with acute pancreatitis. *Eur J Clin Nutr*. 2008 Jul;62(7):923-30.

Qin HL, Zheng JJ, Tong DN, Chen WX, Fan XB, Hang XM, Jiang YQ. Effect of *Lactobacillus plantarum* enteral feeding on the gut permeability and septic complications in the patients with acute pancreatitis. *Eur J Clin Nutr*. 2008 Jul;62(7):923-30.

# REFERENCES AND BIBLIOGRAPHY

Qu C, Srivastava K, Ko J, Zhang TF, Sampson HA, Li XM. Induction of tolerance after establishment of peanut allergy by the food allergy herbal formula-2 is associated with up-regulation of interferon-gamma. *Clin Exp Allergy*. 2007 Jun;37(6):846-55.

Radon K, Danuser B, Iversen M, Jörres R, Monso E, Opravil U, Weber C, Donham KJ, Nowak D. Respiratory symptoms in European animal farmers. *Eur Respir J*. 2001 Apr;17(4):747-54.

Rafter J, Bennett M, Caderni G, Clune Y, Hughes R, Karlsson PC, Klinder A, O'Riordan M, O'Sullivan GC, Pool-Zobel B, Rechkemmer G, Roller M, Rowland I, Salvadori M, Thijs H, Van Loo J, Watzl B, Collins JK. Dietary synbiotics reduce cancer risk factors in polypectomized and colon cancer patients. *Am J Clin Nutr*. 2007 Feb;85(2):488-96.

Raherison C, Pénard-Morand C, Moreau D, Caillaud D, Charpin D, Kopferschmitt C, Lavaud F, Taytard A, Maesano IA. Smoking exposure and allergic sensitization in children according to maternal allergies. *Ann Allergy Asthma Immunol*. 2008 Apr;100(4):351-7.

Rahman MM, Bhattacharya A, Fernandes G. Docosahexaenoic acid is more potent inhibitor of osteoclast differentiation in RAW 264.7 cells than eicosapentaenoic acid. *J Cell Physiol*. 2008 Jan;214(1):201-9.

Raithel M, Weidenhiller M, Abel R, Baenkler HW, Hahn EG. Colorectal mucosal histamine release by mucosa oxygenation in comparison with other established clinical tests in patients with gastrointestinally mediated allergy. *World J Gastroenterol*. 2006 Aug 7;12(29):4699-705.

Raloff J. Ill Winds. *Science News*. 2001;160(14):218.

Rampton DS, Murdoch RD, Sladen GE. Rectal mucosal histamine release in ulcerative colitis. *Clin Sci (Lond)*. 1980 Nov;59(5):389-91.

Rancé F, Kanny G, Dutau G, Moneret-Vautrin DA. Food allergens in children. *Arch Pediatr*. 1999;6(Suppl 1):61S-66S.

Randal Bollinger R, Barbas AS, Bush EL, Lin SS, Parker W. Biofilms in the large bowel suggest an apparent function of the human vermiform appendix. *J Theor Biol*. 2007 Dec 21;249(4):826-31.

Randal Bollinger R, Barbas AS, Bush EL, Lin SS, Parker W. Biofilms in the large bowel suggest an apparent function of the human vermiform appendix. *J Theor Biol*. 2007 Dec 21;249(4):826-31.

Rangavajhyala N, Shahani KM, Sridevi G, Srikumaran S. Nonlipopolysaccharide component(s) of Lactobacillus acidophilus stimulate(s) the production of interleukin-1 alpha and tumor necrosis factor-alpha by murine macrophages. *Nutr Cancer*. 1997;28(2):130-4.

Ranilla LG, Genovese MI, Lajolo FM. Polyphenols and antioxidant capacity of seed coat and cotyledon from Brazilian and Peruvian bean cultivars (Phaseolus vulgaris L.). *J Agric Food Chem*. 2007 Jan 10;55(1):90-8. McCarron DA, Kazaks AG, Geerling JC, Stern JS, Graudal NA. Normal range of human dietary sodium intake: a perspective based on 24-hour urinary sodium excretion worldwide. *Am J Hypertens*. 2013 Oct;26(10):1218-23. doi:10.1093/ajh/hpt139.

Ranilla LG, Genovese MI, Lajolo FM. Polyphenols and antioxidant capacity of seed coat and cotyledon from Brazilian and Peruvian bean cultivars (Phaseolus vulgaris L.). *J Agric Food Chem*. 2007 Jan 10;55(1):90-8.

Ranjbaran Z, Keefer L, Stepanski E, Farhadi A, Keshavarzian A. The relevance of sleep abnormalities to chronic inflammatory conditions. *Inflamm Res*. 2007 Feb;56(2):51-7.

Rankin LC, Groom JR, Chopin M, Herold MJ, Walker JA, Mielke LA, McKenzie AN, Carotta S, Nutt SL, Belz GT. The transcription factor T-bet is essential for the development of NKp46(+) innate lymphocytes via the Notch pathway. Nat Immunol. 2013 Mar 3.

Rao SK, Rao PS, Rao BN. Preliminary investigation of the radiosensitizing activity of guduchi (Tinospora cordifolia) in tumor-bearing mice. *Phytother Res*. 2008 Nov;22(11):1482-9.

Rapin JR, Wiernsperger N. Possible links between intestinal permeablity and food processing: A potential therapeutic niche for glutamine. *Clinics (Sao Paulo)*. 2010 Jun;65(6):635-43.

Rappoport J. Both sides of the pharmaceutical death coin. *Townsend Letter for Doctors and Patients*. 2006 Oct.

Rauha JP, Remes S, Heinonen M, Hopia A, Kähkönen M, Kujala T, Pihlaja K, Vuorela H, Vuorela P. Antimicrobial effects of Finnish plant extracts containing flavonoids and other phenolic compounds. *Int J Food Microbiol*. 2000 May 25;56(1):3-12.

Rauma A. Antioxidant status in vegetarians versus omnivores. *Nutrition*. 2003;16(2): 111-119.

Rautava S, Isolauri E. Cow's milk allergy in infants with atopic eczema is associated with aberrant production of interleukin-4 during oral cow's milk challenge. *J Pediatr Gastroenterol Nutr*. 2004 Nov;39(5):529-35.

Rautava S, Salminen S, Isolauri E. Specific probiotics in reducing the risk of acute infections in infancy – a randomised, double-blind, placebo-controlled study. *Br J Nutr*. 2009 Jun;101(11):1722-6.

Rayes N, Seehofer D, Hansen S, Boucsein K, Müller AR, Serke S, Bengmark S, Neuhaus P. Early enteral supply of lactobacillus and fiber versus selective bowel decontamination: a controlled trial in liver transplant recipients. *Transplantation*. 2002 Jul 15;74(1):123-7.

Rayes N, Seehofer D, Müller AR, Hansen S, Bengmark S, Neuhaus P. Influence of probiotics and fibre on the incidence of bacterial infections following major abdominal surgery – results of a prospective trial. *Z Gastroenterol*. 2002 Oct;40(10):869-76.

Raza S, Graham SM, Allen SJ, Sultana S, Cuevas L, Hart CA, Kaila M, Isolauri E, Saxelin M, Arvilommi H, et al. Lactobacillus GG in acute diarrhea. *Indian Pediatr*. 1995 Oct;32(10):1140-2.

Raza S, Graham SM, Allen SJ, Sultana S, Cuevas L, Hart CA. Lactobacillus GG promotes recovery from acute nonbloody diarrhea in Pakistan. *Pediatr Infect Dis J*. 1995 Feb;14(2):107-11.

Rebhun J. Coexisting immune complex diseases in atopy. *Ann Allergy*. 1980 Dec;45(6):368-71.

Red yeast rice. *Med Lett Drugs Ther*. 2009 Sep 7;51(1320):71-2.

437

Reddy KP, Shahani KM, Kulkarni SM. B-complex vitamins in cultured and acidified yogurt. *J Dairy Sci.* 1976 Feb;59(2):191-5.

Reed KE. Early hominid evolution and ecological change through the African Plio-Pleistocene. *J Hum Evol.* 1997;32:289 – 322.

Reger D, Goode S, Mercer E. *Chemistry: Principles & Practice.* Fort Worth, TX: Harcourt Brace, 1993.

Reger D, Goode S, Mercer E. *Chemistry: Principles & Practice.* Fort Worth, TX: Harcourt Brace, 1993.

Reger MA, Henderson ST, Hale C, Cholerton B, Baker LD, Watson GS, Hyde K, Chapman D, Craft S. Effects of beta-hydroxybutyrate on cognition in memory-impaired adults. Neurobiol Aging. 2004;25:311–314.

Regis E. *Virus Ground Zero.* New York: Pocket, 1996.

Reha CM, Ebru A. Specific immunotherapy is effective in the prevention of new sensitivities. *Allergol Immunopathol (Madr).* 2007 Mar-Apr;35(2):44-51.

Rehm J, Taylor B, Mohapatra S, Irving H, Baliunas D, Patra J, Roerecke M. Alcohol as a risk factor for liver cirrhosis: a systematic review and meta-analysis. Drug Alcohol Rev. 2010 Jul;29(4):437-45.

Reid G, Beuerman D, Heinemann C, Bruce AW. Probiotic Lactobacillus dose required to restore and maintain a normal vaginal flora. *FEMS Immunol Med Microbiol.* 2001 Dec;32(1):37-41.

Reid G, Burton J, Hammond JA, Bruce AW. Nucleic acid-based diagnosis of bacterial vaginosis and improved management using probiotic lactobacilli. *J Med Food.* 2004 Summer;7(2):223-8.

Reid G, Charbonneau D, Erb J, Kochanowski B, Beuerman D, Poehner R, Bruce AW. Oral use of *Lactobacillus rhamnosus* GR-1 and L. fermentum RC-14 significantly alters vaginal flora: randomized, placebo-controlled trial in 64 healthy women. *FEMS Immunol Med Microbiol.* 2003 Mar 20;35(2):131-4.

Rendina E, Hembree KD, Davis MR, Marlow D, Clarke SL, Halloran BP, Lucas EA, Smith BJ. Dried Plum's Unique Capacity to Reverse Bone Loss and Alter Bone Metabolism in Postmenopausal Osteoporosis Model. PLoS One. 2013;8(3):e60569.

Rendina E, Hembree KD, Davis MR, Marlow D, Clarke SL, Halloran BP, Lucas EA, Smith BJ. Dried Plum's Unique Capacity to Reverse Bone Loss and Alter Bone Metabolism in Postmenopausal Osteoporosis Model. PLoS One. 2013;8(3):e60569.

Rendina E, Lim YF, Marlow D, Wang Y, Clarke SL, Kuvibidila S, Lucas EA, Smith BJ. Dietary supplementation with dried plum prevents ovariectomy-induced bone loss while modulating the immune response in C57BL/6J mice. J Nutr Biochem. 2012 Jan;23(1):60-8.

Renkonen R, Renkonen J, Joenväärä S, Mattila P, Parviainen V, Toppila-Salmi S. Allergens are transported through the respiratory epithelium. *Expert Rev Clin Immunol.* 2010 Jan;6(1):55-9.

Renvert S, Lindahl C, Renvert H, Persson GR. Clinical and microbiological analysis of subjects treated with Brånemark or AstraTech implants: a 7-year follow-up study. *Clin Oral Implants Res.* 2008 Apr;19(4):342-7.

Reuter A, Lidholm J, Andersson K, Ostling J, Lundberg M, Scheurer S, Enrique E, Cistero-Bahima A, San Miguel-Moncin M, Ballmer-Weber BK, Vieths S. A critical assessment of allergen component-based in vitro diagnosis in cherry allergy across Europe. *Clin Exp Allergy.* 2006 Jun;36(6):815-23.

Reyna-Villasmil N, Bermúdez-Pirela V, Mengual-Moreno E, Arias N, Cano-Ponce C, Leal-Gonzalez E, Souki A, Inglett GE, Israili ZH, Hernández-Hernández R, Valasco M, Arraiz N. Oat-derived beta-glucan significantly improves HDLC and diminishes LDLC and non-HDL cholesterol in overweight individuals with mild hypercholesterolemia. Am J Ther. 2007 Mar-Apr;14(2):203-12.

Reznik M, Sharif I, Ozuah PO. Rubbing ointments and asthma morbidity in adolescents. *J Altern Complement Med.* 2004 Dec;10(6):1097-9. Uu

Riccia DN, Bizzini F, Perilli MG, Polimeni A, Trinchieri V, Amicosante G, Cifone MG. Anti-inflammatory effects of *Lactobacillus brevis* (CD2) on periodontal disease. *Oral Dis.* 2007 Jul;13(4):376-85.

Riccia DN, Bizzini F, Perilli MG, Polimeni A, Trinchieri V, Amicosante G, Cifone MG. Anti-inflammatory effects of *Lactobacillus brevis* (CD2) on periodontal disease. *Oral Dis.* 2007 Jul;13(4):376-85.

Riccioni G, Barbara M, Bucciarelli T, di Ilio C, D'Orazio N. Antioxidant vitamin supplementation in asthma. *Ann Clin Lab Sci.* 2007 Winter;37(1):96-101.

Riccioni G, Bucciarelli T, Mancini B, Di Ilio C, Della Vecchia R, D'Orazio N. Plasma lycopene and antioxidant vitamins in asthma: the PLAVA study. *J Asthma.* 2007 Jul-Aug;44(6):429-32.

Riccioni G, D'Orazio N. The role of selenium, zinc and antioxidant vitamin supplementation in the treatment of bronchial asthma: adjuvant therapy or not? Expert Opin Investig Drugs. 2005 Sep;14(9):1145-55.

Riccioni G, Di Stefano F, De Benedictis M, Verna N, Cavallucci E, Paolini F, Di Sciascio MB, Della Vecchia R, Schiavone C, Boscolo P, Conti P, Di Gioacchino M. Seasonal variability of non-specific bronchial responsiveness in asthmatic patients with allergy to house dust mites. *Allergy Asthma Proc.* 2001 Jan-Feb;22(1):5-9.

Riccioni G, Scotti L, Di Ilio E, Bucciarelli V, Ballone E, De Girolamo M, D' Orazio N, Martini F, Aceto A, Bucciarelli T. Lycopene and preclinical carotid atherosclerosis. J Biol Regul Homeost Agents. 2011 Jul-Sep;25(3):435-41.

Richardson AJ, Burton JR, Sewell RP, Spreckelsen TF, Montgomery P. Docosahexaenoic Acid for Reading, Cognition and Behavior in Children Aged 7-9 Years: A Randomized, Controlled Trial (The DOLAB Study). PLoS One. 2012;7(9):e43909.

Riedler J, Braun-Fahrländer C, Eder W, Schreuer M, Waser M, Maisch S, Carr D, Schierl R, Nowak D, von Mutius E; ALEX Study Team. Exposure to farming in early life and development of asthma and allergy: a cross-sectional survey. *Lancet.* 2001 Oct 6;358(9288):1129-33.

Rimkiene S, Ragazinskiene O, Savickiene N. The cumulation of Wild pansy (Viola tricolor L.) accessions: the possibility of species preservation and usage in medicine. *Medicina (Kaunas).* 2003;39(4):411-6.

Rinne M, Kalliomaki M, Arvilommi H, Salminen S, Isolauri E. Effect of probiotics and breastfeeding on the bifido-bacterium and lactobacillus/enterococcus microbiota and humoral immune responses. *J Pediatr.* 2005 Aug;147(2):186-91.

Rinne M, Kalliomaki M, Arvilommi H, Salminen S, Isolauri E. Effect of probiotics and breastfeeding on the bifido-bacterium and lactobacillus/enterococcus microbiota and humoral immune responses. *J Pediatr.* 2005 Aug;147(2):186-91.

Rinne M, Kalliomäki M, Salminen S, Isolauri E. Probiotic intervention in the first months of life: short-term effects on gastrointestinal symptoms and long-term effects on gut microbiota. *J Pediatr Gastroenterol Nutr.* 2006 Aug;43(2):200-5.

Río ME, Zago Beatriz L, Garcia H, Winter L. The nutritional status change the effectiveness of a dietary supplement of lactic bacteria on the emerging of respiratory tract diseases in children. *Arch Latinoam Nutr.* 2002 Mar;52(1):29-34.

Río ME, Zago LB, Garcia H, Winter L. Influence of nutritional status on the effectiveness of a dietary supplement of live lactobacillus to prevent and cure diarrhoea in children. *Arch Latinoam Nutr.* 2004 Sep;54(3):287-92.

Riordan NH, Stuard S, Bavera P, Di Renzo A, Kenyon J, Errichi BM. 2003. Prevention of venous thrombosis in long-haul flights with Flite Tabs: the LONFLIT-FLITE randomized, controlled trial. Angiology. Sep-Oct;54(5):531-9.

Riso P, Martini D, Moller P, Loft S, Bonacina G, Moro M, Porrini M. DNA damage and repair activity after broccoli intake in young healthy smokers. Mutagenesis. 2010 Nov;25(6):595-602. doi: 10.1093/mutage/geq045.

Riso P, Vendrame S, Del Bo' C, Martini D, Martinetti A, Seregni E, Visioli F, Parolini M, Porrini M. Effect of 10-day broccoli consumption on inflammatory status of young healthy smokers. Int J Food Sci Nutr. 2013 Sep 2.

Rizos EC, Ntzani EE, Bika E, Kostapanos MS, Elisaf MS. As-sociation between omega-3 fatty acid supplementation and risk of major cardiovascular disease events: a systematic review and meta-analysis. JAMA. 2012 Sep 12;308(10):1024-33.

Robbins KS, Shin EC, Shewfelt RL, Eitenmiller RR, Pegg RB. Update on the Healthful Lipid Constituents of Commercially Im-portant Tree Nuts. J Agric Food Chem. 2011 Oct 27.

Robert AM, Groult N, Six C, Robert L. The effect of procyanidolic oligomers on mesenchymal cells in culture II – Attachment of elastic fibers to the cells. *Pathol Biol.* 1990 Jun;38(6):601-7.

Robert AM, Robert L, Renard G. Protection of cornea against proteolytic damage. Experimental study of procyani-dolic oligomers (PCO) on bovine cornea. *J Fr Ophtalmol.* 2002 Apr;25(4):351-5.

Robert AM, Tixier JM, Robert L, Legeais JM, Renard G. Effect of procyanidolic oligomers on the permeability of the blood-brain barrier. *Pathol Biol.* 2001 May;49(4):298-304.

Roberts G, Lack G. Diagnosing peanut allergy with skin prick and specific IgE testing. *J Allergy Clin Immunol.* 2005 Jun;115(6):1291-6.

Roberts M. Broccoli slows arthritis, researchers think. 2013 Aug. 27. BBC News online http://www.bbc.co.uk/news/health-23847632. Acc. 2013 Sep 4.

Robinson L, Cherewatenko VS, Reeves S. *Epicor: The Key to a Balanced Immune System.* Sherman Oaks, CA: Health Point, 2009.

Rodriguez J, Crespo JF, Burks W, Rivas-Plata C, Fernandez-Anaya S, Vives R, Daroca P. Randomized, double-blind, crossover challenge study in 53 subjects reporting adverse reactions to melon (Cucumis melo). *J Allergy Clin Immunol.* 2000 Nov;106(5):968-72.

Rodriguez-Fragoso L, Reyes-Esparza J, Burchiel SW, Herrera-Ruiz D, Torres E. Risks and benefits of commonly used herbal medicines in Mexico. *Toxicol Appl Pharmacol.* 2008 Feb 15;227(1):125-35.

Rodriguez-Ortiz PG, Muñoz-Mendoza D, Arias-Cruz A, González-Díaz SN, Herrera-Castro D, Vidaurri-Ojeda AC. Epidemiological characteristics of patients with food allergy assisted at Regional Center of Allergies and Clini-cal Immunology of Monterrey. *Rev Alerg Mex.* 2009 Nov-Dec;56(6):185-91.

Roduit C, Scholtens S, de Jongste JC, Wijga AH, Gerritsen J, Postma DS, Brunekreef B, Hoekstra MO, Aalberse R, Smit HA. Asthma at 8 years of age in children born by caesarean section. *Thorax.* 2009 Feb;64(2):107-13.

Roessler A, Friedrich U, Vogelsang H, Bauer A, Kaatz M, Hipler UC, Schmidt I, Jahreis G. The immune system in healthy adults and patients with atopic dermatitis seems to be affected differently by a probiotic intervention. *Clin Exp Allergy.* 2008 Jan;38(1):93-102.

Roessler A, Friedrich U, Vogelsang H, Bauer A, Kaatz M, Hipler UC, Schmidt I, Jahreis G. The immune system in healthy adults and patients with atopic dermatitis seems to be affected differently by a probiotic intervention. *Clin Exp Allergy.* 2008 Jan;38(1):93-102.

Roffman I, Nevo E. Can chimpanzee biology highlight human origin and evolution? Rambam Maimonides Med J. 2010 Jul 2;1(1):e0009. doi: 10.5041/RMMJ.10009.

Roger A, Justicia JL, Navarro LÁ, Eseverri JL, Ferrés J, Malet A, Alvà V. Observational study of the safety of an ultra-rush sublingual immunotherapy regimen to treat rhinitis due to house dust mites. *Int Arch Allergy Immu-nol.* 2011;154(1):69-75. 2010 Jul 27.

Rohrmann S, Zoller D, Hermann S, Linseisen J. Intake of heterocyclic aromatic amines from meat in the European Prospective Investigation into Cancer and Nutrition (EPIC)-Heidelberg cohort. Br J Nutr. 2007 Dec;98(6):1112-5.

Roller M, Clune Y, Collins K, Rechkemmer G, Watzl B. Consumption of prebiotic inulin enriched with oligofruc-tose in combination with the probiotics *Lactobacillus rhamnosus* and *Bifidobacterium lactis* has minor effects on se-lected immune parameters in polypectomised and colon cancer patients. *Br J Nutr.* 2007 Apr;97(4):676-84.

Romaguera D, Ängquist L, Du H, Jakobsen MU, Forouhi NG, Halkjær J, Feskens EJ, van der A DL, Masala G, Steffen A, Palli D, Wareham NJ, Overvad K, Tjonneland A, Boeing H, Riboli E, Sorensen TI. Food composition of the diet in relation to changes in waist circumference adjusted for body mass index. PLoS One. 2011;6(8):e23384. doi: 10.1371/journal.pone.0023384.

Romeo J, Wärnberg J, Nova E, Díaz LE, González-Gross M, Marcos A. Changes in the immune system after moderate beer consumption. *Ann Nutr Metab.* 2007;51(4):359-66.

Romieu I, Barraza-Villarreal A, Escamilla-Núñez C, Texcalac-Sangrador JL, Hernandez-Cadena L, Díaz-Sánchez D, De Batlle J, Del Rio-Navarro BE. Dietary intake, lung function and airway inflammation in Mexico City school children exposed to air pollutants. *Respir Res.* 2009 Dec 10;10:122.

Ronteltap A, van Schaik J, Wensing M, Rynja FJ, Knulst AC, de Vries JH. Sensory testing of recipes masking peanut or hazelnut for double-blind placebo-controlled food challenges. Allergy. 2004 Apr;59(4):457-60. Clark S, Bock SA, Gaeta TJ, Brenner BE, Cydulka RK, Camargo CA; Multicenter Airway Research Collaboration-8 Investigators. Multicenter study of emergency department visits for food allergies. *J Allergy Clin Immunol.* 2004 Feb;113(2):347-52.

Rook GA, Hernandez-Pando R. Pathogenetic role, in human and murine tuberculosis, of changes in the peripheral metabolism of glucocorticoids and antiglucocorticoids. *Psychoneuroendocrinology.* 1997;22 Suppl 1:S109-13.

Ros E, Mataix J. Fatty acid composition of nuts – implications for cardiovascular health. *Br J Nutr.* 2006 Nov;96 Suppl 2:S29-35.

Rosander A, Connolly E, Roos S. Removal of antibiotic resistance gene-carrying plasmids from *Lactobacillus reuteri* ATCC 55730 and characterization of the resulting daughter strain, *L. reuteri* DSM 17938. *Appl Environ Microbiol.* 2008 Oct;74(19):6032-40.

Rosenfeldt V, Benfeldt E, Nielsen SD, Michaelsen KF, Jeppesen DL, Valerius NH, Paerregaard A. Effect of probiotic Lactobacillus strains in children with atopic dermatitis. *J Allergy Clin Immunol.* 2003 Feb;111(2):389-95.

Rosenfeldt V, Benfeldt E, Valerius NH, Paerregaard A, Michaelsen KF. Effect of probiotics on gastrointestinal symptoms and small intestinal permeability in children with atopic dermatitis. *J Pediatr.* 2004 Nov;145(5):612-6.

Rosenfeldt V, Michaelsen KF, Jakobsen M, Larsen CN, Moller PL, Pedersen P, Tvede M, Weyrehter H, Valerius NH, Paerregaard A. Effect of probiotic Lactobacillus strains in young children hospitalized with acute diarrhea. *Pediatr Infect Dis J.* 2002 May;21(5):411-6.

Rosenkranz SK, Swain KE, Rosenkranz RR, Beckman B, Harms CA. Modifiable lifestyle factors impact airway health in non-asthmatic prepubescent boys but not girls. *Pediatr Pulmonol.* 2010 Dec 30.

Rosenlund H, Bergström A, Alm JS, Swartz J, Scheynius A, van Hage M, Johansen K, Brunekreef B, von Mutius E, Ege MJ, Riedler J, Braun-Fahrländer C, Waser M, Pershagen G; PARSIFAL Study Group. Allergic disease and atopic sensitization in children in relation to measles vaccination and measles infection. *Pediatrics.* 2009 Mar;123(3):771-8.

Rossi M, Amaretti A, Raimondi S. Folate production by probiotic bacteria. Nutrients. 2011 Jan;3(1):118-34.

Rousseaux C, Thuru X, Gelot A, Barnich N, Neut C, Dubuquoy L, Dubuquoy C, Merour E, Geboes K, Chamaillard M, Ouwehand A, Leyer G, Carcano D, Colombel JF, Ardid D, Desreumaux P. Lactobacillus acidophilus modulates intestinal pain and induces opioid and cannabinoid receptors. *Nat Med.* 2007 Jan;13(1):35-7

Royer RJ, Schmidt CL. Evaluation of venotropic drugs by venous gas plethysmography. A study of procyanidolic oligomers *Sem Hop.* 1981 Dec 18-25;57(47-48):2009-13.

Rozycki VR, Baigorria CM, Freyre MR, Bernard CM, Zannier MS, Charpentier M. Nutrient content in vegetable species from the Argentine Chaco. *Arch Latinoam Nutr.* 1997 Sep;47(3):265-70.

Rubin E., Farber JL. *Pathology.* 3rd Ed. Philadelphia: Lippincott-Raven, 1999.

Rudders SA, Espinola JA, Camargo CA Jr. North-south differences in US emergency department visits for acute allergic reactions. *Ann Allergy Asthma Immunol.* 2010 May;104(5):413-6.

Ruff C. Body size and body shape in early hominins – implications of the Gona pelvis. J Hum Evol. 2010 Feb;58(2):166-78. doi: 10.1016/j.jhevol.2009.10.003.

Rynard PB, Palij B, Galloway CA, Roughley FR. Resperin inhalation treatment for chronic respiratory diseases. *Can Fam Physician.* 1968 Oct;14(10):70-1.

Saarinen KM, Juntunen-Backman K, Järvenpää AL, Klemetti P, Kuitunen P, Lope L, Renlund M, Siivola M, Vaarala O, Savilahti E. Breast-feeding and the development of cows' milk protein allergy. *Adv Exp Med Biol.* 2000;478:121-30.

Saavedra JM, Abi-Hanna A, Moore N, Yolken RH. Long-term consumption of infant formulas containing live probiotic bacteria: tolerance and safety. *Am J Clin Nutr.* 2004 Feb;79(2):261-7.

Saavedra JM, Bauman NA, Oung I, Perman JA, Yolken RH. Feeding of *Bifidobacterium bifidum* and *Streptococcus thermophilus* to infants in hospital for prevention of diarrhoea and shedding of rotavirus. *Lancet.* 1994 Oct 15;344(8929):1046-9.

Sacco SM, Horcajada MN, Offord E. Phytonutrients for bone health during ageing. Br J Clin Pharmacol. 2013 Mar;75(3):697-707.

Saggioro A. Probiotics in the treatment of irritable bowel syndrome. *J Clin Gastroenterol.* 2004 Jul;38(6 Suppl):S104-6.

Sahagún-Flores JE, López-Peña LS, de la Cruz-Ramírez Jaimes J, García-Bravo MS, Peregrina-Gómez R, de Alba-García JE. Eradication of Helicobacter pylori: triple treatment scheme plus Lactobacillus vs. triple treatment alone. *Cir Cir.* 2007 Sep-Oct;75(5):333-6.

Sahagún-Flores JE, López-Peña LS, de la Cruz-Ramírez Jaimes J, García-Bravo MS, Peregrina-Gómez R, de Alba-García JE. Eradication of *Helicobacter pylori:* triple treatment scheme plus Lactobacillus vs. triple treatment alone. *Cir Cir.* 2007 Sep-Oct;75(5):333-6.

# REFERENCES AND BIBLIOGRAPHY

Sahakian NM, White SK, Park JH, Cox-Ganser JM, Kreiss K. Identification of mold and dampness-associated respiratory morbidity in 2 schools: comparison of questionnaire survey responses to national data. *J Sch Health.* 2008 Jan;78(1):32-7.

Sahin-Yilmaz A, Nocon CC, Corey JP. Immunoglobulin E-mediated food allergies among adults with allergic rhinitis. *Otolaryngol Head Neck Surg.* 2010 Sep;143(3):379-85.

Salazar-Lindo E, Figueroa-Quintanilla D, Caciano MI, Reto-Valiente V, Chauviere G, Colin P; Lacteol Study Group. Effectiveness and safety of Lactobacillus LB in the treatment of mild acute diarrhea in children. *J Pediatr Gastroenterol Nutr.* 2007 May;44(5):571-6.

Salazar-Lindo E, Miranda-Langschwager P, Campos-Sanchez M, Chea-Woo E, Sack RB. *Lactobacillus casei* strain GG in the treatment of infants with acute watery diarrhea: a randomized, double-blind, placebo controlled clinical trial [ISRCTN67363048]. *BMC Pediatr.* 2004 Sep 2;4:18.

Salem N, Wegher B, Mena P, Uauy R. Arachidonic and docosahexaenoic acids are biosynthesized from their 18-carbon precursors in human infants. *Proc Natl Acad Sci.* 1996;93:49-54.

Salib RJ, Howarth PH. Remodelling of the upper airways in allergic rhinitis: is it a feature of the disease? *Clin Exp Allergy.* 2003 Dec;33(12):1629-33.

Salim AS. Sulfhydryl-containing agents in the treatment of gastric bleeding induced by nonsteroidal anti-inflammatory drugs. *Can J Surg.* 1993 Feb;36(1):53-8.

Salmi H, Kuitunen M, Viljanen M, Lapatto R. Cow's milk allergy is associated with changes in urinary organic acid concentrations. *Pediatr Allergy Immunol.* 2010 Mar;21(2 Pt 2):e401-6.

Salminen E, Elomaa I, Minkkinen J, Vapaatalo H, Salminen S. Preservation of intestinal integrity during radiotherapy using live *Lactobacillus acidophilus* cultures. *Clin Radiol.* 1988 Jul;39(4):435-7.

Salminen S, Isolauri E, Salminen E. Clinical uses of probiotics for stabilizing the gut mucosal barrier: successful strains and future challenges. *Antonie Van Leeuwenhoek.* 1996 Oct;70(2-4):347-58.

Salom IL, Silvis SE, Doscherholmen A. Effect of cimetidine on the absorption of vitamin B12. *Scand J Gastroenterol.* 1982;17:129-31.

Salome CM, Marks GB. Sex, asthma and obesity: an intimate relationship? *Clin Exp Allergy.* 2011 Jan;41(1):6-8.

Salpietro CD, Gangemi S, Briuglia S, Meo A, Merlino MV, Muscolino G, Bisignano G, Trombetta D, Saija A. The almond milk: a new approach to the management of cow-milk allergy/intolerance in infants. *Minerva Pediatr.* 2005 Aug;57(4):173-80.

Salvi SS, Barnes PJ. Chronic obstructive pulmonary disease in non-smokers. *Lancet.* 2009 Aug 29;374(9691):733-43.

Samanta M, Sarkar M, Ghosh P, Ghosh J, Sinha M, Chatterjee S. Prophylactic probiotics for prevention of necrotizing enterocolitis in very low birth weight newborns. *J Trop Pediatr.* 2009 Apr;55(2):128-31.

Sanaka M, Yamamoto T, Anjiki H, Nagasawa K, Kuyama Y. Effects of agar and pectin on gastric emptying and post-prandial glycaemic profiles in healthy human volunteers. Clin Exp Pharmacol Physiol. 2007 Nov;34(11):1151-5.

Sancho AI, Hoffmann-Sommergruber K, Alessandri S, Conti A, Giuffrida MG, Shewry P, Jensen BM, Skov P, Vieths S. Authentication of food allergen quality by physicochemical and immunological methods. *Clin Exp Allergy.* 2010 Jul;40(7):973-86.

Sandberg AS. The effect of food processing on phytate hydrolysis and availability of iron and zinc. Adv Exp Med Biol. 1991;289:499-508.

Santos A, Dias A, Pinheiro JA. Predictive factors for the persistence of cow's milk allergy. *Pediatr Allergy Immunol.* 2010 Apr 27.

Sanz Ortega J, Martorell Aragonés A, Michavila Gómez A, Nieto García A; Grupo de Trabajo para el Estudio de la Alergia Alimentaria. Incidence of IgE-mediated allergy to cow's milk proteins in the first year of life. *An Esp Pediatr.* 2001 Jun;54(6):536-9.

Sanz-Penella JM, Frontela C, Ros G, Martinez C, Monedero V, Haros M. Application of bifidobacterial phytases in infant cereals: effect on phytate contents and mineral dializability. J Agric Food Chem. 2012 Nov 28;60(47):11787-92. doi: 10.1021/jf3034013.

Saran S, Gopalan S, Krishna TP. Use of fermented foods to combat stunting and failure to thrive. *Nutrition.* 2002 May;18(5):393-6.

Sato Y, Akiyama H, Matsuoka H, Sakata K, Nakamura R, Ishikawa S, Inakuma T, Totsuka M, Sugita-Konishi Y, Ebisawa M, Teshima R. Dietary carotenoids inhibit oral sensitization and the development of food allergy. *J Agric Food Chem.* 2010 Jun 23;58(12):7180-6.

Satoh A, Tsuji S, Okada Y, Murakami M, Urami M, Nakagawa K, Ishikura M, Katagiri M, Koga Y, Shirasawa T. Preliminary Clinical Evalua-tion of Toxicity and Efficacy of A New Astaxanthin-rich Haematococcus pluvialis Extract. J Clin Biochem Nutr. 2009 May;44(3):280-4.

Satyanarayana S, Sushruta K, Sarma GS, Srinivas N, Subba Raju GV. Antioxidant activity of the aqueous extracts of spicy food additives – evaluation and comparison with ascorbic acid in in-vitro systems. *J Herb Pharmacother.* 2004;4(2):1-10.

Savage JH, Kaeding AJ, Matsui EC, Wood RA. The natural history of soy allergy. *J Allergy Clin Immunol.* 2010 Mar;125(3):683-6.

Savilahti EM, Karinen S, Salo HM, Klemetti P, Saarinen KM, Klemola T, Kuitunen M, Hautaniemi S, Savilahti E, Vaarala O. Combined T regulatory cell and Th2 expression profile identifies children with cow's milk allergy. *Clin Immunol.* 2010 Jul;136(1):16-20.

Savilahti EM, Rantanen V, Lin JS, Karinen S, Saarinen KM, Goldis M, Mäkelä MJ, Hautaniemi S, Savilahti E, Sampson HA. Early recovery from cow's milk allergy is associated with decreasing IgE and increasing IgG4 binding to cow's milk epitopes. *J Allergy Clin Immunol.* 2010 Jun;125(6):1315-1321.e9.

441

Savino F, Pelle E, Palumeri E, Oggero R, Miniero R. *Lactobacillus reuteri* (American Type Culture Collection Strain 55730) versus simethicone in the treatment of infantile colic: a prospective randomized study. Pediatrics. 2007 Jan;119(1):e124-30.

Sazanova NE, Varnacheva LN, Novikova AV, Pletneva NB. Immunological aspects of food intolerance in children during first years of life. *Pediatriia*. 1992;(3):14-8.

Scadding G, Bjarnason I, Brostoff J, Levi AJ, Peters TJ. Intestinal permeability to 51Cr-labelled ethylenediamine-tetraacetate in food-intolerant subjects. *Digestion*. 1989;42(2):104-9.

Scalabrin DM, Johnston WH, Hoffman DR, P'Pool VL, Harris CL, Mitmesser SH. Growth and tolerance of healthy term infants receiving hydrolyzed infant formulas supplemented with Lactobacillus rhamnosus GG: randomized, double-blind, controlled trial. *Clin Pediatr (Phila)*. 2009 Sep;48(7):734-44.

Scarmeas N, Luchsinger JA, Mayeux R, Stern Y. Mediterranean diet and Alzheimer disease mortality. Neurology. 2007 Sep 11;69(11):1084-93.

Scarmeas N, Luchsinger JA, Schupf N, Brickman AM, Cosentino S, Tang MX, Stern Y. Physical activity, diet, and risk of Alzheimer disease. JAMA. 2009 Aug 12;302(6):627-37. Scarmeas N, Stern Y, Tang MX, Mayeux R, Luchsinger JA. Mediterranean diet and risk for Alzheimer's disease. Ann Neurol. 2006 Jun;59(6):912-21.

Scarmeas N, Stern Y, Mayeux R, Luchsinger JA. Mediterranean diet, Alzheimer disease, and vascular mediation. Arch Neurol. 2006 Dec;63(12):1709-17.

Schaafsma G, Meuling WJ, van Dokkum W, Bouley C. Effects of a milk product, fermented by *Lactobacillus acidophilus* and with fructo-oligosaccharides added, on blood lipids in male volunteers. *Eur J Clin Nutr*. 1998 Jun;52(6):436-40.

Schauenberg P, Paris F. *Guide to Medicinal Plants*. New Canaan, CT: Keats Publ, 1977.

Schauss AG, Wu X, Prior RL, Ou B, Huang D, Owens J, Agarwal A, Jensen GS, Hart AN, Shanbrom E. Antioxidant capacity and other bioactivities of the freeze-dried Amazonian palm berry, Euterpe oleraceae mart. (acai). *J Agric Food Chem*. 2006 Nov 1;54(22):8604-10.

Scheiber, M. D., J. H. Liu, *et al*. 2001. Dietary inclusion of whole soy foods results in significant reductions in clinical risk factors for osteoporosis and cardiovascular disease in normal postmenopausal women. Menopause 8(5): 384-92.

Schempp H, Weiser D, Elstner EF. Biochemical model reactions indicative of inflammatory processes. Activities of extracts from Fraxinus excelsior and Populus tremula. *Arzneimittelforschung*. 2000 Apr;50(4):362-72.

Scher JU, Sczesnak A, Longman RS, Segata N, Ubeda C, Bielski C, Rostron T, Cerundolo V, Pamer EG, Abramson SB, Huttenhower C, Littman DR. Expansion of intestinal Prevotella copri correlates with enhanced susceptibility to arthritis. Elife. 2013 Nov 5;2(0). doi:pii: e01202. 10.7554/eLife.01202.

Schillaci D, Arizza V, Dayton T, Camarda L, Di Stefano V. In vitro anti-biofilm activity of Boswellia spp. oleogum resin essential oils. *Lett Appl Microbiol*. 2008 Nov;47(5):433-8.

Schmid B, Kötter I, Heide L. Pharmacokinetics of salicin after oral administration of a standardised willow bark extract. *Eur J Clin Pharmacol*. 2001 Aug;57(5):387-91.

Schmitt DA, Maleki SJ (2004) Comparing the effects of boiling, frying and roasting on the allergenicity of peanuts. *J Allergy Clin Immunol*. 113: S155.

Schnappinger M, Sausenthaler S, Linseisen J, Hauner H, Heinrich J. Fish consumption, allergic sensitisation and allergic diseases in adults. *Ann Nutr Metab*. 2009;54(1):67-74.

Schnappinger M, Sausenthaler S, Linseisen J, Hauner H, Heinrich J. Fish consumption, allergic sensitisation and allergic diseases in adults. *Ann Nutr Metab*. 2009;54(1):67-74.

Schoeninger MJ, Murray S, Bunn HT, Marlett JA. Composition of tubers used by Hadza foragers of Tanzania. J Food Compost Anal. 2001;14:15 – 25.

Scholz-Ahrens KE, Ade P, Marten B, Weber P, Timm W, Açil Y, Glüer CC, Schrezenmeir J. Prebiotics, probiotics, and synbiotics affect mineral absorption, bone mineral content, and bone structure. *J Nutr*. 2007 Mar;137(3 Suppl 2):838S-46S.

Schönfeld P. Phytanic Acid toxicity: implications for the permeability of the inner mitochondrial membrane to ions. *Toxicol Mech Methods*. 2004;14(1-2):47-52.

Schottner M, Gansser D, Spiteller G. Lignans from the roots of Urtica dioica and their metabolites bind to human sex hormone binding globulin (SHBG). *Planta Med*. 1997;65:529-532.

Schouten B, van Esch BC, Hofman GA, Boon L, Knippels LM, Willemsen LE, Garssen J. Oligosaccharide-induced whey-specific CD25(+) regulatory T-cells are involved in the suppression of cow milk allergy in mice. *J Nutr*. 2010 Apr;140(4):835-41.

Schroecksnadel S, Jenny M, Fuchs D. Sensitivity to sulphite additives. *Clin Exp Allergy*. 2010 Apr;40(4):688-9.

Schulick P. *Ginger: Common Spice & Wonder Drug*. Brattleboro, VT: Herbal Free Perss, 1996.

Schulman G. A nexus of progression of chronic kidney disease: charcoal, tryptophan and profibrotic cytokines. *Blood Purif*. 2006;24(1):143-8.

Schulz V, Hansel R, Tyler VE. *Rational Phytotherapy*. Berlin: Springer-Verlag; 1998.

Schulze MB, Manson JE, Willett WC, Hu FB. Processed meat intake and incidence of Type 2 diabetes in younger and middle-aged women. Diabetologia. 2003 Nov;46(11):1465-73.

Schumacher P. *Biophysical Therapy Of Allergies*. Stuttgart: Thieme, 2005.

Schütz K, Carle R, Schieber A. Taraxacum – a review on its phytochemical and pharmacological profile. *J Ethnopharmacol*. 2006 Oct 11;107(3):313-23.

Schwab D, Hahn EG, Raithel M. Enhanced histamine metabolism: a comparative analysis of collagenous colitis and food allergy with respect to the role of diet and NSAID use. *Inflamm Res*. 2003 Apr;52(4):142-7.

# REFERENCES AND BIBLIOGRAPHY

Schwab D, Müller S, Aigner T, Neureiter D, Kirchner T, Hahn EG, Raithel M. Functional and morphologic characterization of eosinophils in the lower intestinal mucosa of patients with food allergy. *Am J Gastroenterol.* 2003 Jul;98(7):1525-34.

Schwelberger HG. Histamine intolerance: a metabolic disease? *Inflamm Res.* 2010 Mar;59 Suppl 2:S219-21.

Schwellenbach LJ, Olson KL. McConnell KJ, Stolepart RS, Nash JD, Merenich JA. The triglyceride-lowering effects of a modest dose of docosahexaenoic acid alone versus in combination with low dose eicosapentaenoic acid in patients with coronary artery disease and elevated triglycerides. *J Am Coll Nutr.* 2006;25(6):480-485.

Scott RS, *et al.* Dental microwear texture analysis reflects diets of living primates and fossil hominins. Nature. 2005;436:693 – 695.

Scott-Taylor TH, O'B Hourihane J, Strobel S. Correlation of allergen-specific IgG subclass antibodies and T lymphocyte cytokine responses in children with multiple food allergies. *Pediatr Allergy Immunol.* 2010 Sep;21(6):935-44.

Scurlock AM, Jones SM. An update on immunotherapy for food allergy. *Curr Opin Allergy Clin Immunol.* 2010 Dec;10(6):587-93.

Sealey-Voyksner JA, Khosla C, Voyksner RD, Jorgenson JW. Novel aspects of quantitation of immunogenic wheat gluten peptides by liquid chromatography-mass spectrometry. *J Chromatog A.* 2010 Jun 18;1217(25):4167-83.

Searing DA, Leung DY. Vitamin D in atopic dermatitis, asthma and allergic diseases. *Immunol Allergy Clin North Am.* 2010 Aug;30(3):397-409.

Sekine K, Toida T, Saito M, Kuboyama M, Kawashima T, Hashimoto Y. A new morphologically characterized cell wall preparation (whole peptidoglycan) from *Bifidobacterium* infantis with a higher efficacy on the regression of an established tumor in mice. *Cancer Res.* 1985 Mar;45(3):1300-7.

Senior F. Fallout. *New York Magazine.* Fall: 2003.

Senna G, Gani F, Leo G, Schiappoli M. Alternative tests in the diagnosis of food allergies. *Recenti Prog Med.* 2002 May;93(5):327-34.

Seo K, Jung S, Park M, Song Y, Choung S. Effects of leucocyanidines on activities of metabolizing enzymes and antioxidant enzymes. *Biol Pharm Bull.* 2001 May;24(5):592-3.

Seo K, Jung S, Park M, Song Y, Choung S. Effects of leucocyanidines on activities of metabolizing enzymes and antioxidant enzymes. *Biol Pharm Bull.* 2001 May;24(5):592-3.

Seo SW, Koo HN, An HJ, Kwon KB, Lim BC, Seo EA, Ryu DG, Moon G, Kim HY, Kim HM, Hong SH. Taraxacum officinale protects against cholecystokinin-induced acute pancreatitis in rats. *World J Gastroenterol.* 2005 Jan 28;11(4):597-9.

Seppo L, Jauhiainen T, Poussa T, Korpela R. A fermented milk high in bioactive peptides has a blood pressure-lowering effect in hypertensive subjects. *Am J Clin Nutr.* 2003 Feb;77(2):326-30.

Seppo L, Korpela R, Lönnerdal B, Metsäniitty L, Juntunen-Backman K, Klemola T, Paganus A, Vanto T. A follow-up study of nutrient intake, nutritional status, and growth in infants with cow milk allergy fed either a soy formula or an extensively hydrolyzed whey formula. *Am J Clin Nutr.* 2005 Jul;82(1):140-5.

Serra A, Cocuzza S, Poli G, La Mantia I, Messina A, Pavone P. Otologic findings in children with gastroesophageal reflux. *Int J Pediatr Otorhinolaryngol.* 2007 Nov;71(11):1693-7. 2007 Aug 22.

Sevar R. Audit of outcome in 455 consecutive patients treated with homeopathic medicines. *Homeopathy.* 2005 Oct;94(4):215-21.

Shahani KM, Ayebo AD. Role of dietary lactobacilli in gastrointestinal microecology. *Am J Clin Nutr.* 1980 Nov;33(11 Suppl):2448-57.

Shahani KM, Chandan RC. Nutritional and healthful aspects of cultured and culture-containing dairy foods. *J Dairy Sci.* 1979 Oct;62(10):1685-94.

Shahani KM, Friend BA. Properties of and prospects for cultured dairy foods. *Soc Appl Bacteriol Symp Ser.* 1983;11:257-69.

Shahani KM, Herper WJ, Jensen RG, Parry RM Jr, Zittle CA. Enzymes in bovine milk: a review. *J Dairy Sci.* 1973 May;56(5):531-43.

Shahani KM, Kwan AJ, Friend BA. Role and significance of enzymes in human milk. *Am J Clin Nutr.* 1980 Aug;33(8):1861-8.

Shahani KM, Meshbesher BF, Mangalampalli V. *Cultivate Health From Within.* Danbury, CT: Vital Health Publ, 2005.

Shaheen S, Potts J, Gnatiuc L, Makowska J, Kowalski ML, Joos G, van Zele T, van Durme Y, De Rudder I, Wöhrl S, Godnic-Cvar J, Skadhauge L, Thomsen G, Zuberbier T, Bergmann KC, Heinzerling L, Gjomarkaj M, Bruno A, Pace E, Bonini S, Fokkens W, Weersink EJ, Loureiro C, Todo-Bom A, Villanueva CM, Sanjuas C, Zock JP, Janson C, Burney P; Selenium and Asthma Research Integration project; GA2LEN. The relation between paracetamol use and asthma: a GA2LEN European case-control study. *Eur Respir J.* 2008 Nov;32(5):1231-6.

Shaheen SO, Newson RB, Rayman MP, Wong AP, Tumilty MK, Phillips JM, Potts JF, Kelly FJ, White PT, Burney PG. Randomised, double blind, placebo-controlled trial of selenium supplementation in adult asthma. *Thorax.* 2007 Jun;62(6):483-90.

Shakib F, Brown HM, Phelps A, Redhead R. Study of IgG sub-class antibodies in patients with milk intolerance. *Clin Allergy.* 1986 Sep;16(5):451-8.

Shalev E, Battino S, Weiner E, Colodner R, Keness Y. Ingestion of yogurt containing *Lactobacillus acidophilus* compared with pasteurized yogurt as prophylaxis for recurrent *Candida* vaginitis and bacterial vaginosis. *Arch Fam Med.* 1996 Nov-Dec;5(10):593-6.

Shamir R, Makhoul IR, Etzioni A, Shehadeh N. Evaluation of a diet containing probiotics and zinc for the treatment of mild diarrheal illness in children younger than one year of age. *J Am Coll Nutr.* 2005 Oct;24(5):370-5.

Sharma P, Sharma BC, Puri V, Sarin SK. An open-label randomized controlled trial of lactulose and probiotics in the treatment of minimal hepatic encephalopathy. *Eur J Gastroent Hepatol.* 2008 Jun;20(6):506-11.

Sharma S, Vik S, Pakseresht M, Shen L, Kolonel LN. Diet impacts mortality from cancer: results from the multiethnic cohort study. *Cancer Causes Control.* 2013 Apr;24(4):685-93. doi: 10.1007/s10552-013-0148-6.

Sharma SC, Sharma S, Gulati OP. Pycnogenol inhibits the release of histamine from mast cells. *Phytother Res.* 2003 Jan;17(1):66-9.

Sharman J, Kumar L, Singh S. Comparison of results of skin prick tests, enzyme-linked immunosorbent assays and food challenges in children with respiratory allergy. *J Trop Pediatr.* 2001 Dec;47(6):367-8.

Shawcross DL, Wright G, Olde Damink SW, Jalan R. Role of ammonia and inflammation in minimal hepatic encephalopathy. *Metab Brain Dis.* 2007 Mar;22(1):125-38.

Shay CM, Van Horn L, Stamler J, Dyer AR, Brown IJ, Chan Q, Miura K, Zhao L, Okuda N, Daviglus ML, Elliott P; INTERMAP Research Group. Food and nutrient intakes and their associations with lower BMI in middle-aged US adults: the International Study of Macro-/Micronutrients and Blood Pressure (INTERMAP). *Am J Clin Nutr.* 2012 Sep;96(3):483-91.

Shea KM, Trucker RT, Weber RW, Peden DB. Climate change and allergic disease. *Clin Rev Allergy Immunol.* 2008;6:443-453.

Shea-Donohue T, Stiltz J, Zhao A, Notari L. Mast Cells. *Curr Gastroenterol Rep.* 2010 Aug 14.

Sheih YH, Chiang BL, Wang LH, Liao CK, Gill HS. Systemic immunity-enhancing effects in healthy subjects following dietary consumption of the lactic acid bacterium *Lactobacillus rhamnosus* HN001. *J Am Coll Nutr.* 2001 Apr;20(2 Suppl):149-56.

Shen CL, von Bergen V, Chyu MC, Jenkins MR, Mo H, Chen CH, Kwun IS. Fruits and dietary phytochemicals in bone protection. *Nutr Res.* 2012 Dec;32(12):897-910.

Shen FY, Lee MS, Jung SK. Effectiveness of pharmacopuncture for asthma: a systematic review and meta-analysis. *Evid Based Complement Alternat Med.* 2011;2011. pii: 678176.

Sheth SS, Waserman S, Kagan R, Alizadehfar R, Primeau MN, Elliot S, St Pierre Y, Wickett R, Joseph L, Harada L, Dufresne C, Allen M, Allen M, Godefroy SB, Clarke AE. Role of food labels in accidental exposures in food-allergic individuals in Canada. *Ann Allergy Asthma Immunol.* 2010 Jan;104(1):60-5.

Shi GX, Liu CZ, Wang LP, Guan LP, Li SQ. Biomarkers of oxidative stress in vascular dementia patients. *Can J Neurol Sci.* 2012 Jan;39(1):65-8.

Shi S, Zhao Y, Zhou H, Zhang Y, Jiang X, Huang K. Identification of antioxidants from Taraxacum mongolicum by high-performance liquid chromatography-diode array detection-radical-scavenging detection-electrospray ionization mass spectrometry and nuclear magnetic resonance experiments. *J Chromatogr A.* 2008 Oct 31;1209(1-2):145-52

Shi S, Zhou H, Zhang Y, Huang K, Liu S. Chemical constituents from Neo-Taraxacum siphonathum. *Zhongguo Zhong Yao Za Zhi.* 2009 Apr;34(8):1002-4.

Shi SY, Zhou CX, Xu Y, Tao QF, Bai H, Lu FS, Lin WY, Chen HY, Zheng W, Wang LW, Wu YH, Zeng S, Huang KX, Zhao Y, Li XK, Qu J. Studies on chemical constituents from herbs of Taraxacum mongolicum. *Zhongguo Zhong Yao Za Zhi.* 2008 May;33(10):1147-57.

Shibata H, Nabe T, Yamamura H, Kohno S. l-Ephedrine is a major constituent of Mao-Bushi-Saishin-To, one of the formulas of Chinese medicine, which shows immediate inhibition after oral administration of passive cutaneous anaphylaxis in rats. *Inflamm Res.* 2000 Aug;49(8):398-403.

Shichinohe K, Shimizu M, Kurokawa K. Effect of M-711 on experimental asthma in rats. *J Vet Med Sci.* 1996 Jan;58(1):55-9.

Shimabukuro M, Higa M, Kinjo R, Yamakawa K, Tanaka H, Kozuka C, Yabiku K, Taira SI, Sata M, Masuzaki H. Effects of the brown rice diet on visceral obesity and endothelial function: the BRAVO study. *Br J Nutr.* 2013 Aug 12:1-11.

Shimauchi H, Mayanagi G, Nakaya S, Minamibuchi M, Ito Y, Yamaki K, Hirata H. Improvement of periodontal condition by probiotics with *Lactobacillus salivarius* WB21: a randomized, double-blind, placebo-controlled study. *J Clin Periodontol.* 2008 Oct;35(10):897-905.

Shimizu K, Ogura H, Goto M, Asahara T, Nomoto K, Morotomi M, Matsushima A, Tasaki O, Fujita K, Hosotsubo H, Kuwagata Y, Tanaka H, Shimazu T, Sugimoto H. Synbiotics decrease the incidence of septic complications in patients with severe SIRS: a preliminary report. *Dig Dis Sci.* 2009 May;54(5):1071-8.

Shimoi T, Ushiyama H, Kan K, Saito K, Kamata K, Hirokado M. Survey of glycoalkaloids content in the various potatoes. *Shokuhin Eiseigaku Zasshi.* 2007 Jun;48(3):77-82.

Shipman P, Harris JM. Habitat preference and paleocecology of Australopithecus boisei in eastern Africa. In: Grine FE, editor. Evolutionary History of the "Robust" Australopithecines. New York: Aldine de Gruyter; 1988. pp. 343 – 381.

Shishehbor F, Behroo L, Ghafouriyan Broujerdnia M, Namjoyan F, Latifi SM. Quercetin effectively quells peanut-induced anaphylactic reactions in the peanut sensitized rats. *Iran J Allergy Asthma Immunol.* 2010 Mar;9(1):27-34.

Shishodia S, Harikumar KB, Dass S, Ramawat KG, Aggarwal BB. The guggul for chronic diseases: ancient medicine, modern targets. *Anticancer Res.* 2008 Nov-Dec;28(6A):3647-64.

Shivpuri DN, Menon MP, Parkash D. Preliminary studies in Tylophora indica in the treatment of asthma and allergic rhinitis. *J Assoc Physicians India.* 1968 Jan;16(1):9-15.

Shivpuri DN, Menon MP, Prakash D. A crossover double-blind study on Tylophora indica in the treatment of asthma and allergic rhinitis. *J Allergy.* 1969 Mar;43(3):145-50.

Shivpuri DN, Singhal SC, Parkash D. Treatment of asthma with an alcoholic extract of Tylophora indica: a cross-over, double-blind study. *Ann Allergy*. 1972; 30:407-12.

Shoaf K, Mulvey GL, Armstrong GD, Hutkins RW. Prebiotic galactooligosaccharides reduce adherence of enteropathogenic *Escherichia coli* to tissue culture cells. *Infect Immun*. 2006 Dec;74(12):6920-8.

Shornikova AV, Casas IA, Isolauri E, Mykkänen H, Vesikari T. *Lactobacillus reuteri* as a therapeutic agent in acute diarrhea in young children. *J Pediatr Gastroenterol Nutr*. 1997 Apr;24(4):399-404.

Shornikova AV, Casas IA, Mykkänen H, Salo E, Vesikari T. Bacteriotherapy with *Lactobacillus reuteri* in rotavirus gastroenteritis. *Pediatr Infect Dis J*. 1997 Dec;16(12):1103-7.

Sicherer SH, Muñoz-Furlong A, Godbold JH, Sampson HA. US prevalence of self-reported peanut, tree nut, and sesame allergy: 11-year follow-up. *J Allergy Clin Immunol*. 2010 Jun;125(6):1322-6.

Sicherer SH, Noone SA, Koerner CB, Christie L, Burks AW, Sampson HA. Hypoallergenicity and efficacy of an amino acid-based formula in children with cow's milk and multiple food hypersensitivities. *J Pediatr*. 2001 May;138(5):688-93.

Sicherer SH, Sampson HA. Food allergy. *J Allergy Clin Immunol*. 2010 Feb;125(2 Suppl 2):S116-25.

Siddiq A, Dembitsky V. Acetylenic anticancer agents. Anticancer Agents Med Chem. 2008 Feb;8(2):132-70.

Sidoroff V, Hyvärinen M, Piippo-Savolainen E, Korppi M. Lung function and overweight in school aged children after early childhood wheezing. Pediatr Pulmonol. 2010 Dec 30.

Sigstedt SC, Hooten CJ, Callewaert MC, Jenkins AR, Romero AE, Pullin MJ, Kornienko A, Lowrey TK, Slambrouck SV, Steelant WF. Evaluation of aqueous extracts of Taraxacum officinale on growth and invasion of breast and prostate cancer cells. *Int J Oncol*. 2008 May;32(5):1085-90.

Silman AJ, MacGregor AJ, Thomson W, Holligan S, Carthy D, Farhan A, Ollier WE. Twin concordance rates for rheumatoid arthritis: results from a nationwide study. *Br J Rheumatol*. 1993 Oct;32(10):903-7.

Silva MF, Kamphorst AO, Hayashi EA, Bellio M, Carvalho CR, Faria AM, Sabino KC, Coelho MG, Nobrega A, Tavares D, Silva AC. Innate profiles of cytokines implicated on oral tolerance correlate with low- or high-suppression of humoral response. *Immunology*. 2010 Jul;130(3):447-57.

Silva MR, Dias G, Ferreira CL, Franceschini SC, Costa NM. Growth of preschool children was improved when fed an iron-fortified fermented milk beverage supplemented with *Lactobacillus acidophilus*. Nutr Res. 2008 Apr;28(4):226-32.

Silvester KR, Bingham SA, Pollock JR, Cummings JH, O'Neill IK. Effect of meat and resistant starch on fecal excretion of apparent N-nitroso compounds and ammonia from the human large bowel. Nutr Cancer. 1997;29(1):13-23.

Simakachorn N, Pichaipat V, Rithipornpaisarn P, Kongkaew C, Tongpradit P, Varavithya W. Clinical evaluation of the addition of lyophilized, heat-killed *Lactobacillus acidophilus* LB to oral rehydration therapy in the treatment of acute diarrhea in children. *J Pediatr Gastroenterol Nutr*. 2000 Jan;30(1):68-72.

Simenhoff ML, Dunn SR, Zollner GP, Fitzpatrick ME, Emery SM, Sandine WE, Ayres JW. Biomodulation of the toxic and nutritional effects of small bowel bacterial overgrowth in end-stage kidney disease using freeze-dried *Lactobacillus acidophilus*. Miner Electrolyte Metab. 1996;22(1-3):92-6.

Simeone D, Miele E, Boccia G, Marino A, Troncone R, Staiano A. Prevalence of atopy in children with chronic constipation. Arch Dis Child. 2008 Dec;93(12):1044-7.

Simões EA, Carbonell-Estrany X, Rieger CH, Mitchell I, Fredrick L, Groothuis JR; Palivizumab Long-Term Respiratory Outcomes Study Group. The effect of respiratory syncytial virus on subsequent recurrent wheezing in atopic and nonatopic children. *J Allergy Clin Immunol*. 2010 Aug;126(2):256-62. 2010 Jul 10.

Simons FER. What's in a name? The allergic rhinitis-asthma connection. Clin Exp All Rev. 2003;3:9-17.

Simonte SJ, Ma S, Mofidi S, Sicherer SH. Relevance of casual contact with peanut butter in children with peanut allergy. *J Allergy Clin Immunol*. 2003 Jul;112(1):180-2.

Simopoulos AP. Essential fatty acids in health and chronic disease. *Am J Clin Nutr*. 1999 Sep;70(3 Suppl):560S-569S.

Simpson A, Tan VY, Winn J, Svensén M, Bishop CM, Heckerman DE, Buchan I, Custovic A. Beyond atopy: multiple patterns of sensitization in relation to asthma in a birth cohort study. *Am J Respir Crit Care Med*. 2010 Jun 1;181(11):1200-6.

Simpson AB, Yousef E, Hossain J. Association between peanut allergy and asthma morbidity. *J Pediatr*. 2010 May;156(5):777-81.

Sin A, Terzioğlu E, Kokuludağ A, Sebik F, Kabakçi T. Serum eosinophil cationic protein (ECP) levels in patients with seasonal allergic rhinitis and allergic asthma. *Allergy Asthma Proc*. 1998 Mar-Apr;19(2):69-73.

Singer P, Shapiro H, Theilla M, Anbar R, Singer J, Cohen J. Anti-inflammatory properties of omega-3 fatty acids in critical illness: novel mechanisms and an integrative perspective. Intensive Care Med. 2008 Sep;34(9):1580-92.

Singh BB, Khorsan R, Vinjamury SP, Der-Martirosian C, Kizhakkeveettil A, Anderson TM. Herbal treatments of asthma: a systematic review. *J Asthma*. 2007 Nov;44(9):685-98.

Singh S, Khajuria A, Taneja SC, Johri RK, Singh J, Qazi GN. Boswellic acids: A leukotriene inhibitor also effective through topical application in inflammatory disorders. *Phytomedicine*. 2008 Jun;15(6-7):400-7.

Singh V, Jain NK. Asthma as a cause for, rather than a result of, gastroesophageal reflux. *J Asthma*. 1983;20(4):241-3. 3.

Sinha R, Cross AJ, Graubard BI, Leitzmann MF, Schatzkin A. Meat intake and mortality: a prospective study of over half a million people. Arch Intern Med. 2009 Mar 23;169(6):562-71.

Sinha R, Cross AJ, Graubard BI, Leitzmann MF, Schatzkin A. Meat in-take and mortality: a prospective study of over half a million people. Arch Intern Med. 2009 Mar 23;169(6):562-71.

Sinn DH, Song JH, Kim HJ, Lee JH, Son HJ, Chang DK, Kim YH, Kim JJ, Rhee JC, Rhee PL. Therapeutic effect of *Lactobacillus acidophilus*-SDC 2012, 2013 in patients with irritable bowel syndrome. *Dig Dis Sci.* 2008 Oct;53(10):2714-8.

Sirvent S, Palomares O, Vereda A, Villalba M, Cuesta-Herranz J, Rodríguez R. nsLTP and profilin are allergens in mustard seeds: cloning, sequencing and recombinant production of Sin a 3 and Sin a 4. *Clin Exp Allergy.* 2009 Dec;39(12):1929-36.

Sistek D, Kelly R, Wickens K, Stanley T, Fitzharris P, Crane J. Is the effect of probiotics on atopic dermatitis confined to food sensitized children? *Clin Exp Allergy.* 2006 May;36(5):629-33.

Skamstrup Hansen K, Vieths S, Vestergaard H, Skov PS, Bindslev-Jensen C, Poulsen LK. Seasonal variation in food allergy to apple. *J Chromatogr B Biomed Sci Appl.* 2001 May 25;756(1-2):19-32.

Skovbjerg S, Roos K, Holm SE, Grahn Håkansson E, Nowrouzian F, Ivarsson M, Adlerberth I, Wold AE. Spray bacteriotherapy decreases middle ear fluid in children with secretory otitis media. *Arch Dis Child.* 2009 Feb;94(2):92-8.

Skripak JM, Nash SD, Rowley H, Brereton NH, Oh S, Hamilton RG, Matsui EC, Burks AW, Wood RA. A randomized, double-blind, placebo-controlled study of milk oral immunotherapy for cow's milk allergy. *J Allergy Clin Immunol.* 2008 Dec;122(6):1154-60.

Sletten GB, Halvorsen R, Egaas E, Halstensen TS. Changes in humoral responses to beta-lactoglobulin in tolerant patients suggest a particular role for IgG4 in delayed, non-IgE-mediated cow's milk allergy. *Pediatr Allergy Immunol.* 2006 Sep;17(6):435-43.

Smecuol E, Hwang HJ, Sugai E, Corso L, Cherñavsky AC, Bellavite FP, González A, Vodánovich F, Moreno ML, Vázquez H, Lozano G, Niveloni S, Mazure R, Meddings J, Mauriño E, Bai JC. Exploratory, randomized, double-blind, placebo-controlled study on the effects of Bifidobacterium infantis natren life start strain super strain in active celiac disease. *J Clin Gastroenterol.* 2013 Feb;47(2):139-47. doi: 10.1097/MCG.0b013e31827759ac.

Smith J. *Genetic Roulette: The Documented Health Risks of Genetically Engineered Foods.* White River Jct, Vermont: Chelsea Green, 2007.

Smith K, Warholak T, Armstrong E, Leib M, Rehfeld R, Malone D. Evaluation of risk factors and health outcomes among persons with asthma. *J Asthma.* 2009 Apr;46(3):234-7.

Smith LJ, Holbrook JT, Wise R, Blumenthal M, Dozor AJ, Mastronarde J, Williams L; American Lung Association Asthma Clinical Research Centers. Dietary intake of soy genistein is associated with lung function in patients with asthma. *J Asthma.* 2004;41(8):833-43.

Smith S, Sullivan K. Examining the influence of biological and psychological factors on cognitive performance in chronic fatigue syndrome: a randomized, double-blind, placebo-controlled, crossover study. *Int J Behav Med.* 2003;10(2):162-73.

Smith TM, Tafforeau P, Reid DJ, Pouech J, Lazzari V, Zermeno JP, Guatelli-Steinberg D, Olejniczak AJ, Hoffman A, Radovcic J, Makaremi M, Toussaint M, Stringer C, Hublin JJ. Dental evidence for ontogenetic differences between modern humans and Neanderthals. *Proc Natl Acad Sci U S A.* 2010 Dec 7;107(49):20923-8. doi: 10.1073/pnas.1010906107.

Snydman DR, Jacobus NV, McDermott LA, Golan Y, Hecht DW, Goldstein EJ, Harrell L, Jenkins S, Newton D, Pierson C, Rihs JD, Yu VL, Venezia R, Finegold SM, Rosenblatt JE, Gorbach SL. Lessons learned from the anaerobe survey: historical perspective and review of the most recent data (2005-2007). Clin Infect Dis. 2010 Jan 1;50 Suppl 1:S26-33. doi: 10.1086/647940.

Sofic E, Denisova N, Youdim K, Vatrenjak-Velagic V, De Filippo C, Mehmedagic A, Causevic A, Cao G, Joseph JA, Prior RL. Antioxidant and pro-oxidant capacity of catecholamines and related compounds. Effects of hydrogen peroxide on glutathione and sphingomyelinase activity in pheochromocytoma PC12 cells: potential relevance to age-related diseases. *J Neural Transm.* 2001;108(5):541-57.

Solá R, Fitó M, Estruch R, Salas-Salvadó J, Corella D, de La Torre R, Muñoz MA, López-Sabater Mdel C, Martínez-González MA, Arós F, Ruiz-Gutierrez V, Fiol M, Casals E, Wärnberg J, Buil-Cosiales P, Ros E, Konstantinidou V, Lapetra J, Serra-Majem L, Covas MI. Effect of a traditional Medi-terranean diet on apolipoproteins B, A-I, and their ratio: a randomized, controlled trial. Atherosclerosis. 2011 Sep;218(1):174-80.

Soleo L, Colosio C, Alinovi R, Guarneri D, Russo A, Lovreglio P, Vimercati L, Birindelli S, Cortesi I, Flore C, Carta P, Colombi A, Parrinello G, Ambrosi L. Immunologic effects of exposure to low levels of inorganic mercury. *Med Lav.* 2002 May-Jun;93(3):225-32.

Solfrizzi V, Frisardi V, Seripa D, Logroscino G, Imbimbo BP, D'Onofrio G, Addante F, Sancarlo D, Cascavilla L, Pilotto A, Panza F. Mediterranean diet in predementia and dementia syndromes. Curr Alzheimer Res. 2011 Aug;8(5):520-42.

Solfrizzi V, Panza F, Frisardi V, Seripa D, Logroscino G, Imbimbo BP, Pilotto A. Diet and Alzheimer's disease risk factors or prevention: the current evidence. Expert Rev Neurother. 2011 May;11(5):677-708.

Solomons NW, Guerrero AM, Torun B. Effective in vivo hydrolysis of milk lactose by beta-galactosidases in the presence of solid foods. *Am J Clin Nutr.* 1985 Feb;41(2):222-7.

Sompamit K, Kukongviriyapan U, Nakmareong S, Pannangpetch P, Kukongviriyapan V. Curcumin improves vascular function and alleviates oxidative stress in non-lethal lipopolysaccharide-induced endotoxaemia in mice. *Eur J Pharmacol.* 2009 Aug 15;616(1-3):192-9.

Sonibare MA, Gbile ZO. Ethnobotanical survey of anti-asthmatic plants in South Western Nigeria. *Afr J Tradit Complement Altern Med.* 2008 Jun 18;5(4):340-5.

Sontag SJ, O'Connell S, Khandelwal S, Greenlee H, Schnell T, Nemchausky B, Chejfec G, Miller T, Seidel J, Sonnenberg A. Asthmatics with gastroesophageal reflux: long term results of a randomized trial of medical and surgical antireflux therapies. *Am J Gastroenterol.* 2003 May;98(5):987-99.

Sosa M, Saavedra P, Valero C, Guañabens N, Nogués X, del Pino-Montes J, Mosquera J, Alegre J, Gómez-Alonso C, Muñoz-Torres M, Quesada M, Pérez-Cano R, Jódar E, Torrijos A, Lozano-Tonkin C, Díaz-Curiel M; GIUMO Study Group. Inhaled steroids do not decrease bone mineral density but increase risk of fractures: data from the GIUMO Study Group. J Clin Densitom. 2006 Apr-Jun;9(2):154-8.

Soyka F, Edmonds A. *The Ion Effect: How Air Electricity Rules your Life and Health.* Bantam, New York: Bantam, 1978.

Spence A. *Basic Human Anatomy.* Menlo Park, CA: Benjamin/Commings, 1986.

Spiller G. *The Super Pyramid.* New York: HRS Press, 1993.

Sponheimer M, *et al.* Diets of Southern African Bovidae: Stable isotope evidence. J Mammal. 2003;84:471 – 479.

Sponheimer M, Lee-Thorp JA. Hominin palaeodiets: The contribution of stable isotopes. In: Henke W, Tattersall I, editors. Handbook of Paleoanthropology. Berlin: Springer-Verlag; 2007. pp. 555 – 586.

Sporik R, Squillace SP, Ingram JM, Rakes G, Honsinger RW, Platts-Mills TA. Mite, cat, and cockroach exposure, allergen sensitisation, and asthma in children: a case-control study of three schools. *Thorax.* 1999 Aug;54(8):675-80.

Srivastava K, Zou ZM, Sampson HA, Dansky H, Li XM. Direct Modulation of Airway Reactivity by the Chinese Anti-Asthma Herbal Formula ASHMI. *J Allergy Clin Immunol.* 2005;115:S7.

Srivastava KD, Qu C, Zhang T, Goldfarb J, Sampson HA, Li XM. Food Allergy Herbal Formula-2 silences peanut-induced anaphylaxis for a prolonged posttreatment period via IFN-gamma-producing CD8+ T cells. *J Allergy Clin Immunol.* 2009 Feb;123(2):443-51.

Srivastava KD, Zhang TF, Qu C, Sampson HA, Li XM. Silencing Peanut Allergy: A Chinese Herbal Formula, FAHF-2, Completely Blocks Peanut-induced Anaphylaxis for up to 6 Months Following Therapy in a Murine Model Of Peanut Allergy. *J Allergy Clin Immunol.* 2006;117:S328.

Stabler SP, Allen RH. Vitamin B12 Deficiency as a Worldwide Problem. Annual Review of Nutrition. Vol. 24: 299-326. July 2004.

Stach A, Emberlin J, Smith M, Adams-Groom B, Myszkowska D. Factors that determine the severity of Betula spp. pollen seasons in Poland (Poznań and Krakow) and the United Kingdom (Worcester and London). *Int J Biometeorol.* 2008 Mar;52(4):311-21.

Stachowska E, Dolegowska B, Chlubek D, Wesolowska T, Ciechanowski K, Gutowski P, Szumilowicz H, Turowski R. Dietary trans fatty acids and composition of human atheromatous plaques. *Eur J Nutr.* 2004 Oct;43(5):313-8.

Staden U, Rolinck-Werninghaus C, Brewe F, Wahn U, Niggemann B, Beyer K. Specific oral tolerance induction in food allergy in children: efficacy and clinical patterns of reaction. *Allergy.* 2007 Nov;62(11):1261-9.

Stadlbauer V, Mookerjee RP, Hodges S, Wright GA, Davies NA, Jalan R. Effect of probiotic treatment on deranged neutrophil function and cytokine responses in patients with compensated alcoholic cirrhosis. *J Hepatol.* 2008 Jun;48(6):945-51.

Stahl SM. Selective histamine H1 antagonism: novel hypnotic and pharmacologic actions challenge classical notions of antihistamines. CNS Spectr. 2008 Dec;13(12):1027-38.

State Pharmacopoeia Commission of The People's Republic of China. *Pharmacopoeia of the People's Republic of China.* Beijing: Chemical Industry Press; 2005.

Steinman HA, Le Roux M, Potter PC. Sulphur dioxide sensitivity in South African asthmatic children. *S Afr Med J.* 1993 Jun;83(6):387-90.

Stenberg JA, Hambäck PA, Ericson L. Herbivore-induced "rent rise" in the host plant may drive a diet breadth enlargement in the tenant. *Ecology.* 2008 Jan;89(1):126-33.

Stengler M. *The Natural Physician's Healing Therapies.* Stamford, CT: Bottom Line Books, 2008.

Stenman SM, Venäläinen JI, Lindfors K, Auriola S, Mauriala T, Kaukovirta-Norja A, Jantunen A, Laurila K, Qiao SW, Sollid LM, Männisto PT, Kaukinen K, Mäki M. Enzymatic detoxification of gluten by germinating wheat proteases: implications for new treatment of celiac disease. Ann Med. 2009;41(5):390-400. doi: 10.1080/07853890902878138.

Stensrud T, Carlsen KH. Can one single test protocol for provoking exercise-induced bronchoconstriction also be used for assessing aerobic capacity? *Clin Respir J.* 2008 Jan;2(1):47-53.

Steurer-Stey C, Russi EW, Steurer J: Complementary and alternative medicine in asthma: do they work? *Swiss Med Wkly.* 2002, 132:338-344.

Stillerman A, Nachtsheim C, Li W, Albrecht M, Waldman J. Efficacy of a novel air filtration pillow for avoidance of perennial allergens in symptomatic adults. Ann Allergy Asthma Immunol. 2010 May;104(5):440-9.

Stirapongsasuti P, Tanglertsampan C, Aunhachoke K, Sangasapaviliya A. Anaphylactic reaction to phuk-waan-ban in a patient with latex allergy. *J Med Assoc Thai.* 2010 May;93(5):616-9.

Stock WD, Chuba CK, Verboom GA. Distribution of South African C3 and C4 species of Cyperaceae in relation to climate and phylogeny. Austral Ecol. 2004;29:313 – 319.

Stordal K, Johannesdottir GB, Bentsen BS, Knudsen PK, Carlsen KC, Closs O, Handeland M, Holm HK, Sandvik L. Acid suppression does not change respiratory symptoms in children with asthma and gastro-oesophageal reflux disease. Arch Dis Child. 2005 Sep;90(9):956-60.

Stratiki Z, Costalos C, Sevastiadou S, Kastanidou O, Skouroliakou M, Giakoumatou A, Petrohilou V. The effect of a bifidobacter supplemented bovine milk on intestinal permeability of preterm infants. *Early Hum Der.* 2007 Sep;83(9):575-9.

Stratiki Z., Costalos C, Sevastiadou S, Kastanidou O, Skouroliakou M, Giakoumatou A, Petrohilou V. The effect of a bifidobacter supplemented bovine milk on intestinal permeability of preterm infants. *Early Hum Dev.* 2007 Sep;83(9):575-9.

Strickland KC, Krupenko NI, Krupenko SA. Molecular mechanisms underlying the potentially adverse effects of folate. Clin Chem Lab Med. 2012 Dec 12:1-10.

Strinnholm A, Brulin C, Lindh V. Experiences of double-blind, placebo-controlled food challenges (DBPCFC): a qualitative analysis of mothers' experiences. *J Child Health Care.* 2010 Jun;14(2):179-88.

Ströhle A, Wolters M, Hahn A. [Human nutrition in the context of evolutionary medicine]. Wien Klin Wochenschr. 2009;121(5-6):173-87. doi: 10.1007/s00508-009-1139-1.

Strozzi GP, Mogna L. Quantification of folic acid in human feces after administration of *Bifidobacterium* probiotic strains. *J Clin Gastroenterol.* 2008 Sep;42 Suppl 3 Pt 2:S179-84.

Stuck BA, Czajkowski J, Hagner AE, Klimek L, Verse T, Hörmann K, Maurer JT. Changes in daytime sleepiness, quality of life, and objective sleep patterns in seasonal allergic rhinitis: a controlled clinical trial. *J Allergy Clin Immunol.* 2004 Apr;113(4):663-8.

Stull DE, Schaefer M, Crespi S, Sandor DW. Relative strength of relationships of nasal congestion and ocular symptoms with sleep, mood and productivity. *Curr Med Res Opin.* 2009 Jul;25(7):1785-92.

Sturtzel B, Mikulits C, Gisinger C, Elmadfa I. Use of fiber instead of laxative treatment in a geriatric hospital to improve the wellbeing of seniors. *J Nutr Health Aging.* 2009 Feb;13(2):136-9.

Stutius LM, Sheehan WJ, Rangsithienchai P, Bharmanee A, Scott JE, Young MC, Dioun AF, Schneider LC, Phipatanakul W. Characterizing the relationship between sesame, coconut, and nut allergy in children. *Pediatr Allergy Immunol.* 2010 Dec;21(8):1114-8.

Su P, Henriksson A, Tandianus JE, Park JH, Foong F, Dunn NW. Detection and quantification of *Bifidobacterium lactis* LAFTI B94 in human faecal samples from a consumption trial. *FEMS Microbiol Lett.* 2005 Mar 1;244(1):99-103.

Sugawara G, Nagino M, Nishio H, Ebata T, Takagi K, Asahara T, Nomoto K, Nimura Y. Perioperative synbiotic treatment to prevent postoperative infectious complications in biliary cancer surgery: a randomized controlled trial. *Ann Surg.* 2006 Nov;244(5):706-14.

Sugnanam KK, Collins JT, Smith PK, Connor F, Lewindon P, Cleghorn G, Withers G. Dichotomy of food and inhalant allergen sensitization in eosinophilic esophagitis. *Allergy.* 2007 Nov;62(11):1257-60.

Sullivan A, Barkholt L, Nord CE. *Lactobacillus acidophilus, Bifidobacterium lactis* and *Lactobacillus* F19 prevent antibiotic-associated ecological disturbances of Bacteroides fragilis in the intestine. *J Antimicrob Chemother.* 2003 Aug;52(2):308-11.

Sulman FG, Levy D, Lunkan L, Pfeifer Y, Tal E. New methods in the treatment of weather sensitivity. Fortschr Med. 1977 Mar 17;95(11):746-52.

Sulman FG. Migraine and headache due to weather and allied causes and its specific treatment. Ups J Med Sci Suppl. 1980;31:41-4.

Sumantran VN, Kulkarni AA, Harsulkar A, Wele A, Koppikar SJ, Chandwaskar R, Gaire V, Dalvi M, Wagh UV. Hyaluronidase and collagenase inhibitory activities of the herbal formulation Triphala guggulu. *J Biosci.* 2007 Jun;32(4):755-61.

Sumiyoshi M, Sakanaka M, Kimura Y. Effects of Red Ginseng extract on allergic reactions to food in Balb/c mice. *J Ethnopharmacol.* 2010 Aug 14.

Sung JH, Lee JO, Son JK, Park NS, Kim MR, Kim JG, Moon DC. Cytotoxic constituents from Solidago virga-aurea var. gigantea MIQ. Arch Pharm Res. 1999 Dec;22(6):633-7.

Suomalainen H, Isolauri E. New concepts of allergy to cow's milk. *Ann Med.* 1994 Aug;26(4):289-96.

Sur R, Nigam A, Grote D, Liebel F, Southall MD. Avenanthramides, polyphenols from oats, exhibit anti-inflammatory and anti-itch activity. Arch Dermatol Res. 2008 May.

Sur S, Camara M, Buchmeier A, Morgan S, Nelson HS. Double-blind trial of pyridoxine (vitamin B6) in the treatment of steroid-dependent asthma. Ann Allergy. 1993 Feb;70(2):147-52.

Sütas Y, Kekki OM, Isolauri E. Late onset reactions to oral food challenge are linked to low serum interleukin-10 concentrations in patients with atopic dermatitis and food allergy. *Clin Exp Allergy.* 2000 Aug;30(8):1121-8.

Suzuki R, Rylander-Rudqvist T, Ye W, Saji S, Adlercreutz H, Wolk A. Dietary fiber intake and risk of postmenopausal breast cancer defined by estrogen and progesterone receptor status – a prospective cohort study among Swedish women. Int J Cancer. 2008 Jan 15;122(2):403-12.

Suzuki R, Ye W, Rylander-Rudqvist T, Saji S, Colditz GA, Wolk A. Alcohol and postmenopausal breast cancer risk defined by estrogen and progesterone receptor status: a prospective cohort study. J Natl Cancer Inst. 2005 Nov 2;97(21):1601-8.

Suzuki Y, Kondo K, Ichise H, Tsukamoto Y, Urano T, Umemura K. Dietary supplementation with fermented soybeans suppresses intimal thickening. *Nutrition.* 2003 Mar;19(3):261-4.

Suzuki Y, Kondo K, Matsumoto Y, Zhao BQ, Otsuguro K, Maeda T, Tsukamoto Y, Urano T, Umemura K. 2003. Dietary supplementation of fermented soybean, natto, suppresses intimal thickening and modulates the lysis of mural thrombi after endothelial injury in rat femoral artery. Life Sci. Jul 25;73(10):1289-98.

Svanes C, Heinrich J, Jarvis D, Chinn S, Omenaas E, Gulsvik A, Künzli N, Burney P. Pet-keeping in childhood and adult asthma and hay fever: European community respiratory health survey. *J Allergy Clin Immunol.* 2003 Aug;112(2):289-300.

Svendsen AJ, Holm NV, Kyvik K, *et al.* Relative importance of genetic effects in rheumatoid arthritis: historical cohort study of Danish nationwide twin population. BMJ 2002;324(7332): 264-266.

# REFERENCES AND BIBLIOGRAPHY

Sweeney B, Vora M, Ulbricht C, Basch E. Evidence-based systematic review of dandelion (Taraxacum officinale) by natural standard research collaboration. *J Herb Pharmacother*. 2005;5(1):79-93.

Swett. JA. *A Treatise on Disease of the Chest*. New York, 1852.

Swiderska-Kielbik S, Krakowiak A, Wiszniewska M, Dudek W, Walusiak-Skorupa J, Krawczyk-Szulc P, Michowicz A, Palczyński C. Health hazards associated with occupational exposure to birds. *Med Pr*. 2010;61(2):213-22.

Szyf M, McGowan P, Meaney MJ. The social environment and the epigenome. *Environ Mol Mutagen*. 2008 Jan;49(1):46-60.

Szymański H, Chmielarczyk A, Strus M, Pejcz J, Jawień M, Kochan P, Heczko PB. Colonisation of the gastrointestinal tract by probiotic L. rhamnosus strains in acute diarrhoea in children. *Dig Liver Dis*. 2006 Dec;38 Suppl 2:S274-6.

Szymański H, Pejcz J, Jawień M, Chmielarczyk A, Strus M, Heczko PB. Treatment of acute infectious diarrhoea in infants and children with a mixture of three *Lactobacillus rhamnosus* strains – a randomized, double-blind, placebo-controlled trial. *Aliment Pharmacol Ther*. 2006 Jan 15;23(2):247-53.

Tabbers MM, de Milliano I, Roseboom MG, Benninga MA. Is Bifidobacterium breve effective in the treatment of childhood constipation? Results from a pilot study. Nutr J. 2011 Feb 23;10:19.

Takada Y, Ichikawa H, Badmaev V, Aggarwal BB. Acetyl-11-keto-beta-boswellic acid potentiates apoptosis, inhibits invasion, and abolishes osteoclastogenesis by suppressing NF-kappa B and NF-kappa B-regulated gene expression. *J Immunol*. 2006 Mar 1;176(5):3127-40.

Takagi A, Ikemura H, Matsuzaki T, Sato M, Nomoto K, Morotomi M, Yokokura T. Relationship between the in vitro response of dendritic cells to *Lactobacillus* and prevention of tumorigenesis in the mouse. *J Gastroenterol*. 2008;43(9):661-9.

Takahashi N, Eisenhuth G, Lee I, Schachtele C, Laible N, Binion S. Nonspecific antibacterial factors in milk from cows immunized with human oral bacterial pathogens. *J Dairy Sci*. 1992 Jul;75(7):1810-20.

Takasaki M, Konoshima T, Tokuda H, Masuda K, Arai Y, Shiojima K, Ageta H. Anti-carcinogenic activity of Taraxacum plant. I. *Biol Pharm Bull*. 1999 Jun;22(6):602-5.

Takata Y, Shu XO, Gao YT, Li H, Zhang X, Gao J, Cai H, Yang G, Xiang YB, Zheng W. Red meat and poultry intakes and risk of total and cause-specific mortality: results from cohort studies of Chinese adults in Shanghai. PLoS One. 2013;8(2):e56963. doi: 10.1371/journal.pone.0056963.

Takeda K, Okumura K. Effects of a fermented milk drink containing *Lactobacillus casei* strain Shirota on the human NK-cell activity. *J Nutr*. 2007 Mar;137(3 Suppl 2):791S-3S.

Takeda K, Suzuki T, Shimada SI, Shida K, Nanno M, Okumura K. Interleukin-12 is involved in the enhancement of human natural killer cell activity by *Lactobacillus casei* Shirota. *Clin Exp Immunol*. 2006 Oct;146(1):109-15.

Tamaoki J, Chiyotani A, Sakai A, Takemura H, Konno K. Effect of menthol vapour on airway hyperresponsiveness in patients with mild asthma. *Respir Med*. 1995 Aug;89(7):503-4.

Tamayo-Ramos JA, Sanz-Penella JM, Yebra MJ, Monedero V, Haros M. Novel phytases from Bifidobacterium pseudocatenulatum ATCC 27919 and Bifidobacterium longum subsp. infantis ATCC 15697. Appl Environ Microbiol. 2012 Jul;78(14):5013-5. doi: 10.1128/AEM.00782-12.

Tamura M, Hori S, Nakagawa H. Lactobacillus rhamnosus JCM 2771: impact on metabolism of isoflavonoids in the fecal flora from a male equol producer. Curr Microbiol. 2011 May;62(5):1632-7.

Tamura M, Shikina T, Morihana T, Hayama M, Kajimoto O, Sakamoto A, Kajimoto Y, Watanabe O, Nonaka C, Shida K, Nanno M. Effects of probiotics on allergic rhinitis induced by Japanese cedar pol-len: randomized double-blind, placebo-controlled clinical trial. *Int Arch Allergy Imml*. 2007;143(1):75-82.

Tang AL, Wilcox G, Walker KZ, Shah NP, Ashton JF, Stojanovska L. Phytase activity from Lactobacillus spp. in calcium-fortified soymilk. J Food Sci. 2010 Aug 1;75(6):M373-6. doi: 10.1111/j.1750-3841.2010.01663.x.

Taniguchi C, Homma M, Takano O, Hirano T, Oka K, Aoyagi Y, Niitsuma T, Hayashi T. Pharmacological effects of urinary products obtained after treatment with saiboku-to, a herbal medicine for bronchial asthma, on type IV allergic reaction. *Planta Med*. 2000 Oct;66(7):607-11.

Tapiero H, Ba GN, Couvreur P, Tew KD. Polyunsaturated fatty acids (PUFA) and eicosanoids in human health and pathologies. *Biomed Pharmacother*. 2002 Jul;56(5):215-22.

Tapola N, Karvonen H, Niskanen L, Mikola M, Sarkkinen E. Glycemic responses of oat bran products in type 2 diabetic patients. Nutr Metab Cardiovasc Dis. 2005 Aug;15(4):255-61.

Tapsell LC, Hemphill I, Cobiac L, Patch CS, Sullivan DR, Fenech M, Roodenrys S, Keogh JB, Clifton PM, Williams PG, Fazio VA, Inge KE. Health benefits of herbs and spices: the past, the present, the future. *Med J Aust*. 2006 Aug 21;185(4 Suppl):S4-24.

Tasli L, Mat C, De Simone C, Yazici H. Lactobacilli lozenges in the management of oral ulcers of Behçet's syndrome. *Clin Exp Rheumatol*. 2006 Sep-Oct;24(5 Suppl 42):S83-6.

Tasli L, Mat C, De Simone C, Yazici H. Lactobacilli lozenges in the management of oral ulcers of Behçet's syndrome. *Clin Exp Rheumatol*. 2006 Sep-Oct;24(5 Suppl 42):S83-6.

Taussig SJ, Batkin S. Bromelain, the enzyme complex of pineapple (Ananas comosus) and its clinical application. An update. *J Ethnopharmacol*. 1988 Feb-Mar;22(2):191-203.

Tavil B, Koksal E, Yalcin SS, Uckan D. Pretransplant nutritional habits and clinical outcome in children undergoing hematopoietic stem cell transplant. Exp Clin Transplant. 2012 Feb;10(1):55-61.

Taylor AB. Feeding behavior, diet, and the functional consequences of jaw form in orangutans, with implications for the evolution of Pongo. J Hum Evol. 2006 Apr;50(4):377-93.

Taylor AL, Dunstan JA, Prescott SL. Probiotic supplementation for the first 6 months of life fails to reduce the risk of atopic dermatitis and increases the risk of allergen sensitization in high-risk children: a randomized controlled trial. *J Allergy Clin Immunol*. 2007 Jan;119(1):184-91.

Taylor AL, Hale J, Wiltschut J, Lehmann H, Dunstan JA, Prescott SL. Effects of probiotic supplementation for the first 6 months of life on allergen- and vaccine-specific immune responses. *Clin Exp Allergy*. 2006 Oct;36(10):1227-35.

Taylor RB, Lindquist N, Kubanek J, Hay ME. Intraspecific variation in palatability and defensive chemistry of brown seaweeds: effects on herbivore fitness. *Oecologia*. 2003 Aug;136(3):412-23.

Teitelbaum J. *From Fatigue to Fantastic*. New York: Avery, 2001.

Terheggen-Lagro SW, Khouw IM, Schaafsma A, Wauters EA. Safety of a new extensively hydrolysed formula in children with cow's milk protein allergy: a double blind crossover study. *BMC Pediatr*. 2002 Oct 14;2:10.

Terracciano L, Bouygue GR, Sarratud T, Veglia F, Martelli A, Fiocchi A. Impact of dietary regimen on the duration of cow's milk allergy: a random allocation study. *Clin Exp Allergy*. 2010 Apr;40(4):637-42.

Tesse R, Schieck M, Kabesch M. Asthma and endocrine disorders: Shared mechanisms and genetic pleiotropy. *Mol Cell Endocrinol*. 2010 Dec 4. [ ahead of print] .

Tevini M, ed. *UV-B Radiation and Ozone Depletion: Effects on humans, animals, plants, microorganisms and materials*. Boca Raton: Lewis Pub, 1993.

Thakkar K, Boatright RO, Gilger MA, El-Serag HB. Gastroesophageal reflux and asthma in children: a systematic review. *Pediatrics*. 2010 Apr;125(4):e925-30. 2010 Mar 29.

Tham KW, Zuraimi MS, Koh D, Chew FT, Ooi PL. Associations between home dampness and presence of molds with asthma and allergic symptoms among young children in the tropics. *Pediatr Allergy Immunol*. 2007 Aug;18(5):418-24.

Thampithak A, Jaisin Y, Meesarapee B, Chongthammakun S, Piyachaturawat P, Govitrapong P, Supavilai P, Sanvarinda Y. Transcriptional regulation of iNOS and COX-2 by a novel compound from Curcuma comosa in lipopolysaccharide-induced microglial activation. *Neurosci Lett*. 2009 Sep 22;462(2):171-5.

Theler B, Brockow K, Ballmer-Weber BK. Clinical presentation and diagnosis of meat allergy in Switzerland and Southern Germany. *Swiss Med Wkly*. 2009 May 2;139(17-18):264-70.

Theofilopoulos AN, Kono DH. The genes of systemic autoimmunity. *Proc Assoc Am Physicians*. 1999;111(3): 228-240.

Theuwissen E, Mensink RP. Water-soluble dietary fibers and cardiovascular disease. Physiol Behav. 2008 May 23;94(2):285-92.

Thibault H, Aubert-Jacquin C, Goulet O. Effects of long-term consumption of a fermented infant formula (with *Bifidobacterium breve* c50 and *Streptococcus thermophilus* 065) on acute diarrhea in healthy infants. *J Pediatr Gastroenterol Nutr*. 2004 Aug;39(2):147-52.

Thiruvengadam KV, Haranath K, Sudarsan S, Sekar TS, Rajagopal KR, Zacharian MG, Devarajan TV. Tylophora indica in bronchial asthma (a controlled comparison with a standard anti-asthmatic drug). *J Indian Med Assoc*. 1978 Oct 1;71(7):172-6.

Thomas M. Are breathing exercises an effective strategy for people with asthma? *Nurs Times*. 2009 Mar 17-23;105(10):22-7.

Thomas Y, Schiff M, Belkadi L, Jurgens P, Kahhak L, Benveniste J. Activation of human neutrophils by electronically transmitted phorbol-myristate acetate. *Med Hypoth*. 2000;54: 33-39.

Thomas, R.G., Gebhardt, S.E. 2008. Nutritive value of pomegranate fruit and juice. *Maryland Dietetic Association Annual Meeting, USDA-ARS*. 2008 April 11.

Thompson D. *On Growth and Form*. Cambridge: Cambridge University Press, 1992.

Thompson T, Lee AR, Grace T. Gluten contamination of grains, seeds, and flours in the United States: a pilot study. *J Am Diet Assoc*. 2010 Jun;110(6):937-40.

Thorp JA, van der Merwe NJ, Brain CK. Diet of Australopithecus robustus at Swartkrans from stable carbon isotopic analysis. J Hum Evol. 1994;27:361 – 372.

Tian JQ, Bae YM, Choi NY, Kang DH, Heu S, Lee SY. Survival and growth of foodborne pathogens in minimally processed vegetables at 4 and 15 °C. J Food Sci. 2012 Jan;77(1):M48-50.

Tien-Huang Lin, Su-Hua Huang, Chien-Chen Wu, Hsin-Ho Liu, Tzyy-Rong Jinn, Yeh Chen, Ching-Ting Lin. Inhibition of Klebsiella pneumoniae Growth and Capsular Polysaccharide Biosynthesis by Fructus mume. Evidence-Based Complementary and Alternative Medicine. Volume 2013 (2013), Article ID 621701, 10 pages http://dx.doi.org/10.1155/2013/621701

Tierra L. *The Herbs of Life*. Freedom, CA: Crossing Press, 1992.

Tierra M. *The Way of Herbs*. New York: Pocket Books, 1990.

Tietze H. *Kombucha: The Miracle Fungus*. Gateway Books: Bath, UK, 1995.

Tieu K, Perier C, Caspersen C, Teismann P, Wu DC, Yan SD, Naini A, Vila M, Jackson-Lewis V, Ramasamy R, Przedborski S. D-beta-hydroxybutyrate rescues mitochondrial respiration and mitigates features of Parkinson disease. J Clin Invest. 2003;112:892–901.

Tisserand R. *The Art of Aromatherapy*. New York: Inner Traditions, 1979.

Tiwari M. *Ayurveda: A Life of Balance*. Rochester, VT: Healing Arts, 1995.

Tlaskalová-Hogenová H, Stepánková R, Hudcovic T, Tucková L, Cukrowska B, Lodinová-Zádníková R, Kozáková H, Rossmann P, Bártová J, Sokol D, Funda DP, Borovská D, Reháková Z, Sinkora J, Hofman J, Drastich P, Kokesová A. Commensal bacteria (normal microflora), mucosal immunity and chronic inflammatory and autoimmune diseases. *Immunol Lett*. 2004 May 15;93(2-3):97-108.

Todd GR, Acerini CL, Ross-Russell R, Zahra S, Warner JT, McCance D. Survey of adrenal crisis associated with inhaled corticosteroids in the United Kingdom. *Arch Dis Child*. 2002 Dec;87(6):457-61.

Tonkal AM, Morsy TA. An update review on Commiphora molmol and related species. *J Egypt Soc Parasitol*. 2008 Dec;38(3):763-96.

Topçu G, Erenler R, Cakmak O, Johansson CB, Celik C, Chai HB, Pezzuto JM. Diterpenes from the berries of Juniperus excelsa. *Phytochemistry*. 1999 Apr;50(7):1195-9.

Toppila-Salmi S, Renkonen J, Joenväärä S, Mattila P, Renkonen R. Allergen interactions with epithelium. *Curr Opin Allergy Clin Immunol*. 2011 Feb;11(1):29-32.

Tordesillas L, Pacios LF, Palacín A, Cuesta-Herranz J, Madero M, Díaz-Perales A. Characterization of IgE epitopes of Cuc m 2, the major melon allergen, and their role in cross-reactivity with pollen profilins. *Clin Exp Allergy*. 2010 Jan;40(1):174-81.

Tormo Carnicer R, Infante Piña D, Roselló Mayans E, Bartolomé Comas R. Intake of fermented milk containing *Lactobacillus casei* DN-114 001 and its effect on gut flora. *An Pediatr*. 2006 Nov;65(5):448-53.

Torrent M, Sunyer J, Muñoz L, Cullinan P, Iturriaga MV, Figueroa C, Vall O, Taylor AN, Anto JM. Early-life domestic aeroallergen exposure and IgE sensitization at age 4 years. *J Allergy Clin Immunol*. 2006 Sep;118(3):742-8.

Touhami M, Boudraa G, Mary JY, Soltana R, Desjeux JF. Clinical consequences of replacing milk with yogurt in persistent infantile diarrhea. *Ann Pediatr*. 1992 Feb;39(2):79-86.

Towers GH. FAHF-1 purporting to block peanut-induced anaphylaxis. *J Allergy Clin Immunol*. 2003 May;111(5):1140; author reply 1140-1.

Towle A. *Modern Biology*. Austin: Harcourt Brace, 1993.

Trenev N. *Probiotics: Nature's Internal Healers*. New York: Avery, 1998.

Tresserra-Rimbau A, Medina-Remón A, Pérez-Jiménez J, Martínez-González MA, Covas MI, Corella D, Salas-Salvadó J, Gómez-Gracia E, Lapetra J, Arós F, Fiol M, Ros E, Serra-Majem L, Pintó X, Muñoz MA, Saez GT, Ruiz-Gutiérrez V, Warnberg J, Estruch R, Lamuela-Raventós RM. Dietary intake and major food sources of polyphenols in a Spanish population at high cardiovascular risk: The PREDIMED study. Nutr Metab Cardiovasc Dis. 2013 Jan 16. doi:pii: S0939-4753(12)00245-1. 10.1016/j.numecd.2012.10.008.

Trois L, Cardoso EM, Miura E. Use of probiotics in HIV-infected children: a randomized double-blind controlled study. *J Trop Pediatr*. 2008 Feb;54(1):19-24.

Trojanová I, Rada V, Kokoska L, Vlková E. The bifidogenic effect of Taraxacum officinale root. *Fitoterapia*. 2004 Dec;75(7-8):760-3.

Troncone R, Caputo N, Florio G, Finelli E. Increased intestinal sugar permeability after challenge in children with cow's milk allergy or intolerance. *Allergy*. 1994 Mar;49(3):142-6.

Trout L, King M, Feng W, Inglis SK, Ballard ST. Inhibition of airway liquid secretion and its effect on the physical properties of airway mucus. *Am J Physiol*. 1998 Feb;274(2 Pt 1):L258-63.

Tsai JC, Tsai S, Chang WC. Comparison of two Chinese medical herbs, Huangbai and Qianniuzi, on influence of short circuit current across the rat intestinal epithelia. *J Ethnopharmacol*. 2004 Jul;93(1):21-5.

Tsong T. Deciphering the language of cells. *Trends in Biochem Sci*. 1989;14:89-92.

Tsuchiya J, Barreto R, Okura R, Kawakita S, Fesce E, Marotta F. Single-blind follow-up study on the effectiveness of a symbiotic preparation in irritable bowel syndrome. *Chin J Dig Dis*. 2004;5(4):169-74.

Tubelius P, Stan V, Zachrisson A. Increasing work-place healthiness with the probiotic *Lactobacillus reuteri*: a randomised, double-blind placebo-controlled study. *Environ Health*. 2005 Nov 7;4:25.

Tucker KL, Olson B, Bakun P, Dallal GE, Selhub J, Rosenberg IH. Breakfast cereal fortified with folic acid, vitamin B-6, and vitamin B-12 increases vitamin concentrations and reduces homocysteine concentrations: a randomized trial. *Am J Clin Nutr*. 2004 May;79(5):805-11.

Tulk HM, Robinson LE. Modifying the n-6/n-3 polyunsaturated fatty acid ratio of a high-saturated fat challenge does not acutely attenuate postprandial changes in inflammatory markers in men with meta-bolic syndrome. *Metabolism*. 2009 Jul 20.

Tunnicliffe WS, Burge PS, Ayres JG. Effect of domestic concentrations of nitrogen dioxide on airway responses to inhaled allergen in asthmatic patients. *Lancet*. 1994 Dec 24-31;344(8939-8940):1733-6.

Tunnicliffe WS, Fletcher TJ, Hammond K, Roberts K, Custovic A, Simpson A, Woodcock A, Ayres JG. Sensitivity and exposure to indoor allergens in adults with differing asthma severity. *Eur Respir J*. 1999 Mar;13(3):654-9.

Tuomilehto J, Lindström J, Hyyrynen J, Korpela R, Karhunen ML, Mikkola L, Jauhiainen T, Seppo L, Nissinen A. Effect of ingesting sour milk fermented using *Lactobacillus helveticus* bacteria producing tripeptides on blood pressure in subjects with mild hypertension. *J Hum Hypertens*. 2004 Nov;18(11):795-802.

Turchet P, Laurenzano M, Auboiron S, Antoine JM. Effect of fermented milk containing the probiotic *Lactobacillus casei* DN-114001 on winter infections in free-living elderly subjects: a randomised, controlled pilot study. *J Nutr Health Aging*. 2003;7(2):75-7.

Tursi A, Brandimarte G, Giorgetti GM, Elisei W. Mesalazine and/or Lactobacillus casei in maintaining long-term remission of symptomatic uncomplicated diverticular disease of the colon. *Hepatogastroenterology*. 2008 May-Jun;55(84):916-20.

Twetman S, Derawi B, Keller M, Ekstrand K, Yucel-Lindberg T, Stecksen-Blicks C. Short-term effect of chewing gums containing probiotic *Lactobacillus reuteri* on the levels of inflammatory mediators in gingival crevicular fluid. *Acta Odontol Scand*. 2009 Feb;67(1):19-24.

U.S. Food and Drug Administration *Guidance for Industry Botanical Drug Products*. CfDEaR. 2000

Uddenfeldt M, Janson C, Lampa E, Leander M, Norbäck D, Larsson L, Rask-Andersen A. High BMI is related to higher incidence of asthma, while a fish and fruit diet is related to a lower- Results from a long-term follow-up study of three age groups in Sweden. *Respir Med*. 2010 Jul;104(7):972-80.

Udupa AL, Udupa SL, Guruswamy MN. The possible site of anti-asthmatic action of Tylophora asthmatica on pituitary-adrenal axis in albino rats. *Planta Med*. 1991 Oct;57(5):409-13.

451

Ueno H, Yoshioka K, Matsumoto T. Usefulness of the skin index in predicting the outcome of oral challenges in children. *J Investig Allergol Clin Immunol.* 2007;17(4):207-10.

Ueno M, Adachi A, Fukumoto T, Nishitani N, Fujiwara N, Matsuo H, Kohno K, Morita E. Analysis of causative allergen of the patient with baker's asthma and wheat-dependent exercise-induced anaphylaxis (WDEIA). *Arerugi.* 2010 May;59(5):552-7.

Ukabam SO, Mann RJ, Cooper BT. Small intestinal permeability to sugars in patients with atopic eczema. *Br J Dermatol.* 1984 Jun;110(6):649-52.

Ulrich RS, Simons RF, Losito BD, Fiorito E, Miles MA, Zelson M. Stress recovery during exposure to natural and urban environments. J Envir Psychol. 1991;11:201-30.

Ungar PS, Grine FE, Teaford MF. Dental microwear and diet of the Plio-Pleistocene hominin Paranthropus boisei. PLoS One. 2008;3:e2044. 10.1371/journal.pone.0002044.

Ungar PS, Krueger KL, Blumenschine RJ, Njau J, Scott RS. Dental microwear texture analysis of hominins recovered by the Olduvai Landscape Paleoanthropology Project, 1995 – 2007. J Hum Evol. 2011.

Ungar PS, Scott RS, Grine FE, Teaford MF. Molar microwear textures and the diets of Australopithecus anamensis and Australopithecus afarensis. Philos Trans R Soc Lond B Biol Sci. 2010;365:3345 – 3354.

Unknown. Proteolytic activity of various lactic acid bacteria. *Japan Jnl Dairy Food Sci.* 1990;39(4).

Uno KT, Cerling TE, Harris JM, Kunimatsu Y, Leakey MG, Nakatsukasa M, Nakaya H. Late Miocene to Pliocene carbon isotope record of differential diet change among East African herbivores. Proc Natl Acad Sci U S A. 2011 Apr 19;108(16):6509-14. doi: 10.1073/pnas.1018435108.

Unsel M, Sin AZ, Ardeniz O, Erdem N, Ersoy R, Gulbahar O, Mete N, Kokuludağ A. New onset egg allergy in an adult. *J Investig Allergol Clin Immunol.* 2007;17(1):55-8.

Upadhyay AK, Kumar K, Kumar A, Mishra HS. Tinospora cordifolia (Willd.) Hook. f. and Thoms. (Guduchi) – validation of the Ayurvedic pharmacology through experimental and clinical studies. *Int J Ayurveda Res.* 2010 Apr;1(2):112-21.

Urata Y, Yoshida S, Irie Y, Tanigawa T, Amayasu H, Nakabayashi M, Akahori K. Treatment of asthma patients with herbal medicine TJ-96: a randomized controlled trial. *Respir Med.* 2002 Jun;96(6):469-74.

USDA National Nutrient Database for Standard Reference, Release 21. NDB 09209. Accessed 10/21/2008.

Vakil JR, Shahani KM. Carbohydrate metabolism of lactic acid cultures. V. Lactobionate and gluconate metabolism of *Streptococcus lactis* UN. *J Dairy Sci.* 1969 Dec;52(12):1928-34.

Valeur N, Engel P, Carbajal N, Connolly E, Ladefoged K. Colonization and immunomodulation by *Lactobacillus reuteri* ATCC 55730 in the human gastrointestinal tract. *Appl Environ Microbiol.* 2004 Feb;70(2):1176-81.

Vally H, Thompson PJ, Misso NL. Changes in bronchial hyperresponsiveness following high- and low-sulphite wine challenges in wine-sensitive asthmatic patients. *Clin Exp Allergy.* 2007 Jul;37(7):1062-6.

van Baarlen P, Troost FJ, van Hemert S, van der Meer C, de Vos WM, de Groot PJ, Hooiveld GJ, Brummer RJ, Kleerebezem M. Differential NF-kappaB pathways induction by *Lactobacillus plantarum* in the duodenum of healthy humans correlating with immune tolerance. *Proc Natl Acad Sci U S A.* 2009 Feb 17;106(7):2371-6

van Beelen VA, Roeleveld J, Mooibroek H, Sijtsma L, Bino RJ, Bosch D, Rietjens IM, Alink GM. A comparative study on the effect of algal and fish oil on viability and cell proliferation of Caco-2 cells. *Food Chem Toxicol.* 2007 May;45(5):716-24.

van Dam RM, Willett WC, Rimm EB, Stampfer MJ, Hu FB. Dietary fat and meat intake in relation to risk of type 2 diabetes in men. Diabetes Care. 2002 Mar;25(3):417-24.

van den Heuvel EG, Schoterman MH, Muijs T. Transgalactooligosaccharides stimulate calcium absorption in postmenopausal women. *J Nutr.* 2000 Dec;130(12):2938-42.

van der Merwe NJ, Masao FT, Bamford MK. Isotopic evidence for contrasting diets of early hominins Homo habilis and Australopithecus boisei of Tanzania. S Afr J Sci. 2008;104:153 – 155.

van Elburg RM, Uil JJ, de Monchy JG, Heymans HS. Intestinal permeability in pediatric gastroenterology. *Scand J Gastroenterol Suppl.* 1992;194:19-24.

van Huisstede A, Braunstahl GJ. Obesity and asthma: co-morbidity or causal relationship? *Monaldi Arch Chest Dis.* 2010 Sep;73(3):116-23.

van Kampen V, Merget R, Rabstein S, Sander I, Bruening T, Broding HC, Keller C, Muesken H, Overlack A, Schultze-Werninghaus G, Walusiak J, Raulf-Heimsoth M. Comparison of wheat and rye flour solutions for skin prick testing: a multi-centre study (Stad 1). *Clin Exp Allergy.* 2009 Dec;39(12):1896-902.

Van Maele-Fabry G, Hoet P, Vilain F, Lison D. Occupational exposure to pesticides and Parkinson's disease: a systematic review and meta-analysis of cohort studies. Environ Int. 2012 Oct 1;46:30-43.

van Odijk J, Peterson CG, Ahlstedt S, Bengtsson U, Borres MP, Hulthén L, Magnusson J, Hansson T. Measurements of eosinophil activation before and after food challenges in adults with food hypersensitivity. *Int Arch Allergy Immunol.* 2006;140(4):334-41.

van Woudenbergh GJ, Kuijsten A, Tigcheler B, Sijbrands EJ, van Rooij FJ, Hofman A, Witteman JC, Feskens EJ. Meat Consumption and Its Asso-ciation With C-Reactive Protein and Incident Type 2 Diabetes: The Rotterdam Study. Diabetes Care. 2012 May 17.

van Zwol A, Moll HA, Fetter WP, van Elburg RM. Glutamine-enriched enteral nutrition in very low birthweight infants and allergic and infectious diseases at 6 years of age. *Paediatr Perinat Epidemiol.* 2011 Jan;25(1):60-6.

Vandenplas Y, De Greef E, Devreker T, Veereman-Wauters G, Hauser B. Probiotics and prebiotics in infants and children. Curr Infect Dis Rep. 2013 Jun;15(3):251-62.

Vanderhoof JA. Probiotics in allergy management. *J Pediatr Gastroenterol Nutr.* 2008 Nov;47 Suppl 2:S38-40.

VanHaitsma TA, Mickleborough T, Stager JM, Koceja DM, Lindley MR, Chapman R. Comparative effects of caffeine and albuterol on the bronchoconstrictor response to exercise in asthmatic athletes. *Int J Sports Med.* 2010 Apr;31(4):231-6.

Vanhatalo A, Fulford J, Bailey SJ, Blackwell JR, Winyard PG, Jones AM. Dietary nitrate reduces muscle metabolic perturbation and improves exercise tolerance in hypoxia. J Physiol. 2011 Nov 15;589(Pt 22):5517-28.

Vanto T, Helppilä S, Juntunen-Backman K, Kalimo K, Klemola T, Korpela R, Koskinen P. Prediction of the development of tolerance to milk in children with cow's milk hypersensitivity. *J Pediatr.* 2004 Feb;144(2):218-22.

Vargas C, Bustos P, Diaz PV, Amigo H, Rona RJ. Childhood environment and atopic conditions, with emphasis on asthma in a Chilean agricultural area. *J Asthma.* 2008 Jan-Feb;45(1):73-8.

Varonier HS, de Haller J, Schopfer C. Prevalence of allergies in children and adolescents. *Helv Paediatr Acta.* 1984;39:129-136.

Varraso R, Fung TT, Barr RG, Hu FB, Willett W, Camargo CA Jr. Prospective study of dietary patterns and chronic obstructive pulmonary disease among US women. *Am J Clin Nutr.* 2007 Aug;86(2):488-95.

Varraso R, Fung TT, Hu FB, Willett W, Camargo CA. Prospective study of dietary patterns and chronic obstructive pulmonary disease among US men. *Thorax.* 2007 Sep;62(9):786-91. 2007 May 15.

Varraso R, Jiang R, Barr RG, Willett WC, Camargo CA Jr. Prospective study of cured meats consumption and risk of chronic obstructive pulmonary disease in men. *Am J Epidemiol.* 2007 Dec 15;166(12):1438-45. 2007 Sep 4. 17785711; .

Vassallo MF, Banerji A, Rudders SA, Clark S, Mullins RJ, Camargo CA Jr. Season of birth and food allergy in children. *Ann Allergy Asthma Immunol.* 2010 Apr;104(4):307-13.

Vassallo N, Scerri C. Mediterranean Diet and Dementia of the Alzheimer Type. Curr Aging Sci. 2012 Sep 27.

Vauthier JM, Lluch A, Lecomte E, Artur Y, Herbeth B. Family resemblance in energy and macronutrient intakes: the Stanislas Family Study. *Int J Epidemiol.* 1996 Oct;25(5):1030-7.

Vaziri F, Najarpeerayeh S, Alebouyeh M, Molaei M, Maghsudi N, Zali MR. Determination of Helicobacter pylori CagA EPIYA types in Iranian isolates with different gastroduodenal disorders. Infect Genet Evol. 2013 Apr 6.

Vempati R, Bijlani RL, Deepak KK. The efficacy of a comprehensive lifestyle modification programme based on yoga in the management of bronchial asthma: a randomized controlled trial. *BMC Pulm Med.* 2009 Jul 30;9:37.

Vendt N, Grünberg H, Tuure T, Malminiemi O, Wuolijoki E, Tillmann V, Sepp E, Korpela R. Growth during the first 6 months of life in infants using formula enriched with Lactobacillus rhamnosus GG: double-blind, randomized trial. *J Hum Nutr Diet.* 2006 Feb;19(1):51-8.

Vendt N, Grünberg H, Tuure T, Malminiemi O, Wuolijoki E, Tillmann V, Sepp E, Korpela R. Growth during the first 6 months of life in infants using formula enriched with *Lactobacillus rhamnosus* GG: double-blind, randomized trial. *J Hum Nutr Diet.* 2006 Feb;19(1):51-8.

Venkatachalam KV. Human 3'-phosphoadenosine 5'-phosphosulfate (PAPS) synthase: biochemistry, molecular biology and genetic deficiency. *IUBMB Life.* 2003 Jan;55(1):1-11.

Venkatesan N, Punithavathi D, Babu M. Protection from acute and chronic lung diseases by curcumin. *Adv Exp Med Biol.* 2007;595:379-405.

Venter C, Hasan Arshad S, Grundy J, Pereira B, Bernie Clayton C, Voigt K, Higgins B, Dean T. Time trends in the prevalence of peanut allergy: three cohorts of children from the same geographical location in the UK. *Allergy.* 2010 Jan;65(1):103-8.

Venter C, Meyer R. Session 1: Allergic disease: The challenges of managing food hypersensitivity. *Proc Nutr Soc.* 2010 Feb;69(1):11-24.

Ventura MT, Polimeno L, Amoruso AC, Gatti F, Annoscia E, Marinaro M, Di Leo E, Matino MG, Buquicchio R, Bonini S, Tursi A, Francavilla A. Intestinal permeability in patients with adverse reactions to food. *Dig Liver Dis.* 2006 Oct;38(10):732-6.

Venturi A, Gionchetti P, Rizzello F, Johansson R, Zucconi E, Brigidi P, Matteuzzi D, Campieri M. Impact on the composition of the faecal flora by a new probiotic preparation: preliminary data on maintenance treatment of patients with ulcerative colitis. *Aliment Pharmacol Ther.* 1999 Aug;13(8):1103-8.

Venturi A, Gionchetti P, Rizzello F, Johansson R, Zucconi E, Brigidi P, Matteuzzi D, Campieri M. Impact on the composition of the faecal flora by a new probiotic preparation: preliminary data on maintenance treatment of patients with ulcerative colitis. *Aliment Pharmacol Ther.* 1999 Aug;13(8):1103-8.

Verhasselt V. Oral tolerance in neonates: from basics to potential prevention of allergic disease. *Mucosal Immunol.* 2010 Jul;3(4):326-33.

Verstege A, Mehl A, Rolinck-Werninghaus C, Staden U, Nocon M, Beyer K, Niggemann B. The predictive value of the skin prick test weal size for the outcome of oral food challenges. Clin Exp Allergy. 2005 Sep;35(9):1220-6.

Rolinck-Werninghaus C, Staden U, Mehl A, Hamelmann E, Beyer K, Niggemann B. Specific oral tolerance induction with food in children: transient or persistent effect on food allergy? *Allergy.* 2005 Oct;60(10):1320-2.

Vidgren HM, Agren JJ, Schwab U, Rissanen T, Hanninen O, Uusitupa MI. Incorporation of n-3 fatty acids into plasma lipid fractions, and erythrocyte membranes and platelets during dietary supplementation with fish, fish oil, and docosahexaenoic acid-rich oil among healthy young men. *Lipids.* 1997 Jul;32(7):697-705.

Vidgren HM, Agren JJ, Schwab U, Rissanen T, Hanninen O, Uusitupa MI. Incorporation of n-3 fatty acids into plasma lipid fractions, and erythrocyte membranes and platelets during dietary supplementation with fish, fish oil, and docosahexaenoic acid-rich oil among healthy young men. *Lipids.* 1997 Jul;32(7):697-705.

Viinanen A, Munhbayarlah S, Zevgee T, Narantsetseg I, Naidansuren Ts, Koskenvuo M, Helenius H, Terho EO. Prevalence of asthma, allergic rhinoconjuctivitis and allergic sensitization in Mongolia. *Allergy*. 2005;60:1370-1377.

Vila R, Mundina M, Tomi F, Furlán R, Zacchino S, Casanova J, Cañigueral S. Composition and antifungal activity of the essential oil of Solidago chilensis. *Planta Med*. 2002 Feb;68(2):164-7.

Viljanen M, Kuitunen M, Haahtela T, Juntunen-Backman K, Korpela R, Savilahti E. Probiotic effects on faecal inflammatory markers and on faecal IgA in food allergic atopic eczema/dermatitis syndrome infants. *Pediatr Allergy Immunol*. 2005 Feb;16(1):65-71.

Viljanen M, Savilahti E, Haahtela T, Juntunen-Backman K, Korpela R, Poussa T, Tuure T, Kuitunen M. Probiotics in the treatment of atopic eczema/dermatitis syndrome in infants: a double-blind placebo-controlled trial. *Allergy*. 2005 Apr;60(4):494-500.

Villarruel G, Rubio DM, Lopez F, Cintioni J, Gurevech R, Romero G, Vandenplas Y. *Saccharomyces boulardii* in acute childhood diarrhoea: a randomized, placebo-controlled study. *Acta Paediatr*. 2007 Apr;96(4):538-41.

Vinson JA, Proch J, Bose P. MegaNatural((R)) Gold Grapeseed Extract: In Vitro Antioxidant and In Vivo Human Supplementation Studies. *J Med Food*. 2001 Spring;4(1):17-26.

Vinson JA, Proch J, Bose P. MegaNatural((R)) Gold Grapeseed Extract: In Vitro Antioxidant and In Vivo Human Supplementation Studies. *J Med Food*. 2001 Spring;4(1):17-26.

Visitsunthorn N, Pacharn P, Jirapongsananuruk O, Weeravejsukit S, Sripramong C, Sookrung N, Bunnag C. Comparison between Siriraj mite allergen vaccine and standardized commercial mite vaccine by skin prick testing in normal Thai adults. *Asian Pac J Allergy Immunol*. 2010 Mar;28(1):41-5.

Visness CM, London SJ, Daniels JL, Kaufman JS, Yeatts KB, Siega-Riz AM, Liu AH, Calatroni A, Zeldin DC. Association of obesity with IgE levels and allergy symptoms in children and adolescents: results from the National Health and Nutrition Examination Survey 2005-2006. *J Allergy Clin Immunol*. 2009 May;123(5):1163-9, 1169.e1-4.

Visness CM, London SJ, Daniels JL, Kaufman JS, Yeatts KB, Siega-Riz AM, Calatroni A, Zeldin DC. Association of childhood obesity with atopic and nonatopic asthma: results from the National Health and Nutrition Examination Survey 1999-2006. *J Asthma*. 2010 Sep;47(7):822-9.

Vivatvakin B, Kowitdamrong E. Randomized control trial of live *Lactobacillus acidophilus* plus *Bifidobacterium infantis* in treatment of infantile acute watery diarrhea. *J Med Assoc Thai*. 2006 Sep;89 Suppl 3:S126-33.

Vlieg-Boerstra BJ, Dubois AE, van der Heide S, Bijleveld CM, Wolt-Plompen SA, Oude Elberink JN, Kukler J, Jansen DF, Venter C, Duiverman EJ. Ready-to-use introduction schedules for first exposure to allergenic foods in children at home. *Allergy*. 2008 Jul;63(7):903-9.

Vlieg-Boerstra BJ, van der Heide S, Bijleveld CM, Kukler J, Duiverman EJ, Wolt-Plompen SA, Dubois AE. Dietary assessment in children adhering to a food allergen avoidance diet for allergy prevention. *Eur J Clin Nutr*. 2006 Dec;60(12):1384-90.

Voicekovska JG, Orlikov GA, Karpov IuG, Teibe U, Ivanov AD, Baidekalne I, Voicehovskis NV, Maulins E. External respiration function and quality of life in patients with bronchial asthma in correction of selenium deficiency. *Ter Arkh*. 2007;79(8):38-41.

Voïtsekhovskaia IuG, Skesters A, Orlikov GA, Silova AA, Rusakova NE, Larmane LT, Karpov IuG, Ivanov AD, Maulins E. Assessment of some oxidative stress parameters in bronchial asthma patients beyond add-on selenium supplementation. *Biomed Khim*. 2007 Sep-Oct;53(5):577-84.

Vojdani A. Antibodies as predictors of complex autoimmune diseases. *Int J Immunopathol Pharmacol*. 2008 Apr-Jun;21(2):267-78.

Volman JJ, Ramakers JD, Plat J. Dietary modulation of immune function by beta-glucans. *Physiol Behav*. 2008 May 23;94(2):276-84.

von Berg A, Filipiak-Pittroff B, Krämer U, Link E, Bollrath C, Brockow I, Koletzko S, Grübl A, Heinrich J, Wichmann HE, Bauer CP, Reinhardt D, Berdel D; GINIplus study group. Preventive effect of hydrolyzed infant formulas persists until age 6 years: long-term results from the German Infant Nutritional Intervention Study (GINI). *J Allergy Clin Immunol*. 2008 Jun;121(6):1442-7.

von Berg A, Koletzko S, Grübl A, Filipiak-Pittroff B, Wichmann HE, Bauer CP, Reinhardt D, Berdel D; German Infant Nutritional Intervention Study Group. The effect of hydrolyzed cow's milk formula for allergy prevention in the first year of life: the German Infant Nutritional Intervention Study, a randomized double-blind trial. *J Allergy Clin Immunol*. 2003 Mar;111(3):533-40.

von Kruedener S, Schneider W, Elstner EF. A combination of Populus tremula, Solidago virgaurea and Fraxinus excelsior as an anti-inflammatory and antirheumatic drug. A short review. *Arzneimittelforschung*. 1995 Feb;45(2):169-71.

von Mutius E, Vercelli D. Farm living: effects on childhood asthma and allergy. *Nat Rev Immunol*. 2010 Dec;10(12):861-8. 2010 Nov 9.

Vuksan V, Whitham D, Sievenpiper JL, Jenkins AL, Rogovik AL, Bazinet RP, Vidgen E, Hanna A. Supplementation of conventional therapy with the novel grain Salba (Salvia hispanica L.) improves major and emerging cardiovascular risk factors in type 2 diabetes: results of a randomized controlled trial. *Diabetes Care*. 2007 Nov;30(11):2804-10.

Vulevic J, Drakoularakou A, Yaqoob P, Tzortzis G and Gibson GR; Modulation of the fecal microflora profile and immune function by a novel trans-galactooligosaccharide mixture (B-GOS) in healthy elderly volunteers. *Am J Clin Nutr*. 1988 88;1438-1446.

Waddell L. Food allergies in children: the difference between cow's milk protein allergy and food intolerance. *J Fam Health Care*. 2010;20(3):104.

Wahler D, Gronover CS, Richter C, Foucu F, Twyman RM, Moerschbacher BM, Fischer R, Muth J, Prufer D. Polyphenoloxidase silencing affects latex coagulation in Taraxacum spp. *Plant Physiol.* 2009 Jul 15.

Waite DA, Eyles EF, Tonkin SL, O'Donnell TV. Asthma prevalence in Tokelauan children in two environments. *Clin Allergy.* 1980;10:71-75.

Waked M, Salameh P. Risk factors for asthma and allergic diseases in school children across Lebanon. *J Asthma Allergy.* 2008 Nov 11;2:1-7.

Walders-Abramson N, Wamboldt FS, Curran-Everett D, Zhang L. Encouraging physical activity in pediatric asthma: a case-control study of the wonders of walking (WOW) program. *Pediatr Pulmonol.* 2009 Sep;44(9):909-16.

Walker S, Wing A. Allergies in children. *J Fam Health Care.* 2010;20(1):24-6.

Walker WA. Antigen absorption from the small intestine and gastrointestinal disease. *Pediatr Clin North Am.* 1975 Nov;22(4):731-46.

Walker WA. Antigen handling by the small intestine. *Clin Gastroenterol.* 1986 Jan;15(1):1-20.

Walle UK, Walle T. Transport of the cooked-food mutagen 2-amino-1-methyl-6-phenylimidazo- 4,5-b pyridine (PhIP) across the human intestinal Caco-2 cell monolayer: role of efflux pumps. *Carcinogenesis.* 1999 Nov;20(11):2153-7.

Walsh MG. Toxocara infection and diminished lung function in a nationally representative sample from the United States population. *Int J Parasitol.* 2010 Nov 8.

Walsh SJ, Rau LM: Autoimmune diseases: a leading cause of death among young and middle-aged women in the United States. *Am J Public Health* 2000, 90(9): 1463-1466.

Walton GE, Lu C, Trogh I, Arnaut F, Gibson GR. A randomised, double-blind, placebo controlled cross-over study to determine the gastrointestinal effects of consumption of arabinoxylanoligosaccharides enriched bread in healthy volunteers. *Nutr J.* 2012 Jun 1;11(1):36.

Walton GE, Lu C, Trogh I, Arnaut F, Gibson GR. A randomised, double-blind, placebo controlled cross-over study to determine the gastrointestinal effects of consumption of arabinoxylanoligosaccharides enriched bread in healthy volunteers. *Nutr J.* 2012 Jun 1;11(1):36.

Wang G, Liu CT, Wang ZL, Yan CL, Luo FM, Wang L, Li TQ. Effects of Astragalus membranaceus in promoting T-helper cell type 1 polarization and interferon-gamma production by up-regulating T-bet expression in patients with asthma. *Chin J Integr Med.* 2006 Dec;12(4):262-7.

Wang H, Chang B, Wang B. The effect of herbal medicine including astragalus membranaceus (fisch) bge, codonpsis pilosula and glycyrrhiza uralensis fisch on airway responsiveness. *Zhonghua Jie He He Hu Xi Za Zhi.* 1998 May;21(5):287-8.

Wang H, Zhai F. Program and Policy Options for Preventing Obesity in China. *Obes Rev.* 2013 Sep 9.

Wang J, Lin J, Bardina L, Goldis M, Nowak-Wegrzyn A, Shreffler WG, Sampson HA. Correlation of IgE/IgG4 milk epitopes and affinity of milk-specific IgE antibodies with different phenotypes of clinical milk allergy. *J Allergy Clin Immunol.* 2010 Mar;125(3):695-702, 702.e1-702.e6.

Wang J, Patil SP, Yang N, Ko J, Lee J, Noone S, Sampson HA, Li XM. Safety, tolerability, and immunologic effects of a food allergy herbal formula in food allergic individuals: a randomized, double-blinded, placebo-controlled, dose escalation, phase 1 study. *Ann Allergy Asthma Immunol.* 2010 Jul;105(1):75-84.

Wang J. Management of the patient with multiple food allergies. *Curr Allergy Asthma Rep.* 2010 Jul;10(4):271-7.

Wang JL, Shaw NS, Kao MD. Magnesium deficiency and its lack of association with asthma in Taiwanese elementary school children. *Asia Pac J Clin Nutr.* 2007;16 Suppl 2:579-84.

Wang JS, Hung WP. The effects of a swimming intervention for children with asthma. *Respirology.* 2009 Aug;14(6):838-42.

Wang KY, Li SN, Liu CS, Perng DS, Su YC, Wu DC, Jan CM, Lai CH, Wang TN, Wang WM. Effects of ingesting Lactobacillus- and Bifidobacterium-containing yogurt in subjects with colonized Helicobacter pylori. *Am J Clin Nutr.* 2004 Sep;80(3):737-41.

Wang KY, Li SN, Liu CS, Perng DS, Su YC, Wu DC, Jan CM, Lai CH, Wang TN, Wang WM. Effects of ingesting *Lactobacillus-* and *Bifidobacterium-*containing yogurt in subjects with colonized *Helicobacter pylori. Am J Clin Nutr.* 2004 Sep;80(3):737-41.

Wang MY, Peng L, Weidenbacher-Hoper V, Deng S, Anderson G, West BJ. Noni juice improves serum lipid profiles and other risk markers in cigarette smokers. *ScientificWorldJournal.* 2012;2012:594657. doi: 10.1100/2012/594657.

Wang X, Govind S, Sajankila SP, Mi L, Roy R, Chung FL. Phenethyl isothiocyanate sensitizes human cervical cancer cells to apoptosis induced by cisplatin. *Mol Nutr Food Res.* 2011 Oct;55(10):1572-81.

Wang XQ, Yan H, Terry PD, Wang JS, Cheng L, Wu WA, Hu SK. Interaction between dietary factors and Helicobacter pylori infection in noncardia gastric cancer: a population-based case-control study in China. *J Am Coll Nutr.* 2012 Oct;31(5):375-84.

Wang YH, Yang CP, Ku MS, Sun HL, Lue KH. Efficacy of nasal irrigation in the treatment of acute sinusitis in children. *Int J Pediatr Otorhinolaryngol.* 2009 Dec;73(12):1696-701. 2009 Sep 27.

Wang YM, Huan GX. *Utilization of Classical Formulas.* Beijing, China: Chinese Medicine and Pharmacology Publishing Co, 1998.

Wang Z, Klipfell E, Bennett BJ, Koeth R, Levison BS, Dugar B, Feldstein AE, Britt EB, Fu X, Chung YM, Wu Y, Schauer P, Smith JD, Allayee H, Tang WH, DiDonato JA, Lusis AJ, Hazen SL. Gut flora metabolism of phosphatidylcholine promotes cardiovascular disease. *Nature.* 2011 Apr 7;472(7341):57-63.

Waring J, Levy D. Challenging adverse reactions in children with food allergies. *Paediatr Nurs.* 2010 Jul;22(6):16-22.

Waser M, Michels KB, Bieli C, Flöistrup H, Pershagen G, von Mutius E, Ege M, Riedler J, Schram-Bijkerk D, Brunekreef B, van Hage M, Lauener R, Braun-Fahrländer C; PARSIFAL Study team. Inverse association of farm milk consumption with asthma and allergy in rural and suburban populations across Europe. *Clin Exp Allergy.* 2007 May;37(5):661-70.

Watkins BA, Hannon K, Ferruzzi M, Li Y. Dietary PUFA and flavonoids as deterrents for environmental pollutants. *J Nutr Biochem.* 2007 Mar;18(3):196-205.

Watson L. *Supernature.* New York: Bantam, 1973.

Watson R. Preedy VR. Botanical Medicine in Clinical Practice. Oxfordshire: CABI, 2008.

Watve MG, Tickoo R, Jog MM, Bhole BD. How many antibiotics are produced by the genus Streptomyces? *Arch Microbiol.* 2001 Nov;176(5):386-90.

Watzl B, Bub A, Blockhaus M, Herbert BM, Lührmann PM, Neuhäuser-Berthold M, Rechkemmer G. Prolonged tomato juice consumption has no effect on cell-mediated immunity of well-nourished elderly men and women. *J Nutr.* 2000 Jul;130(7):1719-23.

Webber CM, England RW. Oral allergy syndrome: a clinical, diagnostic, and therapeutic challenge. *Ann Allergy Asthma Immunol.* 2010 Feb;104(2):101-8; quiz 109-10, 117.

Weber J, Cheinsong-Popov R, Callow D, Adams S, Patou G, Hodgkin K, Martin S, Gotch F, Kingsman A. Immunogenicity of the yeast recombinant p17/p24:Ty virus-like particles (p24-VLP) in healthy volunteers. Vaccine. 1995 Jun;13(9):831-4.

Webster D, Taschereau P, Belland RJ, Sand C, Rennie RP. Antifungal activity of medicinal plant extracts; preliminary screening studies. *J Ethnopharmacol.* 2008 Jan 4;115(1):140-6.

Weekes DJ. Management of Herpes Simplex with Virostatic Bacterial Agent. *EENT Dig.* 1963;25(12).

Weekes DJ. The treatment of aphthous stomatitis with Lactobacillus tablets. *NY State J Med.* 1958 Aug 15;58(16):2672-3.

Wegrowski J, Robert AM, Moczar M. The effect of procyanidolic oligomers on the composition of normal and hypercholesterolemic rabbit aortas. *Biochem Pharmacol.* 1984 Nov 1;33(21):3491-7.

Wei A, Shibamoto T. Antioxidant activities and volatile constituents of various essential oils. *J Agric Food Chem.* 2007 Mar 7;55(5):1737-42.

Wei P, Liu M, Chen Y, Chen DC. Systematic review of soy isoflavone supplements on osteoporosis in women. Asian Pac J Trop Med. 2012 Mar;5(3):243-8.

Weil A. 2004. Dr. Andrew Weil's Self Healing. September, page 6

Weiler JM, Layton T, Hunt M. Asthma in United States Olympic athletes who participated in the 1996 Summer Games. J Allergy Clin Immunol. 1998 Nov;102(5):722-6. 7.

Weiner MA. *Secrets of Fijian Medicine.* Berkeley, CA: Univ. of Calif., 1969.

Weisgerber M, Webber K, Meurer J, Danduran M, Berger S, Flores G. Moderate and vigorous exercise programs in children with asthma: safety, parental satisfaction, and asthma outcomes. Pediatr Pulmonol. 2008 Dec;43(12):1175-82.

Weiss RF. *Herbal Medicine.* Gothenburg, Sweden: Beaconsfield, 1988.

Weizman Z, Asli G, Alsheikh A. Effect of a probiotic infant formula on infections in child care centers: comparison of two probiotic agents. *Pediatrics.* 2005 Jan;115(1):5-9.

Wen MC, Huang CK, Srivastava KD, Zhang TF, Schofield B, Sampson HA, Li XM. Ku-Shen (Sophora flavescens Ait), a single Chinese herb, abrogates airway hyperreactivity in a murine model of asthma. *J Allergy Clin Immunol.* 2004;113:218.

Wen MC, Taper A, Srivastava KD, Huang CK, Schofield B, Li XM. Immunology of T cells by the Chinese Herbal Medicine Ling Zhi (Ganoderma lucidum) *J Allergy Clin Immunol.* 2003;111:S320.

Wen MC, Wei CH, Hu ZQ, Srivastava K, Ko J, Xi ST, Mu DZ, Du JB, Li GH, Wallenstein S, Sampson H, Kattan M, Li XM. Efficacy and tolerability of anti-asthma herbal medicine intervention in adult patients with moderate-severe allergic asthma. *J Allergy Clin Immunol.* 2005;116:517-24.

Wenus C, Goll R, Loken EB, Biong AS, Halvorsen DS, Florholmen J. Prevention of antibiotic-associated diarrhoea by a fermented probiotic milk drink. *Eur J Clin Nutr.* 2008 Feb;62(2):299-301.

Werbach M. *Nutritional Influences on Illness.* Tarzana, CA: Third Line Press, 1996.

West CE, Hammarström ML, Hernell O. Probiotics during weaning reduce the incidence of eczema. *Pediatr Allergy Immunol.* 2009 Aug;20(5):430-7.

West R. Risk of death in meat and non-meat eaters. *BMJ.* 1994 Oct 8;309(6959):955.

Westerholm-Ormio M, Vaarala O, Tiittanen M, Savilahti E. Infiltration of Foxp3- and Toll-like receptor-4-positive cells in the intestines of children with food allergy. *J Pediatr Gastroenterol Nutr.* 2010 Apr;50(4):367-76.

Wexler HM. Bacteroides: the good, the bad, and the nitty-gritty. *Clin Microbiol Rev.* 2007 Oct;20(4):593-621.

Wheeler JG, Bogle ML, Shema SJ, Shirrell MA, Stine KC, Pittler AJ, Burks AW, Helm RM. Impact of dietary yogurt on immune function. *Am J Med Sci.* 1997 Feb;313(2):120-3.

Wheeler JG, Shema SJ, Bogle ML, Shirrell MA, Burks AW, Pittler A, Helm RM. Immune and clinical impact of *Lactobacillus acidophilus* on asthma. *Ann Allergy Asthma Immunol.* 1997 Sep;79(3):229-33.

Wheeler JG, Shema SJ, Bogle ML, Shirrell MA, Burks AW, Pittler A, Helm RM. Immune and clinical impact of *Lactobacillus acidophilus* on asthma. *Ann Allergy Asthma Immunol.* 1997 Sep;79(3):229-33.

White LB, Foster S. The Herbal Drugstore. Emmaus, PA: Rodale, 2000.

White TD, *et al.* Asa Issie, Aramis and the origin of Australopithecus. Nature. 2006;440:883 – 889.

White TD, *et al.* Macrovertebrate paleontology and the Pliocene habitat of Ardipithecus ramidus. Science. 2009;326:87 – 93.

White TD, Suwa G, Simpson S, Asfaw B. Jaws and teeth of Australopithecus afarensis from Maka, Middle Awash, Ethiopia. Am J Phys Anthropol. 2000;111:45 – 68.

# REFERENCES AND BIBLIOGRAPHY

Whitfield KE, Wiggins SA, Belue R, Brandon DT. Genetic and environmental influences on forced expiratory volume in African Americans: the Carolina African-American Twin Study of Aging. *Ethn Dis.* 2004 Spring;14(2):206-11.

WHO. *Guidelines for Drinking-water Quality.* 2nd ed, vol. 2. Geneva: World Health Organization, 1996.

WHO. How trace elements in water contribute to health. *WHO Chronicle.* 1978;32:382-385.

WHO. *INFOSAN Food Allergies. Information Note No. 3.* Geneva, Switzerland: World Health Organization, 2006.

Whorwell PJ, Altringer L, Morel J, Bond Y, Charbonneau D, O'Mahony L, Kiely B, Shanahan F, Quigley EM. Efficacy of an encapsulated probiotic *Bifidobacterium infantis* 35624 in women with irritable bowel syndrome. *Am J Gastroenterol.* 2006 Jul;101(7):1581-90.

Wickens K, Black PN, Stanley TV, Mitchell E, Fitzharris P, Tannock GW, Purdie G, Crane J; Probiotic Study Group. A differential effect of 2 probiotics in the prevention of eczema and atopy: a double-blind, randomized, placebo-controlled trial. *J Allergy Clin Immunol.* 2008 Oct;122(4):788-94.

Widdicombe JG, Ernst E. Clinical cough V: complementary and alternative medicine: therapy of cough. *Handb Exp Pharmacol.* 2009;(187):321-42.

Widmer W. Determination of naringin and neohesperidin in orange juice by liquid chromatography with UV detection to detect the presence of grapefruit juice: Collaborative Study. *J AOAC Int.* 2000 Sep-Oct;83(5):1155-65.

Wildt S, Munck LK, Vinter-Jensen L, Hanse BF, Nordgaard-Lassen I, Christensen S, Avnstroem S, Rasmussen SN, Rumessen JJ. Probiotic treatment of collagenous colitis: a randomized, double-blind, placebo-controlled trial with *Lactobacillus acidophilus* and *Bifidobacterium animalis* subsp. *Lactis. Inflamm Bowel Dis.* 2006 May;12(5):395-401.

Wilkens H, Wilkens JH, Uffmann J, Bövers J, Fröhlich JC, Fabel H. Effect of the platelet-activating factor antagonist BN 52063 on exertional asthma. *Pneumologie.* 1990 Feb;44 Suppl 1:347-8.

Willard T, Jones K. *Reishi Mushroom: Herb of Spiritual Potency and Medical Wonder.* Issaquah, Washington: Sylvan Press, 1990.

Willard T. *Edible and Medicinal Plants of the Rocky Mountains and Neighbouring Territories.* Calgary: 1992.

Willemsen LE, Koetsier MA, Balvers M, Beermann C, Stahl B, van Tol EA. Polyunsaturated fatty acids support epithelial barrier integrity and reduce IL-4 mediated permeability in vitro. *Eur J Nutr.* 2008 Jun;47(4):183-91.

Williams AB, Yu C, Tashima K, Burgess J, Danvers K. Evaluation of two self-care treatments for prevention of vaginal candidiasis in women with HIV. *J Assoc Nurses AIDS Care.* 2001 Jul-Aug;12(4):51-7.

Williams DM. Considerations in the long-term management of asthma in ambulatory patients. *AM J Health Syst Pharm.* 2006;63:S14-21.

Williams LJ, *et al.* Status of Folic Acid Fortification in the United States. Pediatrics 2005; 116; 580-586.

Williamson-Hughes PS, Flickinger BD, Messina MJ, Empie MW. 2006.

Wilson D, Evans M, Guthrie N, Sharma P, Baisley J, Schonlau F, Burki C. A randomized, double-blind, placebo-controlled exploratory study to evaluate the potential of pycnogenol for improving allergic rhinitis symptoms. *Phytother Res.* 2010 Aug;24(8):1115-9.

Wilson K, McDowall L, Hodge D, Chetcuti P, Cartledge P. Cow's milk protein allergy. *Community Pract.* 2010 May;83(5):40-1.

Wilson L. *Nutritional Balancing and Hair Mineral Analysis.* Prescott, AZ: LD Wilson, 1998.

Wilson NM, Charette L, Thomson AH, Silverman M. Gastro-oesophageal reflux and childhood asthma: the acid test. *Thorax.* 1985 Aug;40(8):592-7.

Winchester AM. *Biology and its Relation to Mankind.* New York: Van Nostrand Reinhold, 1969.

Wise M, Doehlert D, McMullen M. Association of Avenanthramide Concentration in Oat (Avena sativa L.) Grain with Crown Rust Incidence and Genetic Resistance. Cereal Chem. 85(5):639-641.

Wiseman H. Vitamin D is a membrane antioxidant. Ability to inhibit iron-dependent lipid peroxidation in liposomes compared to cholesterol, ergosterol and tamoxifen and relevance to anticancer action. FEBS Lett. 1993 Jul 12;326(1-3):285-8.

Witsell DL, Garrett CG, Yarbrough WG, Dorrestein SP, Drake AF, Weissler MC. Effect of *Lactobacillus acidophilus* on antibiotic-associated gastrointestinal morbidity: a prospective randomized trial. *J Otolaryngol.* 1995 Aug;24(4):230-3.

Wittenberg JS. *The Rebellious Body.* New York: Insight, 1996.

Wlodarek D, Glabska D. Influence of the lutein-rich products consumption on its supply in diet of individuals with age-related macular degeneration (AMD). Klin Oczna. 2011;113(1-3):42-6.

Woessner KM, Simon RA, Stevenson DD. Monosodium glutamate sensitivity in asthma. *J Allergy Clin Immunol.* 1999 Aug;104(2 Pt 1):305-10.

Wöhrl S, Hemmer W, Focke M, Rappersberger K, Jarisch R. Histamine intolerance-like symptoms in healthy volunteers after oral provocation with liquid histamine. *Allergy Asthma Proc.* 2004 Sep-Oct;25(5):305-11.

Wolvers DA, van Herpen-Broekmans WM, Logman MH, van der Wielen RP, Albers R. Effect of a mixture of micronutrients, but not of bovine colostrum concentrate, on immune function parameters in healthy volunteers: a randomized placebo-controlled study. *Nutr J.* 2006 Nov 21;5:28.

Wolverton BC. *How to grow fresh air: 50 houseplants that purify your home or office.* New York: Penguin, 1997.

Wong GWK, Hui DSC, Chan HH, Fox TF, Leung R, Zhong NS, Chen YZ, Lai CKW. Prevalence of respiratory and atopic disorders in Chinese schoolchildren. *Clinical and Experimental Allergy.* 2001;31:1125-1231.

Wong WM, Lai KC, Lam KF, Hui WM, Hu WH, Lam CL, Xia HH, Huang JQ, Chan CK, Lam SK, Wong BC. Prevalence, clinical spectrum and health care utilization of gastro-oesophageal reflux disease in a Chinese population: a population-based study. *Aliment Pharmacol Ther.* 2003 Sep 15;18(6):595-604.

Wood M. *The Book of Herbal Wisdom.* Berkeley, CA: North Atlantic, 1997.

Wood RA, Kraynak J. *Food Allergies for Dummies.* Hoboken, NJ: Wiley Publ, 2007.

Woods RK, Abramson M, Bailey M, Walters EH. International prevalences of reported food allergies and intolerances. Comparisons arising from the European Community Respiratory Health Survey (ECRHS) 1991-1994. *Eur J Clin Nutr* 2001;55:298-304.

Woods RK, Abramson M, Raven JM, Bailey M, Weiner JM, Walters EH. Reported food intolerance and respiratory symptoms in young adults. *Eur Respir J.* 1998;11: 151-155.

Wouters EF, Reynaert NL, Dentener MA, Vernooy JH. Systemic and local inflammation in asthma and chronic obstructive pulmonary disease: is there a connection? *Proc Am Thorac Soc.* 2009 Dec;6(8):638-47.

Wright GR, Howieson S, McSharry C, McMahon AD, Chaudhuri R, Thompson J, Donnelly I, Brooks RG, Lawson A, Jolly L, McAlpine L, King EM, Chapman MD, Wood S, Thomson NC. Effect of improved home ventilation on asthma control and house dust mite allergen levels. *Allergy.* 2009 Nov;64(11):1671-80.

Wright RJ. Epidemiology of stress and asthma: from constricting communities and fragile families to epigenetics. *Immunol Allergy Clin North Am.* 2011 Feb;31(1):19-39.

Wu B, Yu J, Wang Y. Effect of Chinese herbs for tonifying Shen on balance of Th1 /Th2 in children with asthma in remission stage. *Zhongguo Zhong Xi Yi Jie He Za Zhi.* 2007 Feb;27(2):120-2.

Wu GD, Chen J, Hoffmann C, Bittinger K, Chen YY, Keilbaugh SA, Bewtra M, Knights D, Walters WA, Knight R, Sinha R, Gilroy E, Gupta K, Baldassano R, Nessel L, Li H, Bushman FD, Lewis JD. Linking long-term dietary patterns with gut microbial enterotypes. Science. 2011 Oct 7;334(6052):105-8. doi: 10.1126/science.1208344.

Wu Q, Wu K, Ye Y, Dong X, Zhang J. Quorum sensing and its roles in pathogenesis among animal-associated pathogens – a review. *Wei Sheng Wu Xue Bao.* 2009 Jul 4;49(7):853-8.

Wu ZC, Yu JT, Li Y, Tan L. Clusterin in Alzheimer's disease. Adv Clin Chem. 2012;56:155-73.

Würsch P, Pi-Sunyer FX. The role of viscous soluble fiber in the metabolic control of diabetes. A review with special emphasis on cereals rich in beta-glucan. Diabetes Care. 1997 Nov;20(11):1774-80.

Wyka J. [Nutritional factors in prevention of Alzheimer's disease]. Rocz Panstw Zakl Hig. 2012;63(2):135-40.

Wylie LJ, Mohr M, Krustrup P, Jackman SR, Ermidis G, Kelly J, Black MI, Bailey SJ, Vanhatalo A, Jones AM. Dietary nitrate supplementation improves team sport-specific intense intermittent exercise performance. Eur J Appl Physiol. 2013 Feb 1.

Xi L, Han DM, Lü XF, Zhang L. Psychological characteristics in patients with allergic rhinitis and its associated factors analysis.. *Zhonghua Er Bi Yan Hou Tou Jing Wai Ke Za Zhi.* 2009 Dec;44(12):982-5.

Xiao D, Srivastava SK, Lew KL, Zeng Y, Hershberger P, Johnson CS, Trump DL, Singh SV. Allyl isothiocyanate, a constituent of cruciferous vegetables, inhibits proliferation of human prostate cancer cells by causing G2/M arrest and inducing apoptosis. Carcinogenesis. 2003 May;24(5):891-7.

Xiao JZ, Kondo S, Takahashi N, Miyaji K, Oshida K, Hiramatsu A, Iwatsuki K, Kokubo S, Hosono A. Effects of milk products fermented by *Bifidobacterium longum* on blood lipids in rats and healthy adult male volunteers. *J Dairy Sci.* 2003 Jul;86(7):2452-61.

Xiao JZ, Kondo S, Yanagisawa N, Miyaji K, Enomoto K, Sakoda T, Iwatsuki K, Enomoto T. Clinical efficacy of probiotic *Bifidobacterium longum* for the treatment of symptoms of Japanese cedar pollen allergy in subjects evaluated in an environmental exposure unit. *Allergol Int.* 2007 Mar;56(1):67-75.

Xiao JZ, Kondo S, Yanagisawa N, Takahashi N, Odamaki T, Iwabuchi N, Miyaji K, Iwatsuki K, Togashi H, Enomoto K, Enomoto T. Probiotics in the treatment of Japanese cedar pollinosis: a double-blind placebo-controlled trial. *Clin Exp Allergy.* 2006 Nov;36(11):1425-35.

Xiao JZ, Kondo S, Yanagisawa N, Takahashi N, Odamaki T, Iwabuchi N, Iwatsuki K, Kokubo S, Togashi H, Enomoto K, Enomoto T. Effect of probiotic *Bifidobacterium longum* BB536 in relieving clinical symptoms and modulating plasma cytokine levels of Japanese cedar pollinosis during the pollen season. A randomized double-blind, placebo-controlled trial. *J Investig Allergol Clin Immunol.* 2006;16(2):86-93.

Xiao P, Kubo H, Ohsawa M, Higashiyama K, Nagase H, Yan YN, Li JS, Kamei J, Ohmiya S. kappa-Opioid receptor-mediated antinociceptive effects of stereoisomers and derivatives of (+)-matrine in mice. *Planta Med.* 1999 Apr;65(3):230-3.

Xiao SD, Zhang DZ, Lu H, Jiang SH, Liu HY, Wang GS, Xu GM, Zhang ZB, Lin GJ, Wang GL. Multicenter, randomized, controlled trial of heat-killed *Lactobacillus acidophilus* LB in patients with chronic diarrhea. *Adv Ther.* 2003 Sep-Oct;20(5):253-60.

Xie JY, Dong JC, Gong ZH. Effects on herba epimedii and radix Astragali on tumor necrosis factor-alpha and nuclear factor-kappa B in asthmatic rats. *Zhongguo Zhong Xi Yi Jie He Za Zhi.* 2006 Aug;26(8):723-7.

Xu X, Cui S, Zhang F, Luo Y, Gu Y, Yang B, Li F, Chen Q, Zhou G, Wang Y, Pang L, Lin L. Prevalence and Characterization of Cefotaxime and Ciprofloxacin Co-Resistant Escherichia coli Isolates in Retail Chicken Carcasses and Ground Pork, China. Microb Drug Resist. 2013 Aug 17.

Xu X, Zhang D, Zhang H, Wolters PJ, Killeen NP, Sullivan BM, Locksley RM, Lowell CA, Caughey GH. Neutrophil histamine contributes to inflammation in mycoplasma pneumonia. *J Exp Med.* 2006 Dec 25;203(13):2907-17.

Yadav H, Jain S, Sinha PR. Antidiabetic effect of probiotic dahl containing *Lactobacillus acidophilus* and *Lactobacillus casei* in high fructose fed rats. *Nutrition.* 2007 Jan;23(1):62-8.

Yadav RK, Ray RB, Vempati R, Bijlani RL. Effect of a comprehensive yoga-based lifestyle modification program on lipid peroxidation. *Indian J Physiol Pharmacol.* 2005 Jul-Sep;49(3):358-62.

Yadav VS, Mishra KP, Singh DP, Mehrotra S, Singh VK. Immunomodulatory effects of curcumin. *Immunopharmacol Immunotoxicol.* 2005;27(3):485-97.

Yadzir ZH, Misnan R, Abdullah N, Bakhtiar F, Arip M, Murad S. Identification of Ige-binding proteins of raw and cooked extracts of Loligo edulis (white squid). *Southeast Asian J Trop Med Public Health*. 2010 May;41(3):653-9.

Yamamura S, Morishima H, Kumano-go T, Suganuma N, Matsumoto H, Adachi H, Sigedo Y, Mikami A, Kai T, Masuyama A, Takano T, Sugita Y, Takeda M. The effect of *Lactobacillus helveticus* fermented milk on sleep and health perception in elderly subjects. *Eur J Clin Nutr*. 2009 Jan;63(1):100-5.

Yang Y, Luo Y, Millner P, Turner E, Feng H. Assessment of Escherichia coli O157:H7 transference from soil to iceberg lettuce via a contaminated field coring harvesting knife. Int J Food Microbiol. 2012 Feb 15;153(3):345-50.

Yang Z. Are peanut allergies a concern for using peanut-based formulated foods in developing countries? *Food Nutr Bull*. 2010 Jun;31(2 Suppl):S147-53.

Yao Y, Sang W, Zhou M, Ren G. Phenolic composition and antioxidant activities of 11 celery cultivars. J Food Sci. 2010 Jan-Feb;75(1):C9-13.

Yasuda T, Takeyama Y, Ueda T, Shinzeki M, Sawa H, Nakajima T, Kuroda Y. Breakdown of Intestinal Mucosa Via Accelerated Apoptosis Increases Intestinal Permeability in Experimental Severe Acute Pancreatitis. *J Surg Res*. 2006 Apr 4.

Yeager S, ed. 1998. Doctor's Book of Food Remedies. Rodale Press, p. 494.

Yeager S. Food Remedies. Rodale Press, 1998.

Yeager S. *The Doctor's Book of Food Remedies*. Emmaus, PA: Rodale Press, 1998.

Yeager S. The Doctor's Book of Food Remedies. Emmaus, PA: Rodale Press, 1998.

Ye Q, Huang B, Zhang X, Zhu Y, Chen X. Astaxanthin protects against MPP+-induced oxidative stress in PC12 cells via the HO-1/NOX2 axis. BMC Neurosci. 2012 Dec 29;13:156. doi: 10.1186/1471-2202-13-156.

Yeh CC, Lin CC, Wang SD, Chen YS, Su BH, Kao ST. Protective and anti-inflammatory effect of a traditional Chinese medicine, Xia-Bai-San, by modulating lung local cytokine in a murine model of acute lung injury. *Int Immunopharmacol*. 2006 Sep;6(9):1506-14.

Yeh CT, Yen GC. Effect of vegetables on human phenolsulfotransferases in relation to their antioxidant activity and total phenolics. Free Radic Res. 2005 Aug;39(8):893-904.

Yonekura S, Okamoto Y, Okawa T, Hisamitsu M, Chazono H, Kobayashi K, Sakurai D, Horiguchi S, Hanazawa T. Effects of daily intake of Lactobacillus paracasei strain KW3110 on Japanese cedar pollinosis. *Allergy Asthma Proc*. 2009 Jul-Aug;30(4):397-405.

Yu L, Zhang Y, Chen C, Cui HF, Yan XK. Meta-analysis on randomized controlled clinical trials of acupuncture for asthma. *Zhongguo Zhen Jiu*. 2010 Sep;30(9):787-92.

Yu LC. The epithelial gatekeeper against food allergy. *Pediatr Neonatol*. 2009 Dec;50(6):247-54.

Yun CH, Estrada A, Van Kessel A, Gajadhar A, Redmond M, Laarveld B. Immunomodulatory effects of oat beta-glucan administered intragastrically or parenterally on mice infected with Eimeria vermiformis. Microbiol Immunol. 1998;42(6):457-65.

Yusoff NA, Hampton SM, Dickerson JW, Morgan JB. The effects of exclusion of dietary egg and milk in the management of asthmatic children: a pilot study. *J R Soc Promot Health*. 2004 Mar;124(2):74-80.

Zamora-Ros R, Agudo A, Luján-Barroso L, Romieu I, Ferrari P, Knaze V, Bueno-de-Mesquita HB, Leenders M, Travis RC, Navarro C, Sánchez-Cantalejo E, Slimani N, Scalbert A, Fedirko V, Hjartåker A, Engeset D, Skeie G, Boeing H, Förster J, Li K, Teucher B, Agnoli C, Tumino R, Mattiello A, Saieva C, Johansson I, Stenling R, Redondo ML, Wallström P, Ericson U, Khaw KT, Mulligan AA, Trichopoulou A, Dilis V, Katsoulis M, Peeters PH, Igali L, Tjønneland A, Halkjær J, Touillaud M, Perquier F, Fagherazzi G, Amiano P, Ardanaz E, Bredsdorff L, Overvad K, Ricceri F, Riboli E, González CA. Dietary flavonoid and lignan intake and gastric adenocarcinoma risk in the European Prospective Investigation into Cancer and Nutrition (EPIC) study. Am J Clin Nutr. 2012 Dec;96(6):1398-408.

Zand J, Lanza F, Garg HK, Bryan NS. All-natural nitrite and nitrate containing dietary supplement promotes nitric oxide production and reduces triglycerides in humans. Nutr Res. 2011 Apr;31(4):262-9.

Zanjanian MH. The intestine in allergic diseases. *Ann Allergy*. 1976 Sep;37(3):208-18.

Zarate G, Gonzalez S, Chaia AP. *Assessing survival of dairy propionibacteria in gastrointestinal conditions and adherence to intestinal epithelia. Centro de Referencia para Lactobacilos-CONICET. Tucuman, Argentina: Humana Press. 2004.*

Zarkadas M, Scott FW, Salminen J, Ham Pong A. Common Allergenic Foods and Their Labelling in Canada. *Can J Allerg Clin Immun*. 1999; 4:118-141.

Zarnowski R, Suzuki Y, Yamaguchi I, Pietr SJ. Alkylresorcinols in barley Hordeum vulgare L. distichon) grains. Z Naturforsch. 2002 Jan-Feb;57(1-2):57-62.

Zarnowski R, Suzuki Y. 5-n-Alkylresorcinols from grains of winter barley (Hordeum vulgare L.). Z Naturforsch. 2004 May-Jun;59(5-6):315-7.

Zeiger RS, Heller S. The development and prediction of atopy in high-risk children: follow-up at age seven years in a prospective randomized study of combined maternal and infant food allergen avoidance. *J Allergy Clin Immunol*. 1995 Jun;95(6):1179-90.

Zeng J, Li YQ, Zuo XL, Zhen YB, Yang J, Liu CH. Clinical trial: effect of active lactic acid bacteria on mucosal barrier function in patients with diarrhoea-predominant irritable bowel syndrome. *Aliment Pharmacol Ther*. 2008 Oct 15;28(8):994-1002.

Zhan S, Ho SC. 2005. Meta-analysis of the effects of soy protein containing isoflavones on the lipid profile. Am J Clin Nutr. Feb;81(2):397-408.

Zhang CS, Yang AW, Zhang AL, Fu WB, Thien FU, Lewith G, Xue CC. Ear-acupressure for allergic rhinitis: a systematic review. *Clin Otolaryngol*. 2010 Feb;35(1):6-12.

Zhang J, Sun C, Yan Y, Chen Q, Luo F, Zhu X, Li X, Chen K. Purification of naringin and neohesperidin from Huyou (Citrus changshanensis) fruit and their effects on glucose consumption in human HepG2 cells. Food Chem. 2012 Dec 1;135(3):1471-8.

Zhang QH, Zhang L, Shang LX, Shao CL, Wu YX. Studies on the chemical constituents of flowers of Prunus mume. Zhong Yao Cai. 2008 Nov;31(11):1666-8.

Zhang T, Srivastava K, Wen MC, Yang N, Cao J, Busse P, Birmingham N, Goldfarb J, Li XM. Pharmacology and immunological actions of a herbal medicine ASHMI on allergic asthma. Phytother Res. 2010 Jul;24(7):1047-55.

Zhang X, Shu XO, Xiang YB, Yang G, Li H, Gao J, Cai H, Gao YT, Zheng W. Cruciferous vegetable consumption is associated with a reduced risk of total and cardiovascular disease mortality. Am J Clin Nutr. 2011 Jul;94(1):240-6.

Zhang Z, Lai HJ, Roberg KA, Gangnon RE, Evans MD, Anderson EL, Pappas TE, Dasilva DF, Tisler CJ, Salazar LP, Gern JE, Lemanske RF Jr. Early childhood weight status in relation to asthma development in high-risk children. J Allergy Clin Immunol. 2010 Dec;126(6):1157-62. 2010 Nov 4.

Zhao FD, Dong JC, Xie JY. Effects of Chinese herbs for replenishing shen and strengthening qi on some indexes of neuro-endocrino-immune network in asthmatic rats. Zhongguo Zhong Xi Yi Jie He Za Zhi. 2007 Aug;27(8):715-9.

Zhao HY, Wang HJ, Lu Z, Xu SZ. Intestinal microflora in patients with liver cirrhosis. Chin J Dig Dis. 2004;5(2):64-7.

Zhao J, Bai J, Shen K, Xiang L, Huang S, Chen A, Huang Y, Wang J, Ye R. Self-reported prevalence of childhood allergic diseases in three cities of China: a multicenter study. BMC Public Health. 2010 Sep 13;10:551.

Zheng M. Experimental study of 472 herbs with antiviral action against the herpes simplex virus. Zhong Xi Yi Jie He Za Zhi. 1990 Jan;10(1):39-41, 6.

Zheng X, Gessel MM, Wisniewski ML, Viswanathan K, Wright DL, Bahr BA, Bowers MT. Z-Phe-Ala-diazomethylketone (PADK) disrupts and remodels early oligomers states of the Alzheimer disease Aβ42 protein. J Biol Chem. 2012 Feb 24;287(9):6084-8.

Zhou B, Luo Y, Millner P, Feng H. Sanitation and Design of Lettuce Coring Knives for Minimizing Escherichia coli O157:H7 Contamination. J Food Prot. 2012 Mar;75(3):563-6.

Zhou Q, Zhang B, Verne GN. Intestinal membrane permeability and hypersensitivity in the irritable bowel syndrome. Pain. 2009 Nov;146(1-2):41-6.

Zhu DD, Zhu XW, Jiang XD, Dong Z. Thymic stromal lymphopoietin expression is increased in nasal epithelial cells of patients with mugwort pollen sensitive-seasonal allergic rhinitis. Chin Med J (Engl). 2009 Oct 5;122(19):2303-7.

Zhu HH, Chen YP, Yu JE, Wu M, Li Z. Therapeutic effect of Xincang Decoction on chronic airway inflammation in children with bronchial asthma in remission stage. Zhong Xi Yi Jie He Xue Bao. 2005 Jan;3(1):23-7.

Ziaei Kajbaf T, Asar S, Alipoor MR. Relationship between obesity and asthma symptoms among children in Ahvaz, Iran:A cross sectional study. Ital J Pediatr. 2011 Jan 6;37(1):1.

Zielen S, Kardos P, Madonini E. Steroid-sparing effects with allergen-specific immunotherapy in children with asthma: a randomized controlled trial. J Allergy Clin Immunol. 2010 Nov;126(5):942-9. 2010 Jul 10.

Zielińska-Przyjemska M, Olejnik A, Kostrzewa A, Luczak M, Jagodziński PP, Baer-Dubowska W. The beetroot component betanin modulates ROS production, DNA damage and apoptosis in human polymorphonuclear neutrophils. Phytother Res. 2012 Jun;26(6):845-52.

Ziemniak W. Efficacy of Helicobacter pylori eradication taking into account its resistance to antibiotics. J Physiol Pharmacol. 2006 Sep;57 Suppl 3:123-41.

Ziment I, Tashkin DP. Alternative medicine for allergy and asthma. J Allergy Clin Immunol. 2000 Oct;106(4):603-14.

Ziment I. Alternative therapies for asthma. Curr Opin Pulm Med. 1997 Jan;3(1):61-71.

Zizza, C. The nutrient content of the Italian food supply 1961-1992. Euro J Clin Nutr. 1997;51: 259-265.

Zoccatelli G, Pokoj S, Foetisch K, Bartra J, Valero A, Del Mar San Miguel-Moncin M, Vieths S, Scheurer S. Identification and characterization of the major allergen of green bean (Phaseolus vulgaris) as a non-specific lipid transfer protein (Pha v 3). Mol Immunol. 2010 Apr;47(7-8):1561-8.

Zschäbitz S, Cheng TY, Neuhouser ML, Zheng Y, Ray RM, Miller JW, Song X, Maneval DR, Beresford SA, Lane D, Shikany JM, Ulrich CM. B vitamin intakes and incidence of colorectal cancer: results from the Women's Health Initiative Observational Study cohort. Am J Clin Nutr. 2012 Dec 19.

Zwolińska-Wcisło M, Brzozowski T, Mach T, Budak A, Trojanowska D, Konturek PC, Pajdo R, Drozdowicz D, Kwiecień S. Are probiotics effective in the treatment of fungal colonization of the gastrointestinal tract? Experimental and clinical studies. J Physiol Pharmacol. 2006 Nov;57 Suppl 9:35-49.

# Index

*(Foods and nutrients are too numerous to index —
refer to ebook search for complete index ability)*

# INDEX